Primary and Secondary Immunodeficiency

Jonathan A. Bernstein
Editor

Primary and Secondary Immunodeficiency

A Case-Based Guide to Evaluation and Management

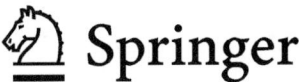

Editor
Jonathan A. Bernstein
College of Medicine
University of Cincinnati
Cincinnati, OH
USA

ISBN 978-3-030-57156-6   ISBN 978-3-030-57157-3 (eBook)
https://doi.org/10.1007/978-3-030-57157-3

© Springer Nature Switzerland AG 2021

This work is subject to copyright. All rights are reserved by the Publisher, whether the whole or part of the material is concerned, specifically the rights of translation, reprinting, reuse of illustrations, recitation, broadcasting, reproduction on microfilms or in any other physical way, and transmission or information storage and retrieval, electronic adaptation, computer software, or by similar or dissimilar methodology now known or hereafter developed.

The use of general descriptive names, registered names, trademarks, service marks, etc. in this publication does not imply, even in the absence of a specific statement, that such names are exempt from the relevant protective laws and regulations and therefore free for general use.

The publisher, the authors and the editors are safe to assume that the advice and information in this book are believed to be true and accurate at the date of publication. Neither the publisher nor the authors or the editors give a warranty, expressed or implied, with respect to the material contained herein or for any errors or omissions that may have been made. The publisher remains neutral with regard to jurisdictional claims in published maps and institutional affiliations.

This Springer imprint is published by the registered company Springer Nature Switzerland AG
The registered company address is: Gewerbestrasse 11, 6330 Cham, Switzerland

*I carry your heart with me (I carry it in
my heart) I am never without it (anywhere
I go you go, my dear; and whatever is done
by only me is your doing, my darling)
From "I carry your heart with me," by
E. E. Cummings
This book is dedicated in loving memory of
Liv Rose Meisterman
(daughter of Ali and Danny Meisterman)
4/22/2019 to 7/11/2019
The specialty of immunodeficiency requires
that we appreciate the complexity of the
human body and the fragility of life. Liv was
a blessing and will always be in our hearts.*

Contents

1	**An Overview of Primary Immunodeficiencies** .... Jonathan A. Bernstein	1

Part I B-Lymphocyte Immunodeficiency

2	**Common Variable Immunodeficiency, Hypogammaglobulinemia, and Specific Antibody Deficiency** .... Heather K. Lehman and Parteet Sandhu	15
3	**Agammaglobulinemia** .... Camile Ortega and Vivian Hernandez-Trujillo	37
4	**Class-Switch Defects** .... Ramsay L. Fuleihan	49
5	**Transient Immunodeficiency of Infancy** .... Kristin C. Sokol	59
6	**Selective Isotype Immunodeficiency** .... Robert Tamayev and Jenny Shliozberg	69
7	**Common Variable Immunodeficiency-Like Disorders** .... Rohan Ameratunga, Caroline Allan, and See-Tarn Woon	91

Part II T-Cell Immunodeficiency

8	**Severe Combined Immunodeficiency** .... Jessica Galant-Swafford and Bob Geng	107
9	**Idiopathic CD4 Lymphopenia** .... Yuliya Afinogenova and Joel P. Brooks	139

10	**Hyper IgE Syndrome**	149
	Taha Al-Shaikhly	
11	**Genetic Syndromes with Associated Immunodeficiencies**	169
	Rebecca A. Marsh and Andrew W. Lindsley	

Part III Immune Dysregulation Syndromes

12	**Autoimmune Lymphoproliferative Syndrome**	187
	David T. Yang	
13	**Autoinflammatory Syndromes**	203
	James M. Fernandez, John McDonnell, and Christine A. Royer	
14	**Immune Dysregulation Leading to Autoimmunity**	221
	Melissa D. Gans and Rachel Eisenberg	
15	**Dendritic Cells in Primary Immunodeficiency**	255
	Justin Greiwe	

Part IV Innate Immune Defects

16	**Congenital Neutropenia and Migration Defects**	271
	Thomas F. Michniacki, Saara Kaviany, and Kelly Walkovich	
17	**Chronic Granulomatous Disease**	289
	Danielle E. Arnold and Jennifer R. Heimall	
18	**Primary Immunodeficiencies of Complement**	313
	Peter D. Arkwright	
19	**Natural Killer Cell Defects**	331
	Natalia S. Chaimowitz and Lisa R. Forbes	
20	**Mucocutaneous Candidiasis**	349
	William K. Dolen, Laura S. Green, and Betty B. Wray	

Part V Secondary Immunodeficiency

21	**Immunodeficiency Secondary to Malignancies and Biologics**	363
	S. Shahzad Mustafa	
22	**Immunodeficiency Secondary to Prematurity, Pregnancy, and Aging**	381
	Irina Dawson and Mark Ballow	
23	**Vaccinations in Primary and Secondary Immunodeficiencies Including Asplenia**	397
	Lauren Fine and Nofar Kimchi	

Index 411

Contributors

Yuliya Afinogenova, MD Department of Rheumatology, Allergy & Immunology, Yale New Haven Hospital and Yale School of Medicine, New Haven, CT, USA

Caroline Allan, MBChB Department of Immunology, Auckland City Hospital, Auckland, New Zealand

Taha Al-Shaikhly, MBChB Department of Medicine, Penn State College of Medicine, Hershey, PA, USA

Rohan Ameratunga, BHB, MBChB, PhD Department of Clinical Immunology, Auckland City Hospital, Auckland, New Zealand

Peter D. Arkwright, MB BS, D Phil Department of Pediatric Allergy and Immunology, Lydia, Manchester, UK

Becker Institute, Manchester, Lancashire, UK

Danielle E. Arnold, MD Immune Deficiency – Cellular Therapy Program, National Cancer Institute, National Institutes of Health, Bethesda, MD, USA

Mark Ballow, MD Division of Allergy and Immunology, Johns Hopkins All Children's Hospital/USF Department of Pediatrics, St. Petersburg, FL, USA

Jonathan A. Bernstein, MD College of Medicine, University of Cincinnati, Cincinnati, OH, USA

Joel P. Brooks, DO, MPH Department of Allergy and Immunology, George Washington University School of Medicine and Health Sciences, Children's National Health System, Washington, DC, USA

Natalia S. Chaimowitz, MD, PhD Section of Immunology, Allergy and Retrovirology, Department of Pediatrics, Texas Children's Hospital, Houston, TX, USA

Irina Dawson, MD Division of Allergy and Immunology, Johns Hopkins All Children's Hospital/USF Department of Pediatrics, St. Petersburg, FL, USA

William K. Dolen, MD Medical College of Georgia at Augusta University, Augusta, GA, USA

Rachel Eisenberg, MD Children's Hospital at Montefiore, Division of Allergy and Immunology, Montefiore Medicial Center, Bronx, NY, USA

James M. Fernandez, MD, PhD Department of Allergy and Clinical Immunology, Cleveland Clinic Foundation, Cleveland, OH, USA

Lauren Fine, MD Department of Medicine, VA Medical Center Miami, Miami, FL, USA

Lisa R. Forbes, MD Texas Children's Hospital, Section of Immunology, Allergy and Retrovirology, Department of Pediatrics, Baylor College of Medicine, Houston, TX, USA

Ramsay L. Fuleihan, MD Department of Allergy and Immunology, Ann and Robert H. Lurie Children's Hospital of Chicago, Chicago, IL, USA

Jessica Galant-Swafford, MD Department of Medicine, Division of Rheumatology, Allergy and Immunology, University of California, San Diego, San Diego, CA, USA

Melissa D. Gans, MD Children's Hospital at Montefiore, Division of Allergy and Immunology, Montefiore Medicial Center, Bronx, NY, USA

Bob Geng, MD University of California, San Diego, and Rady Children's Hospital, Division of Allergy and Immunology, San Diego, CA, USA

Laura S. Green, MD The Allergy, Asthma and Sinus Center, Knoxville, TN, USA

Justin Greiwe, MD Division of Immunology, Allergy, and Rheumatology, University of Cincinnati, Cincinnati, OH, USA

Jennifer R. Heimall, MD Immune Deficiency – Cellular Therapy Program, National Cancer Institute, National Institutes of Health, Bethesda, MD, USA

Vivian Hernandez-Trujillo, MD Allergy and Immunology Care Center of South Florida, Nicklaus Children's Hospital, Miami Lakes, FL, USA

Saara Kaviany, BS, DO Monroe Carell Jr. Children's Hospital at Vanderbilt, Nashville, TN, USA

Nofar Kimchi, MD Ruth and Bruce Rappaport Faculty of Medicine, Technion Israel Institute of Technology, Haifa, Israel

Heather K. Lehman, MD University of Buffalo Jacobs School of Medicine and Biomedical Sciences, Department of Pediatric Allergy and Immunology, Buffalo, NY, USA

Contributors

Andrew W. Lindsley, MD, PhD Department of Allergy and Immunology, University of Cincinnati, Cincinnati Children's Hospital Medical Center, Cincinnati, OH, USA

Rebecca A. Marsh, MD Bone Marrow Transplantation and Immune Deficiency, University of Cincinnati, Cincinnati Children's Hospital Medical Center, Cincinnati, OH, USA

John McDonnell, MD Department of Allergy and Clinical Immunology, Cleveland Clinic Foundation, Cleveland, OH, USA

Thomas F. Michniacki, MD Division of Pediatric Hematology/Oncology, C.S. Mott Children's Hospital/University of Michigan, Ann Arbor, MI, USA

S. Shahzad Mustafa, MD Division of Allergy, Immunology, Rheumatology, Rochester Regional Health, University of Rochester School of Medicine and Dentistry, Rochester, NY, USA

Camile Ortega, DO Department of Medical Education, Nicklaus Children's Hospital, Miami, FL, USA

Christine A. Royer, MD Department of Allergy and Clinical Immunology, Cleveland Clinic Foundation, Cleveland, OH, USA

Parteet Sandhu, MD Division of Allergy and Clinical Immunology, University of Buffalo Jacobs School of Medicine and Biomedical Sciences, Buffalo, NY, USA

Jenny Shliozberg, MD Department of Allergy and Immunology, Montefiore Medical Center/Albert Einstein College of Medicine, Bronx, NY, USA

Kristin C. Sokol, MD, MS, MPH Schreiber Allergy, Rockville, MD, USA

Robert Tamayev, MD, PhD New York Allergy and Sinus Center, Glendale, NY, USA

Kelly Walkovich, MD Division of Pediatric Hematology/Oncology, C.S. Mott Children's Hospital/University of Michigan, Ann Arbor, MI, USA

Betty B. Wray, MD Medical College of Georgia at Augusta, Augusta, GA, USA

David T. Yang, MD Department of Pathology and Laboratory Medicine, University of Wisconsin, Madison, WI, USA

Chapter 1
An Overview of Primary Immunodeficiencies

Jonathan A. Bernstein

Introduction

Immunodeficiency, whether primary or secondary, is a serious disorder that requires early diagnosis and intervention to prevent comorbidities and potential death. The majority of primary immunodeficiency (PID) cases are rare monogenic defects that present in infancy or early childhood. However, with improved screening recommendations (e.g., T-cell receptor excision circle (TREC) screening for severe combined immunodeficiency (SCID)) and diagnostic testing as well as advanced therapies, these patients are surviving longer into adulthood, requiring systems that allow transitioning to adult care more seamless. However, some of the more common PID (IgA deficiency, common variable immunodeficiency (CVID)) and secondary immunodeficiencies (SID) present in adults but often go unrecognized as uneventful recurrent sinus infections or chronic bronchitis with intermittent pneumonia. Early warning signs of possible PID such as recurrent otitis media, recurrent sinusitis or pneumonia, severe infections requiring intravenous antibiotics, failure to thrive or growth retardation in an infant or a child, recurrent skin or organ abscesses, persistent oral or skin candidiasis, severe infections leading to septicemia, or a family history of PID should alert additional workup or referral to an immunodeficiency specialist. However, many cases are identified serendipitously, such as when a patient being evaluated for celiac disease is found to have an undetectable IgA level, prompting referral to an immunologist for further assessment. As most patients with PID and SID present to their primary care physician or a community specialist without specialized immunodeficiency training, it is imperative that resources like this casebook are available that can provide guidance for their initial clinical evaluation and management.

J. A. Bernstein (✉)
College of Medicine, University of Cincinnati, Cincinnati, OH, USA
e-mail: bernstja@ucmail.uc.edu

Ultimately, it is hoped that the clinician will develop a fundamental knowledge of immunodeficiency conditions outlined in this book so they can become more comfortable in the diagnosis and treatment of these disorders. For those interested in a more in-depth understanding of the immune system, *Stiehm's Immune Deficiencies* is a useful reference.

Overview of Casebook

This book uses a case-based approach that focuses on our current understanding of specific B- and T-cell immunodeficiencies, immune dysregulation syndromes, innate immune defects, and secondary immunodeficiencies. Although there may be some rarer disorders that have been omitted or topics not discussed in sufficient detail, the major conditions encountered by clinicians and their appropriate management are reviewed clearly and succinctly in each chapter.

The first section of this book addresses B-cell immunodeficiency conditions, which include common variable immunodeficiency (CVID), hypogammaglobulinemia, specific antibody deficiency, agammaglobulinemia, immunoglobulin class-switch defects, transient immunodeficiency of infancy, selective isotype immunodeficiency, and CVID-like disorders. The second section focuses on T-cell immunodeficiency, which includes severe combined immunodeficiency, idiopathic CD4 lymphopenia, hyper-IgE syndromes, and genetic syndromes with associated immunodeficiencies. The third section centers on immune dysregulation syndromes including autoimmune lymphoproliferative syndrome, auto-inflammatory syndromes, immune dysregulation leading to autoimmunity, and dendritic cell immunodeficiency conditions. The fourth section addresses innate immune defects and includes congenital neutropenia and migration defect disorders, chronic granulomatous disease, primary immunodeficiencies of complement, natural killer cell defects, and mucocutaneous candidiasis. Finally, the fifth section addresses immunodeficiency secondary to malignancies and biologics, immunodeficiency secondary to prematurity, pregnancy, and aging as well as the appropriate approach to vaccinations in primary and secondary immunodeficiencies, including in asplenic patients. Each chapter provides two case presentations nested with a discussion of the essential elements of a proper medical history, differential diagnosis, diagnostic testing, treatment options, and long-term management. Each chapter concludes with a "Clinical Pearls and Pitfalls" summary that emphasizes the important take-home messages for the reader. It is clear from each chapter that evaluation of PID requires much more than ordering a Complete blood count (CBC) with differential, quantitative immunoglobulins, and B- and T-cell vaccination responses. Therefore, it is advisable to involve a clinical immunologist, who may be trained in hematology or allergy, to determine whether a more in-depth evaluation is required.

Immunodeficiency Comorbidities

Some notable important observations can be gleaned from reading the various chapters in this book that are worth emphasizing. In addition to severe life-threatening infections which can affect multiple organ systems, primary immunodeficiency patients are at increased risk for several comorbid conditions including malignancies and autoimmune diseases. Therefore, careful monitoring of these patients over time is a necessary component of their management. For example, DNA breakage disorders such as ataxia telangiectasia, Bloom's syndrome, and Nijmegen breakage syndrome are all at increased risk for leukemias and lymphomas [1]. However, carcinomas and brain tumors can also occur in Bloom's syndrome and Nijmegen breakage syndrome, respectively [1]. CVID patients are at increased risk for lymphoma, gastric, thyroid, and skin cancers, whereas patients with immune dysregulation syndromes like Autoimmune lymphoproliferative syndrome (ALPS) are at increased risk for Hodgkin's and non-Hodgkin's lymphoma. In addition, GATA2 patients are at increased risk for myelodysplastic syndrome (MDS), acute myelogenous leukemia (AML), as well as Epstein Barr Virus (EBV)- and Human Papillomavirus (HPV)-induced tumors [1, 2]. Patients with other immunodeficiencies such as Wiskott-Aldrich syndrome are at increased risk for MDS, lymphomas, and acute lymphocytic leukemia [1, 2]. It is important to note that while many of these malignancies occur in children and adolescents, they also are known to occur in adult CVID patients [2].

Autoimmune disorders are the most frequent noninfectious complications occurring in 20–30% of CVID patients [3]. In one registry study, autoimmune cytopenias were 700 times more common in CVID patients than in the general population [3]. The most common autoimmune cytopenias are immune thrombocytopenia and hemolytic anemia and less commonly autoimmune neutropenia which in up to 60% of the time precede the onset of CVID [3]. CVID patients with interstitial lung disease are more likely to have autoimmune cytopenias [3]. CVID patients are also at increased risk for splenomegaly, granulomatous and lymphoproliferative disease, organ-specific autoimmune disease, and malignancy. In addition, other autoimmune disorders reported in less than 5% of CVID patients include inflammatory arthritis, systemic lupus erythematosus, Sjogren's, Behcet's, psoriasis, alopecia areata, vitiligo, type I diabetes mellitus, inflammatory bowel disease, autoimmune enteropathy, and gastritis [3].

Technological Advancements in Immunodeficiency

Another important observation worth discussing is the rapidity with which the specialty of immunodeficiency has evolved. Since 1971, when the term "common variable immunodeficiency" was first proposed to describe a heterogeneous group of patients with recurrent infections characterized primarily by late-onset antibody failure unrelated to any other underlying cause, it has expanded exponentially as a direct result of immunophenotyping and genotyping technologies [4]. As patient phenotyping has improved, it has been possible to use cellular and molecular techniques such as flow cytometry, next-generation sequencing (NGS), whole exome sequencing (WES), and gene editing to identify monogenic defects in many of these patients never previously characterized [1, 3–6]. By 2016, the International Union of Immunological Societies (IUIS) has classified more than 400 inborn errors of immunity (IEI), which have doubled since 2009 [5]. For example, NGS has identified monogenic defects such as transmembrane activator and calcium-modulator and cyclophilin ligand interactor (TACI), signal transducer and activator of transcription 3 gene (STAT3) and phosphatidylinositol-4, 5-bisphosphate 3-kinase, catalytic subunit delta gene (PIK3CD), gain-of-function (GOF) mutations, nuclear factor kappa beta (NFkB), lipopolysaccharide (LPS)-responsive and beige-like anchor protein (LRBA) and cytotoxic T-lymphocyte-associated protein 4 (CTLA-4) and their associated risk for autoimmune or malignancy complications [1, 3, 7]. In addition, deep intronic mutations such as UNC13D-associated hemophagocytic lymphohistiocytosis (HLH), IL-7R and Janus kinase 3 for severe combined immunodeficiency (SCID), zeta chain–associated protein kinase (ZAP70) in children with T-cell immunodeficiencies, signal transducer and activator of transcription-3 (STAT3) in hyper-IgE syndrome, and NF-kB essential modulator (NEMO) in ectodermal dysplasia and immunodeficiency have been identified [5]. RNA sequencing has been useful for identifying partial or complete loss of gene expression in probands compared to controls which otherwise never would have been recognized using older methodologies [5]. Furthermore, flow cytometric assays are now routinely being used to assess for hemophagocytic lymphohistiocytosis (HLH) which can be a primary IEI (i.e., perforin deficiency) or secondary to infections, malignancies, or autoimmune disease without a genetic cause [6]. Specifically, functional flow cytometric 107a assays have been found to be increasingly useful to measure whether NK and cytotoxic T-lymphocytes (CTLs) can release lysosomes after stimulation with K562 cells (NK cells), anti-CD16 antibodies (NK cells), or anti-CD3 antibodies (CTLs) to evaluate for primary and secondary HLH [6].

Novel Therapeutic Advancements

Intravenous immunoglobulin replacement therapy has been the mainstay of treatment for immunodeficiencies with impaired B-cell function resulting in hypogammaglobulinemia. However, this treatment is frequently associated with systemic side effects that require pretreatment with H1-antihistamines, nonsteroidal anti-inflammatory agents, or glucocorticoids. Even with these pretreatment approaches and changing from one preparation to another, these therapies are still intolerable for many patients. The development of subcutaneous immunoglobulin products has made it possible for patients to self-administer immunoglobulin treatment in their home and is associated with significantly fewer side effects [8].

Not surprisingly, advancements in molecular technology have also led to the development of novel biologic therapies and small molecules that target very

Table 1.1 Targeted therapies for primary immunodeficiencies [7]

Molecular structure	Molecular target	Drug	Indication
Macrolide compound	mTOR	Sirolimus	NLCR4 GOF POMP deficiency CTLA-4 Haploinsufficiency APDS
CTLA-4 IgG fusion protein	B7-1 (CD80), B7-2 (CD86)	Abatacept Belatacept	CTLA-4 haploinsufficiency, LRBA deficiency CTLA-4 haploinsufficiency
Antihuman IL-1 IgG1 mAb IgG1 linked to IL-1R and IL-1R accessory protein	IL-1beta	Canakinumab Rilonacept	CAPS FCAS MWS DIRA
IgG1k recombinant humanized mAb	IL-6R	Tocilizumab	STAT3 GOF
Fusion protein Chimeric mAb Humanized mAb	TNF-alpha	Etanercept Infliximab Adalimumab	SAVI CANDLE syndrome POMP deficiency
Small molecule inhibitor	JAK1 and JAK2 JAK1 and JAK3 P110	Ruxolitinib, Tofacitinib Baricitinib Tofacitinib Leniolisib	STAT3 GOF STAT1 GOF CANDLE syndrome APDS
Recombinant IL-18 binding protein	IL-18 binding protein	Tadekinig-alpha	NLCR4 GOF

CTLA4 cytotoxic T-lymphocyte–associated antigen 4, *STAT* signal transducer and activator of transcription, *GOF* gain of function, *APD* activated phosphoinositide 3-kinase delta syndrome, *CAPS* cryopyrin-associated periodic syndrome, *CANDLE* chronic atypical neutrophilic dermatosis with lipodystrophy and elevated temperature, *POMP* proteasome maturation protein, *FCAS* familial cold autoinflammatory syndrome, *LRBA* lipopolysaccharide (LPS)-responsive and beige-like anchor protein, *MWS* Muckle-Wells syndrome, *DIRA* deficiency of IL-1 receptor antagonist, *SAVI* STING-associated vasculopathy with onset in infancy

specific checkpoints important for regulating immunity, inflammation, and cancer (Table 1.1) [5, 9]. Genetic sequencing has been successful in identifying point mutations that have led to precision, targeted therapies such as the CTLA-4 immunoglobulin fusion proteins, Abatacept and Belatacept, used as replacement therapy for CTLA-4 haploinsufficient and LRBA-deficient patients. These therapies have also been effective for treating their associated autoimmune complications [9]. Other cytokine therapies such as Tocilizumab, an anti-IL6 receptor antagonist, have been effective for treating STAT3 GOF mutations [9].

In addition, hematopoietic stem cell transplantation and novel forms of conditioning strategies, which are gradually replacing conventional chemotherapies, have been curative for many of these IEI disorders [5, 10]. Even more astonishing are the advancements in gene therapy to cure IEIs, which has become more feasible as safer lentiviral vectors are being used to correct the molecular defect in vitro by gene addition [5]. This has reduced the risk for graft versus host disease after autologous stem cell infusion and is currently being used in clinical trials to treat Recombination activating gene (RAG)-SCID, X-linked lymphoproliferative disease, and perforin deficiency [5]. Gene editing using CRISPR/Cas9 technology appears promising; however, due to lower transfection efficiency as a result of increased cell mortality compared to gene editing methods, this technique still requires further refinement [5, 10]. Early trials using CRISPR/Cas9 technology to treat gain-of-function (GOF) mutations associated with X-linked SCID and agammaglobulinemia, chronic granulomatous disease (CGD), and hyper-IgM syndrome are ongoing [5, 10]. Other approaches, such as T-cell gene therapy and base editing for use in correcting T-cell defects and single point mutations, also appear promising [5].

As a result of the advancements achieved in patient phenotyping and subsequent identification of specific monogenic defects, strong consideration should be given to obtain a limited immunology exome sequencing panel for all confirmed CVID patients that includes primers for known mutations so they can be risk-stratified for future complications like malignancy and autoimmune diseases which require closer monitoring so precision therapies can be implement if and when they manifest.

Conclusion

The management of patients with immunodeficiencies involves many stakeholders, including the patient's families and friends, primary care clinicians, patient advocacy groups and foundations, insurance companies, specialty pharmacies, hospitals, immunodeficiency centers of excellence for patient care and research, immunodeficiency reference laboratories, and immunodeficiency professional organizations. In many instances, finding resources in one's community to refer a patient for an immunodeficiency workup can be very challenging and may require travel for many of these patients because not all academic centers have this expertise. The Jeffrey Modell Foundation (http://www.info4pi.org/village/patient-organizations) and the Immune Deficiency Foundation (https://primary-immune.org/about-primary-immunodeficiencies) have many available patient resources, physician referral information, and research initiatives. Table 1.2 lists many of the immunodeficiency centers primarily at major university medical centers that have immunodeficiency specialists where patients can be sent for consultation. Many of these centers also have immunodeficiency laboratories where specialized testing can be performed.

Ultimately, it is hoped that this casebook illustrates the great strides made in understanding and treating PID and SID disorders. However, while reading the cases and current algorithms for management for many of these conditions, it should become increasingly clear that amidst all of the technical and therapeutic advancements made over the past 50 years, diagnoses of immunodeficiency disorders are still frequently delayed, and there remain many knowledge gaps that require further investigation.

1 An Overview of Primary Immunodeficiencies

Table 1.2 List of transplant centers with immunodeficiency laboratories in the United States, Canada, and United Kingdom (from the Rare Disease Network Organization; https://www.rarediseasesnetwork.org/cms/pidtc/Learn-More/Participating-Clinical-Centers)

State	Center	Immunologist	Transplanter	Address
UNITED STATES				
Alabama	The Children's Hospital of Alabama	Prescott Atkinson	Fred Goldman	Children's Hospital of Alabama ACC 512 1600 7th Ave S Birmingham AL 35233
Arizona	Phoenix Children's Hospital Center for Cancer and Blood Disorders	Holly Miller	Roberta H. Adams	1919 E. Thomas Rd. Phoenix, AZ 85016
California				
	Children's Hospital LA	Michael Pulsipher	Neena Kapoor	Division of Research Immunology and Bone Marrow Transplant 4650 Sunset Boulevard - Mail Stop 62 Los Angeles, CA 90027
	Lucile Packard Children's Hospital Stanford	Katja Weinacht	Matthew Porteus	265 Campus Drive Building G3040B MC 5462 Stanford, CA 94305
	Mattel Children's Hospital UCLA	Caroline Kuo	Theodore Moore	Division of Hematology/Oncology 10833 Le Conte Avenue; Rm A2-410 MDCC Los Angeles, CA 90095-1752
	UCSF Benioff Children's Hospital	Jennifer Puck	Christopher Dvorak	505 Parnassus Ave, Rm M674 San Francisco, CA 94143-1278
Colorado	Children's Hospital Colorado	Ralph Quinones	John Craddock	13123 East 16th Avenue, B115 Aurora, CO 80045
Washington, D.C.	Children's National Medical Center	Michael Keller	Blachy Davila Saldana	Center for Cancer and Blood Disorders 111 Michigan Avenue, NW Washington DC 20010-2970

(continued)

Table 1.2 (continued)

State	Center	Immunologist	Transplanter	Address
Delaware	Alfred I. duPont Hospital for Children/ Nemours	Magee DeFelice	Emi Caywood	1600 Rockland Road Wilmington, DE 19803
Florida	Johns Hopkins All Children's Hospital	Jennifer Leiding	Benjamin Oshrine	Blood and Marrow Transplant Program All Children's Hospital 601 5th Street South 3rd Floor St. Petersburg, FL 33701
Georgia	Children's Healthcare of Atlanta	Lisa Kobrinski	Elizabeth Stenger	AFLAC Cancer Center 4th Floor, Tower 1 1405 Clifton Road NE Atlanta, GA 30322
Illinois	Ann & Robert H. Lurie Children's Hopsital of Chicago	Ramsay Fuleihan	Morris Kletzel	Ann & Robert H. Lurie Children's Hopsital of Chicago Division of Pediatric Hem, Onc and Stem Cell Transplant 2300 Children's Plaza, Box 30 Chicago, IL 60614
Louisiana	Children's Hospital, LSUHSC	Ken Paris	Lolie Yu	200 Henry Clay, Suite 4109 New Orleans, LA 70118
Massachusetts	Boston Children's Hospital	Craig Platt	Sung-Yun Pai	Karp Family Research Labs, Rm 08214 300 Longwood Avenue Boston, MA 02115
Maryland	NIAID/NIH	Harry Malech	Elizabeth Kang	Building 10-CRC, Room 6W-3752 9000 Rockville Pike: 10 Center Drive MSC 1456 Bethesda MD 20892-1456
Michigan	University of Michigan Health System	Mark Vander Lugt	Gregory Yanik	1500 E Medical Center Drive SPC 57 Ann Arbor, MI 48109
Minnesota	University of Minnesota Medical Center		Angela Smith	Pediatric Blood and Marrow Transplant 420 Delaware Street SE, MMC 484 Minneapolis, MN 55455
Missouri				

Table 1.2 (continued)

State	Center	Immunologist	Transplanter	Address
	Cardinal Glennon Children's Medical Center	Deepika Bhatla	Alan P. Knutsen	1465 South Grand Blvd. St. Louis, MO 63104
	Washington University School of Medicine	Jeffrey Bednarski	Shalini Shenoy	Box 8116 1 Children's Place St. Louis, MO 63110
North Carolina	Duke University Medical Center	Rebecca Buckley	Suhag Parikh	Pediatric Stem Cell Transplant Program Duke University Medical Center Box 3350, Durham, NC 27710
New Jersey	Hackensack University Medical Center	Alfred P. Gilli		Pediatric BMT Program 30 Prospect Avenue Hackensack, NJ 07601
New York				
	Memorial Sloan Kettering Cancer Center	Susan Prockop		1275 York Avenue New York, NY 10065
	Maria Fareri Children's Hospital/ NYMC	Subhadra Siegel	Cori Abikoff	40 Sunshine Cottage Road Skyline IN-H09 Valhalla, NY 10595
	University of Rochester Medical Center	Maria Slack	Jeffrey Andolina	601 Elmwood Avenue, Rochester, NY 14642
Ohio	Cincinnati Children's Hospital Medical Center University of Cincinnati and Bernstein Allergy Group	Jack Bleesing Jonathan Bernstein	Rebecca Marsh	3333 Burnet Avenue, MLC 11027 Cincinnati, OH 45229-3039 8444 Winton Road, Cincinnati, Ohio 45231
Oregon	Oregon Health & Science University Doernbecher Children's Hospital		Evan Shereck	3181 SW Sam Jackson Park Road, CDRC-P Portland, OR 97239
Pennsylvania				
	The Children's Hospital of Pennsylvania	Kathleen Sullivan Jennifer Heimall Soma Jyonouchi		3615 Civic Center Blvd. Philadelphia, PA 19104
	Children's Hospital of Pittsburgh of UPMC	Hey Jin Chong	Paul Szabolcs	4401 AOB Suite 3300 Pittsburgh, PA 15232

(continued)

Table 1.2 (continued)

State	Center	Immunologist	Transplanter	Address
Tennessee	St. Jude Children's Research Hospital	Jay Lieberman	Ewelina Mamcarz	262 Danny Thomas Place, Memphis, TN 38105
Texas				
	Texas Children's Hospital/Baylor	Imelda Celine Hanson	William Shearer	1102 Bates Street, Suite 330 Houston, TX 77030-2399
	Methodist Children's Hospital of South Texas		Troy C. Quigg	Pediatric Blood and Marrow Transplantation Program Texas Transplant Institute, Methodist Physician Practices, PLLC 4410 Medical Drive, Suite 550 San Antonio, TX 78229
	University of Texas Southwestern Medical Center Dallas		Victor Aquino	Pediatric Hematology Oncology 5323 Harry Hines Blvd Dallas, TX 75390-9263
Utah	Primary Children's Medical Center University of Utah School of Medicine	David Shyr	Michael Boyer	100 N. Mario Capecchi Drive Salt Lake City, UT 84113
Washington	Seattle Children's Hospital Fred Hutchinson Cancer Research Center		Lauri Burroughs Aleksandra Petrovic	1100 Fairview Avenue North Mailstop D1-100 Seattle, WA 98109
Wisconsin				
	Medical College of Wisconsin Children's Hospital of Wisconsin	John M. Routes	Monica Thakar	8701 Watertown Plank Road Milwaukee, WI 53226
	University of Wisconsin, American Family Children's Hospital	Christine Seroogy	Ken Desantes	1111 Highland Ave, 4103 WIMR Madison, WI 53705-2275
CANADA				
Alberta	Alberta Children's Hospital	Nicola Wright	Victor Lewis	2888 Shaganappi Trail NW Calgary, AB, Canada T3B 6A8

Table 1.2 (continued)

State	Center	Immunologist	Transplanter	Address
British Columbia	Children's & Women's Health Centre of British Columbia	Stuart Turvey	Jeffrey H. Davis	4480 Oak Street Vancouver BC, Canada V6H 3V4
Manitoba	CancerCare Manitoba		Geoff Cuvelier	675 McDermot Avenue Winnipeg, MB, Canada R3E 0V9
Quebec	CHU Sainte-Justine		Elie Haddad	Centre de Cancérologie Charles-Bruneau, A484 3175, chemin de la Côte-Sainte-Catherine Montréal, QC (Canada) H3T 1C5
Toronto	SickKids/The Hospital for Sick Children	Eyal Grunebaum		555 University Avenue Toronto Ontario, Canada M5G 1X8
UNITED KINGDOM				
Tyne and Wear	The Great North Children's Hospital, Newcastle		Andrew Gennery	

References

1. Renzi S, Langenberg-Ververgaert KPS, Waespe N, Ali S, Bartram J, Michaeli O, et al. Primary immunodeficiencies and their associated risk of malignancies in children: an overview. Eur J Pediatr. 2020;179(5):689–97.
2. Kebudi R, Kiykim A, Sahin MK. Primary immunodeficiency and cancer in children; a review of the literature. Curr Pediatr Rev. 2019;15(4):245–50.
3. Gereige JD, Maglione PJ. Current understanding and recent developments in common variable immunodeficiency associated autoimmunity. Front Immunol. 2019;10:2753.
4. Ameratunga R, Woon ST. Perspective: evolving concepts in the diagnosis and understanding of Common Variable Immunodeficiency Disorders (CVID). Clin Rev Allergy Immunol. 2019. https://doi.org/10.1007/s12016-019-08765-6. Online ahead of print.
5. Bucciol G, Meyts I. Recent advances in primary immunodeficiency: from molecular diagnosis to treatment. F1000Res. 2020;9:F1000.
6. Chiang SCC, Bleesing JJ, Marsh RA. Current flow cytometric assays for the screening and diagnosis of primary HLH. Front Immunol. 2019;10:1–11.
7. Aggarwal V, Banday AZ, Jindal AK, Das J, Rawat A. Recent advances in elucidating the genetics of common variable immunodeficiency. Genes Dis. 2020;7(1):26–37.
8. Sriaroon P, Ballow M. Immunoglobulin replacement therapy for primary immunodeficiency. Immunol Allergy Clin North Am. 2015;35:713–30.
9. Delmonte OM, Notarangelo LD. Targeted therapy with biologicals and small molecules in primary immunodeficiencies. Med Princ Pract. 2020;29(2):101–12.
10. Gennery AR, Albert MH, Slatter MA, Lankester A. Hematopoietic stem cell transplantation for primary immunodeficiencies. Front Pediatr. 2019;7:445.

Part I
B-Lymphocyte Immunodeficiency

Chapter 2
Common Variable Immunodeficiency, Hypogammaglobulinemia, and Specific Antibody Deficiency

Heather K. Lehman and Parteet Sandhu

Introduction

Antibody deficiencies are a group of primary immune deficiencies caused by defects in B-cell development, B-cell activation, or antibody synthesis. They account for more than half of all diagnosed cases of primary immune deficiencies [1, 2]. Immune deficiencies that are considered primarily antibody deficiencies include agammaglobulinemia (X-linked and autosomal recessive), combined variable immunodeficiency (CVID), specific antibody deficiency (SAD), unspecified hypogammaglobulinemia, transient hypogammaglobulinemia of infancy, selective IgA deficiency, and immunoglobulin class-switch defects. While IgG subclass deficiency has also been recognized as an antibody deficiency, there is some controversy regarding its significance in the absence of associated functional defects in specific antibody production [3]. The focus of this chapter will be on the diagnosis and management of CVID, SAD, and unspecified hypogammaglobulinemia.

There is uncertainty regarding the exact prevalence of CVID; however, it is agreed that it affects at least one in 30,000 persons worldwide [2]. The prevalence of SAD differs between different populations; it has been found to be present in 6–23% of children with recurrent infections [4–7]. In adults, SAD was diagnosed in 12–24% of patients with chronic rhinosinusitis and 8% of patients with recurrent pneumonia [8]. Females have a higher prevalence of antibody deficiencies as compared with males [1]. Complicating prevalence estimates of these conditions is the concern that primary

---

H. K. Lehman (✉)
University of Buffalo Jacobs School of Medicine and Biomedical Sciences, Department of Pediatrics, Division of Allergy and Clinical Immunology, Buffalo, NY, USA
e-mail: hkm@buffalo.edu

P. Sandhu
Division of Allergy and Clinical Immunology, University of Buffalo Jacobs School of Medicine and Biomedical Sciences, Buffalo, NY, USA

immune deficiencies are likely underdiagnosed [1]. Diagnostic delay also occurs, with multiple studies of patients with CVID demonstrating a mean delay ranging from 5 to 9 years between the onset of symptoms and disease diagnosis [9–12].

Classification schema for antibody deficiencies has evolved over time, beginning in 1966 when Rosen and Janeway grouped them by their mode of inheritance [13]. Currently, there has been a focus on classifying CVID subgroups based on B-cell phenotype via flow cytometry [12].

Antibody deficiencies can have infectious and noninfectious disease presentations. While infectious complications are common in all three diseases discussed in this chapter, noninfectious features are common in CVID and are rare in SAD and hypogammaglobulinemia. Overall, these antibody deficiencies have a good prognosis. Morbidity related to infectious complications has decreased drastically after the introduction of immunoglobulin (Ig) replacement [11]. However, noninfectious complications remain a burden and are the major cause of morbidity and mortality in CVID (Table 2.1). These noninfectious symptoms require close monitoring and a multidisciplinary approach.

Table 2.1 Noninfectious complications of CVID

Pulmonary
Lymphocytic interstitial pneumonitis
Nodular lymphoid hyperplasia
Granulomatous lymphocytic interstitial lung disease (GLILD)
Dermatologic
Psoriasis
Vitiligo
Lichen planus
Alopecia
Gastrointestinal
Atrophic gastritis
Gastric carcinoma
Pernicious anemia
Autoimmune enteropathy
Small bowel villous flattening
Primary biliary cirrhosis
Primary sclerosing cholangitis
Rheumatologic
Lupus
Rheumatoid arthritis
Vasculitis
Hematologic
Immune thrombocytopenia
Hemolytic anemia
Autoimmune neutropenia
Evan's syndrome
Lymphoid
Lymphoid hyperplasia
Splenomegaly
Non-Hodgkin's lymphoma

Case Presentation 1

A 2-year-old male with a history of controlled allergic rhinitis and mild intermittent asthma presented to immunology clinic for the evaluation of frequent infections. He had been suffering from frequent upper respiratory infections, including bilateral otitis media, sinusitis, and pharyngitis. His symptoms started when he was 6 months old, and he required antibiotic courses every 2–4 weeks. He had bilateral tympanostomy tubes placed without improvement in symptoms. He did not have a history of pneumonia or skin infections. On physical exam, he was a well-nourished male with bilateral tympanostomy tubes present, pink nasal mucosa without turbinate swelling, and normal lung exam. There was no lymphadenopathy or organomegaly present. His laboratory evaluation showed normal complete blood count (CBC) with differential. He had a low IgA level (<5 mg/dL) but had normal levels of IgG (850 mg/dL) and IgM (29 mg/dL) for his age. His baseline pneumococcal titers (following primary pneumococcal conjugate vaccine series) showed 4 out of 23 serotypes protective (≥ 1.3 µg/mL), and he had protective titers against tetanus. He received pneumococcal polysaccharide vaccine, and repeat pneumococcal titers 1 month following vaccination were protective against only 8 out of 23 serotypes. A diagnosis of specific antibody deficiency (SAD) was made. He took trimethoprim-sulfamethoxazole prophylaxis for 3 months, and the frequency of infection improved; however, he continued to have a significant burden from infections. Subsequently, he was started on 0.5 g/kg of intravenous immunoglobulin (IVIG) every 4 weeks with control of infections.

Clinical Presentation

Differentiating frequent infections due to common risk factors such as day-care attendance or passive smoke exposure from primary immune deficiency should be based on a detailed history and physical examination. It is crucial to determine the location, timeline, and severity of the infections. On average, a healthy child will have four to six upper respiratory infections per year, and it is typical for children attending day care to have an increased number of infections [14]. Children with intact immune systems typically handle these infections well, either without antibiotics or with rapid resolution of bacterial infections using appropriate antibiotics.

The clinical presentation of hypogammaglobulinemia and specific antibody deficiency consists mostly of increased frequency and severity of sinopulmonary infections as seen in the case above. In contrast, common variable immune deficiency (CVID) is a clinical disease label that encompasses a heterogeneous group of disease presentations. A substantial subset of patients with CVID have noninfectious complications that drive much of the morbidity and mortality related to the diagnosis, while others may have isolated infectious complications without evidence of immune dysregulation. Patients with hypogammaglobulinemia and specific antibody deficiency will generally present with mild bacterial infections, including sinusitis, bronchitis, and otitis media. Severe infections such as meningitis, sepsis, osteomyelitis, and skin abscesses are rare in SAD. In contrast, patients with CVID are at higher risk of developing pneumonia and invasive infections such as meningitis and sepsis.

Common respiratory organisms implicated in upper and lower respiratory infections in CVID, SAD, and hypogammaglobulinemia include encapsulated bacteria (e.g., *Haemophilus influenzae, Streptococcus pneumoniae*) and atypical bacteria (*Mycoplasma* sp.) [9, 15, 16]. These patients are also at risk for recurrent viral infections with common pathogens such as human rhinovirus [17]. Ten to fifteen percent of patients with CVID may have symptoms consistent with allergic asthma, despite negative specific IgE to common aeroallergens [18].

Patients with antibody deficiencies also have an increased incidence of gastrointestinal infections, sometimes resulting in chronic diarrhea and malabsorption. The most common pathogens include *Giardia* spp., *Campylobacter jejuni*, and *Salmonella* spp. However, *Helicobacter pylori*, *Shigella* spp., *Norovirus*, and *Parechovirus* can also be implicated in these diseases [9]. Rarely, patients with CVID can also have recurrent urinary tract infections with *Ureaplasma* spp. [16, 19].

Physical appearance can provide clues regarding disease syndromes that may be associated with antibody deficiencies. These include Down syndrome, Kabuki syndrome, trichohepatoenteric syndrome, and Wolf-Hirschhorn syndrome [20–23]. Structural abnormalities in the nasal, otic, and respiratory pathways should be assessed on physical exam, as may be underlying causes of recurrent sinusitis, otitis media, or pneumonia. On examination of the lungs, localized inspiratory or expiratory wheezes may reveal bronchial obstruction, while crackles or rhonchi may elucidate lung parenchymal damage. Lymphadenopathy or organomegaly are found in some CVID patients. Imaging should be obtained when the diagnosis of bacterial infection is unclear, when structural abnormalities are suspected, and as baseline evaluation for bronchiectasis or interstitial disease in CVID, but it should be used judiciously as patients with CVID have been found to be radiosensitive [24].

Diagnostic Criteria

CVID is largely a clinical diagnosis, and the diagnostic criteria have varied over time and from different sources. The widely accepted definition of CVID is proposed by the International Consensus Document (ICON). It defines CVID as low IgG (compared to age-specific norms) along with either low IgA or IgM (low IgA preferred), and an impaired vaccine response, with other causes of hypogammaglobulinemia being excluded [25]. Clinical manifestations such as infections or autoimmunity are not required for the diagnosis, though most patients will have at least one characteristic manifestation of CVID at the time of diagnosis.

Low functional antibody response to vaccines has to be present for a patient to be diagnosed with CVID, SAD, or hypogammaglobulinemia. The exception to the rule is when a patient is found to have an extremely low IgG level of <100 to 300 mg/dL in the absence of protein-losing enteropathy. Given such low IgG levels, there is a high likelihood of these patients having a clinically significant antibody deficiency and being at risk of severe invasive infections. It is recommended to start immunoglobulin replacement without waiting for the evaluation of immune response to vaccines when the IgG level is extremely low [26, 27].

Hypogammaglobulinemia diagnoses include both transient hypogammaglobulinemia of infancy (THI) and unspecified hypogammaglobulinemia that can persist through adulthood. Maternal IgG is transferred to infants transplacentally and has a half-life of 21 days [28]. Maternally acquired IgG remains in an infant for the first 3–6 months of their life [29]. In some children, there is delayed antibody production and do not develop a normal humoral immune system until early childhood. Due to this delay, they have recurrent upper respiratory infections in infancy and early childhood. The diagnosis of THI is a diagnosis of exclusion and is made after immunoglobulin levels have normalized. In patients with THI, IgG levels normalize at 27 months of age on average, and all THI patients reach normal levels by 59 months. Those patients that have persistent infections and low immunoglobulins past this age are given alternative diagnoses of CVID or unspecified hypogammaglobulinemia. Generally, patients with THI can produce specific antibodies to antigens; however, some may have a suppressed response until 36–48 months [30]. Hypogammaglobulinemia beyond 60 months of age is termed unspecified hypogammaglobulinemia. For this diagnosis, the patient needs to have increased infections consistent with antibody deficiency, along with low IgG levels (normal IgA and IgM levels) and abnormal vaccine response [31].

A patient with recurrent respiratory infections, normal immunoglobulin levels, and abnormal vaccine response to the unconjugated polysaccharide *Streptococcus pneumoniae* vaccine is diagnosed with SAD. Patients with SAD will have a normal response to protein and protein-conjugated polysaccharide vaccines [27]. SAD is often identified in children and may represent a subtle developmental delay of the humoral immune system. As seen with other humoral immune deficiencies, these patients develop infections sometime after 7–9 months of age, once maternal IgG has been lost by the infant [32]. However, the diagnosis cannot be given to patients younger than two years of age as the immune system is unable to respond to polysaccharide antigens before this age. In a study of pediatric patients with SAD by Wolpert et al., 44% outgrew the immune defect, developing normal antibody responses after an average of 3.1 years [33]. Ruuskanen et al. reported eight of ten children with initial diagnosis of SAD eventually responded to revaccination with pneumococcal vaccine [34]. However, SAD has also been described in adult patients [35].

The presence of low total immunoglobulins but intact functional responses to vaccines is not indicative of a primary immune deficiency, and the immunoglobulin levels should be repeated. These patients should be evaluated for other causes of low immunoglobulins such as medications, AIDS/HIV, protein-losing enteropathy, and nephrotic syndrome. Stool testing for alpha-1-antitrypsin is used to screen for protein-losing enteropathy, and urinalysis is performed when nephrotic syndrome is suspected. Medications commonly known to lead to hypogammaglobulinemia include, among others, anticonvulsants (carbamazepine, phenytoin, valproic acid), antimalarials, chemotherapeutics (gold salts, thiopurines), and anti-B–cell monoclonal antibodies [25, 36]. RT-PCR should be used to evaluate HIV/AIDS, and referral to hematology should be made when bone marrow failure or B-cell lymphoma are suspected.

Laboratory Findings

Initial evaluation for antibody deficiency includes complete blood count (CBC) with differential to screen for lymphopenia, and serum immunoglobulin IgA, IgM, and IgG concentrations along with measurement of T-cell–dependent and –independent vaccine response. If the patient has lymphopenia on CBC with differential or extremely low total serum immunoglobulins, flow cytometry for lymphocyte subsets should be obtained. As mentioned earlier, to be diagnosed with CVID, patients must present with low IgG concentrations associated with either low IgA or IgM concentration. Patients with nonspecific hypogammaglobulinemia have low IgG concentrations with normal IgA and IgM concentrations, while patients with SAD have normal total immunoglobulin levels. It is critical to compare immunoglobulin concentrations to age-specific norms during evaluation [37]. In the EUROclass trial, 24% of the patients diagnosed with CVID had a low IgA level, and 50% had an undetectable level. Low and undetectable IgM levels were present in 49% and 30% of patients with CVID, respectively [12]. Some patients with CVID may also present with elevated IgM levels, and this may be associated with poorer prognosis. In one series, for every 100 mg/dL increase in IgM concentration, there was 16% and 31% higher risk of developing polyclonal lymphocytic infiltrate and lymphoid malignancy, respectively [38].

Vaccine Response

Vaccines are used to gain insight into the functional capacity of the adaptive immune system. Vaccines containing protein, polysaccharide, and protein-conjugated polysaccharide antigens are used for this evaluation. The humoral immune response to a protein vaccine, such as tetanus or diphtheria, and to a polysaccharide vaccine, such as 23-valent unconjugated pneumococcal polysaccharide vaccine, should be assessed during evaluation for immune deficiency. Protein and protein-conjugated polysaccharide vaccines produce T-cell–dependent antibody responses, while polysaccharide vaccines produce T-cell–independent immune responses, which are weaker and more short-lived.

Protein antigens in protein and protein-conjugated polysaccharide vaccines are presented by dendritic cells to CD4+ T cells via major histocompatibility complex (MHC) class II, leading to helper T-cell activation. These antigens are also recognized by B-cell receptors (BCRs), leading to receptor-mediated endocytosis of the antigen by B cells. These B cells then engage with antigen-specific helper T cells via CD40:CD40L interactions. This T:B cell interaction leads to isotype switching, affinity maturation, and production of memory B cells. Polysaccharides, glycolipids, and nucleic acids cannot be presented to T cells via MHC molecules; hence, T-cell help is not engaged when developing an antibody response to these antigens. These non-protein antigens are multivalent and instead lead to B-cell activation through BCR crosslinking. B-cell activation can be further enhanced by complement proteins and toll-like receptors in this T-cell–independent antibody response, there are low levels of isotype switching: no affinity maturation and limited memory B-cell production [39].

There are two types of pneumococcal vaccines: 23-valent unconjugated pneumococcal polysaccharide vaccine (PPV23) and pneumococcal conjugate vaccine (PCV13). PPV23 formulation contains 23 serotypes of pneumococcal polysaccharide capsule: 1, 2, 3, 4, 5, 6B, 7F, 8, 9N, 9V, 10A, 11A, 12F, 14, 15B, 17F, 18C, 19A, 19F, 20, 22F, 23F, and 33F. The PCV13 vaccine includes serotypes 1, 3, 4, 5, 6A, 6B, 7F, 9V, 14, 18C, 19A, and 19F. Conventionally, unconjugated polysaccharide vaccines such as PPV23 are reserved for ages 2 and older [40]. However, some data suggest that infants over the age of 6 months can produce an adequate response to polysaccharide antigens [41, 42].

Specific antibody responses are measured 4–8 weeks following vaccination. When using PPV23, specific antibodies to at least six serotypes only present in PPV23 (not common to PCV13) should be checked. There have been controversies surrounding what constitutes an adequate response to PPV23 vaccination. An adequate serotype-specific titer to prevent invasive pneumococcal disease following PPV is considered to be ≥ 1.3 µg/mL [27]. Most immunocompetent patients will have a twofold increase in antibody titers from baseline in response to vaccination. However, the higher the pre-vaccination titers, the lesser the magnitude of increase after vaccination. Expert opinion suggests that a normal response to PPV23 for children 2–5 years old is conversion of 50% or more serotypes with at least a twofold increase in the titers. For patients ages 6–65 years, a normal response is considered to be conversion of at least 70% of serotypes with at least a twofold increase in the titers [27]. If normal response is not achieved, repeat doses of PPV23 vaccine in close succession are not recommended as it can lead to a diminished response to the vaccine [27].

SAD can be classified into phenotypes based on degree of response to the unconjugated PPV23 vaccine. For patients less than 6 years of age, a response of ≤ 2 protective antibody titers is considered to be a severe phenotype, <50% of serotypes protective is considered a moderate phenotype, and failure of a twofold increase in 50% of serotypes is considered mild phenotype. For patients over 6 years of age, a response of ≤ 2 protective titers is considered severe, <70% of serotypes protective is considered moderate, and failure of a twofold increase in 70% of serotypes is considered mild. For all patients, loss of response within 6 months following vaccination is considered to be a memory-deficient phenotype of specific antibody deficiency [27].

Other vaccines can also be used in the assessment of humoral immune deficiency in place of pneumococcal and tetanus vaccines. *Haemophilus influenzae* type b conjugate, meningococcal conjugate, pneumococcal conjugate, and rabies vaccines can be used to assess T-cell–dependent responses. The coupling of saccharides to proteins converts the polysaccharides to T-cell–dependent antigens, which are capable of eliciting a more robust B-cell immune response. In contrast, unconjugated meningococcal polysaccharide vaccine can be used to assess T-cell–independent responses. Alternatively, isohemagglutinin titer concentrations can also be used to check for IgG and IgM polysaccharide-specific antibody responses [43]. It is also possible to measure antibody function in an opsonophagocytic assay as wells as antibody avidity; however, these tests are not commercially available [44, 45].

Case Presentation 2

A 6-year-old female with a history of asthma and chronic rhinitis developed chronic vomiting, iron deficiency anemia, and hypoalbuminemia. Endoscopy and colonoscopy demonstrated nodularity in the gastric bulb, gastric antrum, esophagus, ileum, and colon. Pathology was significant for multiple lymphoid nodules in the GI tract and eosinophils in the distal esophagus and stomach. She had an infectious history of frequent otitis media, bronchitis, sinusitis, and pneumonia, but never exhibited severe enough infections that warranted hospitalization.

Her CBC with differential was significant only for microcytic anemia. Immunoglobulin levels were IgG 239 (nl 591–1597), IgA 22.6 (nl 52–329), and IgM 38 (nl 28–115). She had protective antibody responses against rubella and tetanus but was not protected against measles, despite being up-to-date on vaccinations. Her baseline pneumococcal titers were 0/23 protective, and her titers 1-month post-PPV23 were again 0/23 protective. Flow cytometry for lymphocyte subsets showed normal numbers of CD4, CD8, CD3, CD19, and NK cells, but B-cell phenotyping revealed low switched memory B cells (1.8%) (Table 2.2). She was diagnosed with CVID and was started on IVIG 0.6 g/kg every 4 weeks, with the improvement of

Table 2.2 B-cell subpopulation surface markers

B-Cell Subpopulation	B-Cell Surface Markers
Mature naïve B cell	CD27−
Activated B cell	$CD21^{lo}CD38^{lo}$
Marginal zone B cell	CD27+ IgM+ IgD+
Switched memory B cell	CD27+ IgG+ IgM− IgD−
Transitional B cell	$CD38^{hi}IgM^{hi}$
Plasmablast	$CD38^{hi}IgM−$
Plasma cell	CD27+, CD138+

Data from [12, 39]

infections. Her gastrointestinal symptoms also improved, with resolution of vomiting, and her laboratory abnormalities including anemia and hypoalbuminemia normalized. Due to clinical improvement in the gastrointestinal symptoms, her family declined further colonoscopy. A commercial genetic testing panel for genes implicated in CVID and CVID-like diseases showed a known pathogenic heterozygous mutation in *TNFRSF13B* (TACI).

Clinical Presentation

Although recurrent or persistent infections are the most common presentation of antibody deficiencies, noninfectious diseases cause a higher morbidity. In the case above, the evaluation of immune deficiency was prompted by nodular lymphoid hyperplasia in the gastrointestinal tract. The patient suffered from sinopulmonary infections as well, but her significant disease burden was resultant of gastrointestinal pathology. Noninfectious complications can include autoimmune, lymphoproliferative, and granulomatous diseases (see Table 2.1). These noninfectious diseases are common in CVID, and though they can also occur in SAD, THI, or hypogammaglobulinemia, these occurrences are relatively rare [46, 47]. Pulmonary, gastrointestinal, or hematologic manifestations are the most common noninfectious complications in CVID. Since these complications might be the presenting symptoms in some cases of CVID, it is essential they are recognized. It has been noted that patients presenting with only autoimmune disorders have a greater delay in the diagnosis of CVID than those presenting with recurrent infections [38].

Respiratory Disease

Thirty percent of patients with CVID suffer from noninfectious respiratory disease. This occurs equally in males and females [48]. Noninfectious pulmonary complications are challenging to treat and persist after the resolution of infections post-initiation of immunoglobulin replacement therapy.

Bronchiectasis occurs in 11% of patients with CVID and is associated with reduced survival. It is thought to be secondary to recurrent lower respiratory tract infections as opposed to immune dysregulation [38, 48]. Recurrent respiratory infections can also lead to restrictive or obstructive pulmonary disease. On computed tomography (CT) scans, patients with CVID can have nodular, reticular, fibrotic, or ground glass changes. These nodules could be scars, lymphoid collections, or granulomatous infiltrates [49].

Granulomatous and lymphocytic interstitial lung disease (GLILD) is a serious pulmonary manifestation of CVID characterized by granulomatous and lymphoproliferative histopathologic patterns. These include noncaseating granulomas, lymphoproliferative interstitial pneumonia, follicular bronchiolitis, and lymphoid hyperplasia. Patients with GLILD usually present with cough, sputum production, and dyspnea. The pulmonary function test shows a restrictive pattern with decreased CO diffusion capacity. GLILD is also found to be associated with splenomegaly [50]. In a small study of nine patients with GLILD, the human herpesvirus 8 genome was detected in biopsies of 80% of the patients with GLILD versus 5% in the control group [51].

Gastrointestinal Disease

Gastrointestinal complications in CVID can include abnormal liver function tests, chronic gastritis, nodular lymphoid hyperplasia, chronic liver disease, villous atrophy, and inflammatory bowel disease. Chronic gastritis in CVID can be associated with *H. pylori* infection or atrophic gastritis [52, 53]. A T-cell–mediated process is implicated in the pathogenesis of atrophic gastritis in CVID instead of autoantibodies to parietal cells or intrinsic factor [53]. Patients with CVID suffer from enteropathy, which is similar to celiac sprue; however, it is insensitive to gluten withdrawal. These patients have villous atrophy on biopsy, and it is associated with malabsorption, weight loss, diarrhea, hypoalbuminemia, anemia, and low CD4+ T cells [54].

Chronic diarrhea is the most common gastrointestinal manifestation of CVID, and while some cases can be related to infection with *Giardia*, Norovirus, or other pathogens, diarrhea in CVID may also be noninfectious. Findings can include steatorrhea, achlorhydria, pernicious anemia, or small intestinal abnormalities [55]. Eight percent of patients with CVID have intestinal nodular lymphoid hyperplasia [11]. Along with malabsorption, diarrhea, and weight loss, nodular lymphoid hyperplasia is associated with mucosal flattening and can cause intestinal obstruction due to large nodules. The etiology is unknown but is thought to be a compensatory mechanism to the antibody deficiency [52].

Around 40% of the patients with CVID have abnormal liver function tests, with an increased level of alkaline phosphatase being the most common abnormality. Liver pathology in CVID can occur secondary to viral infection, granulomatous infiltrative disease, or nodular regenerative hyperplasia, leading to non-icteric portal hypertension [56]. Some patients with CVID have also been found to have unexplained hepatomegaly [38].

Autoimmune Disease

It has been estimated that 22–29% of the patients with CVID have one or more autoimmune manifestations. The most common manifestations are autoimmune cytopenias [9, 10, 25, 48]. Cytopenias are present in 12–20% of the patients with CVID [12, 38], and idiopathic thrombocytopenia, autoimmune hemolytic anemia, or both (Evan syndrome) are present in 64%, 25%, and 11% of these patients, respectively. Other autoimmune manifestations include vitiligo, psoriasis, pernicious anemia, atrophic gastritis, hypothyroidism, thyroiditis, seronegative arthritis, antinuclear antibody-positive connective tissue like disease, and diabetes [12]. Some patients with THI have also been noted to exhibit autoimmunity [46].

Lymphoproliferative Disease

Patients with CVID are susceptible to neoplastic and non-neoplastic lymphoproliferative disease. Non-neoplastic lymphoproliferative disease is secondary to polyclonal lymphocytic infiltration in lymph nodes, the spleen, lungs, and gastrointestinal tract but may manifest as unexplained granulomas [38]. Splenomegaly can be present in 40% of patients, while lymphadenopathy is present in 26% of the patients with non-neoplastic lymphoproliferative disease. There is no difference in sex, age at onset, or age at diagnosis in patients with or without splenomegaly or lymphadenopathy [12]. Splenomegaly is associated with many other complications of CVID, including cytopenia, hepatomegaly, granulomas, and solid organ autoimmunity [38]. Granulomatous disease can present in the lungs, bone marrow, spleen, liver, and gastrointestinal tract. It is often associated with an increased incidence of autoimmune disease and is often confused with sarcoidosis [12, 57].

Malignancies

Patients with antibody deficiency have increased incidence of hematologic and solid organ malignancies. Common hematologic malignancies associated with CVID includes non-Hodgkin's lymphoma and lymphoma of mucosal-associated lymphoid tissue. Solid organ tumors can include breast, prostate, ovary, skin, and colon cancers [9]. Non-neoplastic lymphoproliferative disease is a risk factor for developing B-cell malignancies. In 1985, the incidence of stomach cancer in patients with CVID was thought to be 47-fold higher than in the general population [47]. However, recent studies show that the relative risk in patients with CVID is closer to 10-fold greater than in the general population. This risk is independent of pernicious anemia or *H. pylori* infection [58, 59].

Good Syndrome

In the differential diagnosis of CVID and unspecified hypogammaglobulinemia, it is important to recognize a subset of patients with Good syndrome, who have adult-onset hypogammaglobulinemia or agammaglobulinemia associated with thymoma. Along with low IgG levels, it is common for these patients to have low IgA and IgM levels. These patients present with sinopulmonary infections similar to CVID; however, they are also at risk for opportunistic infections including mucocutaneous candidiasis, severe varicella infection, *Pneumocystis carinii*, cytomegalovirus, and recurrent herpes simplex virus. CT of the chest is required for the diagnosis. Similar to CVID, Good syndrome also presents with noninfectious complications, including autoimmune diseases, which are mostly cytopenias. These patients also suffer from chronic diarrhea of unknown etiology. However, unlike CVID, Good syndrome is not associated with lymphadenopathy or splenomegaly [60, 61].

Laboratory Findings

Flow Cytometry

Flow cytometry for lymphocyte subsets is not part of the typical evaluation of unspecified hypogammaglobulinemia or SAD. However, it is an important tool for CVID subclassification. In patients with CVID, most have B cells within the normal limits. However, <10% of patients diagnosed with CVID can have <1% B cells, and in these patients, evaluation for mutations associated with X-linked or autosomal recessive agammaglobulinemia is essential. While the majority of patients with CVID have a normal number of T cells and NK cells, about 20% of patients do have some degree of CD4 T-lymphopenia, and decreased naïve T-cell subsets have been demonstrated in patients with CVID [9, 12, 62]. Patients with Good syndrome present with absent or very low B cells, low CD4+ T cells, and reduced in vitro T-cell response to mitogens [61]. While patients with SAD and unspecified hypogammaglobulinemia have normal lymphocyte subsets, rarely patients with THI can have low levels of T cells [63].

In recent years, several CVID classification schemes based on B-cell immunophenotyping have emerged. There are six basic populations of circulating B cells: naive B cells (IgM+ IgD+ CD27−), marginal zone-like B cells (IgM+ IgD+ CD27+), switched memory B cells (IgM− IgD− CD27+), transitional B cells (CD38^{hi}IgM^{hi}), activated B cells (CD21^{lo}CD38^{lo}), and switched plasmablasts (CD38^{hi}IgM−) (see Table 2.2). Their role in pathogenesis of CVID has not been defined, but some associations with different phenotypes have been observed. More than 80% of the patients with CVID have a percentage of switched memory B cells below the normal range (nl 6.5–29.2% of total B cells), with 58% of CVID patients having very low switched memory B cells (≤2% of total B cells; smB−). About 15% of the patients had expansion of transitional B cells (≥9% of total B cells; tr^{hi}), and most of these were associated with low marginal zone-like B cells. About 76% of the patients with CVID had increased levels of CD21^{lo} B cells [12].

The EUROclass classification (Fig. 2.1) is the most recent CVID classification schema utilizing B-cell subsets. It incorporates features from previous classifications (Freiburg and Paris) [12, 64, 65], and identified associations between

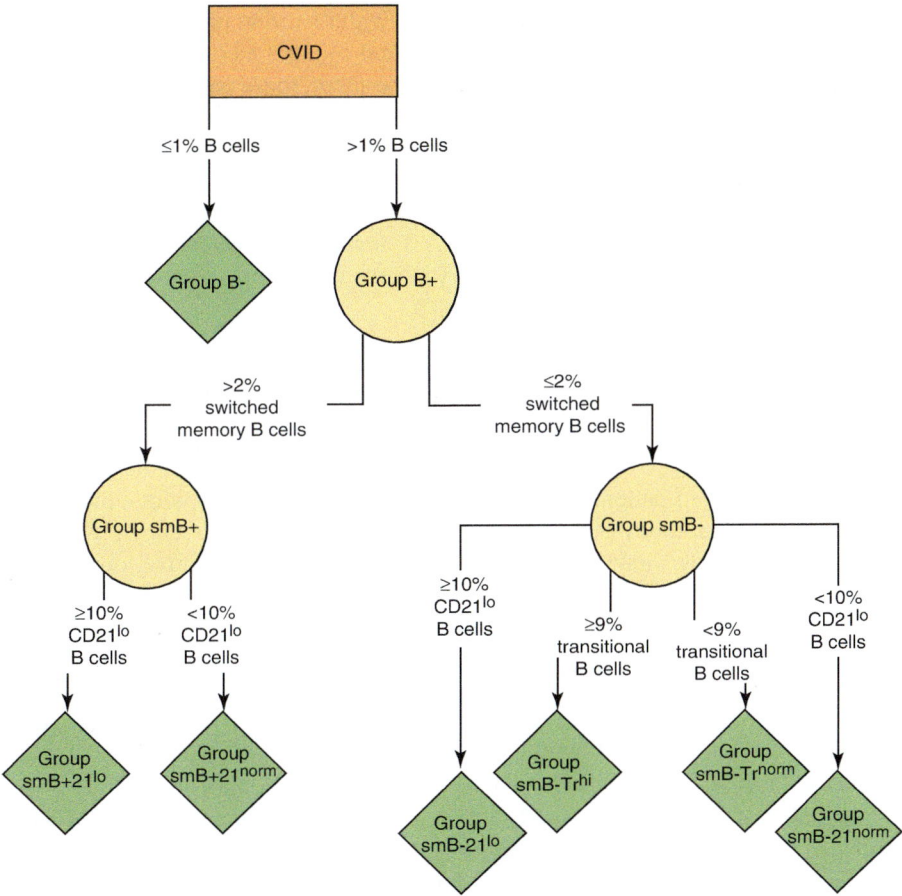

Fig. 2.1 B-cell subsets in CVID. EUROclass classification divides patients into the following subgroups: B- (<1% B-cells), group smB+ 21^{lo} (>2% switched memory B cells and ≥10% $CD21^{lo}$ B cells), smB+ 21^{norm} (>2% switched memory B cells and <10% $CD21^{lo}$ B cells), smB-21^{lo} (≤2% switched memory B cells and ≥10% $CD21^{lo}$ B cells), smB–21^{norm} (≤2% switched memory B cells and <10% $CD21^{lo}$ B-cells), smB-Tr^{hi} (≤2% memory B cells and ≥9% transitional) and smB-Tr^{norm} (≤2% switched memory B cells and <9% transitional) [12]

clinical parameters and various imbalances in B-cell subsets. Incidence of splenomegaly and granulomatous disease was higher in the group of patients with ≤2% switched memory B cells (smB−) versus >2% switched memory B cells (smB+). In the smB− group, splenomegaly and granulomatous diseases were seen in 52% and 17% of patients, respectively. Furthermore, a subgroup of patients with ≥10% B cells with low expression of CD21 activated B cells ($CD21^{lo}$) had increased incidence of splenomegaly, independent of whether they were in the smB− or smB+ group. The incidence of lymphadenopathy was highest (57%) in patients with low switched memory B cells and high transitional B cells (smB−tr^{hi}) [12].

A study by Carsetti et al. compared patients with recurrent pneumonia and bronchiectasis with patients without lung disease and found a lack of IgM memory B cells in patients with recurrent infections. Furthermore, these patients were not able to develop anti-pneumococcal polysaccharide IgM. Evident from this study is that IgM memory B cells are required for immune response to encapsulated bacteria and seem to be decreased in patients with increased infections [66].

Decreased switched memory B cells have been observed in patients with SAD as well [46, 67]. In a study of patients with THI, Moschese et al. found that children with lower IgM levels or switched memory B cells were more likely to have persistence of immune deficiency [46].

Genetic Testing

The majority of patients with CVID have no history of affected family members. However, 10–20% of patients have one or more family members with either CVID or a more subtle antibody deficiency, such as selective IgA deficiency [68]. There are currently no known mutations for SAD or unspecified hypogammaglobulinemia. The genetic cause of CVID is unknown in a majority of cases. However, broader availability of genetic testing has recently led to increasing identification of causative mutations in patients with CVID-like disease. The most common genetic mutation in CVID includes mutation in one of the alleles of *TNFRSF13B*. It has been found to occur in 9–21% of patients with CVID [64, 65]. *TNFRSF13B* encodes TNF receptor superfamily 13B that encodes transmembrane activator and CAML interactor (TACI). TACI is involved in class-switch recombination to IgG and IgA. B-cell activating factor (BAFF) and a proliferating inducing ligand (APRIL), produced by monocytes and dendritic cells, bind to TACI and BAFF-R, leading to isotype switching. Patients with TACI polymorphism have been found to have either IgA deficiency or CVID [64]. After genetic analysis, some patients with symptoms initially attributed to CVID are found to have X-linked agammaglobulinemia, X-linked lymphoproliferative disorder, or immunoglobulin class-switch defects.

Patients with predominantly noninfectious complications may have a genetic defect causing a CVID-like primary immune regulatory disease (PIRD). PIRDs present with immune dysregulation including immune cytopenias, enteropathy or colitis, interstitial lung disease, and nonmalignant lymphoproliferation, mirroring many of the noninfectious complications seen in CVID, and hypogammaglobulinemia is a more variable feature of many of these defects. Heterozygous *CTLA-4* mutations cause a disease of immune dysregulation and infectious susceptibility. CTLA-4 is an inhibitory receptor which competes with the CD28 costimulatory receptor on T cells for the binding of CD80/CD86 on antigen-presenting cells (APC), preventing APC activation of conventional T cells. It is also essential for the function of regulatory T cells [69]. The clinical presentation of CTLA-4 often includes severe autoimmune cytopenias, lymphoproliferation and increased risk of lymphoma, enteropathy or inflammatory bowel disease, GLILD, and recurrent infections, with an immune phenotype that may include hypogammaglobulinemia and CD4 T-lymphopenia [70]. Homozygous *LRBA* mutations result in a phenotype similar to that of CTLA-4 haploinsufficiency. LRBA is a scaffold protein controlling movement of CTLA-4 from endosomes to the cell membrane of T cells. When LRBA is deficient, CTLA-4 is not adequately expressed on the T-cell membrane [71]. The clinical phenotype of LRBA deficiency is variable but may include hypogammaglobulinemia with recurrent infections, hepatosplenomegaly and lymphoproliferation, immune cytopenias, enteropathy, GLILD, and Type I diabetes [72]. Autosomal dominant gain-of-function mutations in *PIK3CD* and *PIK3R1* are the causes of activated phosphoinositide 3-kinase delta syndrome-1 and -2 (APDS-1 and APDS-2), respectively. APDS-1 and -2 present with variable humoral immune deficiency, respiratory infections often with bronchiectasis, herpes virus infections, splenomegaly and lymphadenopathy with increased risk of lymphomas, nodular lymphoid hyperplasia, and frequent autoimmunity [73]. Numerous other rare genetic mutations associated with CVID are summarized in Table 2.3.

Table 2.3 Genetic mutations in CVID

Gene	Inheritance	Notable features
CVID-causing mutations		
ICOS	AR	Autoimmunity, granulomas
TNFRSF13B (TACI)	AD or AR	Variable clinical expression
TNFRSF13C (BAFF-R)	AR	Variable clinical expression
CD19	AR	Possible glomerulonephritis
CD81	AR	Only one identified patient, glomerulonephritis
CR2 (CD21)	AR	Respiratory tract infections
MS4A1 (CD20)	AR	Respiratory tract infections
TNFSF12 (TWEAK)	AD	Only one patient identified
IKZF1 (IKAROS)	AD	Risk of acute lymphocytic leukemia
IRF2BP2	AD	Autoimmunity, inflammatory disease
NFKB1	AD	Alopecia, immune cytopenias, EBV-induced lymphoproliferation
NFKB2	AD (LOF)	Alopecia, endocrinopathies
Primary immune regulatory diseases		
LRBA	AR	Organomegaly, immune cytopenias, enteropathy, hypogammaglobulinemia, GLILD, Type I diabetes
CTLA4	AD	Severe immune cytopenias, hypogammaglobulinemia, lymphoproliferation and risk of lymphoma, enteropathy/colitis, GLILD
PIK3CD	AD	Respiratory bacterial infections, herpesvirus infections, lymphoproliferation and risk of lymphoma, nodular lymphoid hyperplasia

continued

Table 2.3 (continued)

Gene	Inheritance	Notable features
PIK3R1	AD	Respiratory bacterial infections, herpesvirus infections, lymphoproliferation and risk of lymphoma, nodular lymphoid hyperplasia
IL21	AR	Early-onset inflammatory bowel disease
IL21R	AR	Cholangitis, liver disease, *Cryptosporidium*
PRKCD	AR	Multiple autoimmune conditions, lymphoproliferation, variable immunoglobulin levels
PLCG2	AD	Cold urticaria, granulomatous disease, autoimmunity, hypogammaglobulinemia

Data from [64, 70, 72, 73, 82–90]

Management

Standard of care for treatment of CVID is lifelong routine replacement of immunoglobulin (Ig) via intravenous or subcutaneous routes. Most US and international guidelines recommend a starting dose of 400–500 mg/kg/month for intravenous immunoglobulin (IVIG) or 400–600 mg/kg/month for subcutaneous immunoglobulin (SCIG). In patients with bronchiectasis, dosing at 600 mg/kg/month may give better outcomes. Some experts also recommend higher doses of 600–800 mg/kg/month for patients with enteropathy or splenomegaly. There is recent research supporting the consideration of individualization of the Ig dose, focusing on the incidence of breakthrough infections, rather than a standard IgG trough or weight-based Ig dose [74, 75]. Unfortunately, replacement Ig has not been shown to prevent or treat noninfectious inflammatory complications of CVID such autoimmunity, granulomatous disease, or malignancy.

Treatment with prophylactic antibiotics may be trialed as first-line therapy of specific antibody deficiency or hypogammaglobulinemia, before moving on to Ig replacement therapy. However, in addition to the response to antibiotic prophylaxis, severity of infections should be an important factor in the decision to provide Ig replacement therapy. In patients with SAD, a recent AAAAI Work Group paper recommended the following as indications for Ig therapy: difficult-to-manage recurrent otitis media at risk for permanent hearing loss, bronchiectasis, recurrent infections necessitating IV antibiotics, failed antibiotic prophylaxis, impaired quality of life due to recurrent infections despite antibiotic prophylaxis, and multiple antibiotic hypersensitivities interfering with treatment [76]. Patients with initial poor response to the pneumococcal polysaccharide vaccine may clinically benefit from immunization with the conjugate vaccine, though it does not play a role in the diagnosis of SAD.

Dysregulatory features of CVID are often not responsive to treatment with conventional Ig replacement and represent a major challenge in the treatment of patients with CVID. High-dose IVIG is often successful in treating immune thrombocytopenic purpura associated with CVID, but rituximab (anti-CD20 mAb) is the preferred treatment for CVID-associated autoimmune hemolytic anemia [77]. Rituximab has been trialed for other lymphoproliferative complications of CVID, with variable results, but rituximab combined with azathioprine has become the standard treatment for GLILD [78]. For several CVID-like PIRDs, targeted treatment with biologic therapies have offered new opportunities for treating the dysregulatory complications that are major features of these diseases.

Prognosis

Specific antibody deficiency and unspecified hypogammaglobulinemia are often not lifelong diagnoses, especially when presentation occurs in childhood. Several groups have observed that young children may outgrow specific antibody deficiency and, therefore, recommended holding immunoglobulin (if started) and revaccinating 6–24 months after the initial diagnosis [33, 79]. However, there are also patients that have been found to progress from these milder humoral defects to a more dramatic CVID phenotype.

The prognosis for patients with CVID has improved dramatically in the last 50 years, and these improvements are felt to be due in large part to increasing standard replacement doses of Ig therapy. In a 1971 report, survival to 12 years after diagnosis only occurred in 30% of patients with hypogammaglobulinemia [80]. Twenty-year survival following diagnosis improved to 64% for males and 67% for females by the late 1990s [9]. In some of the most recent literature, there is an expected survival rate of 58% 45 years after diagnosis [38]. Individual prognosis depends on the clinical phenotype of the patient. Those without noninfectious complications have an almost normal life expectancy. However, patients with enteropathy, chronic lung disease, lymphoproliferation, or cytopenias have reduced survival. In a large Italian cohort, overall survival was 35% at 40 years following diagnosis. While no patients with cancer survived beyond 35 years after diagnosis, patients without malignancy had an overall survival of 65% at 40 years [81].

> **Clinical Pearls and Pitfalls**
> - Patients with antibody deficiencies can present with infectious or noninfectious complications. Noninfectious complications occur in a substantial subset of patients with CVID and are rare in SAD and non-specific hypogammaglobulinemia.
> - Common sites of infection include the sinopulmonary and gastrointestinal tracts. Bacterial respiratory infections are caused by encapsulated and atypical bacteria, while gastrointestinal infections are most commonly caused by *Giardia* sp., *Campylobacter jejuni*, and *Salmonella* sp.
> - Noninfectious complications seen in CVID can include chronic lung disease, gastrointestinal disease, autoimmune disease, and lymphoproliferative disease.

- Diagnosis of antibody deficiencies is based on the clinical picture, immunoglobulin levels, and functional immune response to vaccines.
- In patients with CVID, low levels of class-switched memory B cells are associated with increased incidence of splenomegaly, autoimmunity, and granulomatous disease.
- Initial treatment for SAD and hypogammaglobulinemia includes prophylactic antibiotics before immunoglobulin replacement therapy, while immunoglobulin replacement therapy is the first-line treatment for CVID.
- Recommended starting dose of immunoglobulin replacement is 400–500 mg/kg/month for intravenous immunoglobulin (IVIG) or 400–600 mg/kg/month for subcutaneous immunoglobulin (SCIG). Doses may then be adjusted to minimize significant breakthrough infections.
- Immunoglobulin replacement therapy has improved survival for patients with antibody deficiency. Patients with isolated infectious symptoms have a good prognosis, yet patients with noninfectious complications still experience reduced life expectancy.

References

1. Kobrynski L, Powell RW, Bowen S. Prevalence and morbidity of primary immunodeficiency diseases, United States 2001–2007. J Clin Immunol. 2014;34(8):954–61.
2. Stray-Pedersen A, Abrahamsen TG, Frøland SS. Primary immunodeficiency diseases in Norway. J Clin Immunol. 2000;20(6):477–85.
3. Buckley RH. Immunoglobulin G subclass deficiency: fact or fancy? Curr Allergy Asthma Rep. 2002;2(5):356–60.
4. Bossuyt X, Moens L, Van Hoeyveld E, Jeurissen A, Bogaert G, Sauer K, et al. Coexistence of (partial) immune defects and risk of recurrent respiratory infections. Clin Chem. 2007;53(1):124–30.
5. Epstein MM, Gruskay F. Selective deficiency in pneumococcal antibody response in children with recurrent infections. Ann Allergy Asthma Immunol. 1995;75(2):125–31.
6. Jeurissen A, Moens L, Raes M, Wuyts G, Willebrords L, Sauer K, et al. Laboratory diagnosis of specific antibody deficiency to pneumococcal capsular polysaccharide antigens. Clin Chem. 2007;53(3):505–10.
7. Boyle R, Le C, Balloch A, Tang MLK. The clinical syndrome of specific antibody deficiency in children. Clin Exp Immunol. 2006;146(3):486–92.
8. Perez E, Bonilla FA, Orange JS, Ballow M. Specific antibody deficiency: controversies in diagnosis and management. Front Immunol. 2017;8:586.
9. Cunningham-Rundles C, Bodian C. Common variable immunodeficiency: clinical and immunological features of 248 patients. Clin Immunol. 1999;92(1):34–48.
10. Gathmann B, Mahlaoui N, Gérard L, Oksenhendler E, Warnatz K, Schulze I, et al. Clinical picture and treatment of 2212 patients with common variable immunodeficiency. J Allergy Clin Immunol. 2014;134(1):116–26. e11.
11. Quinti I, Soresina A, Spadaro G, Martino S, Donnanno S, Agostini C, et al. Long-term follow-up and outcome of a large cohort of patients with common variable immunodeficiency. J Clin Immunol. 2007;27(3):308–16.
12. Wehr C, Kivioja T, Schmitt C, Ferry B, Witte T, Eren E, et al. The EUROclass trial: defining subgroups in common variable immunodeficiency. Blood. 2008;111(1):77–85.

13. Rosen FS, Janeway CA. The gamma globulins: the antibody deficiency syndromes. N Engl J Med. 1966;275(14):769–75.
14. Adkinson NF Jr, Bochner BS, Burks AW, Busse WW, Holgate ST, Lemanske RF, et al. Middleton's allergy E-Book: principles and practice. Philadelphia: Elsevier Health Sciences; 2013.
15. Gelfand EW. Unique susceptibility of patients with antibody deficiency to mycoplasma infection. Clin Infect Dis. 1993;17 Suppl 1:S250–S3.
16. Roifman CM, Rao CP, Lederman HM, Lavi S, Quinn P, Gelfand EW. Increased susceptibility to mycoplasma infection in patients with hypogammaglobulinemia. Am J Med. 1986;80(4):590–4.
17. Kainulainen L, Vuorinen T, Rantakokko-Jalava K, Österback R, Ruuskanen O. Recurrent and persistent respiratory tract viral infections in patients with primary hypogammaglobulinemia. J Allergy Clin Immunol. 2010;126(1):120–6.
18. Agondi R, Barros M, Rizzo L, Kalil J, Giavina Bianchi P. Allergic asthma in patients with common variable immunodeficiency. Allergy. 2010;65(4):510–5.
19. Webster A, Taylor-Robinson D, Furr P, Asherson G. Chronic cystitis and urethritis associated with ureaplasmal and mycoplasmal infection in primary hypogammaglobulinaemia. Br J Urol. 1982;54(3):287–91.
20. Hoffman JD, Ciprero KL, Sullivan KE, Kaplan PB, McDonald-McGinn DM, Zackai EH, et al. Immune abnormalities are a frequent manifestation of Kabuki syndrome. Am J Med Genet Part A. 2005;135(3):278–81.
21. Fabre A, André N, Breton A, Broué P, Badens C, Roquelaure B. Intractable diarrhea with "phenotypic anomalies" and tricho-hepato-enteric syndrome: two names for the same disorder. Am J Med Genet Part A. 2007;143(6):584–8.
22. Hanley-Lopez J, Estabrooks LL, Stiehm ER. Antibody deficiency in Wolf-Hirschhorn syndrome. J Pediatr. 1998;133(1):141–3.
23. Costa-Carvalho BT, Martinez RMA, Dias ATN, Kubo CA, Barros-Nunes P, Leiva L, et al. Antibody response to pneumococcal capsular polysaccharide vaccine in Down syndrome patients. Braz J Med Biol Res. 2006;39(12):1587–92.
24. Palanduz S, Palanduz A, Yalcin I, Somer A, Ones U, Ustek D, et al. In VitroChromosomal Radiosensitivity in common variable immune deficiency. Clin Immunol Immunopathol. 1998;86(2):180–2.
25. Bonilla FA, Barlan I, Chapel H, Costa-Carvalho BT, Cunningham-Rundles C, de la Morena MT, et al. International Consensus Document (ICON): common variable immunodeficiency disorders. J Allergy Clin Immunol In Pract. 2016;4(1):38–59.
26. Agarwal S, Cunningham-Rundles C. Assessment and clinical interpretation of reduced IgG values. Ann Allergy Asthma Immunol. 2007;99(3):281–3.
27. Orange JS, Ballow M, Stiehm ER, Ballas ZK, Chinen J, De La Morena M, et al. Use and interpretation of diagnostic vaccination in primary immunodeficiency: a working group report of the Basic and Clinical Immunology Interest Section of the American Academy of Allergy, Asthma & Immunology. J Allergy Clin Immunol. 2012;130(3):S1–S24.
28. Waldmann TA, Strober W. Metabolism of immunoglobulins. Prog Allergy. 1969;13:1–110. Elsevier.
29. Berg T. Serum immunoglobulin development during the first year of life: a longitudinal study. Acta Paediatr. 1969;58(3):229–36.
30. Dorsey MJ, Orange JS. Impaired specific antibody response and increased B-cell population in transient hypogammaglobulinemia of infancy. Ann Allergy Asthma Immunol. 2006;97(5):590–5.
31. Keles S, Artac H, Kara R, Gokturk B, Ozen A, Reisli I. Transient hypogammaglobulinemia and unclassified hypogammaglobulinemia: 'similarities and differences'. Pediatr Allergy Immunol. 2010;21(5):843–51.
32. Ballow M. Primary immunodeficiency disorders: antibody deficiency. J Allergy Clin Immunol. 2002;109(4):581–91.
33. Wolpert J, Knutsen AP. Natural history of selective antibody deficiency to bacterial polysaccharide antigens in children. Pediatr Asthma Allergy Immunol. 1998;12(3):183–91.

34. Ruuskanen O, Nurkka A, Helminen M, Viljanen MK, Kayhty H, Kainulainen L. Specific antibody deficiency in children with recurrent respiratory infections: a controlled study with follow-up. Clin Exp Immunol. 2013;172(2):238–44.
35. Cheng YK, Decker PA, O'Byrne MM, Weiler CR. Clinical and laboratory characteristics of 75 patients with specific polysaccharide antibody deficiency syndrome. Ann Allergy Asthma Immunol. 2006;97(3):306–11.
36. Compagno N, Malipiero G, Cinetto F, Agostini C. Immunoglobulin replacement therapy in secondary hypogammaglobulinemia. Front Immunol. 2014;5:626.
37. Buckley RH, Dees SC, O'Fallon WM. Serum immunoglobulins: I. Levels in normal children and in uncomplicated childhood allergy. Pediatrics. 1968;41(3):600–11.
38. Chapel H, Lucas M, Lee M, Bjorkander J, Webster D, Grimbacher B, et al. Common variable immunodeficiency disorders: division into distinct clinical phenotypes. Blood. 2008;112(2):277–86.
39. Abbas AK, Lichtman AH, Pillai S, Baker DL, Baker A. Cellular and molecular immunology. 9th ed. Philadelphia: Elsevier Health Sciences; 2018.
40. Leinonen M, Säkkinen A, Kalliokoski R, Luotonen J, Timonen M, Mäkelä P. Antibody response to 14-valent pneumococcal capsular polysaccharide vaccine in pre-school age children. Pediatr Infect Dis. 1986;5(1):39–44.
41. Balloch A, Licciardi PV, Russell FM, Mulholland EK, Tang ML. Infants aged 12 months can mount adequate serotype-specific IgG responses to pneumococcal polysaccharide vaccine. J Allergy Clin Immunol. 2010;126(2):395–7.
42. Riley I, Alpers M, Gratten H, Lehmann D, Marshall TD, Smith D. Pneumococcal vaccine prevents death from acute lower-respiratory-tract infections in Papua New Guinean children. Lancet. 1986;328(8512):877–81.
43. Tiller TL Jr, Buckley RH. Transient hypogammaglobulinemia of infancy: review of the literature, clinical and immunologic features of 11 new cases, and long-term follow-up. J Pediatr. 1978;92(3):347–53.
44. Licciardi PV, Balloch A, Russell FM, Burton RL, Lin J, Nahm MH, et al. Pneumococcal polysaccharide vaccine at 12 months of age produces functional immune responses. J Allergy Clin Immunol. 2012;129(3):794–800.e2.
45. Fried AJ, Altrich ML, Liu H, Halsey JF, Bonilla FA. Correlation of pneumococcal antibody concentration and avidity with patient clinical and immunologic characteristics. J Clin Immunol. 2013;33(4):847–56.
46. Moschese V, Graziani S, Avanzini M, Carsetti R, Marconi M, La Rocca M, et al. A prospective study on children with initial diagnosis of transient hypogammaglobulinemia of infancy: results from the Italian Primary Immunodeficiency Network. Int J Immunopathol Pharmacol. 2008;21(2):343–52.
47. Alachkar H, Taubenheim N, Haeney MR, Durandy A, Arkwright PD. Memory switched B cell percentage and not serum immunoglobulin concentration is associated with clinical complications in children and adults with specific antibody deficiency and common variable immunodeficiency. Clin Immunol. 2006;120(3):310–8.
48. Resnick ES, Moshier EL, Godbold JH, Cunningham-Rundles C. Morbidity and mortality in common variable immune deficiency over 4 decades. Blood. 2012;119(7):1650–7.
49. Cunningham-Rundles C. How I treat common variable immune deficiency. Blood. 2010;116(1):7–15.
50. Park JH, Levinson AI. Granulomatous-lymphocytic interstitial lung disease (GLILD) in common variable immunodeficiency (CVID). Clin Immunol. 2010;134(2):97–103.
51. Wheat WH, Cool CD, Morimoto Y, Rai PR, Kirkpatrick CH, Lindenbaum BA, et al. Possible role of human herpesvirus 8 in the lymphoproliferative disorders in common variable immunodeficiency. J Exp Med. 2005;202(4):479–84.
52. Agarwal S, Mayer L. Pathogenesis and treatment of gastrointestinal disease in antibody deficiency syndromes. J Allergy Clin Immunol. 2009;124(4):658–64.
53. Twomey J, Jordan P, Jarrold T, Trubowitz S, Ritz N, Conn H. The syndrome of immunoglobulin deficiency and pernicious anemia: a study of ten cases. Am J Med. 1969;47(3):340–50.

54. Luzi G, Zullo A, Iebba F, Rinaldi V, Mete LS, Muscaritoli M, et al. Duodenal pathology and clinical-immunological implications in common variable immunodeficiency patients. Am J Gastroenterol. 2003;98(1):118.
55. Hermans PE, Diaz-Buxo JA, Stobo JD. Idiopathic late-onset immunoglobulin deficiency: clinical observations in 50 patients. Am J Med. 1976;61(2):221–37.
56. Fuss IJ, Friend J, Yang Z, He JP, Hooda L, Boyer J, et al. Nodular regenerative hyperplasia in common variable immunodeficiency. J Clin Immunol. 2013;33(4):748–58.
57. Mechanic LJ, Dikman S, Cunnigham-Rundles C. Granulomatous disease in common variable immunodeficiency. Ann Intern Med. 1997;127(8_Part_1):613–7.
58. Dhalla F, Da Silva S, Lucas M, Travis S, Chapel H. Review of gastric cancer risk factors in patients with common variable immunodeficiency disorders, resulting in a proposal for a surveillance programme. Clin Exp Immunol. 2011;165(1):1–7.
59. Kinlen L, Webster A, Bird A, Haile R, Peto J, Soothill J, et al. Prospective study of cancer in patients with hypogammaglobulinaemia. Lancet. 1985;325(8423):263–6.
60. Federico P, Imbimbo M, Buonerba C, Damiano V, Marciano R, Serpico D, et al. Is hypogammaglobulinemia a constant feature in Good's syndrome? Int J Immunopathol Pharmacol. 2010;23(4):1275–9.
61. Kelesidis T, Yang O. Good's syndrome remains a mystery after 55 years: a systematic review of the scientific evidence. Clin Immunol. 2010;135(3):347–63.
62. Bateman E, Ayers L, Sadler R, Lucas M, Roberts C, Woods A, et al. T cell phenotypes in patients with common variable immunodeficiency disorders: associations with clinical phenotypes in comparison with other groups with recurrent infections. Clin Exp Immunol. 2012;170(2):202–11.
63. Siegel RL, Issekutz T, Schwaber J, Rosen FS, Geha RS. Deficiency of T helper cells in transient hypogammaglobulinemia of infancy. N Engl J Med. 1981;305(22):1307–13.
64. Castigli E, Wilson SA, Garibyan L, Rachid R, Bonilla F, Schneider L, et al. TACI is mutant in common variable immunodeficiency and IgA deficiency. Nat Genet. 2005;37(8):829.
65. Salzer U, Bacchelli C, Buckridge S, Pan-Hammarström Q, Jennings S, Lougaris V, et al. Relevance of biallelic versus monoallelic TNFRSF13B mutations in distinguishing disease-causing from risk-increasing TNFRSF13B variants in antibody deficiency syndromes. Blood. 2009;113(9):1967–76.
66. Carsetti R, Rosado MM, Donnanno S, Guazzi V, Soresina A, Meini A, et al. The loss of IgM memory B cells correlates with clinical disease in common variable immunodeficiency. J Allergy Clin Immunol. 2005;115(2):412–7.
67. Leiva LE, Monjure H, Sorensen RU. Recurrent respiratory infections, specific antibody deficiencies, and memory B cells. J Clin Immunol. 2013;33(1):57–61.
68. Vořechovský I, Zetterquist H, Paganelli R, Koskinen S, David A, Webster B, et al. Family and linkage study of selective IgA deficiency and common variable immunodeficiency. Clin Immunol Immunopathol. 1995;77(2):185–92.
69. Walker LS, Sansom DM. Confusing signals: recent progress in CTLA-4 biology. Trends Immunol. 2015;36(2):63–70.
70. Schwab C, Gabrysch A, Olbrich P, Patiño V, Warnatz K, Wolff D, et al. Phenotype, penetrance, and treatment of 133 cytotoxic T-lymphocyte antigen 4–insufficient subjects. J Allergy Clin Immunol. 2018;142(6):1932–46.
71. Lo B, Zhang K, Lu W, Zheng L, Zhang Q, Kanellopoulou C, et al. Patients with LRBA deficiency show CTLA4 loss and immune dysregulation responsive to abatacept therapy. Science. 2015;349(6246):436–40.
72. Gámez-Díaz L, August D, Stepensky P, Revel-Vilk S, Seidel MG, Noriko M, et al. The extended phenotype of LPS-responsive beige-like anchor protein (LRBA) deficiency. J Allergy Clin Immunol. 2016;137(1):223–30.
73. Coulter TI, Chandra A, Bacon CM, Babar J, Curtis J, Screaton N, et al. Clinical spectrum and features of activated phosphoinositide 3-kinase δ syndrome: a large patient cohort study. J Allergy Clin Immunol. 2017;139(2):597–606.e4.

74. Bonagura VR, Marchlewski R, Cox A, Rosenthal DW. Biologic IgG level in primary immunodeficiency disease: the IgG level that protects against recurrent infection. J Allergy Clin Immunol. 2008;122(1):210.
75. Lucas M, Lee M, Lortan J, Lopez-Granados E, Misbah S, Chapel H. Infection outcomes in patients with common variable immunodeficiency disorders: relationship to immunoglobulin therapy over 22 years. J Allergy Clin Immunol. 2010;125(6):1354–60.e4.
76. Perez EE, Orange JS, Bonilla F, Chinen J, Chinn IK, Dorsey M, et al. Update on the use of immunoglobulin in human disease: a review of evidence. J Allergy Clin Immunol. 2017;139(3):S1–S46.
77. Gobert D, Bussel JB, Cunningham Rundles C, Galicier L, Dechartres A, Berezne A, et al. Efficacy and safety of rituximab in common variable immunodeficiency-associated immune cytopenias: a retrospective multicentre study on 33 patients. Br J Haematol. 2011;155(4):498–508.
78. Chase NM, Verbsky JW, Hintermeyer MK, Waukau JK, Tomita-Mitchell A, Casper JT, et al. Use of combination chemotherapy for treatment of granulomatous and lymphocytic interstitial lung disease (GLILD) in patients with common variable immunodeficiency (CVID). J Clin Immunol. 2013;33(1):30–9.
79. Ortigas A, Leiva L, Moore C, Bradford N, Sorensen R. Natural history of specific antibody deficiency after IgG replacement therapy. Ann Allergy Asthma Immunol. 1999;82:71.
80. Healy M, for the Medical Research Council working party on hypogammaglobulinaemia. Hypogammaglobulinaemia in the United Kingdom: XII statistical analyses: prevalence, mortality and effects of treatment. Spec Rep Ser Med Res Counc (G B). 1971;310:115–23.
81. Quinti I, Agostini C, Tabolli S, Brunetti G, Cinetto F, Pecoraro A, et al. Malignancies are the major cause of death in patients with adult onset common variable immunodeficiency. Blood. 2012;120(9):1953–4.
82. Online Mendelian Inheritance in Man, OMIM®. McKusick-Nathans Institute of Genetic Medicine, Johns Hopkins University (Baltimore, MD), 2019. World Wide Web URL: https://omim.org/. Accessed November 3, 2019.
83. Picard C, Gaspar HB, Al-Herz W, Bousfiha A, Casanova J-L, Chatila T, et al. International union of immunological societies: 2017 primary immunodeficiency diseases committee report on inborn errors of immunity. J Clin Immunol. 2018;38(1):96–128.
84. Kotlarz D, Ziętara N, Uzel G, Weidemann T, Braun CJ, Diestelhorst J, et al. Loss-of-function mutations in the IL-21 receptor gene cause a primary immunodeficiency syndrome. J Exp Med. 2013;210(3):433–43.
85. Salzer E, Santos-Valente E, Klaver S, Ban SA, Emminger W, Prengemann NK, et al. B-cell deficiency and severe autoimmunity caused by deficiency of protein kinase C δ. Blood. 2013;121(16):3112–6.
86. Ombrello MJ, Remmers EF, Sun G, Freeman AF, Datta S, Torabi-Parizi P, et al. Cold urticaria, immunodeficiency, and autoimmunity related to PLCG2 deletions. N Engl J Med. 2012;366(4):330–8.
87. Chen K, Coonrod EM, Kumánovics A, Franks ZF, Durtschi JD, Margraf RL, et al. Germline mutations in NFKB2 implicate the noncanonical NF-κB pathway in the pathogenesis of common variable immunodeficiency. Am J Hum Genet. 2013;93(5):812–24.
88. Kuehn HS, Boisson B, Cunningham-Rundles C, Reichenbach J, Stray-Pedersen A, Gelfand EW, et al. Loss of B cells in patients with heterozygous mutations in IKAROS. N Engl J Med. 2016;374(11):1032–43.
89. Keller MD, Pandey R, Li D, Glessner J, Tian L, Henrickson SE, et al. Mutation in IRF2BP2 is responsible for a familial form of common variable immunodeficiency disorder. J Allergy Clin Immunol. 2016;138(2):544–50.e4.
90. Kuehn HS, Niemela JE, Rangel-Santos A, Zhang M, Pittaluga S, Stoddard JL, et al. Loss-of-function of the protein kinase C δ (PKCδ) causes a B-cell lymphoproliferative syndrome in humans. Blood. 2013;121(16):3117–25.

Chapter 3
Agammaglobulinemia

Camile Ortega and Vivian Hernandez-Trujillo

Case Presentation 1

A 2-year-old partially vaccinated Hispanic male with a history of febrile seizures presented to the emergency department with fever, oliguria, watery diarrhea, lethargy, meningismus, ecthyma gangrenosum, and lower abdominal tenderness. Eight days prior to presentation, he was evaluated by his pediatrician for facial rash and low grade temperature and was diagnosed with hand-foot-and-mouth disease. He was prescribed amoxicillin, with subsequent worsening of symptoms and was switched to cefdinir. He had a history of respiratory synctial virus (RSV) infection associated with febrile seizures 5 months prior to presentation. He had no history of sinopulmonary infections, but he did not attend day care and did not have siblings. Family history was significant for recurrent sinopulmonary infections in his mother and maternal aunts. His vaccines were delayed due to parental choice, and he had not yet received live vaccines including MMR, VZV, or Rotavirus. A full sepsis evaluation was performed in the emergency department. Cerebral spinal fluid (CSF) demonstrated pleocytosis, and he was started on empiric antibiotics and transferred to the intensive care unit for further evaluation and management. Due to worsening abdominal pain, computed tomography of the abdomen was performed. He was found to have a ruptured appendix and septic emboli at the lung bases. Viral encephalitis PCR panel of CSF was positive for HHV-6, and he was started on ganciclovir. CSF and blood cultures grew *Pseudomonas aeruginosa*. He was found to have undetectable immunoglobulins, and lymphocyte subsets revealed profound B-cell

---

C. Ortega
Department of Medical Education, Nicklaus Children's Hospital, Miami, FL, USA

V. Hernandez-Trujillo (✉)
Allergy and Immunology Care Center of South Florida, Nicklaus Children's Hospital, Miami Lakes, FL, USA
e-mail: office@sfallergy.com

lymphopenia (5 cells/uL). In addition to IV antibiotics, he received 500 mg/kg intravenous immunoglobulin (IVIG). BTK protein analysis demonstrated hemizygous BTK pathogenic variant confirming the diagnosis of X-linked agammaglobulinemia (XLA). The patient's hospital course was complicated by brain abscesses and pyoventriculitis. He was followed closely by Immunology and Infectious Disease and treated with three more doses of IVIG and IV antibiotics. Repeat brain MRI nearly 4 weeks later demonstrated significant improvement. He had remarkable clinical recovery and was discharged home at his baseline neurological status. His IgG level upon discharge was 605 mg/dL, with a plan to increase the dose to 600 mg/kg per month. At the time of presentation, the patient's mother was 24 weeks pregnant and was not aware of the sex of the baby. As advised, she had a fetal ultrasound and male sex was identified. Upon birth, lymphocyte subsets and genetic testing were performed confirming BTK mutation and XLA diagnosis. Both brothers receive monthly IVIG and have remained in good health.

Diagnosis/Assessment

XLA is the most common cause of agammaglobulinemia. It was first described in 1952 and comprises approximately 85% of patients who present with early-onset infections, profound hypogammaglobulinemia, and less than 2% CD19+ B cells in peripheral circulation [1]. Only males are affected, and every male who has a mutant copy of Btk has symptoms of the disease [2]. Bruton tyrosine kinase (BTK) is the gene affected in XLA and plays a critical role in B-cell development [1]. There is an arrest of maturation of B lymphocytes in blood and tissue. Therefore, there is no generation of plasma cells, which results in absent or severely decreased production of all classes of immunoglobulins with markedly defective antibody responses [1]. Btk is a member of a family of cytoplasmic tyrosine kinases, called Tec kinases, which are activated by growth, differentiation, and survival signals and are characterized by a C-terminal kinase domain preceded by SH2 and SH3 domains, a proline-rich region, and an NH2-terminal PH (pleckstrin homology) domain. Btk is activated through the BCR (B-cell receptor) and pre-BCR [3]. Cross-linking of a number of cell-surface receptors, including the BCR, the high-affinity IgE receptor on mast cells, and the collagen VI receptor on platelets, results in the recruitment of cytosolic Btk to the plasma membrane and activation of Btk by tyrosine phosphorylation [4–8]. Upon activation, Btk moves to the inner side of the plasma membrane where it is phosphorylated and partially activated by an src family member (Fig. 3.1) [9]. Btk then undergoes autophosphorylation [10]. Src family members also phosphorylate the immunoreceptor tyrosine-based activation motifs (ITAMs) on Igα and Igβ, the signal transduction molecules that escort the μ heavy chain to the cell surface [2]. The two phosphorylated tyrosines in the ITAMs act as docking sites for syk, a cytoplasmic tyrosine kinase with two SH2 domains [11]. Syk is then able to phosphorylate downstream targets including the

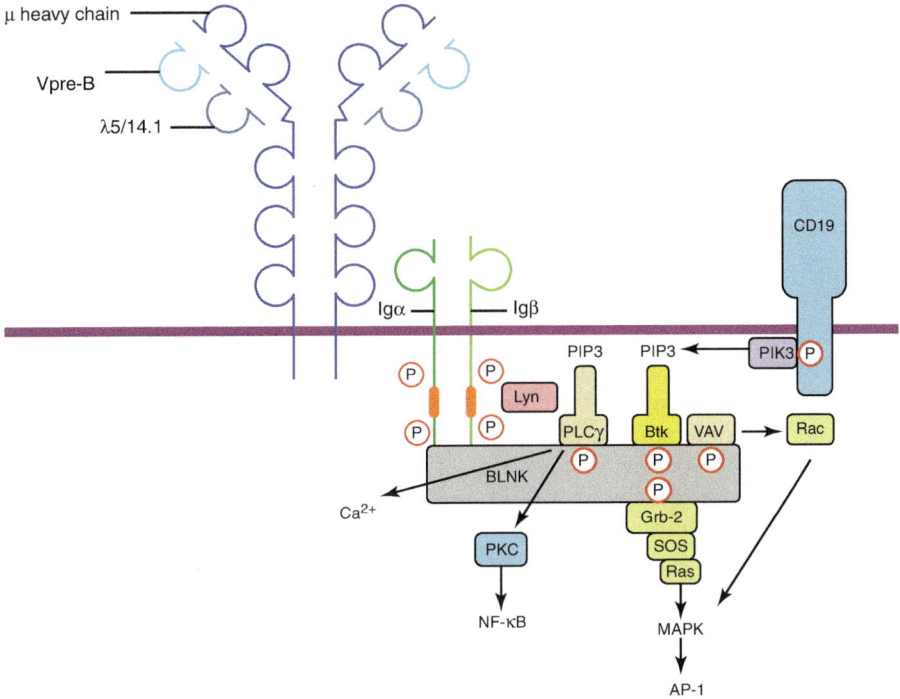

Fig. 3.1 B-cell receptor signaling. The phosphorylation and activation of Btk by an src family member (depicted as Lyn) trigger a downstream signaling cascade, which ultimately leads to the production of transcription factors

tyrosine-rich adapter protein BLNK (B-cell linker protein). At the cell membrane, activated Btk interacts with phospholipase gamma (PLCγ), leading to enhanced tyrosine phosphorylation of PLCγ and resulting in accumulation of inositol 1,4,5-triphosphate (IP3) and mobilization of extracellular calcium [4] and activation of mitogen activating protein (MAP) kinases, extracellular-signal-regulated kinase (ERK) and c-Jun N-terminal kinase (JNK) [12]. Btk is expressed in myeloid cells, platelets, and B cells. Over 90% of mutations in Btk are associated with the absence of Btk in monocytes [13]. B-lineage cells in all organs are affected, resulting in reduced sizes of lymphoid tissue and absent tonsils [1]. XLA is maintained in the population by new mutations, similar to other X-linked disorders that are lethal without medical intervention. In many families, it is possible to identify the source of a new mutation in Btk [3]. The mother of a patient with sporadic XLA has an 80% chance of being a carrier, but the maternal grandmother is a carrier only 25% of the time [14].

XLA is estimated to occur at an incidence from 1:100,000 to 1:200,000 live births [1]. Patients with XLA are usually healthy in the newborn period, and the onset of recurrent bacterial infections appears after transferred maternal IgG antibodies decline from 4 to 6 months of age [15]. Although the majority of patients are diagnosed as having immunodeficiency at less than 5 years of age, there are rare adults who are recognized to have hypogammaglobulinemia, markedly reduced numbers of B cells, and a mutation in Btk, when a nephew or grandson is found to have XLA [16, 17]. Before diagnosis and instigation of treatment, patients experience recurrent, often life-threatening infections, particularly those caused by encapsulated bacteria, most commonly such as *Streptococcus pneumonia* and *Haemophilus influenza*, as well as *Giardia lamblia* [15]. There is considerable variation in site of infection, with sinusitis, otitis media, and lower respiratory tract infections being the most common [4]. Most patients are recognized to have immunodeficiency when they are hospitalized for a severe infection such as sepsis, meningitis, or pneumonia with empyema [3]. A history of hospitalization for a common viral infection, such as croup, diarrhea, or RSV pneumonia, is not common although these infections are not generally considered worrisome in XLA [3]. Although the disease has been considered to be limited to the B-lymphocyte compartment, up to 25% of patients with XLA have profound neutropenia at the time of diagnosis [4]. It seems likely that an antecedent viral infection precipitates neutropenia in these patients, which then leads to susceptibility to pseudomonas or staphylococcal infection [18]. In the case of XLA, in particular, neutropenia may be considered to be transient and secondary to infectious episodes [19]. T-lymphocyte function is normally maintained, and they are able to eliminate fungi and most viruses competently. The notable exception to this is the enterovirus family. Patients with XLA are particularly susceptible to both wild type and vaccine-associated polio, ECHO 11, and Coxsackie, which may be life-threatening [15]. These agents can cause a dermatomyositis-like syndrome or fatal chronic encephalitis [20–24]. The modifying factors that confer susceptibility to severe enteroviral infections in patients with XLA have not been identified [3]. As many as one-third of patients are evaluated for immunodeficiency when they are hospitalized for a dramatic constellation of findings, including (a) pyoderma gangrenosum, perirectal abscess, cellulitis, or impetigo; (b) pseudomonas or staphylococcal sepsis; and (c) neutropenia [3], which was the scenario for the present case which prompted the clinician to obtain an immunoglobulin panel at the time of presentation. When compared to immunocompetent individuals, hypogammaglobulinemic patients are found to have increased mycoplasma and ureaplasma at mucosal sites obtained by culture [25]. Therefore, any acute nontraumatic joint swelling, pain, or erythema in XLA patients should prompt investigation into possible mycoplasma or ureaplasma, as these infections are often difficult to isolate and treat [25].

The mean age of diagnosis of XLA in North America is 3 years, but the median is 26 months, despite being a congenital form of agammaglobulinemia [7]. XLA can be diagnosed soon after birth through kappa-deleting recombination excision circle- (KREC-) level quantification [26], although this is not standard practice. Newborn screening would allow the early diagnosis of XLA and initiation of treatment at a pre-symptomatic phase [15].

Management/Outcome

As the case above highlights, the early diagnosis and treatment with immunoglobulin replacement therapy are essential in order to prevent sequelae of infections [26], particularly when coupled with aggressive use of antibiotics [2]. The prognosis of XLA appears to be excellent if diagnosed and treated before long-term complications of infection occur [27]. Immunoglobulin may be administered intravenously (IVIG) or subcutaneously (SCIG) at intervals of 2–4 weeks for the intravenous route and 1–14 days for the subcutaneous route [1]. A new formulation for the administration of SCIG, using recombinant human hyaluronidase to facilitate the administration of large volumes of SCIG on a monthly basis, is also available [1]. The IgG trough levels, obtained just prior to infusion, in association with the clinical course determine the adequacy of the IgG replacement dose. Adjustments may be needed for excessive infections, growth, enteric loss, or increased metabolism [1]. The frequency of monitoring depends on age, with more frequent monitoring in younger growing children, patients with breakthrough infections, and the clinical considerations of the individual patient [1]. The most commonly reported adverse reactions occurring with IVIG infusions are headaches, nausea, vomiting, flushing, and myalgia. Only experienced practitioners should supervise IVIG administration, and appropriate education should be provided to patients on home therapy for recognizing and managing adverse reactions [4]. The most common sides effects from subcutaneous IG administration include local reactions and itching. Immunoglobulin is a blood product prepared from cold alcohol fractionation of pooled human plasma. There is a risk of virus transmission, albeit very low, as with all blood product preparations. Improvements in the fractionation process have been effective in removal and inactivation of most viruses [4]. Although XLA patients on replacement immunoglobulin are generally healthy, unusual infections, unexpected inflammatory complications, and clonal CD8+ T-cell lymphomas have been reported, suggesting the possibility of discrete cellular defects [28]. The lack of IgA and IgM in current treatment and the subsequent risk of recurrent respiratory tract infections are also of concern, as they do appear to be leading to a significant burden of bronchiectasis [15]. Additionally, current treatment makes no attempt to replace the other lost functions of B lymphocytes or on other deficits on the immune system caused by Btk deficiency [15]. Quality-of-life studies have shown that patients report treatment placed a greater burden on their quality of life than the disease itself [29]. An increasing number of patients with XLA are living past middle age. Despite adequate doses of gamma globulin, many of these patients still develop chronic lung disease, persistent sinusitis, joint pains, or liver disease [30, 31]. Relatively few patients with XLA have survived into their fifties or sixties; therefore, it is difficult to predict how they will be affected by common comorbid diseases of adulthood such as hypertension, cardiac disease, diabetes, and malignancy [10]. Hematopoietic stem cell transplantation (HSCT) is not routinely offered for treatment of XLA, due to lack of consistent benefit, the risks of GvHD, and the associated mortality of 10–15% [15]. However, curative gene therapy in XLA may be on the horizon as it has shown promising results in murine models from gene therapy trials for other primary immunodeficiencies.

Case Presentation 2

A 1-year-old female with a history of recurrent otitis and fevers since 3 months of age presented for the evaluation of frequent foul-smelling stools. Parents reported 2–3 soft foul-smelling stools per day. A review of systems was also pertinent for chronic cough, chronic conjunctivitis characterized by yellowish discharge, and episodes of emesis 1–2 times per month (not associated with nausea or coughing). Family history was significant for a maternal uncle and a female maternal cousin with immunodeficiency. Both height and weight were considerably below the 3rd percentile. Physical exam was notable for matted eyelashes, erythematous conjunctiva, dry papular rash over the elbows, and abdominal distention without hepatosplenomegaly or tenderness. Complete blood cell count was unremarkable. Chemistries demonstrated severe hypoproteinemia with a total protein of 4.8 g (nl 6–8.3 g/dL) and albumin of 2.5 g (nl 3.5–5.5 g/dL). Other chemistries were consistent with hypoproteinemia and included low BUN, low calcium, and low liver function tests. Lymphocyte subsets were significant for 0% CD19+ B cells, 95% CD3+ T cells, 53% CD4+ T cells, 42% CD8+ T cells, and 5% NK cells, and her response to mitogens (PHA, Con A, and PWM) were normal. The serum IgA was <6 mg/dL, IgM was <5 mg/dL, and IgG was 88 mg/dL. The chest radiograph showed peribronchial thickening, and the sinus films demonstrated bilateral opacification of the maxillary antrum. The stool exam was positive for *Giardia*. Genotyping revealed a homozygous μ heavy-chain defect. The patient was started on treatment with IVIG and antibiotic prophylaxis with trimethoprim- sulfamethoxazole, which was effective for the conjunctivitis as well as the chronic bronchitis. The patient was also treated with a course of metronidazole for the *Giardia* infection.

Diagnosis/Assessment

Autosomal recessive forms of congenital agammaglobulinemia were initially described in the 1970s, nearly two decades after XLA was first described, following several reports of females with a clinically indistinguishable disorder from XLA [18, 32, 33]. Hematopoietic stem cells in the bone marrow develop into B cells and mature into antibody-secreting plasma cells in peripheral lymphoid tissues in a complex and tightly regulated manner [4]. Successful assembly and functional signaling through pre-B and B-cell receptor (BCR) complexes determine B-cell development from the pre-B cell stage onwards [4]. Central to this process is the

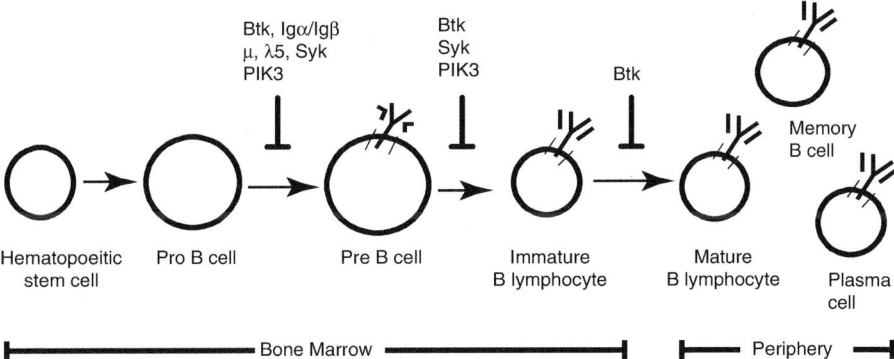

Fig. 3.2 B-cell development. A block in any of the components of the pre-BCR causes an arrest of the developing B cell, most commonly from the pre-B to the pro-B stage in the bone marrow, which leads to an absence of B cells in the periphery and agammaglobulinemia

expression of individual components of the receptor and also the molecules that transduce signals from the receptor to initiate cellular events [4] (Fig. 3.2). Pre-B cell receptor (pre-BCR) assembly is a pivotal step for the progression of B-cell development in the bone marrow [34]. The pre-BCR complex is expressed transiently and at a very low cell density on the surface of developing B cells [33]. The transition of the pro-B stage to the pre-B stage of differentiation marks the successful expression of the pre-BCR [33]. The pre-BCR is composed of the membrane form of the μ heavy chain, the surrogate light chain composed of VpreB and λ5/14.1, and the immunoglobulin-associated, signal-transducing chains, Igα and Igβ [35]. Before the rearrangement of the light chain genes, the surrogate light chains are responsible for determining the ability of the rearranged μ heavy chain to bind conventional light chain [35]. The Igα/Igβ heterodimer escorts the μ heavy chain to the cell surface by masking the hydrophilic transmembrane domain [35]. Prior to the completion of V-DJ rearrangement, the components of the surrogate light chain and the Igα/Igβ heterodimer are expressed in the cytoplasm of B-cell precursors [36, 37]. The genes for surrogate light chains are expressed exclusively in pro-B cells and pre-B cells and can act as markers for these stages of differentiation [38, 39]. Early B-cell development is dependent on the sequential immunoglobulin gene rearrangements and selective expansion of cells that have successfully passed checkpoint controls [40, 41]. Mutations in components of the pre-BCR or in the downstream signaling cascade have been reported to result in the rare forms of autosomal recessive agammaglobulinemia (ARA) [34]. This rare condition is characterized by absent peripheral B cells and severe hypogammaglobulinemia due to a developmental arrest at the pro-B stage to pre-B stage. It has been estimated that approximately 10% of agammaglobulinemic syndromes are autosomally inherited [4]. In some affected families, there is known consanguinity, and in others, the parents or grandparents are from an isolated community [2]. Mutations in the μ heavy chain account for approximately 5% of patients with defects in early B-cell development [3] and have a clinical picture that is similar to that seen in XLA [42].

Table 3.1 Types of agammaglobulinemia

–	X-Linked Agammaglobulinemia	Autosomal Recessive Agammaglobulinemia
Protein affected	Btk	μ heavy chain, Igα (CD79A), Igβ (CD79B), λ5/14.1, BLNK, and p85α (PI3K)
Sex affected	Males only	Males and females
Approximate percentage of agammaglobulinemic patients	85% [1, 2, 4, 15]	10% [4]
Average age at diagnosis	35 months [3]	11 months [3]
Severity of infections	Severe	More severe
Immunoglobulin levels	Low [1]	Severely low [4]
Peripheral CD19+ B lymphocytes	Low (<2%) [2]	Absent (0%) [17, 20]
Treatment	Immunoglobulin replacement	Immunoglobulin replacement

Defects in the genes encoding for Igα, Igβ, λ5, BLNK, and p85α (PI3K) have been identified as other, rarer, causes for ARA in humans [34]. These patients generally have clinical findings that are indistinguishable from those seen in mutations in Btk. Similar to patients with defects in μ heavy chain, patients with other forms of ARA tend to have the onset of severe infections within the first year of life [3]. All the reported mutations have been associated with the complete absence of CD19+ B cells in peripheral circulation, as seen in the second case presented [3]. This can serve as a distinguishing feature from XLA when evaluating a young male with recurrent infections and agammaglobulinemia (Table 3.1). Although there is considerable overlap, patients with μ heavy chain mutations tend to have a more severe phenotype than that seen in patients with BTK mutations [43]. These findings suggest the protective value of the small amount of immunoglobulin produced by patients with XLA. This may contribute to the earlier diagnosis of ARA who are recognized at a mean age of 11 months rather than 35 months in patients with XLA. Although the patient in the present case had not developed dramatic problems secondary to her immune deficiency, she did have some related complications. Although hypoproteinemia is invariably a result of hypogammaglobulinemia, the degree of hypoproteinemia, in this case, may have been a result of the superimposed *Giardia* infection. There also was an apparent element of failure to thrive. A higher incidence of enteroviral infections and pseudomonas sepsis with neutropenia has also been reported in ARA [3]. These findings imply that the enteroviral infections and neutropenia in patients with XLA result from hypogammaglobulinemia rather than solely due to requirements for Btk in myeloid cells [3].

It is also worth mentioning that an autosomal dominant form of agammaglobulinemia was identified in patients with the unusual phenotype characterized by an increased expression of CD19, but the absence of the BCR [44]. BCR expression and signaling is necessary for positive selection of B cells and prevention of death by apoptosis [4]. Genetic studies demonstrated a de novo mutation in the broadly expressed transcription factor E47, which plays a critical role in the quality control mechanism of enforcing a block to prevent cells that lack a pre-BCR from further development [44].

Management/Outcome

The mainstay of treatment for patients with ARA is identical to that for patients with XLA: immunoglobulin and aggressive use of antibiotics [2]. Unlike BTK gene defects in XLA, for which laboratory assays are commercially available and more than 600 different mutations have been described to date [45], identifying a genetic cause of ARA remains a challenge [46]. A better understanding of susceptibility genes and modifying genetic factors as well as the identification of mutant genes in patients who do not appear to have defects in the genes already associated with immunodeficiency should be the goals of further areas of investigation [3]. Advances in whole-genome sequencing will greatly facilitate the molecular diagnosis of genetic defects in additional genes that can cause ARA [44]. It is unlikely that gene therapy will be an option for these patients in the near future, due to the complexity of the μ heavy chain locus and the rarity of the other autosomal recessive forms of agammaglobulinemia [2].

> **Clinical Pearls and Pitfalls**
> - Developmental arrest of B cells in the bone marrow leads to the absence of B cells in the peripheral blood, resulting in agammaglobulinemia from defects in any components of the pre-BCR or downstream signaling cascade [19].
> - Antibody deficiencies are associated with an increased susceptibility to infection with encapsulated bacteria, particularly *Streptococcus pneumoniae* and *Haemophilus influenza* [3].
> - Unusual invasive infections should lead to an immunological workup [32].
> - A patient's risk of infectious exposures should be considered when severe, refractory sinopulmonary infections occur or if they do not have a typical disease course.
> - X-linked inheritance, severely decreased numbers of peripheral B lymphocytes, and decreased immunoglobulin production make a clinical diagnosis of XLA very likely [4].
> - The autosomal recessive forms of agammaglobulinemia have been reported to present with a more severe and earlier onset of disease than XLA [32].
> - Although family history of immunodeficiency can alert the clinician to evaluate for primary immunodeficiency, de novo mutations are known to occur.
> - Acute nontraumatic joint swelling, pain, or erythema in XLA patients should prompt investigation into possible mycoplasma or ureaplasma.

- In patients phenotypically similar to patients with XLA without a mutation in BTK, either male or female, screening for defects in the components of the B cell or pre-B cell receptor complex should be considered [4].
- Early diagnosis of primary immunodeficiencies is important in order to provide optimal treatment and limit possible complications that may compromise the patient's quality of life [47].
- The mainstay of treatment for all congenital agammaglobulinemia regardless of molecular defect is immunoglobulin replacement therapy [4].
- Dose and frequency should be tailored to the patient's clinical health status. Individuals who continue to have recurrent infections may need higher or more frequent doses [4].
- Despite the excellent clinical response of most patients to immunoglobulin replacement therapy, monitoring patients on a regular basis is essential.
- *Giardia* infections are common and may cause hypoproteinemia and poor weight gain in the absence of a history of abdominal pain or diarrhea [48].
- Chronic lung disease may develop in the absence of acute infection [2].
- Enteroviral disease, and especially chronic meningoencephalitis, remains one of the greatest dangers to agammaglobulinemic patients.

References

1. El-Sayed ZA, Abramova I, Aldave JC, Al-Herz W, Bezrodnik L, Boukari R, et al. X-linked agammaglobulinemia (XLA): phenotype, diagnosis, and therapeutic challenges around the world. World Allergy Organ J. 2019;12(3):100018. https://doi.org/10.1016/j.waojou.2019.100018.eCollection2019.
2. Conley ME, Broides A, Hernandez-Trujillo V, Howards V, Kanegane H, Miyawaki T, et al. Genetic analysis of patients with defects in early B-cell development. Immunol Rev. 2005;203:216.
3. Conley ME, Dobbs AK, Farmer DM, Kilic S, Paris K, Grigoriadou S, et al. Primary B cell immunodeficiencies: comparisons and contrasts. Annu Rev Immunol. 2009;27:199–227.
4. Gaspar HB, Conley ME. Early B cell defects. Clin Exp Immunol. 2000;119(3):383.
5. de Weers M, Brouns GS, Hinshelwood S, Kinnon C, Schuurman RK, Hendriks RW, et al. B-cell antigen receptor stimulation activates the human Bruton's tyrosine kinase, which is deficient in X-linked agammaglobulinemia. J Biol Chem. 1994;269:23857–60.
6. Aoki Y, Isselbacher KJ, Pillai S. Bruton tyrosine kinase is tyrosine phosphorylated and activated in pre-B lymphocytes and receptor-ligated B cells. Proc Natl Acad Sci U S A. 1994;91:10606–9.
7. Kawakami Y, Yao L, Miura T, Tsukada S, Witte ON, Kawakami T. Tyrosine phosphorylation and activation of Bruton tyrosine kinase upon Fc epsilon RI cross-linking. Mol Cell Biol. 1994;14:5108–13.
8. Oda A, Ikeda Y, Ochs HD, Druker BJ, Ozaki K, Handa M, et al. Rapid tyrosine phosphorylation and activation of Bruton's tyrosine/Tec kinases in platelets induced by collagen binding or CD32 cross-linking. Blood. 2000;95:1663–70.
9. Rawlings DJ, Scharenberg AM, Park H, Wahl MI, Lin S, Kato RM, et al. Activation of BTK by a phosphorylation mechanism initiated by SRC family kinases. Science. 1996;271(5250):822–5.

10. Park H, Wahl MI, Afar DE, Turck CW, Rawlings DJ, Tam C, et al. Regulation of BTK function by a major autophosphorylation site within the SH3 domain. Immunity. 1996;4(5):515–25.
11. Bu JY, Shaw AS, Chan AC. Analysis of the interaction of ZAP-70 and syk protein tyrosine kinases with the T-cell antigen receptor by plasmon resonance. Proc Natl Acad Sci U S A. 1995;92:5106–10.
12. Rawlings DJ. Bruton's tyrosine kinase controls a sustained calcium signal essential for B lineage development and function. Clin Immunol. 1999;91(3):243–53.
13. Nonoyama S, Tsukada S, Yamadori T, Miyawaki T, Jin YZ, Watanabe C, et al. Functional analysis of peripheral blood B cells in patients with X-linked agammaglobulinemia. J Immunol. 1998;134:3070–4.
14. Conley ME, Mathias D, Treadaway J, Minegishi Y, Rohrer J. Mutations in BTK in patients with presumed X-linked agammaglobulinemia. Am J Hum Genet. 1998;62(5):1034–43.
15. Shillitoe B, Gennery A. X-linked agammaglobulinemia: outcome in the modern era. Clin Immunol. 2017;183:54–62.
16. Kornfeld SJ, Haire RN, Strong SJ, Tang H, Sung SS, Fu SM, et al. A novel mutation (Cys145-stop) in Bruton's tyrosine kinase is associated with newly diagnosed X-linked agammaglobulinemia in a 51-year-old male. Mol Med. 1996;2:619–23.
17. Conley ME, Howard V. Clinical findings leading to the diagnosis of X-linked agammaglobulinemia. J Pediatr. 2002;141:566–71.
18. Aiuti F, Fontana L, Gatti RA. Membrane-bound immunoglobulin (Ig) and in vitro production of Ig by lymphoid cells from patients with primary immunodeficiencies. Scand J Immunol. 1973;2(1):9–16.
19. Lougaris V, Massimilliano V, Baronio M, Moratto D, Tampella G, Biasini A, et al. Autosomal recessive agammaglobulinemia: the third case of Igβ deficiency due to a novel non-sense mutation. J Clin Immunol. 2014;34(4):425–7.
20. Wilfert CM, Buckley RH, Mohanakumar T, Griffith JF, Katz SL, Whisnant JK, et al. Persistent and fatal central nervous system ECHOvirus infections in patients with agammaglobulinemia. N Engl J Med. 1977;296:1485–9.
21. Wyatt HV. Poliomyelitis in hypogammaglobulinemics. J Infect Dis. 1973;128:802–6.
22. Bardelas JA, Winkelstein JA, Seto DS, Tsai T, Rogol AD. Fatal ECHO 24 infection in a patient with hypogammaglobulinemia: relationship to dermatomyositis-like syndrome. J Pediatr. 1977;90:396–9.
23. McKinney RE Jr, Katz SL, Wilfert CM. Chronic enteroviral meningoencephalitis in agammaglobulinemic patients. Rev Infect Dis. 1987;9:334–56.
24. Hidalgo S, Garcia EM, Cisterna D, Freire MC. Paralytic poliomyelitis caused by a vaccine derived polio virus in an antibody-deficient Argentinean child. Pediatr Infect Dis J. 2003;22:570–2.
25. Furr PM, Taylor-Robinson D, Webster AD. Mycoplasmas and ureaplasmas in patients with hypogammaglobulinaemia and their role in arthritis: microbiological observations over twenty years. Ann Rheum Dis. 1994;53:183–7.
26. King J, Borte S, Brodszki N, von Dobeln U, Smith CIE, Hammartrom L. Kappa-deleting recombination excision circle levels remain low or undetectable throughout life in patients with X-linked agammaglobulinemia. Pediatr Allergy Immunol. 2018;29(4):453–6.
27. Winkelstein JA, Marino MC, Lederman HM, Jones SM, Sullivan K, Burks AW, et al. X-linked agammaglobulinemia report on a United States registry of 201 patients. Medicine. 2006;85(4):193–202.
28. Ramesh M, Simchoni N, Hamm D, Cunningham-Rundles C. High-throughput sequencing reveals an altered T cell repertoire in X-linked agammaglobulinemia. Clin Immunol. 2015;161(2):190–6.
29. Howard V, Greene JM, Pahwa S, Winkelstein JA, Boyle JM, Kocak M, et al. The health status and quality of life of adults with X-linked agammaglobulinemia. Clin Immunol. 2006;118(2–3):201–8. Epub 2005 Dec 22.

30. Quartier P, Debré M, De Blic J, de Sauverzac R, Sayegh N, Jabado N, et al. Early and prolonged intravenous immunoglobulin replacement therapy in childhood agammaglobulinemia: a retrospective survey of 31 patients. J Pediatr. 1999;134:589–96.
31. Plebani A, Soresina A, Rondelli R, Amato GM, Azzari C, Cardinale F, et al. Clinical, immunological, and molecular analysis in a large cohort of patients with X-linked agammaglobulinemia: an Italian multicenter study. Clin Immunol. 2002;104:221–30.
32. Hoffman T, Winchester R, Schulkind M, Frias JL, Ayoub EM, Good RA. Hypoimmunoglobulinemia with normal T cell function in female siblings. Clin Immunol Immunopathol. 1977;7:364–71.
33. Conley ME, Sweinberg SK. Females with a disorder phenotypically identical to X-linked agammaglobulinemia. J Clin Immunol. 1992;12(2):139–43.
34. Khalili A, Plebani A, Massimiliano V, Abolhassani H, Lougaris V, Mirminachi B, et al. Autosomal recessive agammaglobulinemia: a novel non-sense mutation in CD79a. J Clin Immunol. 2014;34(2):138–41.
35. Minegishi Y, Coustan-Smith E, Rapalus L, Ersoy F, Campana D, Conley ME. Mutations in Igα (CD79a) result in a complete block in B-cell development. J Clin Invest. 1999;104(8):1115.
36. Karasuyama H, Rolink A, Shinkai Y, Young F, Alt FW, Melchers F. The expression of Vpre-B/lambda 5 surrogate light chain in early bone marrow precursor B cells of normal and B cell-deficient mutant mice. Cell. 1994;77(1):133–43.
37. Lassoued K, Illges H, Benlagha K, Cooper MD. Fate of surrogate light chains in B lineage cells. J Exp Med. 1996;183(2):421–9.
38. Kudo A, Melchers F. A second gene, VpreB in the lambda 5 locus of the mouse, which appears to be selectively expressed in pre-B lymphocytes. EMBO J. 1987;6(8):2267–72.
39. Sakaguchi N, Melchers F. Lambda 5, a new light-chain–related locus selectively expressed in pre–B lymphocytes. Nature. 1986;324(6097):579–82.
40. Spanopoulou E, Roman CA, Corcoran LM, Schlissel MS, Silver DP, Nemazee D, et al. Functional immunoglobulin transgenes guide ordered B-cell differentiation in Rag-1–deficient mice. Genes Dev. 1994;8(9):1030–42.
41. Young F, Ardman B, Shinkai Y, Lansford R, Blackwell TK, Mendelsohn M, et al. Influence of immunoglobulin heavy- and light-chain expression on B-cell differentiation. Genes Dev. 1994;8(9):1043–57.
42. Yel L, Minegishi Y, Coustan-Smith E, Buckley RH, Trübel H, Pachman LM, et al. Mutations in the mu heavy chain gene in patients with agammaglobulinemia. N Engl J Med. 1996;335(20):1486–93.
43. Lopez-Granados E, Porpiglia AS, Hogan MB, Matamoros N, Krasovec S, Pignata C, et al. Clinical and molecular analysis of patients with defects in mu heavy chain gene. J Clin Invest. 2002;110(7):1029–35.
44. Boisson B, Wang YD, Bosompem A, Ma CS, Lim A, Kochetkov T, et al. A recurrent dominant negative E47 mutation causes agammaglobulinemia and BCR-B cells. J Clin Invest. 2013;123(11):4781–5.
45. Valiaho J, Smith CI, Vihinen M. BTKbase: the mutation database for X-linked agammaglobulinemia. Hum Mutat. 2006;27:1209e1217.
46. Gemayel KT, Litman GW, Sriaroon P. Autosomal recessive agammaglobulinemia associated with an IGLL1 gene missense mutation. Ann Allergy Asthma Immunol. 2016;117(4):439–41.
47. Routes J, Abinun M, Al-Herz W, Bustamante J, Condino-Neto A, De La Morena MT, et al. ICON: the early diagnosis of congenital immunodeficiencies. J Clin Immunol. 2014;34:398–424.
48. LoGalbo PR, Sampson HA, Buckley RH. Symptomatic giardiasis in three patients with X-linked agammaglobulinemia. J Pediatr. 1982;101:78–80.

Chapter 4
Class-Switch Defects

Ramsay L. Fuleihan

Introduction

Immunoglobulin class switching is a mechanism by which B lymphocytes switch from producing IgM and IgD antibodies to IgG, IgA, or IgE antibodies to generate diverse antibody effector functions while retaining the same antigen specificity [1]. Class switching is dependent on antigen recognition and requires interaction between CD40 ligand (CD40L, CD154) on activated CD4 T cells and CD40 present on the surface of B cells. This signaling process is also required for somatic hypermutation, a mechanism by which the affinity of antibody molecules to antigens is increased. A variety of inherited defects along the CD40L/CD40 signaling pathway result in antibody deficiency with or without defects in somatic hypermutation and in some cases T-cell dysfunction, malignancy, or autoimmunity [2]. A high index of suspicion is important in diagnosing these diseases, and identifying the underlying genetic defect confirms the type of class-switch defect and helps decide on optimal therapy for the patient.

Case Presentation 1

A 33-month-old boy presented with a history of recurrent episodes of otitis media since 6 months of age despite myringotomy tube placement and adenoidectomy. His infections started with a febrile upper respiratory infection, and he was found to have otitis media on examination by his pediatrician. He had more than 20 different episodes diagnosed and treated. He has been treated with albuterol during these

---

R. L. Fuleihan (✉)
Department of Allergy and Immunology, Ann and Robert H. Lurie Children's Hospital of Chicago, Chicago, IL, USA
e-mail: rlf2151@cumc.columbia.edu

episodes for cough, but there was no history of wheezing. There is no history of pneumonia and a CXR done before his visit was normal with no evidence of an infiltrate or any other specific finding. He had no history of thrush, abscesses, or other infections except for one episode of hand-foot-and-mouth disease with tonsillar enlargement. There is no history of eczema or food or drug allergy. There is no family history of immunodeficiency, but there is a history of a maternal aunt who died at 3 months of age. His father is allergic to cats, his mother has photosensitivity, and his maternal grandmother developed allergy to fruits. Review of systems was positive for frequent loose stools. Physical examination was normal except for the presence of myringotomy tubes in both ears.

Diagnosis/Assessment

The differential diagnosis of recurrent otitis media includes allergic diseases as well as immunodeficiency. Skin testing was performed in clinic and was negative to molds, dust mites, cockroach, dog and feather. Laboratory results showed a normal CBC with differential except for a low percentage and absolute number of neutrophils (404 cells/mcl), a markedly low serum IgG level (43 mg/dl) with a normal IgM level (104 mg/dl) but undetectable IgA level (<2 mg/dl), low CD8 (3%, 155 cells/mm^3) and NK cells (2%, 103 cells/mm^3), but normal T-cell proliferation to mitogens. Naïve and memory T-cell percentages were essentially normal, but he had severely reduced total (1.3%, nl 5.6–33%) and class-switched (3.3%, nl 28.7–65.6%) memory B cells. Flow cytometry for CD40L on activated CD4+ T cells using a monoclonal antibody to CD40L showed normal expression (Fig. 4.1). Expression of CD40 on B cells was also normal. Genetic testing done at another institution showed a point mutation in the *CD40L* gene. Subsequently, staining for CD40L on activated CD4+ T cells was normal using a monoclonal antibody but severely reduced using a chimeric soluble CD40 reagent consistent with the point mutation found in his *CD40L* gene and with the diagnosis of X-linked hyper IgM (see Fig. 4.1). Because some point mutations do not affect the expression of the CD40L molecule on the surface of activated CD4+ T cells [3], using a chimeric CD40 receptor reagent will help determine whether the expressed CD40L molecule is able to bind to CD40. In this patient, the inability to bind to CD40 confirmed that the point mutation in the *CD40L* gene was pathogenic and the cause of his immunodeficiency.

X-linked hyper IgM is a severe immunodeficiency disease resulting from mutations in the *CD40L* gene, affecting the ability of CD40L to bind and activate CD40 [2]. CD40L is expressed on activated CD4+ T cells, which then binds to CD40 on B cells or other antigen-presenting cells such as monocytes, macrophages, and dendritic cells as well as a variety of other cell types. In B cells, the signaling pathway activates the class-switch and somatic hypermutation pathways involving signaling via NF-κB and activation of activation-induced cytidine deaminase (AID) and uracyl-*N*-glycosylase (UNG) as well as mismatch repair enzymes (Fig. 4.2). Defects along this pathway result in a hyper-IgM phenotype. Activation of CD40 by CD40L

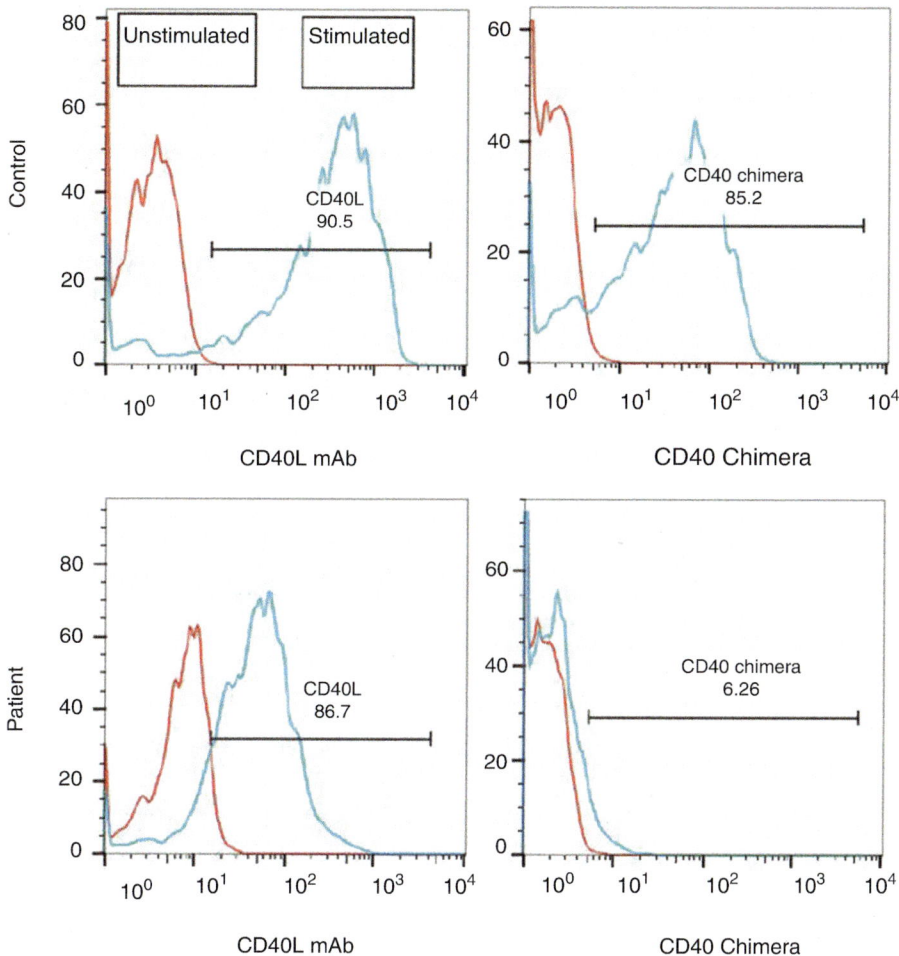

Fig. 4.1 Flow cytometry of CD40L expression in patient (bottom panels) and control (upper panels), with and without stimulation, measured by a monoclonal antibody (mAb, left panels) and soluble CD40 chimeric molecule (right panels) showing that the patient has detectable but reduced-intensity expression of CD40L but markedly reduced binding to CD40

also results in expression of costimulatory molecules on all antigen-presenting cells as well as cytokine secretion that plays a role in T-cell differentiation. As a result, defects in *CD40L* (X-linked) and *CD40* (autosomal recessive, AR) result in a severe immunodeficiency disease with susceptibility to opportunistic infections (pneumocystis jirovicii pneumonia (PJP) and cryptosporidium), fungal infections [4], neutropenia, and an increased risk of cancer of the pancreas, liver, and biliary tree [5] as well as neuroectodermal adenocarcinoma [6, 7]. These patients also have small lymph nodes with absent germinal centers [8]. However, this patient did not have a typical presentation of X-linked hyper IgM. He had a history of recurrent infections

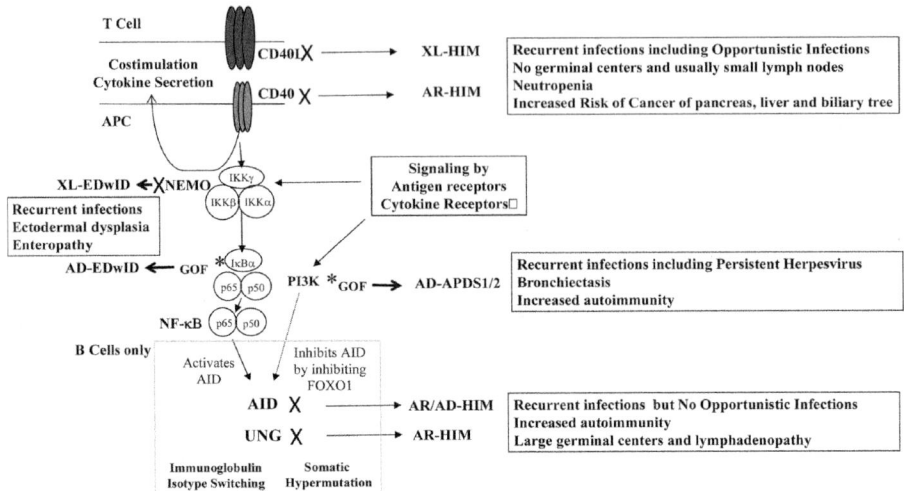

Fig. 4.2 Schematic diagram of the CD40L/CD40 signaling pathway in antigen-presenting cells (APC) and all CD40 expressing cells, leading to class switching and somatic hypermutation, which occur in B cells only. Loss of function defects demarcated by an X; gain-of-function mutations by *GOF. The main clinical consequences of gene defects are also shown. (XL X-linked, AR autosomal recessive, AD autosomal dominant)

but no opportunistic infections. He also had a history of adenoidal hypertrophy requiring adenoidectomy. There is a report of two patients with defects in *CD40L* from the Latin American Registry with lymphadenopathy [4]. This may be an aberration in response to chronic infections. However, he did have neutropenia, a typical feature of X-linked hyper IgM, that became profound with less than 100 cells/mcl for an extended period of time.

In addition to defects in *CD40L* and *CD40*, hypomorphic defects in the NF-κB essential modulator (*NEMO*) gene in boys (X-linked) results in ectodermal dysplasia with immunodeficiency and many but not all of the patients have a hyper-IgM phenotype [9]. Because NF-κB plays an important role in a variety of signaling pathways including the TNF receptors (CD40), antigen receptors, and toll-like receptors, patients with defects in *NEMO* have a susceptibility to a wide spectrum of infectious agents. An autosomal dominant gain-of-function mutation in the inhibitor of NF-κB, *IκB*, results in a similar phenotype [10].

Management/Outcome

Our patient was started on immunoglobulin replacement intravenously (IVIG) with 500 mg/kg every 4 weeks because of his low serum IgG level and continued once the diagnosis of X-linked hyper-IgM syndrome was confirmed. He was also started on PJP prophylaxis with oral trimethoprim-sulfamethoxazole. He remained well on this treatment regimen with no serious infections but had persistent neutropenia. Therefore, his PJP prophylaxis was switched to IV pentamidine (4 mg/kg IV) every 4 weeks. Stem cell transplantation has become a therapeutic option for X-linked hyper-IgM patients, particularly with their susceptibility to opportunistic infections and cancer, which indicates that the disease is a combined immunodeficiency and not simply an antibody deficiency. Unlike patients with severe combined immunodeficiency, patients with X-linked hyper IgM usually survive beyond the first 2 years of life but few survive beyond 30 years of age [4, 11–13]. This raises a dilemma about embarking on a potentially fatal procedure but one that has the promise of a cure. Two international reviews of the outcome of stem cell transplantation in X-linked hyper IgM found no overall improvement in survival [14, 15]. However, results from transplantation performed in more recent years showed improved survival, better quality of life, and none of the transplanted patients developed cancer. A stem cell transplant was considered for this patient, but finding a matching donor was difficult. Finally, the search yielded a well-matched unrelated donor. Our patient underwent a stem cell transplant with reduced-intensity conditioning but had a primary graft failure with no donor cells detected. His own cell counts recovered with resolution of his neutropenia. He continues to receive IVIG and PJP prophylaxis. He has frequent episodes of diarrhea but repeated testing for cryptosporidium has always been negative. He has never had a PJP infection. Neutropenia can be treated with granulocyte colony-stimulating factor (G-CSF) [16]; however, despite very low neutrophil counts, our patient never developed symptoms or infections related to his neutropenia and thus did not require G-CSF.

Gene therapy has become a potential therapy for several primary immunodeficiency diseases including ADA-SCID and X-linked SCID [17]. It is intriguing to consider gene therapy for X-linked hyper IgM but unlike SCID, there is no selective growth advantage for corrected cells and CD40L expression is tightly regulated [18, 19]. Overexpression of CD40L in animal models resulted in lymphoproliferation [20], and CD40L has been found to be overexpressed in active systemic lupus erythematosus [21]. Therefore, gene therapy models would require strict regulation of expression of CD40L, which is very difficult to achieve with gene addition techniques. Novel techniques of gene correction in situ offer the potential for gene therapy of X-linked hyper IgM but require further testing and evaluation [22, 23]. Of concern is that gene correction needs to be achieved in stem cells or in thymic precursors, because CD40L may play an important role in thymic selection as has been shown in animal models [24].

Case Presentation 2

A 6-month-old girl with a past medical history of failure to thrive presented with upper airway obstruction. Her illness began with decreased oral intake and spitting up food. The following day, she began to have a fever with nasal discharge. She saw her pediatrician, who noted a right-sided neck mass. She was sent to a local hospital for further evaluation, where she had respiratory distress with agitation and positional desaturations. CT scan revealed a right-sided collection impinging on the airway. She was transferred to our hospital and underwent incision and drainage of a retropharyngeal abscess, which provided 15 ml of pus. Cultures were positive for methicillin-sensitive *Staphylococcus aureus*, and the patient responded to trimethoprim-sulfamethoxazole treatment. She had a past history of snoring. Flexible laryngoscopy revealed laryngomalacia, and thus, reflux medications and precautions were initiated. The patient was born at term with no complications before or at birth, and she went home with her mother. Review of systems was negative other than what is described in the history above. There is no family history of immunodeficiency. Physical examination was normal except for being small for age.

Diagnosis/Assessment

The presence of a retropharyngeal abscess on presentation raised the concern of a neutrophil defect such as autosomal recessive chronic granulomatous disease [25]. CBC with differential was normal and a neutrophil oxidative burst was normal. Her immunoglobulin levels showed an elevated IgM (464 mg/dL), decreased IgG (137 mg/dL), and normal IgA (10.3 mg/dL). Immunoglobulin levels were repeated at 8 months of age and showed that her serum IgM remained elevated (418 mg/dL), but her IgG and IgA were below detection (<33.3 and <6.67 mg/dL, respectively). Tetanus antibody levels were very low (0.02 IU/ml) and lymphocyte subsets showed slightly low CD8 percentage and a high absolute CD4 count but were otherwise normal including CD40 expression on B cells. T-cell proliferation to mitogens was normal. Genetic sequencing for the *AID* gene showed a homozygous missense mutation, which was pathogenic and consistent with autosomal recessive hyper-IgM syndrome.

Autosomal recessive hyper-IgM syndrome can result from defects along the CD40L/CD40 pathway including *CD40*, *AID*, and *UNG* as well as defects in missense repair enzymes [2]. *CD40* defects, as described earlier, result in autosomal recessive hyper-IgM syndrome that is very similar to *CD40L* defects, and affected patients are susceptible to opportunistic infections and cancer. However, defects in AID and *UNG* only affect class switching and somatic hypermutation, resulting in an antibody deficiency without susceptibility to opportunistic infections. All other signaling via CD40 occurs normally, including upregulation of costimulatory molecules and cytokine secretion (see Fig. 4.2). Patients with *AID* defects are more likely to develop autoimmunity than patients with defects in *CD40L* or *CD40* [26]. In addition, unlike patients with *CD40L* or *CD40* defects, who normally have small lymph nodes, patients with defects in AID have large germinal centers and develop lymphoid hyperplasia.

Another cause of a hyper-IgM phenotype includes patients with gain-of-function mutations in *PIK3CD* or *PIK3R1* [27]. Phosphoinositide 3-kinase (PI3K), which is activated by a variety of signaling pathways including antigen receptors and cytokine receptors, inhibits expression of the AID gene, *AICDA*, by inhibiting the transcription factor FOXO1. Therefore, gain-of-function mutations in *PIK3CD* or *PIK3R1* result in decreased class-switch recombination. Many but not all patients have elevated IgM levels with variable IgG levels. These patients are susceptible to viral infections but not opportunistic infections and have an increased risk of lymphoma. A hyper-IgM phenotype also develops in some but not all patients with autosomal recessive defects in DNA mismatch repair enzymes including ataxia telangiectasia mutated (*ATM*), *PMS2*, and *NBS1*. *ATM* is responsible for ataxia telangiectasia [28], *PMS2* is associated with gastrointestinal adenocarcinomas [29], and *NBS1* is the gene responsible for Nijmegen breakage syndrome [30]. However, these diseases usually have additional features specific to their gene defects, and because of the defect in DNA repair, they are also susceptible to the development of cancer.

Management/Outcome

Our second patient was started on immunoglobulin replacement therapy intravenously at 500 mg/kg per dose every 4 weeks. She continued to have upper respiratory symptoms until we learned through a translator that she was having snoring and sleep apnea. She was referred to otorhinolaryngology and was found to have markedly enlarged adenoids that were removed surgically. After surgery, her upper airway congestion resolved and her appetite improved and she gained weight and caught up with her weight percentile for age. Because these defects mainly affect antibody production and there is no increased susceptibility to opportunistic infections or cancer, stem cell transplantation was not considered. She is currently thriving and doing well on IVIG replacement therapy. Her mother delivered another daughter, who was tested at birth and found to be a carrier of the disease and is healthy and growing well.

Clinical Pearls and Pitfalls
- A hyper-IgM phenotype may result from defects of a number of genes in the CD40L/CD40 signaling pathway, leading to class-switch recombination including DNA mismatch repair enzymes.
- Available clinical laboratory tests may not identify a defect in *CD40L*, and testing the ability of the CD40L molecule to bind to CD40 is important in making the diagnosis in some patients.
- Aggressive therapy with immunoglobulin replacement therapy in all types of hyper IgM and prophylaxis for opportunistic infections by antimicrobials as well as boiling drinking water to prevent infection by cryptosporidium is necessary for optimal management.
- Stem cell therapy for X-linked hyper-IgM and *CD40* defects when there is a good HLA-matched donor should be considered.
- Genetic testing will help differentiate between the different forms of hyper IgM as well as rule out other immunodeficiency diseases that may present with a hyper-IgM phenotype.

References

1. Stavnezer J, Schrader CE. IgH chain class switch recombination: mechanism and regulation. J Immunol. 2014;193(11):5370–8.
2. Qamar N, Fuleihan RL. The hyper IgM syndromes. Clin Rev Allergy Immunol. 2014;46(2):120–30.
3. Seyama K, Nonoyama S, Gangsaas I, Hollenbaugh D, Pabst HF, Aruffo A, et al. Mutations of the CD40 ligand gene and its effect on CD40 ligand expression in patients with X-linked hyper IgM syndrome. Blood. 1998;92(7):2421–34.
4. Cabral-Marques O, Klaver S, Schimke LF, Ascendino EH, Khan TA, Pereira PV, et al. First report of the Hyper-IgM syndrome Registry of the Latin American Society for Immunodeficiencies: novel mutations, unique infections, and outcomes. J Clin Immunol. 2014;34(2):146–56.
5. Hayward AR, Levy J, Facchetti F, Notarangelo L, Ochs HD, Etzioni A, et al. Cholangiopathy and tumors of the pancreas, liver, and biliary tree in boys with X-linked immunodeficiency with hyper-IgM. J Immunol. 1997;158(2):977–83.
6. Erdos M, Garami M, Rakoczi E, Zalatnai A, Steinbach D, Baumann U, et al. Neuroendocrine carcinoma associated with X-linked hyper-immunoglobulin M syndrome: report of four cases and review of the literature. Clin Immunol. 2008;129(3):455–61.
7. Malhotra RK, Li W. Poorly differentiated gastroenteropancreatic neuroendocrine carcinoma associated with X-linked hyperimmunoglobulin M syndrome. Arch Pathol Lab Med. 2008;132(5):847–50.
8. Facchetti F, Appiani C, Salvi L, Levy J, Notarangelo LD. Immunohistologic analysis of ineffective CD40-CD40 ligand interaction in lymphoid tissues from patients with X-linked immunodeficiency with hyper-IgM. Abortive germinal center cell reaction and severe depletion of follicular dendritic cells. J Immunol. 1995;154(12):6624–33.
9. Hanson EP, Monaco-Shawver L, Solt LA, Madge LA, Banerjee PP, May MJ, et al. Hypomorphic nuclear factor-kappaB essential modulator mutation database and reconstitution system identifies phenotypic and immunologic diversity. J Allergy Clin Immunol. 2008;122(6):1169–77.e16.
10. Courtois G, Smahi A, Reichenbach J, Doffinger R, Cancrini C, Bonnet M, et al. A hypermorphic IkappaBalpha mutation is associated with autosomal dominant anhidrotic ectodermal dysplasia and T cell immunodeficiency. J Clin Invest. 2003;112(7):1108–15.
11. Levy J, Espanol-Boren T, Thomas C, Fischer A, Tovo P, Bordigoni P, et al. Clinical spectrum of X-linked hyper-IgM syndrome. J Pediatr. 1997;131(1 Pt 1):47–54.
12. Winkelstein JA, Marino MC, Ochs H, Fuleihan R, Scholl PR, Geha R, et al. The X-linked hyper-IgM syndrome: clinical and immunologic features of 79 patients. Medicine (Baltimore). 2003;82(6):373–84.
13. Leven EA, Maffucci P, Ochs HD, Scholl PR, Buckley RH, Fuleihan RL, et al. Hyper IgM syndrome: a report from the USIDNET Registry. J Clin Immunol. 2016;36:490–501.
14. de la Morena MT, Leonard D, Torgerson TR, Cabral-Marques O, Slatter M, Aghamohammadi A, et al. Long-term outcomes of 176 patients with X-linked hyper-IgM syndrome treated with or without hematopoietic cell transplantation. J Allergy Clin Immunol. 2017;139(4):1282–92.
15. Ferrua F, Galimberti S, Courteille V, Slatter MA, Booth C, Moshous D, et al. Hematopoietic stem cell transplantation for CD40 ligand deficiency: results from an EBMT/ESID-IEWP-SCETIDE-PIDTC study. J Allergy Clin Immunol. 2019;143(6):2238–53.
16. Wang WC, Cordoba J, Infante AJ, Conley ME. Successful treatment of neutropenia in the hyper-immunoglobulin M syndrome with granulocyte colony-stimulating factor. Am J Pediatr Hematol Oncol. 1994;16(2):160–3.
17. Thrasher AJ, Williams DA. Evolving gene therapy in primary immunodeficiency. Mol Ther. 2017;25(5):1132–41.
18. Fuleihan R, Ahern D, Geha RS. Expression of the CD40 ligand in T lymphocytes and induction of IgE isotype switching. Int Arch Allergy Immunol. 1995;107(1–3):43–4.

19. Vavassori S, Covey LR. Post-transcriptional regulation in lymphocytes: the case of CD154. RNA Biol. 2009;6(3):259–65.
20. Brown MP, Topham DJ, Sangster MY, Zhao J, Flynn KJ, Surman SL, et al. Thymic lymphoproliferative disease after successful correction of CD40 ligand deficiency by gene transfer in mice. Nat Med. 1998;4(11):1253–60.
21. Desai-Mehta A, Liangjun L, Ramsey-Goldman R, Datta SK. Hyperexpression of CD40 ligand by B and T cells in human lupus and its role in pathogenic autoantibody production. J Clin Invest. 1996;97:2063–73.
22. Hubbard N, Hagin D, Sommer K, Song Y, Khan I, Clough C, et al. Targeted gene editing restores regulated CD40L function in X-linked hyper-IgM syndrome. Blood. 2016;127(21):2513–22.
23. Kuo CY, Long JD, Campo-Fernandez B, de Oliveira S, Cooper AR, Romero Z, et al. Site-specific gene editing of human hematopoietic stem cells for X-linked hyper-IgM syndrome. Cell Rep. 2018;23(9):2606–16.
24. Foy TM, Page DM, Waldschmidt TJ, Schoneveld A, Laman JD, Masters SR, et al. An essential role for gp39, the ligand for CD40, in thymic selection. J Exp Med. 1995;182:1377–88.
25. Holland SM. Chronic granulomatous disease. Hematol Oncol Clin North Am. 2013;27(1):89–99, viii.
26. Quartier P, Bustamante J, Sanal O, Plebani A, Debre M, Deville A, et al. Clinical, immunologic and genetic analysis of 29 patients with autosomal recessive hyper-IgM syndrome due to activation-induced cytidine deaminase deficiency. Clin Immunol. 2004;110(1):22–9.
27. Jhamnani RD, Nunes-Santos CJ, Bergerson J, Rosenzweig SD. Class-switch recombination (CSR)/hyper-IgM (HIGM) syndromes and phosphoinositide 3-kinase (PI3K) defects. Front Immunol. 2018;9:2172.
28. Pan-Hammarstrom Q, Dai S, Zhao Y, van Dijk-Hard IF, Gatti RA, Borresen-Dale AL, et al. ATM is not required in somatic hypermutation of VH, but is involved in the introduction of mutations in the switch mu region. J Immunol. 2003;170(7):3707–16.
29. Gologan A, Sepulveda AR. Microsatellite instability and DNA mismatch repair deficiency testing in hereditary and sporadic gastrointestinal cancers. Clin Lab Med. 2005;25(1):179–96.
30. Piatosa B, van der Burg M, Siewiera K, Pac M, van Dongen JJ, Langerak AW, et al. The defect in humoral immunity in patients with Nijmegen breakage syndrome is explained by defects in peripheral B lymphocyte maturation. Cytometry A. 2012;81(10):835–42.

Chapter 5
Transient Immunodeficiency of Infancy

Kristin C. Sokol

Introduction

Transient immunodeficiency of infancy, or transient hypogammaglobulinemia of infancy (THI), is a rare disorder in which there is an exaggeration or extension of the physiologic nadir of immunoglobulin G (IgG). The typical nadir occurs around 3–6 months of life, consistent with the loss of transplacentally acquired maternal IgG, and before adequate IgG production by the infant [1]. Most children are prone to increased infections during this time of prolonged hypogammaglobulinemia. THI can often present with concomitant atopy and/or autoimmunity. Sixty percent of patients are male [1]. The time to recovery is different for every patient, and there is no consensus on a definitive age of recovery for diagnosis. THI should have no other explanation for reversible hypogammaglobulinemia. Hypogammaglobulinemia associated with a reduction in circulating B cells, abnormal cellular immunity, and syndromic features is excluded from the definition of THI. The prevalence of THI is difficult to ascertain, as many cases likely remain undetected. The cause of THI remains unknown despite various proposed pathogenic mechanisms [2]. In addition, there is no known genetic basis for this disorder, although an increased incidence of THI has been documented in family members of patients with other immunodeficiencies [1, 3].

K. C. Sokol (✉)
Schreiber Allergy, Rockville, MD, USA

© Springer Nature Switzerland AG 2021
J. A. Bernstein (ed.), *Primary and Secondary Immunodeficiency*,
https://doi.org/10.1007/978-3-030-57157-3_5

Case Presentation 1

A 10-month-old baby boy presented to the allergy/immunology clinic referred by his pediatrician for moderate atopic dermatitis. He was born vaginally at 39 weeks with no problems during or after birth. The parents described the baby's skin as constantly dry, itchy, and inflamed, especially in hot weather, present since the age of 2 months. They could not identify any other triggers. They described the baby as being otherwise healthy. He has not had any symptoms consistent with IgE-mediated food allergy, was exclusively breastfed until 6 months of age, and had been introduced to a variety of different solid foods including dairy, egg, wheat, soy, peanut, and fish. Upon further questioning, the parents mentioned that he seems to get sick with upper respiratory illnesses frequently. He has required three courses of antibiotics in the past 4 months for acute otitis media and was hospitalized for dehydration once on a separate occasion. Family history was significant for a mother with seasonal allergy symptoms and atopic dermatitis, and a sister with recurrent ear and sinus infections and one episode of pneumonia as a young toddler who is now a healthy 7-year-old. There were no other family members with recurrent infections, immunodeficiencies, or autoimmune conditions. Social history was unremarkable as the patient lives with his parents, sister, and a dog. He stays at home with his mother during the day and does not attend day care. He is not exposed to tobacco smoke. At the visit, his vital signs were normal, and his weight and height were both in the 40th percentile, consistent with his parameters at birth. His physical examination revealed dry skin with several areas of erythematous patches consistent with atopic dermatitis on his torso and flexural areas of his legs, as well as his cheeks. Bilateral tympanic membranes were dull, without erythema or bulging. Eye, nose, throat, heart, lung, and abdominal examination were within normal limits. Given his history, labs were drawn and revealed a normal CBC with differential. His total serum IgE was 10 kU/L, his total serum IgG was 150 mg/dL, his total serum IgM was 60 mg/dL, and his total serum IgA was 30 mg/dL (normal immunoglobulin values and reference ranges with 95% confidence intervals for a 10-month-old: IgG 594 (294–1069); IgM 82 (41–149); IgA 40 (16–84)) [4]. Repeat serum IgG remained low. Measurement of specific antibody production and enumeration of lymphocyte subsets by means of flow cytometry were within normal limits. He had normal vaccine responses. He was started on prophylactic antibiotic therapy for his recurrent bacterial upper respiratory infections. His parents were given advice regarding the management of his atopic dermatitis, including bathing nightly with an immediate application of ointment, and liberal application of cream and/or ointment throughout the daytime. At a follow-up visit 3 months later, the parents reported that the baby had been doing well. He had experienced only one mild upper respiratory tract infection with rhinorrhea at the same time his older sister had common cold symptoms. He had not required any additional antibiotic therapy. He was eating well and gaining weight. He was subsequently followed yearly by the allergy/immunology clinic, and his prophylactic antibiotics were eventually discontinued. His repeat serum IgG level at 4 years of age was 950 mg/dL.

Diagnosis/Assessment

The child in this clinical vignette has transient immunodeficiency of infancy (THI). Serum IgG levels must be recorded at more than two standard deviations below age-matched controls with or without decreased levels of other serum immunoglobulins on at least two separate occasions for a diagnosis of THI. A definitive diagnosis of THI is only possible after normalization of IgG levels (usually during childhood) and the exclusion of other disorders and syndromes that can present with hypogammaglobulinemia [5]. This case highlights a pediatric patient with no other physical or laboratory features of a syndromic or immunodeficiency disorder. The main clinical features in patients with THI are respiratory infections and allergic disorders, and most follow a benign clinical course (Table 5.1) [5]. Some infants can present with atopic conditions, including moderate to severe atopic dermatitis [6]. More severe, albeit rare, manifestations of THI include urinary tract infections, gastroenteritis, and invasive infections. Physical exam findings are consistent with the specific type of infection. Some infants and children do remain asymptomatic and are diagnosed following immunological evaluation for other reasons, including family history.

The laboratory investigation for evaluation of transient hypogammaglobulinemia of infancy includes a complete blood count with differential count, quantitative assessment of immunoglobulin levels, B-cell quantitative assessment, antibody testing (detection of isohemagglutinins and post-exposure/post-immunization IgG antibodies), immunophenotyping (CD+ 3, CD+ 4, and CD+ 8 T-cell percentages and absolute numbers by flow cytometry), and T-cell function [1, 10]. In THI, IgG is at least 2 standard deviations below expected controls. The Ig levels must be carefully interpreted as there is marked variability with age. At birth, IgG of the newborn is

Table 5.1 Clinical features of THI

Clinical feature	Prevalence
Infections	~91%
Upper respiratory infections	34–95%
Lower respiratory infections	12–81%
Gastrointestinal infections	8–23%
Urinary infections	14–27%
Severe infections (abscess, sepsis, HZV, etc.)	0–11%
Atopic disease	24–65%
Asthma	18–55%
Atopic dermatitis	10–33%
Food allergy/intolerance	38–66%
Growth delay/failure to thrive	2–18%
Autoimmune disease	4%
Family history of immunodeficiency	11–24%
Asymptomatic	39%

Data from [3, 7–13]

virtually all maternally derived. The levels of maternally derived IgG decline rapidly, and serum IgG levels reach their lowest point between 6 and 12 months of age [14]. More than half of children with THI have IgG levels as low as 200 mg/dL. IgA and IgM may not be abnormal. Children with low serum IgG and low serum IgA levels but with elevated IgM serum levels should always be suspected for hyper-IgM syndrome [14]. IgG levels less than 100 mg/dL and/or pan-hypogammaglobulinemia may suggest a permanent immunodeficiency. Most infants with THI produce normal antibodies to vaccines including diphtheria, tetanus, hepatitis A and B, conjugated Haemophilus influenza, measles, mumps, and rubella, and this can differentiate a diagnosis of THI from a more permanent immunodeficiency like common variable immunodeficiency (CVID) [14]. Children undergoing evaluation for THI should be vaccinated with the conjugated pneumococcal vaccine and most respond well. If a lack of response is found to any of the above-listed vaccines, the child should then be evaluated for another immunodeficiency disorder. T- and B-cell function is also normal in most children evaluated for and diagnosed with THI. Additional testing such as microbiological studies, DNA testing, or imaging studies may be necessary as clinically indicated to exclude other causes.

Management/Outcome

As there are no clinical features or diagnostic tests to differentiate self-limiting hypogammaglobulinemia from permanent immune defects, it is important to monitor symptomatic patients with hypogammaglobulinemia periodically [5]. Of note, for asymptomatic infants and young children, no treatment is required. Clinical observation and supportive counseling may be all that is necessary. Advising longer duration of breastfeeding to mothers that are able to do so could be beneficial. One study from Turkey revealed that a longer duration of breastfeeding may shorten time to recovery of IgG. This study showed that breastfeeding less than 10 months put children with THI at a higher risk of late recovery which was defined as after 36 months of age [15]. IgG levels should be repeated every 4–6 months [1]. Since the 10-month-old baby in this clinical vignette has a history of recurrent upper respiratory tract infections, supportive measures such as reducing exposure to infections by minimizing exposure to other children, and timely and appropriate treatment of respiratory infections is warranted. Some patients may be treated with prophylactic antibiotic therapy during respiratory infection season or year-round. Inactivated vaccines should be given as scheduled and live viral vaccines should be postponed. Immunoglobulin replacement therapy is not usually necessary except in rare instances when infections are severe and the child has concomitant failure to thrive. Newer reports reveal that improvement in AD and normalization of IgG occurs in infants with severe atopic dermatitis and hypogammaglobulinemia treated with replacement immunoglobulin [6]. However, there has been concern that IVIG replacement therapy can delay endogenous specific antibody production and one study does indicate that this therapy can actually prolong time to recovery [15]. This therapy should be reserved for those suffering from frequent and severe infections. Like most children with THI, the baby in the clinical vignette developed age-appropriate levels of IgG by age 3 [16].

Case Presentation 2

A 6-year-old boy presented to the allergy/immunology clinic with a history of recurrent respiratory tract infections, including several episodes of pneumonia. He had also had numerous episodes of diarrhea lasting several weeks at a time. He had been hospitalized twice for IV antibiotics for pneumonia. He had his tonsils and adenoids removed, as well as tympanostomy tubes placed for recurrent infections at the age of 2.5. Despite these interventions, he continued to have recurrent ear, sinus, and throat infections, especially in the late fall and winter seasons. He had a history of egg and peanut allergy, and currently avoids both these foods in his diet. He had accidental exposure to peanut 2 years ago with subsequent anaphylaxis which required administration of epinephrine. He had no other chronic illnesses and did not take any medications on a regular basis. He lived at home with his mother and father as an only child and attended elementary school. He was not exposed to second-hand smoke. His family owned a cat. His father had a history of recurrent ear and sinus infections as a young child and also had surgery to remove his tonsils and adenoids. In the office, his vital signs were normal except for a temperature of 100.4 degrees. His weight and height were in the 5th percentile, which was lower than previous parameters. His physical examination revealed a thin appearing boy with clear rhinorrhea, and bulging erythematous tympanic membranes. The rest of his physical examination, including skin, lung, and abdominal examination, was normal. Skin prick testing to common environmental inhalant allergens was all negative except for the histamine control. Skin prick testing to both egg and peanut allergens was positive. Blood work revealed a normal CBC with normal differential, low total serum IgG (230 mg/dL), low serum IgM (15 mg/dL), and low serum IgA (20 mg/dL) (normal immunoglobulin values and reference ranges with 95% confidence intervals for a 6 year old boy: IgG 780 [463–1236]; IgM 99 [43–196]; IgA 68 [25–154]) [4]. Serum total IgE was elevated at 2000 kU/L. Vaccine responses were suboptimal to pneumococcal titers but normal for Hib and tetanus titers. Enumeration of lymphocyte subsets by means of flow cytometry was within normal limits. Genetic studies evaluating for X-linked and other forms of autosomal recessive agammaglobulinemia were negative. Due to his clinical presentation and laboratory findings, he was started on immunoglobulin replacement therapy. He was followed closely and maintained on this therapy for several years with a dramatic reduction in infection frequency and severity. At age 11, his IVIG was discontinued for 6 months, and repeat immunoglobulin levels were found to be normal. He was subsequently followed in the clinic yearly thereafter with an absence of recurrent infections and normal laboratory findings.

Diagnosis/Assessment

Although this patient's clinical course is significantly different, and more severe, than the patient in the prior clinical vignette, a diagnosis of THI can still be made in his childhood due to improvement in his infections, normalization of IgG level as well as other normal laboratory findings. Since hypogammaglobulinemia is a finding in other cellular or combined immunodeficiencies, additional laboratory workup must be done, especially if the patient presents with severe and recurrent infections. The complete blood count, including differential count, is a very simple, low-cost laboratory tool for differentiating pure humoral immunodeficiencies from combined immunodeficiencies as the presence of lymphopenia is seen in the latter [14]. The enumeration of T-cell subsets is a useful tool for the identification of some forms of combined immunodeficiencies presenting with a normal lymphocyte count. In addition, the evaluation of the ability of the patient's lymphocytes to proliferate in vitro upon stimulation with antigens, allogenic cells, and mitogens can be an additional useful tool in the identification of cellular immunodeficiencies [14]. Typically, THI can be differentiated from X-linked agammaglobulinemia as the latter is characterized by a severe deficiency of all Ig isotypes, an inability to produce antibodies, absence of normal peripheral lymphoid tissues, absence or a very low number of circulating B cells, and the presence of severe pyogenic infections starting in the first or second year of life [6]. The patient in this clinical vignette was found to have a normal CBC with a normal differential, normal T-cell subsets, and negative genetic testing.

Although familial cases of THI have been described, no genetic marker has been identified at this time [3, 7]. Genetic testing as an infant, if negative, can rule out X-linked or autosomal causes of hypogammaglobulinemia [17]. Genetic testing with next-generation sequencing (NGS) could be considered for those patients with persistent severe hypogammaglobulinemia, particularly if symptomatic. The presence of a causative mutation of CVID or CVID-like disorder would effectively rule out THI.

Many patients with transient hypogammaglobulinemia of infancy are also diagnosed with atopic disease, including asthma, allergic rhinitis, atopic dermatitis, and food allergy. It is suggested that subclinical protein loss from the gut due to allergic inflammation may be a contributing factor to the development of THI in some patients with food allergy [13]. Otherwise, the underlying mechanism for this link is not yet understood [2].

Management/Outcome

Most patients with THI can be observed and treated for infections as needed. However, patients with more severe and frequent infections, like the boy in this clinical vignette, can be treated with subcutaneous or intravenous immune globulin replacement therapy. As this is an expensive treatment and a blood product, the risks and benefits of therapy should be weighed before the decision is made to treat a patient with THI. Most patients with THI that receive subcutaneous or intravenous immune globulin replacement therapy are treated for short periods of time. Therapy is discontinued when the frequency and severity of infections has decreased significantly and IgG, as well as IgM and IgA, normalize or increase [18, 19]. After therapy is stopped, patients require periodic follow-up to ensure complete clinical and laboratory resolution is sustained [18]. Patients with severe disease may be affected with opportunistic infections, atopy, or autoimmunity, associated with a more complicated course but, by definition, THI should completely resolve.

Tonsillectomy, adenoidectomy, and tympanostomy tube placement can reduce the frequency and severity of upper respiratory tract infections. If atopic patients are sensitized to environmental allergens, they can undergo allergen-specific immunotherapy later in childhood, which has been shown to reduce both upper respiratory tract allergies and infections [7].

From case reports, it is known that THI is slower to resolve when IgA or IgM, along with IgG, are low on initial presentation [11]. Children who do not normalize their IgG levels within the first 24 months of age show a higher frequency of severe infections and sometimes autoimmunity, often sharing a clinical and immunological profile with other primary immunodeficiencies. Similar to the patient in this clinical vignette, some children may not spontaneously correct their immunoglobulin abnormalities until later in their first decade of life, usually resembling a more severe primary immunodeficiency like common variable immune deficiency (CVID) [11]. One study indicated that invasive infection or low tetanus antibodies at presentation could be associated with the development of a significant humoral immunodeficiency [8]. Other studies have attempted to identify a prognostic factor that could predict the outcome of hypogammaglobulinemia in early childhood. For example, increased levels of T regulatory cells were demonstrated to be predictive but this is not used as a routine clinical test [2, 20]. A more recent study notes that THI is a misnomer, as the majority of patients do not recover in infancy [7]. Recovery from THI can extend into adulthood, and Ameratunga et al. conclude that THI must even be considered in the differential diagnosis of adolescents or young adults presenting with primary hypogammaglobulinemia [7].

Conclusion

Transient hypogammaglobulinemia or immunodeficiency of infancy is a rare disorder that can present as a spectrum of disease, from asymptomatic to severe infection, atopy, and/or autoimmunity. Since identification of this disorder requires full recovery of immunoglobulin levels, diagnosis cannot be made until after this occurs. Diagnosis also requires exclusion of any other condition that causes diminished immunoglobulin levels, including other immunodeficiencies like common variable immunodeficiency (CVID). Most patients fully recover their immunoglobulin levels and become asymptomatic before the age of 4 without any interventions. Some patients require management with prophylactic antibiotics or replacement immunoglobulin therapy. More recent data have shown that there is a small subset of patients who do not fully recover their immunoglobulin levels until adolescence or early adulthood. These patients tend to have more severe infections at initial presentation and other laboratory abnormalities in addition to a decreased IgG level. The two patients in the clinical vignettes presented in this chapter depict two very different presentations of THI, both with eventual full recovery of symptoms and laboratory abnormalities.

Clinical Pearls and Pitfalls
- THI can present with a variety of clinical manifestations, including benign and severe infections, atopic conditions, and autoimmunity.
- Compared to SCID or CVID, THI is a relatively benign disorder.
- Patients with THI may or may not have a family history of immunodeficiency.
- Atopic disorders, including food allergy, asthma, and atopic dermatitis, are commonly seen in patients with THI.
- Immunoglobulin levels and infectious manifestations typically reverse by age 3 but rarely will not recover until adolescence or early adulthood.
- Prophylactic antibiotics or replacement immunoglobulin therapy can be used in symptomatic patients for management of infections until normalization of IgG.
- A definitive diagnosis of THI is only possible once IgG levels normalize.
- Differential diagnosis of THI includes other immunodeficiency disorders such as X-linked agammaglobulinemia, specific IgA deficiency, and CVID.
- In older children with unresolved hypogammaglobulinemia, the main differential cause is CVID.

References

1. Bonilla FA, Khan DA, Ballas ZK, Chinen J, Frank MM, Hsu JT, et al. Practice parameter for the diagnosis and management of primary immunodeficiency. J Allergy Clin Immunol. 2015;136(5):1186–1205.e78.
2. Ovadia A, Dalal I. Transient hypogammaglobulinemia of infancy. Lymphosign. 2014;1(1):1–9.
3. Moschese V, Graziani S, Avanzini MA, Carsetti R, Marconi M, La Rocca M, et al. A prospective study on children with initial diagnosis of transient hypogammaglobulinemia of infancy: results from the Italian Primary Immunodeficiency Network. Int J Immunopathol Pharmacol. 2008;21(2):343.
4. Kjellman NM, Johansson SG, Roth A. Serum IgE levels in healthy children quantified by a sandwich technique (PRIST). Clin Allergy. 1976;6:51.
5. Ricci G, Piccinno V, Giannetti A, Miniaci A, Specchia F, Masi M. Evolution of hypogammaglobulinemia in premature and full-term infants. Int J Immunopathol Pharmacol. 2011;24:721–6.

6. Breslin ME, Lin JH, Roberts R, Lim KJ, Stiehm ER. Transient hypogammaglobulinemia and severe atopic dermatitis: open-label treatment with immunoglobulin in a case series. Allergy Rhinol (Providence). 2016;7(2):69–73.
7. Ameratunga R, Ahn Y, Steele R, Woon ST. Transient hypogammaglobulinaemia of infancy: many patients recover in adolescence and adulthood. Clin Exp Immunol. 2019;198(2):224–32.
8. Dalal I, Reid B, Nisbet-Brown E, Roifman CM. The outcome of patients with hypogammaglobulinemia in infancy and early childhood. J Pediatr. 1998;133(1):144.
9. Keles S, Artac H, Kara R, Gokturk B, Ozen A, Reisli I. Transient hypogammaglobulinemia and unclassified hypogammaglobulinemia: 'similarities and differences. Pediatr Allergy Immunol. 2010;21(5):843–51.
10. Kidon MI, Handzel ZT, Schwartz R, Altboum I, Stein M, Zan-Bar I. Symptomatic hypogammaglobulinemia in infancy and childhood - clinical outcome and in vitro immune responses. BMC Fam Pract. 2004;5:23.
11. Kutukculer N, Gulez N. The outcome of patients with unclassified hypogammaglobulinemia in early childhood. Pediatr Allergy Immunol. 2009;20(7):693.
12. Tiller TL Jr, Buckley RH. Transient hypogammaglobulinemia of infancy: review of the literature, clinical and immunologic features of 11 new cases, and long-term follow-up. J Pediatr. 1978;92(3):347–53.
13. Walker AM, Kemp AS, Hill DJ, Shelton MJ. Features of transient hypogammaglobulinemia in infants screened for immunological abnormalities. Arch Dis Child. 1994;70(3):183.
14. Plebani A, Palumbo L, Dotta L, Lougaris V. Diagnostic approach of hypogammaglobulinemia in infancy. Pediatr Allergy Immunol. 2020;31 Suppl 24:11–2.
15. Sütçü M, Akturk H, Salman N, Ozceker D, Gulumser-Sisko S, Acar M, et al. Transient hypogammaglobulinemia of infancy: predictive factors for late recovery. Turk J Pediatr. 2015;57(6):592–8.
16. Whelan MA, Hwan WH, Beausoleil J, Hauck WW, McGeady SJ. Infants presenting with recurrent infections and low immunoglobulins: characteristics and analysis of normalization. J Clin Immunol. 2006;26(1):7–11.
17. Kornfeld SJ, Kratz J, Haire RN, Litman GW, Good RA. X-linked agammaglobulinemia presenting as transient hypogammaglobulinemia of infancy. JACI. 1995;95(4):915–7.
18. Cano F, Mayo DR, Ballow M. Absent specific viral antibodies in patients with transient hypogammaglobulinemia if infancy. J Allergy Clin Immunol. 1990;85(2):510.
19. Duse M, Iacobini M, Leonardi L, Smacchia P, Antonetti L, Giancane G. Transient hypogammaglobulinemia of infancy: intravenous immunoglobulin as first line therapy. Int J Immunopathol Pharmacol. 2010;23:349–53.
20. Rutowska M, Lenart M, Bukowska-Strakova K, Szaflarska A, Pituch-Noworolska A, Kobylarz K, et al. The number of circulating CD4+CD25high Foxp3+ T lymphocytes is transiently elevated in the early childhood of transient hypogammaglobulinemia of infancy patients. Clin Immunol. 2011;140:307–10.

Chapter 6
Selective Isotype Immunodeficiency

Robert Tamayev and Jenny Shliozberg

Case Presentation 1

An 11-year-old female is referred to an immunologist, by her pulmonologist, for worsening respiratory status due to bronchiectasis and recurrent sinusitis, for an immunologic evaluation. She has a history of severe-persistent, allergic asthma treated with high-dose inhaled corticosteroids, a long-acting beta-agonist combination inhaler, a leukotriene antagonist, and an oral second-generation H1-antihistamine. Due to the bronchiectasis and numerous episodes of sinusitis, the pulmonologist initiated an immunodeficiency work-up which found a total IgG level of 1780 mg/dL (normal 844–1912 mg/dL), IgM of 54 mg/dL (normal 50–300 mg/dL), and IgA of 238 mg/dL (normal 40–350 mg/dL). Lymphocyte enumeration showed slightly decreased T cells with normal T-cell percentages. The patient had a negative chloride sweat test. Laboratory evaluation in the immunology clinic confirmed normal total levels of immunoglobulins; however, a decreased level of IgG2 of 15 mg/dL (normal 81–500 mg/dL) with an increased level of IgG1 of 1370 mg/dL (normal 350–965 mg/dL), normal level of IgG3 of 114 mg/dL (normal 16–130 mg/dL), and a decreased level of IgG4 of less than 0.2 mg/dL (normal 6–220 mg/dL) was found. The patient had decreased pneumococcal IgG 23 titers which did not show an adequate response to revaccination with Pneumovax 23. Her CT of the thorax showed tree-in-bud opacities in the lower lung base along with significant bronchiectasis in both lungs. Treatment was initiated with 0.5 mg/kg of intravenous immunoglobulins (IVIG) every 4 weeks. After 6 months, the patient was transitioned to subcutaneous

R. Tamayev (✉)
New York Allergy and Sinus Center, Glendale, NY, USA

J. Shliozberg
Department of Allergy and Immunology, Montefiore Medical Center/Albert Einstein College of Medicine, Bronx, NY, USA

immunoglobulins (SCIG) 12 g weekly. Her sinusitis infections decreased from over 4 per year to 1 per year, over the next 3 years, and there was a significant decrease in flares of her upper and lower respiratory diseases as well.

Diagnosis/Assessment

The patient in the above case had a normal total immunoglobulin G level upon initial evaluation, but due to a history of recurrent infections required a more extensive immunodeficiency assessment, which included checking of IgG subclass levels. Measuring IgG subclass levels is controversial among immunologists as they have been found to be decreased in patients without any clinical consequence and thus are not routinely recommended to be part of the initial immunologic evaluation [1]. However, as in this patient, if a patient is noted to have poor responses to antigens, specifically to previously administered vaccines, measuring IgG subclasses may be of utility. IgG subclass deficiency is only relevant if there is a clinical history of recurrent infections; otherwise, it can frequently represent an incidental laboratory finding.

Selective immunoglobulin deficiency is defined as a decrease in one immunoglobulin without a decrease in others, which includes selective IgA, selective IgG subclasses, and selective IgM deficiencies. Selective IgG subclass deficiency refers to a decrease in the levels of one of the IgG subclasses with a normal level of total IgG [2, 3]. Total immunoglobulin levels vary with age (Table 6.1), as do normal serum levels for each IgG subclass (Table 6.2) [2–9]. The levels of IgG1 and IgG3 reach adult levels earlier than IgG2 and IgG4 [10]. In adults, IgG1 encompasses 60–72% of the total IgG, followed by IgG2 at 19–31%, IgG3 at 5–8.5%, and IgG4 at 0.5–4.5% [11]. The lower limit of IgG1 is 250–300 mg/dL, IgG2 is 50 mg/dL, IgG3 is 1425 mg/dL, and IgG4 is 0.5 mg/dL. Any individual level below the lower limit would be considered an IgG subclass deficiency if the patient's total IgG level is normal. In children, the most common IgG subclass deficiency is an IgG2 deficiency, while in adults it is an IgG3 deficiency [3, 12]. In a group of patients with frequent recurrent infections, IgG subclass deficiency was as high as 21% [4, 13].

Table 6.1 Normal serum immunoglobulin levels by age

Age	IgG	IgA	IgM
1–6 months	427 ± 160	25 ± 15	35 ± 15
7–12 months	660 ± 220	35 ± 15	55 ± 25
1–2 years	760 ± 205	50 ± 25	60 ± 20
2–3 years	890 ± 180	70 ± 35	60 ± 20
3–8 years	925 ± 240	110 ± 35	60 ± 20
9–16 years	1050 ± 180	140 ± 60	70 ± 27
Adults	1150 ± 300	200 ± 60	100 ± 25

Modified from [8]. Data presented as mean (mg/dl) ± 1SD

Table 6.2 Normal IgG subclass levels by age

Age (year)	IgG1	IgG2	IgG3	IgG4
0–1	350 ± 150	65 ± 35	30 ± 20	19 ± 18
1–4	500 ± 250	120 ± 70	35 ± 25	20 ± 15
4–8	600 ± 275	160 ± 95	45 ± 30	40 ± 30
8–18	650 ± 300	250 ± 100	60 ± 40	50 ± 35
Adults	650 ± 300	350 ± 130	65 ± 35	55 ± 40

Modified from [2–9]. Data presented as mean (mg/dl) ± 2SD

If the patient has a low level of a selective IgG subclass, which was confirmed on a separate occasion 4 weeks after the initial test, and the patient has a history of recurrent infections, the diagnosis of selective IgG deficiency can be made. Care must be taken to exclude alternative causes of low levels, such as acute and chronic illnesses, including EBV, CMV, and HIV, malignancies, and medications [14]. Medications that lower IgG levels include glucocorticoids, anti-epileptics, and sulfasalazine [15–18]. Patients with diseases that lead to a loss of proteins, such as protein-losing enteropathy and nephrotic syndromes, may also have decreased levels of immunoglobulins.

Individual IgG subclass deficiencies have slightly distinct clinical presentations and pathogenic susceptibilities. The increase in IgG subclass levels to adult ranges varies between subclasses; IgG1 and IgG3 increase earlier than IgG2 and IgG4, with IgG1 reaching adult levels by the age of 5–7 years of age and IgG3 by 7–9 years of age [11]. Meanwhile, IgG2 achieves adult levels by the age of 8–10 years and IgG4 by 9–11 years. All IgG subclasses cross the placenta from the mother to the fetus, but IgG2 is generally less effective than the other three subclasses. IgG1 deficiency is sometimes found concomitantly with IgG3 deficiency, while IgG2 deficiency is more commonly found along with IgG4 deficiency, which was seen in the patient described. IgG1 and IgG3 activate the complement system more vigorously compared to IgG2, while IgG4 does not.

Since IgG1 makes up over 50% of the total quantity of immunoglobulin G, in most situations, the total IgG level is low if IgG1 levels are substantially reduced [19]. However, to make a diagnosis of CVID, levels of IgM or IgA must be diminished as well as the total IgG level. In selective IgG1 disease, only IgG1 is decreased, without decreases in IgA, IgM, or total IgG levels [20, 21]. The total IgG level remains in normal range due to increases in the other IgG subclasses, which is likely secondary to repeated infections and chronic inflammation [22]. Under the age of 5 years, a low level of IgG1 is most likely transient hypogammaglobulinemia. The most common infections seen with isolated IgG1 deficiency include sinusitis, pneumonia, bronchitis, otitis media, pharyngitis, tonsillitis, and bronchiectasis. The most common pathogens include *Streptococcus pneumoniae* and *Haemophilus influenzae* type b. Since IgG1 plays an important role in protection against protein antigens, including viral proteins, viral infections are also increased in IgG1 deficiency [10, 11]. Patients are also at a higher risk of autoimmune conditions, hypothyroidism, allergic rhinoconjunctivitis, atopic dermatitis, and asthma. The most common autoimmune manifestations include systemic lupus erythematosus, Sjogren's disease, Hashimoto's thyroiditis, mixed connective tissue disease, and rheumatoid arthritis (Table 6.3).

The patient described in the case above had an IgG2 deficiency. An IgG2 deficiency has been described to be as common as 17% in children with recurrent infections and may be seen together with IgG4 deficiency and IgA deficiency; the patient above also had concomitant IgG4 deficiency [23–25]. IgG2 is the subclass specifically responsible for responses to polysaccharide encapsulated organisms, and thus, in IgG2 deficiency, patients demonstrate poor responses to polysaccharide antigens, resulting in increased susceptibility to *Streptococcus pneumoniae*, *Haemophilus influenzae* type b, and *Neisseria meningitidis* [10, 20, 26–28]. These pathogens lead to recurrent episodes of sinusitis, pneumonia, otitis media, bronchitis, and meningitis. Recurrent pulmonary infections may lead to bronchiectasis [29]. IgG2 deficiency has been reported to progress to more severe immunodeficiency, including CVID. Reactivity to protein antigens is unchanged in patients with selective IgG2 deficiency, since IgG1 and IgG3 play a more significant role in protein antigens [10]. IgG2 subclass deficiency is associated with numerous autoimmune disorders, such as SLE, Sjogren's, and vasculitis (see Table 6.3), as well as with other clinical scenarios including HIV and influenza infections, bone marrow transplant, cystic fibrosis, and Hodgkin's lymphoma [22, 30–32]. IgG subclass deficiency has been reported post-bone marrow transplantation, with 1 study showing 23 patients having low subclass levels, which tended to be lower after an infection [33]. Vaccination post-transplant to *Haemophilus influenzae* type b and pneumococcal polysaccharide vaccine led to appropriate levels of IgG subclasses [34].

Selective IgG3 deficiency is the most common selective immunoglobulin deficiency in adults. IgG3 antibodies are the first ones to appear during an acute infection [11, 35]. Patients with this deficiency are more susceptible to infections by *Moraxella catarrhalis* and *Streptococcus pyogenes* [36]. The types of infections are generally similar to the other selective IgG deficiencies including sinusitis, pneumonia, diarrhea, and meningitis [37, 38]. Responses to polysaccharide antigens may be impaired, however, not as frequently as in IgG2 deficiency [37]. In addition, patients with IgG3 deficiency have an increased rate of hypothyroidism, asthma, sinusitis, chronic bronchitis, pneumonia, otitis media, pharyngitis, and tonsillitis [13, 37]. Autoimmune conditions are also increased including rheumatoid arthritis, SLE, Hashimoto's thyroiditis, and Sjogren's disease. Patients with any of the selective immunoglobulin deficiencies have a higher rate of atopy, but it is more pronounced in IgG3 deficiency [22].

Normal levels of IgG4 are lower than the other IgG subclasses, and thus an IgG4 deficiency leading to an immune aberration is controversial [22]. IgG4 levels tend to be higher in males and have been found to play a role as blocking antibodies,

Table 6.3 Autoimmune conditions associated with selective IgG deficiencies

Systemic lupus erythematous	Hashimoto's thyroiditis
Mixed connective tissue disease	Rheumatoid arthritis
Vasculitis	Sjogren's syndrome

specifically in allergies and parasites due to persistent antigenic stimulation [11, 22]. As was seen in the patient discussed, IgG4 deficiency may accompany IgG2 deficiency and may also coincide with IgA deficiency [39]. The clinical consequences of a selective IgG4 deficiency, if any symptoms exist, tend to be recurrent respiratory infections and bronchiectasis [39, 40]. Responses to polysaccharide antigens are normal; however, rarely poor responses to protein antigens have been noted [40].

Also included in the differential for the above patient during the initial evaluation is specific antibody deficiency (SAD). Patients are diagnosed with specific antibody deficiency, a primary immunodeficiency, when they experience recurrent infections but have normal levels of total immunoglobulins, normal levels of IgG subclasses, normal responses to protein antigens, but poor responses to polysaccharide antigens [41–43]. The titers to the 23-valent pneumococcal polysaccharide vaccine are usually found to be less than 1.3 μg/mL, but some studies may have reported titers less than 0.35 μg/mL [44]. These patients are at an increased risk for atopic diseases, including asthma and allergic rhinitis, and infections to encapsulated microbes, such as *Streptococcus pneumoniae*, *Haemophilus influenzae*, *Moraxella catarrhalis*, and *Staphylococcus aureus*, leading to sinusitis, otitis media, pneumonia, and bronchitis [42, 43]. The prevalence of SAD may be as high as 25% in patients with recurrent infections. The diagnosis of SAD is a diagnosis of exclusion as many patients with the clinical presentation have identifiable immunodeficiencies, such as CVID or IgG2 subclass deficiency, which also have poor polysaccharide responses. Although having a poor response to polysaccharide antigens predisposes to recurrent infections, up to 10% of patients may have poor responses without a clinical history of infections [45]. In addition, a diagnosis of specific antibody deficiency should not be made until after the age of 2 years since children under 2 years of age may not mount a strong enough response to polysaccharide vaccines [42]. Patients with SAD should be managed similar to an IgG subclass deficiency, including revaccination once with Pneumovax 23, and if the patient continues to have a poor response, then consider administrating a conjugated vaccine if available (e.g., such as the 13-valent pneumococcal conjugate vaccine). Patients with severe recurrent infections should be considered for prophylactic antibiotics, and possibly antibody replacement therapy, though this is not universally agreed upon [42, 46, 47]. Most cases have no identifiable molecular cause; however, a defect in Bruton's tyrosine kinase, usually responsible for X-linked agammaglobulinemia, has been implicated [48]. Other causes for poor responses to polysaccharide antigens include other primary immunodeficiencies, such as 22q11 deficiency, hyper-IgE syndrome, Wiskott-Aldrich, and ataxiatelangiectasia, malignancies, asplenia, and immunosuppressive medications.

Selective IgM deficiency is another primary immunodeficiency that should be in the differential for a patient with recurrent infections. The prevalence is unknown; however, studies have shown that healthy patients may have selective IgM deficiency ranging from at 0.03% to 1.68%, while in an immunology clinic, immunodeficient patients had rates from 0.07% to 2.1% [49–53]. The diagnosis is made when there is a significantly decreased level of IgM, while IgG and IgA levels are normal [49, 50, 54]. Infections include meningococcal meningitis, otitis media, sinusitis, bronchitis, pneumonia, urinary tract infections, cellulitis, and sepsis [49, 55]. These

Table 6.4 Autoimmune conditions associated with selective IgM deficiency

Crohn's disease	Celiac disease
Myasthenia gravis	Rheumatoid arthritis
Systemic lupus erythematous	Hashimoto's thyroiditis
Autoimmune glomerulonephritis	Vitiligo
Autoimmune hemolytic anemia	Polymyositis
Addison's disease	Sjogren's syndrome

infections are usually caused by *Streptococcus pneumoniae, Haemophilus influenzae, Neisseria meningitides, Pseudomonas aeruginosa, Aspergillus fumigatus,* and *Giardia lamblia* [50]. Patients with selective IgM deficiency have normal levels of IgG but have been demonstrated to exhibit decreased specific IgG responses to polysaccharide antigens, low isohemagglutinin titers, and increased levels of IgE [54, 56]. In addition, these patients have a higher rate of allergic and autoimmune diseases. Allergies and asthma have been seen in almost half of the reported cases. The associated autoimmune conditions include celiac disease, Crohn's disease, myasthenia gravis, rheumatoid arthritis, systemic lupus erythematosus, and autoimmune glomerulonephritis, among others (Table 6.4) [49, 53]. A genetic basis is unknown for most cases; however, an association with 22q11.2 deletion has been reported, and a few familial cases have also been described [49, 50]. Treatment should include management of the comorbid diseases. The immunodeficiency may benefit from prophylactic antibiotics and/or immunoglobulin replacement therapy [50].

The cause and mechanism for an IgG subclass deficiency are unknown. Mutations and deletions in structural and regulatory genes have been shown to play a role in rare cases, such as deletions of sections of the immunoglobulin gene [11, 22]. One such example is a deletion in the gene encoding the γ-2 heavy chain constant region, leading to an IgG2 deficiency; however, not all of these patients have evidence of a clinically significant immunodeficiency [10, 22, 57]. Similarly, mutations and deletions on chromosome 14q32, which encodes the common γ-chain, have led to IgG subclass deficiencies [58, 59]. A homozygous deletion leads to the absence of a single IgG subclass [60]. Activated PI3Kδ mutations, which is an autosomal dominant gain-of-function mutation, leads to a decrease in IgG2 levels with impaired responses to polysaccharide antigens [61, 62]. Low IgG subclass levels, as well as low IgA levels, were seen in both Nijmegen breakage syndrome and ataxia-telangiectasia (ATM) though the exact mechanism is unknown [63, 64]. ATM shares the PI3K domain mentioned above. VICI syndrome, a multisystem disorder characterized by agenesis (failure to develop) of the corpus callosum, cataracts, hypopigmentation of the eyes and hair, and cardiomyopathy, is also characterized by immunodeficiency, in which levels of IgG2 as well as CD4+ T-lymphocytes are low [65].

Symptoms and Comorbidities

As mentioned, levels of IgG subclasses may be low, or even absent, in healthy adults and are thus not always pathogenic [22, 64]. For those patients who are symptomatic, the most common symptoms are recurrent ear, sinus, and pulmonary infections [22].

More serious infections may include meningitis, osteomyelitis, and cellulitis [3]. Prolonged and recurrent pulmonary infections may lead to bronchiectasis, just as repeated episodes of otitis media may lead to hearing loss. This is particularly more common when a selective IgG deficiency accompanies an IgA deficiency [41, 66, 67]. In these circumstances, the infections are usually due to bacterial encapsulated pathogens such as *Streptococcus pneumoniae* and *Haemophilus influenzae* [68].

Testing

Patients presenting with recurrent infections, including pneumonia, sinusitis, and otitis media, require an immunological assessment. The initial evaluation should include a detailed history of each infection and appropriate treatment with antibiotics. A physical exam should be performed, focusing on auscultation of the lungs and lymph node evaluation. The laboratory evaluation should begin with a complete blood count with a differential, total levels of immunoglobulins, complement evaluation with a total hemolytic complement, an alternative hemolytic complement level and complement C2 levels, as well as monitoring for antibody titer levels to protein and polysaccharide antigens to which the patient had previously been vaccinated with. If antibody titers are decreased, then IgG subclass levels should be measured. The patient should be vaccinated to a vaccine to which they do not have protective titers, with a reassessment of the levels in 4–6 weeks. If levels of IgG subclasses are low, they should be repeated to confirm the abnormality, especially at a young age when the levels are still rising [11]. As it pertains to IgG subclass deficiency, the two bacteria to which revaccination should be addressed are *Streptococcus pneumoniae* and *Haemophilus influenzae*. If a patient has had recurrent sinus or pulmonary infections, then imaging of the sinuses, with a sinus CT, and lungs, with either a chest X-ray or chest CT, should be performed to assess for sinusitis and bronchiectasis, respectively. If the patient is young and has recurrent sinusitis, pneumonia, and gastrointestinal symptoms, a sweat test and possibly genetics to rule out cystic fibrosis should be performed. Physicians should be aware that immunoglobulin levels, both total and subclasses, may be reduced with prolonged use of systemic corticosteroids [69, 70].

Management/Outcome

Management of confirmed selective IgG deficiency depends on the severity and degree of the recurrent infections and the comorbidities. For patients who also have asthma or allergic rhinitis, these diseases need to be managed and optimized accordingly. If allergen immunotherapy is being considered, a selective IgG deficiency is not a contraindication, and immunotherapy may be initiated. As stated previously, patients should be revaccinated to polysaccharide vaccines as well as conjugated vaccines [71–73]. During acute infections, antibiotics need to be initiated as early as possible. The decision to use prophylactic antibiotics needs to be individualized but should be considered for patients who have frequent and prolonged infectious courses, especially in patients with known bronchiectasis [44, 74]. Cultures should be obtained when possible to help determine appropriate antibiotic therapy. For severe cases, immunoglobulin replacement therapy also needs to be considered especially when the patient exhibits an extremely poor response to polysaccharide antigens [75–77].

The prognosis of selective IgG deficiency varies with age. Those patients diagnosed with selective IgG deficiency under the age of 6 generally have a good prognosis as most of their deficiencies will resolve with age, including a lack of response to polysaccharide antigens [46]. After 6 years of age, their disease generally persists but the severity is variable and difficult to discern. Some patients may progress to CVID.

Monitoring Control

Patients with selective IgG deficiency should have regular visits with their primary care physician and at least once yearly with an immunologist to reassess their immunoglobulin levels. No specific ongoing workup, other than re-evaluating the abnormal IgG subclass levels and rechecking of other immunoglobulin levels, are currently recommended. Any signs of infection should quickly prompt the patient to get a complete medical evaluation. If a patient is on immunoglobulin replacement therapy, discontinuation can be considered once patient is free of bacterial infections for a year. An immunological evaluation should be deferred for 4–6 months after discontinuation [46, 77].

Case Presentation 2

A 20-year-old woman is referred by her gastroenterologist for an immunologic work-up. She initially presented with 9 months of intermittent, cramping abdominal pain and non-abating, non-bloody diarrhea. Her evaluation was negative for any infectious causes; however, serology was positive for a tissue transglutaminase IgG greater than 100 U/mL. Her tissue transglutaminase IgA was less than 4 U/mL and total IgA was less than 5 mg/dL (normal 60–400 mg/dL). Gastroenterology performed an esophagogastroduodenoscopy (EGD) with biopsies of the duodenum, which found intraepithelial lymphocytes, increased crypt hyperplasia, and mild villous atrophy (Marsh IIIa), confirming the diagnosis of celiac disease. Due to a decreased level of IgA, she was referred to the immunology clinic for further evaluation. Her past medical history includes mild-intermittent asthma, atopic dermatitis, food allergies, and allergic rhinitis. Upon further review of her history, she states she had a chest X-ray confirming pneumonia at the age of 8 years and has had recurrent acute sinusitis 3–4 times a year for the past few years, which responded well to antibiotics each time. Her physical exam and family history as well as her complete blood count, liver function tests, and basic metabolic panel were all unremarkable. An immunologic evaluation confirmed a low serum IgA level, a normal IgM level of 92 mg/dL (normal 50–300 mg/dL), a normal total IgG level of 885 mg/dL, an IgE of less than 2 mg/dL, and normal lymphocyte subsets. IgG subclass evaluation revealed a decreased IgG2 level of 55 mg/dL (normal 240–700 mg/dL), with normal IgG1 (594 mg/dL), IgG3 (58 mg/dL), and IgG4 (6 mg/dL) levels. IgA subclasses were decreased with a low IgA1 subclass of 10 mg/dL (normal 46–378 mg/dL) and a low IgA2 subclass of less than 1 mg/dL (normal 13–91 mg/dL). She had no anti-IgA antibodies present. Thus, she was found to have a low total IgA level as well as a low IgG2 level with recurrent acute sinusitis and celiac disease. Antibody titers showed adequate immunity against tetanus and diphtheria toxoids, mumps, rubella, and varicella, with inadequate response to *Streptococcus pneumoniae* (only 2 out of 23 antibodies above 0.3 μg/mL) and *Haemophilus influenzae* type b, demonstrating a poor response to polysaccharide antigens. The patient was vaccinated with the Pneumovax vaccine and placed on a gluten-free diet resulting in improvement of her abdominal symptoms.

Diagnosis/Assessment

The case above described a patient with two selective antibody deficiencies—IgG2 and IgA deficiency. IgG2 deficiency was discussed in the first case and selective IgA deficiency will be discussed here. IgA is the antibody isotype produced in greater abundance by our immune system [78–80]. Selective IgA deficiency is defined as a low or absent serum IgA level in a patient over 4 years of age with normal levels of IgM and total IgG and in whom other causes of hypogammaglobulinemia are excluded [78, 81]. An IgA level below 7 mg/dL is labelled as selective IgA deficiency, whereas level 2 standard deviations below normal, but above 7 mg/dl, are called partial IgA deficiency. Selective IgA deficiency is the most common primary immunodeficiency with an incidence of 1 in 600, though this may not fully capture the true prevalence since most patients are asymptomatic [79, 82, 83]. Selective IgA deficiency may have variable clinical manifestations which range from no clinical symptoms to significant recurrent infections and autoimmune diseases. Over 85% of patients with an IgA deficiency are believed to be asymptomatic [78, 81]. Blood levels of IgA measure only the serum IgA levels and not the secreted levels, so patients may have low levels of circulating IgA in the blood but normal levels of mucosal IgA [78, 84]. This may explain why certain patients with low levels of IgA may not exhibit any symptoms. In addition, it has been shown that in patients with selective IgA deficiency, levels of IgM are increased, which may act as a compensatory mechanism.

The molecular defects that cause IgA deficiency are not well characterized, but several genetic mutations have been found to likely play a role. The first such mutation was in transmembrane activator and calcium-modulator and cyclophilin ligand interactor (TACI), which is involved in isotype switching in B cells. A mutation in TACI is also one of the causes of CVID; thus, defective isotype switching may also play a pathogenic role leading to IgA deficiency [85–87]. Numerous other mutations, including in chromosomes 14, 16, and 18, and cytokine abnormalities lead to immature and dysfunctional IgA, pointing to a maturation defect of B cells to make IgA as a possible cause for IgA deficiency [78, 79, 88]. A deletion of the heavy chain encoding IgA on chromosome 14 may lead to low levels of IgA [89]. In addition, a genetic association has been found between autoimmunity and selective IgA deficiency [90].

Symptoms

Most cases of selective IgA deficiency are asymptomatic; however, as with the patient in the second case, there may be a broad range of clinical manifestations [83]. These include recurrent sinopulmonary infections; intestinal infections, such as *Giardia*; allergic disorders; autoimmune disorders; malignancies; and complications, including anaphylaxis, with blood product transfusions [78, 91–94].

In children, the most common infectious manifestations of selective IgA deficiency are recurrent sinusitis, pneumonia, and otitis media [78]. In adults, the same infections are common with a lesser chance of otitis media compared to sinusitis and pneumonia [95]. The prevalent infectious agents are encapsulated bacteria such as *Streptococcus pneumoniae* and *Haemophilus influenzae* [79, 93, 94]. The risks of viral upper and lower respiratory infections are increased in patients with selective IgA deficiency. Recurrent infections may lead to bronchiectasis, especially when combined with an IgG or IgM deficiency [96].

Patients with selective IgA deficiency may first present with gastrointestinal manifestations, as in the patient in case 2 who was found to have celiac disease, which is found in nearly 10% of selective IgA deficiency [97, 98]. Of all patients with confirmed celiac disease, up to 2% have IgA deficiency [99]. Gastrointestinal infectious diseases in selective IgA deficiency are predominantly *Giardia lamblia* [100, 101]. Selective IgA deficiency is also associated with nodular lymphoid hyperplasia, as in CVID, malabsorption, lactose intolerance, and, rarely, inflammatory bowel disease [78, 93, 102, 103].

Some patients with selective IgA deficiency make autoantibodies against IgA. These patients, usually those with undetectable levels of IgA, are at increased risk of anaphylactic reactions to blood products when the anti-IgA antibodies react against the IgA found in the plasma of blood products being administered, including whole blood, fresh frozen plasma, packed red blood cells, platelets, cryoprecipitate, and intravenous immunoglobulins [104, 105]. These reactions happen in as much as 1 in 20,000 transfusion reactions, and they cannot be differentiated from other causes of anaphylaxis, other than findings of anti-IgA antibodies. The patient in the case above had undetectable levels of anti-IgA antibodies, but that finding on its own does not ensure the safe administration of blood products.

Comorbidities

IgA deficiency is associated with numerous conditions including CVID, IgG2 subclass deficiency, DiGeorge syndrome, ataxia-telangiectasia, and RAG1 and RAG2 immunodeficiency. A case has been described of a RAG1 deficiency which presented as a selective IgA deficiency [106]. Some cases of selective IgA deficiency progress to CVID, though this is not well understood [107, 108]. Studies have showed an increase in the development of cancer, particularly gastrointestinal and lymphoid malignancies, in adult patients with IgA deficiency [93, 109].

Young patients with selective IgA deficiency were found to be at a higher risk of allergic disease. This includes increased risks of food allergies, allergic rhinitis, atopic dermatitis, urticaria, and allergic asthma and is more prominent in patients with significantly reduced levels of IgA [87, 94, 95]. Those that had asthma generally had a more severe form [95]. Up to 30% of patients with selective IgA deficiency develop autoimmune disorders, which are the second most common clinical manifestation after respiratory infections [93]. A wide spectrum of autoimmune disorders have been documented, including rheumatoid arthritis, systemic lupus erythematosus (SLE), Graves' disease, psoriasis, polymyalgia rheumatica, type I diabetes mellitus, vitiligo, idiopathic thrombocytopenia purpura (ITP), hemolytic anemia, pemphigus, celiac disease, and myasthenia gravis (Table 6.5) [91, 93, 95, 98, 110]. Patients with selective IgA deficiency were also more likely to have autoantibodies without autoimmune disease [111].

Testing

Evaluation of IgA deficiency should be considered in those patients with recurrent sinusitis and pneumonias and otitis media in children. The evaluation should also be performed for those patients with celiac disease; those with diarrhea caused by

Table 6.5 Autoimmune conditions associated with selective IgA deficiency

Idiopathic thrombocytopenia purpura	Celiac disease
Autoimmune hemolytic anemia	Psoriasis
Juvenile rheumatoid arthritis	Pemphigus
Systemic lupus erythematous	Grave's disease
Polymyalgia rheumatica	Rheumatoid arthritis
Type I diabetes mellitus	Myasthenia gravis

Giardia lamblia, any family history of CVID, or selective IgA deficiency; or any patient who has had an anaphylactic reaction to any blood product.

If a patient is suspected to have an IgA deficiency, levels of IgA, IgG, and IgM should be measured. All three levels are necessary to differentiate selective IgA deficiency from other disorders, such as CVID or other diseases in which levels are decreased. If the levels return low, a repeat test should be performed to confirm the level and exclude lab error. A diagnosis of selective IgA deficiency should not be made in children under the age of 4, and after that age, levels need to be closely monitored, as they may normalize, which in most cases happens between the ages of 9 and 16 years [112]. Selective IgA deficiency needs to be characterized based on its severity, with a distinction made between severe deficiency, in which levels are below 7 mg/dL, and partial deficiency, where levels are below normal but above 7 mg/dL. In both cases, serum levels of IgG and IgM should be in normal range and other causes of hypogammaglobulinemia excluded [81].

The evaluation of IgA deficiency should further include a complete blood count with differential, basic metabolic panel; evaluation of autoimmune disorders based on symptoms, such as thyroid levels and autoantibodies; evaluation of allergies with either skin prick tests or serum total and specific IgE levels; and screening for inflammation and chronic infections with a C-reactive protein and erythrocyte sedimentation rate. As discussed previously, patients with selective IgA deficiency are at an increased risk for blood product transfusion reactions and autoimmunity. Anti-IgA antibodies may be measured, but a lack of these antibodies does not rule out a risk of anaphylaxis with blood products. Clinicians should have a low threshold for autoimmune evaluations if the appropriate symptoms are seen [95, 98]. If performing screening testing for celiac disease, an IgG-anti-gliadin antibody or tissue transglutaminase IgG should be measured as testing with an IgA-based assay will result in false negatives [97, 113]. Patients may also require an EGD with biopsies for a confirmed diagnosis of celiac disease, as was performed in the patient in case 2.

Further testing is necessary for patients with recurrent infections, which should include imaging. Patients with recurrent pulmonary infections should be evaluated with chest radiographs and CT of the chest to ensure there is no chronic damage, such as bronchiectasis, and to rule out other potential causes of the pulmonary disease [114]. CT of the sinuses should be performed in patients with recurrent sinusitis. In addition, due to the nature of the recurrent infections, levels of other arms of the immune system, such as total complement levels (CH50), alternative complement levels (AH50), and lymphocyte enumeration, should be measured. If patients have a history of recurrent sinopulmonary infections, but a normal total IgG level, then IgG subclass levels should be measured, which may show an IgG subclass deficiency as seen in our patient. In these cases, evaluation of responses to vaccine antigens should be considered. Patients with poor responses should be followed closely as they may progress to CVID [107, 108]. Patients with IgA deficiency combined with either IgG2 or IgG3 deficiency have more severe sinopulmonary infections [67, 115, 116].

Alternate causes of low IgA need to be excluded prior to giving a diagnosis of IgA deficiency, including protein-losing pathologies and medications. These medications include phenytoin, lamotrigine, sodium valproate, carbamazepine, captopril, sulfasalazine, cyclosporine, thyroxine, and NSAIDs [16, 18, 117–123]. All of these have been reported as reversible, except cyclosporine and lamotrigine [119, 122]. Infants may have transient hypogammaglobulinemia of infancy, and thus, as described earlier, a diagnosis of selective IgA deficiency should not be made at a young age.

Management/Outcome

IgA deficiency should be managed by close observation and patient education. In most situations, patients with IgA deficiency are asymptomatic and have no significant burden of disease. Recently, more patients are being referred for evaluation due to increased evaluation for celiac disease, which is tested with IgG and IgA to transglutaminase, and the test generally includes a total IgA level [113]. Asymptomatic patients should be educated about the possible complications of a deficiency including infections, autoimmune diseases, and reactions to blood products, but no treatment is recommended aside from wearing a medical alert bracelet in case of an urgent need of a transfusion. Avoiding exposure to *Giardia* may be discussed. If a patient recently received blood products, consider checking for anti-IgA antibodies. Clinicians could perform periodic monitoring of IgA, IgG, and IgM levels to ensure the patient is not progressing to CVID. Medications, as listed above, should be decreased or discontinued, if possible, to ensure there is no further drop in IgA levels.

Clinicians should ensure that patients with low serum levels of IgA and a history of infections be vaccinated to pneumococcal vaccines, Prevnar and Pneumovax, to reduce the number of sinopulmonary infections [87]. Patients with IgA levels below 7 mg/dL should avoid live viral vaccines, such as oral polio, yellow fever, and bacille Calmette-Guérin (BCG). Patients with selective IgA deficiency and associated diseases, such as celiac disease and other autoimmune diseases, allergic diseases, and/or asthma, should be evaluated and treated for those diseases. It is up to the physician's discretion to consider prophylactic antibiotics for patients with recurrent infections. Patients who continue to have infections can be treated with immunoglobulin replacement, which is more likely in patients who also have an IgG subclass deficiency. Immunoglobulin replacement can be done via an intravenous route or subcutaneous route, but care must be taken since these may lead to anaphylaxis due to the presence of small amounts of IgA [124, 125]. Therefore, it is best to use immunoglobulin replacement preparations, and other blood products, that are IgA depleted, if possible. It should be noted that patients improve due to the introduction of IgG antibodies and not due to IgA replacement, since the amount of IgA in IVIG and SCIG is minimal and does not significantly increase IgA levels in the blood. Patients may consider wearing a medical allergy bracelet stating that they need IgA-depleted blood in case of emergencies. Desensitization to IgA in blood products has been successfully performed [126].

As mentioned previously, patients with IgA deficiency are at a slightly increased risk of malignancy, particularly gastrointestinal, but no monitoring recommendations are available at this time [93, 109].

Conclusion

Selective immunoglobulin deficiency is a decreased level of IgA, IgM, or one of the four subclasses of IgG, while the total level of IgG is within normal range. It is different from CVID, a more severe form of immunodeficiency, which is associated with a decrease in total IgG and a decrease in either IgA or IgM. Prevalence of IgG subclass deficiency is unknown but believed to be one of the more common antibody deficiencies. Measuring levels of IgG subclasses is controversial but should be considered in the evaluation of a patient with recurrent infections, especially if the patient is having poor responses to vaccinations. Patient presentations vary from asymptomatic to severe immunodeficiency requiring prophylactic antibiotics or immunoglobulin replacement. IgA deficiency is the most common immunodeficiency with over 80% of patients being asymptomatic. Symptomatic patients may have recurrent sinopulmonary infections, allergic disease, gastrointestinal disorders, autoimmune diseases, and, rarely, anaphylaxis to blood products. Patients with selective immunoglobulin deficiency require close monitoring as their values may either normalize or progress to more severe immunodeficiency. In conclusion, selective isotype immunodeficiency is relatively common in the general population with a broad clinical spectrum ranging from asymptomatic to significant immunodeficiency and autoimmune disease.

> **Clinical Pearls and Pitfalls**
> - Patients with recurrent sinopulmonary infections with poor responses to protein or polysaccharide antigens should have levels for IgG subclass deficiency measured.
> - A finding of a low level of an IgG subclass does not necessarily indicate an immunodeficiency.
> - Patients with IgG subclass deficiency have a higher rate of associated allergic disease, autoimmune disorders, and poor response to vaccinations and may suffer from recurrent infections.
> - Specific antibody deficiency is marked by normal levels of immunoglobulins, including IgG subclasses, with poor responses to polysaccharide antigens.
> - IgA deficiency is the most common immunodeficiency and may be asymptomatic; however, patients may have recurrent sinopulmonary infections, autoimmune disorders, and gastrointestinal disorders and are at risk for transfusion reactions.

- The mainstay of IgA deficiency treatment is patient education and close clinical monitoring. For patients who have associated diseases, such as allergies or autoimmune disorders, treatment for these disorders is required. Patients should be advised to wear a medical bracelet in case a transfusion is necessary.
- The management of immunoglobulin subclass deficiency includes treating associated diseases, patient education, close clinical monitoring, and, in rare cases, prophylactic antibiotics or immunoglobulin replacement therapy.

References

1. Nahm MH, Macke K, Kwon OH, Madassery JV, Sherman LA, Scott MG. Immunologic and clinical status of blood donors with subnormal levels of IgG2. J Allergy Clin Immunol. 1990;85(4):769–77.
2. Herrod HG. IgG subclass deficiency. Allergy Proc. 1992;13(6):299–302.
3. Hanson LA, Söderström R, Avanzini A, Bengtsson U, Björkander J, Söderström T. Immunoglobulin subclass deficiency. Pediatr Infect Dis J. 1988;7(5 Suppl):S17–21.
4. Aucouturier P, Mariault M, Lacombe C, Preud'homme JL. Frequency of selective IgG subclass deficiency: a reappraisal. Clin Immunol Immunopathol. 1992;63(3):289–91.
5. Schur PH, Rosen F, Norman ME. Immunoglobulin subclasses in normal children. Pediatr Res. 1979;13(3):181–3.
6. Oxelius VA. IgG subclass levels in infancy and childhood. Acta Paediatr Scand. 1979;68(1):23–7.
7. Plebani A, Ugazio AG, Avanzini MA, Massimi P, Zonta L, Monafo V, et al. Serum IgG subclass concentrations in healthy subjects at different age: age normal percentile charts. Eur J Pediatr. 1989;149(3):164–7.
8. Stiehm ER, Fudenberg HH. Serum levels of immune globulins in health and disease: a survey. Pediatrics. 1966;37(5):715–27.
9. Nieuwenhuys EJ, Out TA. Comparison of normal values of IgG subclasses. Protides of the Biological Fluids, Elsevier. 1989;36:71–9.
10. Jefferis R, Kumararatne DS. Selective IgG subclass deficiency: quantification and clinical relevance. Clin Exp Immunol. 1990;81(3):357–67.
11. Hamilton RG. Human IgG subclass measurements in the clinical laboratory. Clin Chem. 1987;33(10):1707–25.
12. Söderström T, Söderström R, Avanzini A, Brandtzaeg P, Karlsson G, Hanson LA. Immunoglobulin G subclass deficiencies. Int Arch Allergy Appl Immunol. 1987;82(3–4):476–80.
13. Aucouturier P, Lacombe C, Bremard C, Lebranchu Y, Seligmann M, Griscelli C, et al. Serum IgG subclass levels in patients with primary immunodeficiency syndromes or abnormal susceptibility to infections. Clin Immunol Immunopathol. 1989;51(1):22–37.
14. Zenone T, Souquet PJ, Cunningham-Rundles C, Bernard JP. Hodgkin's disease associated with IgA and IgG subclass deficiency. J Intern Med. 1996;240(2):99–102.
15. Klaustermeyer WB, Gianos ME, Kurohara ML, Dao HT, Heiner DC. IgG subclass deficiency associated with corticosteroids in obstructive lung disease. Chest. 1992;102(4):1137–42.
16. Leickly FE, Buckley RH. Development of IgA and IgG2 subclass deficiency after sulfasalazine therapy. J Pediatr. 1986;108(3):481–2.
17. Ishizaka A, Nakanishi M, Kasahara E, Mizutani K, Sakiyama Y, Matsumoto S. Phenytoin-induced IgG2 and IgG4 deficiencies in a patient with epilepsy. Acta Paediatr. 1992;81(8):646–8.

18. Kato Z, Watanabe M, Kondo N. IgG2, IgG4 and IgA deficiency possibly associated with carbamazepine treatment. Eur J Pediatr. 2003;162(3):209–11.
19. Schauer U, Stemberg F, Rieger CH, Borte M, Schubert S, Riedel F, et al. IgG subclass concentrations in certified reference material 470 and reference values for children and adults determined with the binding site reagents. Clin Chem. 2003;49(11):1924–9.
20. Barton JC, Bertoli LF, Barton JC, Acton RT. Selective subnormal IgG1 in 54 adult index patients with frequent or severe bacterial respiratory tract infections. J Immunol Res. 2016;2016:1405950.
21. Morgan G, Levinsky RJ. Clinical significance of IgG subclass deficiency. Arch Dis Child. 1988;63(7):771–322.
22. Lacombe C, Aucouturier P, Preud'homme JL. Selective IgG1 deficiency. Clin Immunol Immunopathol. 1997;84(2):194–201.
23. Javier FC 3rd, Moore CM, Sorensen RU. Distribution of primary immunodeficiency diseases diagnosed in a pediatric tertiary hospital. Ann Allergy Asthma Immunol. 2000;84(1):25–30.
24. Braconier JH, Nilsson B, Oxelius VA, Karup-Pedersen F. Recurrent pneumococcal infections in a patient with lack of specific IgG and IgM pneumococcal antibodies and deficiency of serum IgA, IgG2 and IgG4. Scand J Infect Dis. 1984;16(4):407–10.
25. Bruyn GA, Hiemstra PS, Rijkers GT. Type-specific anti-pneumococcal antibodies in a vaccinated patient with combined immunoglobulin A and IgG2 deficiency and invasive pneumococcal infections. J Infect Dis. 1992;166(6):1460–1.
26. Siber GR, Schur PH, Aisenberg AC, Weitzman SA, Schiffman G. Correlation between serum IgG-2 concentrations and the antibody response to bacterial polysaccharide antigens. N Engl J Med. 1980;303(4):178–82.
27. Bass JL, Nuss R, Mehta KA, Morganelli P, Bennett L. Recurrent meningococcemia associated with IgG2-subclass deficiency. N Engl J Med. 1983;309(7):430.
28. Escobar-Pérez X, Dorta-Contreras AJ, Interián-Morales MT, Noris-García E, Ferrá-Valdés M. IgG2 immunodeficiency: association to pediatric patients with bacterial meningoencephalitis. Arq Neuropsiquiatr. 2000;58(1):141–5.
29. Schatorjé EJ, de Jong E, van Hout RW, García Vivas Y, de Vries E. The challenge of immunoglobulin-G subclass deficiency and specific polysaccharide antibody deficiency--a Dutch Pediatric Cohort Study. J Clin Immunol. 2016;36(2):141–8.
30. Bussel J, Morell A, Skvaril F. IgG2 deficiency in autoimmune cytopenias. Monogr Allergy. 1986;20:116–8.
31. Eriksson P, Almroth G, Denneberg T, Lindström FD. IgG2 deficiency in primary Sjögren's syndrome and hypergammaglobulinemic purpura. Clin Immunol Immunopathol. 1994;70(1):60–5.
32. Jiménez A, López-Trascasa M, Fontán G. Incidence of selective IgG2 deficiency in patients with vasculitis. Clin Exp Immunol. 1989;78(2):149–52.
33. Aucouturier P, Barra A, Intrator L, Cordonnier C, Schulz D, Duarte F, Vernant JP, Preud'homme JL. Long lasting IgG subclass and antibacterial polysaccharide antibody deficiency after allogeneic bone marrow transplantation. Blood. 1987;70(3):779–85.
34. Parkkali T, Käyhty H, Anttila M, Ruutu T, Wuorimaa T, Soininen A, et al. IgG subclasses and avidity of antibodies to polysaccharide antigens in allogeneic BMT recipients after vaccination with pneumococcal polysaccharide and Haemophilus influenzae type b conjugate vaccines. Bone Marrow Transplant. 1999;24(6):671–8.
35. Skvaril F. IgG subclasses in viral infections. Monogr Allergy. 1986;19:134–43.
36. de Moraes LC, Oliveira LC, Diogo CL, Kirschfink M, Grumach AS. Immunoglobulin G subclass concentrations and infections in children and adolescents with severe asthma. Pediatr Allergy Immunol. 2002;13(3):195–202.
37. Barton JC, Bertoli LF, Barton JC, Acton RT. Selective subnormal IgG3 in 121 adult index patients with frequent or severe bacterial respiratory tract infections. Cell Immunol. 2016;299:50–7.
38. Snowden JA, Milford-Ward A, Cookson LJ, McKendrick MW. Recurrent lymphocytic meningitis associated with hereditary isolated IgG subclass 3 deficiency. J Infect. 1993;27(3):285–9.

39. Heiner DC, Myers A, Beck CS. Deficiency of IgG4: a disorder associated with frequent infections and bronchiectasis that may be familial. Clin Rev Allergy. 1983;1(2):259–66.
40. Moss RB, Carmack MA, Esrig S. Deficiency of IgG4 in children: association of isolated IgG4 deficiency with recurrent respiratory tract infection. J Pediatr. 1992;120(1):16–21.
41. Picard C, Bobby Gaspar H, Al-Herz W, Bousfiha A, Casanova JL, Chatila T, et al. International Union of Immunological Societies: 2017 Primary Immunodeficiency Diseases Committee Report on inborn errors of immunity. J Clin Immunol. 2018;38(1):96–128.
42. Perez E, Bonilla FA, Orange JS, Ballow M. Specific antibody deficiency: controversies in diagnosis and management. Front Immunol. 2017;8:586.
43. Ambrosino DM, Umetsu DT, Siber GR, Howie G, Goularte TA, Michaels R, et al. Selective defect in the antibody response to Haemophilus influenzae type b in children with recurrent infections and normal serum IgG subclass levels. J Allergy Clin Immunol. 1988;81(6):1175–9.
44. Go ES, Ballas ZK. Anti-pneumococcal antibody response in normal subjects: a meta-analysis. J Allergy Clin Immunol. 1996;98(1):205–15.
45. Ekdahl K, Braconier JH, Svanborg C. Immunoglobulin deficiencies and impaired immune response to polysaccharide antigens in adult patients with recurrent community-acquired pneumonia. Scand J Infect Dis. 1997;29(4):401–7.
46. Wolpert J, Knutsen AP. Natural history of selective antibody deficiency to bacterial polysaccharide antigens in children. Pediatr Asthma Allergy Immunol. 1998;12:183.
47. Cohn JA, Skorpinski E, Cohn JR. Prevention of pneumococcal infection in a patient with normal immunoglobulin levels but impaired polysaccharide antibody production. Ann Allergy Asthma Immunol. 2006;97(5):603–5.
48. Wood PM, Mayne A, Joyce H, Smith CI, Granoff DM, Kumararatne DS. A mutation in Bruton's tyrosine kinase as a cause of selective anti-polysaccharide antibody deficiency. J Pediatr. 2001;139(1):148–51.
49. Gupta S, Gupta A. Selective IgM deficiency-an underestimated primary immunodeficiency. Front Immunol. 2017;8:1056.
50. Louis AG, Gupta S. Primary selective IgM deficiency: an ignored immunodeficiency. Clin Rev Allergy Immunol. 2014;46(2):104–11.
51. Cassidy JT, Nordby GL. Human serum immunoglobulin concentrations: prevalence of immunoglobulin deficiencies. J Allergy Clin Immunol. 1975;55(1):35–48.
52. Entezari N, Adab Z, Zeydi M, Saghafi S, Jamali M, Kardar GA, et al. The prevalence of Selective Immunoglobulin M Deficiency (SIgMD) in Iranian volunteer blood donors. Hum Immunol. 2016;77(1):7–11.
53. Goldstein MF, Goldstein AL, Dunsky EH, Dvorin DJ, Belecanech GA, Shamir K. Selective IgM immunodeficiency: retrospective analysis of 36 adult patients with review of the literature. Ann Allergy Asthma Immunol. 2006;97(6):717–30.
54. Chovancova Z, Kralickova P, Pejchalova A, Bloomfield M, Nechvatalova J, Vlkova M, et al. Selective IgM deficiency: clinical and laboratory features of 17 patients and a review of the literature. J Clin Immunol. 2017;37(6):559–74.
55. Hobbs JR, Milner RD, Watt PJ. Gamma-M deficiency predisposing to meningococcal septicaemia. Br Med J. 1967;4(5579):583–6.
56. Yel L, Ramanuja S, Gupta S. Clinical and immunological features in IgM deficiency. Int Arch Allergy Immunol. 2009;150(3):291–8.
57. Lefranc MP, Lefranc G, Rabbitts TH. Inherited deletion of immunoglobulin heavy chain constant region genes in normal human individuals. Nature. 1982;300(5894):760–2.
58. Oxelius VA, Pandey JP. Human immunoglobulin constant heavy G chain (IGHG) (Fcγ) (GM) genes, defining innate variants of IgG molecules and B cells, have impact on disease and therapy. Clin Immunol. 2013;149(3):475–86.
59. Rabbani H, Kondo N, Smith CI, Hammarström L. The influence of gene deletions and duplications within the IGHC locus on serum immunoglobulin subclass levels. Clin Immunol Immunopathol. 1995;76(3 Pt 2):S214–8.
60. Carbonara AO, Demarchi M. Ig isotypes deficiency caused by gene deletions. Monogr Allergy. 1986;20:13–7.

61. Coulter TI, Chandra A, Bacon CM, Babar J, Curtis J, Screaton N, et al. Clinical spectrum and features of activated phosphoinositide 3-kinase δ syndrome: a large patient cohort study. J Allergy Clin Immunol. 2017;139(2):597–606.e4.
62. Lucas CL, Chandra A, Nejentsev S, Condliffe AM, Okkenhaug K. PI3Kδ and primary immunodeficiencies. Nat Rev Immunol. 2016;16(11):702–14.
63. Maciejczyk M, Heropolitanska-Pliszka E, Pietrucha B, Sawicka-Powierza J, Bernatowska E, Wolska-Kusnierz B, et al. Antioxidant defense, redox homeostasis, and oxidative damage in children with ataxia telangiectasia and Nijmegen Breakage syndrome. Front Immunol. 2019;10:2322.
64. Shiloh Y. Ataxia-telangiectasia and the Nijmegen breakage syndrome: related disorders but genes apart. Annu Rev Genet. 1997;31:635–62.
65. Finocchi A, Angelino G, Cantarutti N, Corbari M, Bevivino E, Cascioli S, et al. Immunodeficiency in Vici syndrome: a heterogeneous phenotype. Am J Med Genet A. 2012;158A(2):434–9.
66. Plebani A, Ugazio AG, Meini A, Ruggeri L, Negrini A, Albertini A, et al. Extensive deletion of immunoglobulin heavy chain constant region genes in the absence of recurrent infections: when is IgG subclass deficiency clinically relevant? Clin Immunol Immunopathol. 1993;68(1):46–50.
67. Björkander J, Bake B, Oxelius VA, Hanson LA. Impaired lung function in patients with IgA deficiency and low levels of IgG2 or IgG3. N Engl J Med. 1985;313(12):720–4.
68. Umetsu DT, Ambrosino DM, Quinti I, Siber GR, Geha RS. Recurrent sinopulmonary infection and impaired antibody response to bacterial capsular polysaccharide antigen in children with selective IgG-subclass deficiency. N Engl J Med. 1985;313(20):1247–51.
69. Settipane GA, Pudupakkam RK, McGowan JH. Corticosteroid effect on immunoglobulins. J Allergy Clin Immunol. 1978;62(3):162–6.
70. Milburn HJ, Poulter LW, Dilmec A, Cochrane GM, Kemeny DM. Corticosteroids restore the balance between locally produced Th1 and Th2 cytokines and immunoglobulin isotypes to normal in sarcoid lung. Clin Exp Immunol. 1997;108(1):105–13.
71. Sorensen RU, Leiva LE, Giangrosso PA, Butler B, Javier FC 3rd, Sacerdote DM, et al. Response to a heptavalent conjugate Streptococcus pneumoniae vaccine in children with recurrent infections who are unresponsive to the polysaccharide vaccine. Pediatr Infect Dis J. 1998;17(8):685–91.
72. Briere EC, Rubin L, Moro PL, Cohn A, Clark T, Messonnier N, Division of Bacterial Diseases, National Center for Immunization and Respiratory Diseases, CDC. Prevention and control of haemophilus influenzae type b disease: recommendations of the advisory committee on immunization practices (ACIP). MMWR Recomm Rep. 2014;63(RR-01):1–14.
73. Rubin LG, Levin MJ, Ljungman P, Davies EG, Avery R, Tomblyn M, et al. Infectious Diseases Society of America. 2013 IDSA clinical practice guideline for vaccination of the immunocompromised host. Clin Infect Dis. 2014;58(3):309–18.
74. Karaca NE, Karadeniz C, Aksu G, Kutukculer N. Clinical and laboratory evaluation of periodically monitored Turkish children with IgG subclass deficiencies. Asian Pac J Allergy Immunol. 2009;27(1):43–8.
75. Abdou NI, Greenwell CA, Mehta R, Narra M, Hester JD, Halsey JF. Efficacy of intravenous gammaglobulin for immunoglobulin G subclass and/or antibody deficiency in adults. Int Arch Allergy Immunol. 2009;149(3):267–74.
76. Edgar JDM, Richter AG, Huissoon AP, Kumararatne DS, Baxendale HE, Bethune CA, United Kingdom Primary Immunodeficiency Network (UKPIN) Immunoglobulin Decision to Treat Study Group, et al. Prescribing immunoglobulin replacement therapy for patients with non-classical and secondary antibody deficiency: an analysis of the practice of clinical immunologists in the UK and Republic of Ireland. J Clin Immunol. 2018;38(2):204–13.
77. Olinder-Nielsen AM, Granert C, Forsberg P, Friman V, Vietorisz A, Björkander J. Immunoglobulin prophylaxis in 350 adults with IgG subclass deficiency and recurrent respiratory tract infections: a long-term follow-up. Scand J Infect Dis. 2007;39(1):44–50.
78. Yel L. Selective IgA deficiency. J Clin Immunol. 2010;30(1):10–6.

79. Cunningham-Rundles C. Physiology of IgA and IgA deficiency. J Clin Immunol. 2001;21(5):303–9.
80. Woof JM, Kerr MA. The function of immunoglobulin A in immunity. J Pathol. 2006;208(2):270–82.
81. Conley ME, Notarangelo LD, Etzioni A. Diagnostic criteria for primary immunodeficiencies. Representing PAGID (Pan-American Group for Immunodeficiency) and ESID (European Society for Immunodeficiencies). Clin Immunol. 1999;93:190–7.
82. Stiehm ER. The four most common pediatric immunodeficiencies. J Immunotoxicol. 2008;5(2):227–34.
83. Koistinen J. Selective IgA deficiency in blood donors. Vox Sang. 1975;29(3):192–202.
84. Brandtzaeg P, Karlsson G, Hansson G, Petruson B, Björkander J, Hanson LA. The clinical condition of IgA-deficient patients is related to the proportion of IgD- and IgM-producing cells in their nasal mucosa. Clin Exp Immunol. 1987;67(3):626–36.
85. Pan-Hammarström Q, Salzer U, Du L, Björkander J, Cunningham-Rundles C, Nelson DL, et al. Reexamining the role of TACI coding variants in common variable immunodeficiency and selective IgA deficiency. Nat Genet. 2007;39(4):429–30.
86. Castigli E, Wilson SA, Garibyan L, Rachid R, Bonilla F, Schneider L, et al. TACI is mutant in common variable immunodeficiency and IgA deficiency. Nat Genet. 2005;37(8):829–34.
87. Yazdani R, Azizi G, Abolhassani H, Aghamohammadi A. Selective IgA deficiency: epidemiology, pathogenesis, clinical phenotype, diagnosis, prognosis and management. Scand J Immunol. 2017;85(1):3–12.
88. Plebani A, Carbonara AO, Bottaro A, Gallina R, Boccazzi C, Crispino P, et al. Gene deletion as a cause of associated deficiency of IgA1, IgG2, IgG4 and IgE. Immunodeficiency. 1993;4(1–4):245–8.
89. Suzuki H, Kaneko H, Fukao T, Jin R, Kawamoto N, Asano T, et al. Various expression patterns of alpha1 and alpha2 genes in IgA deficiency. Allergol Int. 2009;58(1):111–7.
90. Ferreira RC, Pan-Hammarström Q, Graham RR, Gateva V, Fontán G, Lee AT, et al. Association of IFIH1 and other autoimmunity risk alleles with selective IgA deficiency. Nat Genet. 2010;42(9):777–80.
91. Koskinen S. Long-term follow-up of health in blood donors with primary selective IgA deficiency. J Clin Immunol. 1996;16(3):165–70.
92. Domínguez O, Giner MT, Alsina L, Martín MA, Lozano J, Plaza AM. Clinical phenotypes associated with selective IgA deficiency: a review of 330 cases and a proposed follow-up protocol. An Pediatr (Barc). 2012;76(5):261–7.
93. Edwards E, Razvi S, Cunningham-Rundles C. IgA deficiency: clinical correlates and responses to pneumococcal vaccine. Clin Immunol. 2004;111(1):93–7.
94. Janzi M, Kull I, Sjöberg R, Wan J, Melén E, Bayat N, et al. Selective IgA deficiency in early life: association to infections and allergic diseases during childhood. Clin Immunol. 2009;133(1):78–85.
95. Jorgensen GH, Gardulf A, Sigurdsson MI, Sigurdardottir ST, Thorsteinsdottir I, Gudmundsson S, et al. Clinical symptoms in adults with selective IgA deficiency: a case-control study. J Clin Immunol. 2013;33(4):742–7.
96. Hodkinson JP, Bangs C, Wartenberg-Demand A, Bauhofer A, Langohr P, Buckland MS, et al. Low IgA and IgM is associated with a higher prevalence of bronchiectasis in primary antibody deficiency. J Clin Immunol. 2017;37(4):329–31.
97. Meini A, Pillan NM, Villanacci V, Monafo V, Ugazio AG, Plebani A. Prevalence and diagnosis of celiac disease in IgA-deficient children. Ann Allergy Asthma Immunol. 1996;77(4):333–6.
98. Wang N, Shen N, Vyse TJ, Anand V, Gunnarson I, Sturfelt G, et al. Selective IgA deficiency in autoimmune diseases. Mol Med. 2011;17(11–12):1383–96.
99. Cataldo F, Marino V, Bottaro G, Greco P, Ventura A. Celiac disease and selective immunoglobulin A deficiency. J Pediatr. 1997;131(2):306–8.
100. Langford TD, Housley MP, Boes M, Chen J, Kagnoff MF, Gillin FD, et al. Central importance of immunoglobulin A in host defense against Giardia spp. Infect Immun. 2002;70(1):11–8.

101. Zinneman HH, Kaplan AP. The association of giardiasis with reduced intestinal secretory immunoglobulin A. Am J Dig Dis. 1972;17(9):793–7.
102. Atarod L, Raissi A, Aghamohammadi A, Farhoudi A, Khodadad A, Moin M, et al. A review of gastrointestinal disorders in patients with primary antibody immunodeficiencies during a 10-year period (1990–2000), in children hospital medical center. Iran J Allergy Asthma Immunol. 2003;2(2):75–9.
103. Iizuka M, Itou H, Sato M, Yukawa M, Shirasaka T, Chiba M, et al. Crohn's disease associated with selective immunoglobulin a deficiency. J Gastroenterol Hepatol. 2001;16(8):951–2.
104. Ferreira A, Garcia Rodriguez MC, Lopez-Trascasa M, Pascual Salcedo D, Fontan G. Anti-IgA antibodies in selective IgA deficiency and in primary immunodeficient patients treated with gamma-globulin. Clin Immunol Immunopathol. 1988;47(2):199–207.
105. Sandler SG, Mallory D, Malamut D, Eckrich R. IgA anaphylactic transfusion reactions. Transfus Med Rev. 1995;9(1):1–8.
106. Kato T, Crestani E, Kamae C, Honma K, Yokosuka T, Ikegawa T, et al. RAG1 deficiency may present clinically as selective IgA deficiency. J Clin Immunol. 2015;35(3):280–8.
107. Español T, Catala M, Hernandez M, Caragol I, Bertran JM. Development of a common variable immunodeficiency in IgA-deficient patients. Clin Immunol Immunopathol. 1996;80(3 Pt 1):333–5.
108. Aghamohammadi A, Mohammadi J, Parvaneh N, Rezaei N, Moin M, Espanol T, et al. Progression of selective IgA deficiency to common variable immunodeficiency. Int Arch Allergy Immunol. 2008;147(2):87–92.
109. Ludvigsson JF, Neovius M, Ye W, Hammarström L. IgA deficiency and risk of cancer: a population-based matched cohort study. J Clin Immunol. 2015;35(2):182–8.
110. Abolhassani H, Gharib B, Shahinpour S, Masoom SN, Havaei A, Mirminachi B, et al. Autoimmunity in patients with selective IgA deficiency. J Investig Allergol Clin Immunol. 2015;25(2):111–9.
111. Barka N, Shen GQ, Shoenfeld Y, Alosachie IJ, Gershwin ME, Reyes H, et al. Multireactive pattern of serum autoantibodies in asymptomatic individuals with immunoglobulin A deficiency. Clin Diagn Lab Immunol. 1995;2(4):469–72.
112. Lim CK, Dahle C, Elvin K, Andersson BA, Rönnelid J, Melén E, et al. Reversal of immunoglobulin A deficiency in children. J Clin Immunol. 2015;35(1):87–91.
113. McGowan KE, Lyon ME, Butzner JD. Celiac disease and IgA deficiency: complications of serological testing approaches encountered in the clinic. Clin Chem. 2008;54(7):1203–9.
114. Gomez-Carrasco JA, Barrera-Gómez MJ, García-Mouriño V, Alvarez de Mon M, García de Frías E. Selective and partial IgA deficiency in an adolescent male with bronchiectasis. Allergol Immunopathol (Madr). 1994;22(6):261–3.
115. Oxelius VA, Laurell AB, Lindquist B, Golebiowska H, Axelsson U, Björkander J, et al. IgG subclasses in selective IgA deficiency: importance of IgG2-IgA deficiency. N Engl J Med. 1981;304(24):1476–7.
116. French MA, Denis KA, Dawkins R, Peter JB. Severity of infections in IgA deficiency: correlation with decreased serum antibodies to pneumococcal polysaccharides and decreased serum IgG2 and/or IgG4. Clin Exp Immunol. 1995;100(1):47–53.
117. Braconier JH. Reversible total IgA deficiency associated with phenytoin treatment. Scand J Infect Dis. 1999;31(5):515–6.
118. Ashrafi M, Hosseini SA, Abolmaali S, Biglari M, Azizi R, Farghadan M, et al. Effect of anti-epileptic drugs on serum immunoglobulin levels in children. Acta Neurol Belg. 2010;110(1):65–70.
119. Maruyama S, Okamoto Y, Toyoshima M, Hanaya R, Kawano Y. Immunoglobulin A deficiency following treatment with lamotrigine. Brain and Development. 2016;38(10):947–9.
120. Hammarström L, Smith CI, Berg CI. Captopril-induced IgA deficiency. Lancet. 1991;337(8738):436.
121. Farr M, Kitas GD, Tunn EJ, Bacon PA. Immunodeficiencies associated with sulphasalazine therapy in inflammatory arthritis. Br J Rheumatol. 1991;30(6):413–7.

122. Murphy EA, Morris AJ, Walker E, Lee FD, Sturrock RD. Cyclosporine A induced colitis and acquired selective IgA deficiency in a patient with juvenile chronic arthritis. J Rheumatol. 1993;20(8):1397–8.
123. Seager J. IgA deficiency during treatment of infantile hypothyroidism with thyroxine. Br Med J (Clin Res Ed). 1984;288(6430):1562–3.
124. Cunningham-Rundles C, Zhou Z, Mankarious S, Courter S. Long-term use of IgA-depleted intravenous immunoglobulin in immunodeficient subjects with anti-IgA antibodies. J Clin Immunol. 1993;13(4):272–8.
125. Björkander J, Hammarström L, Smith CI, Buckley RH, Cunningham-Rundles C, Hanson LA. Immunoglobulin prophylaxis in patients with antibody deficiency syndromes and anti-IgA antibodies. J Clin Immunol. 1987;7(1):8–15.
126. Kiani-Alikhan S, Yong PF, Grosse-Kreul D, Height SE, Mijovic A, Suddle AR, et al. Successful desensitization to immunoglobulin A in a case of transfusion-related anaphylaxis. Transfusion. 2010;50(9):1897–901.

Chapter 7
Common Variable Immunodeficiency-Like Disorders

Rohan Ameratunga, Caroline Allan, and See-Tarn Woon

Case Presentation 1

Initial Presentation of the Index Patient with CVID [1]

The proband (II.2), aged 63, presented with symptomatic hypogammaglobulinemia in her teenage years and was diagnosed with CVID at age 33 (Fig. 7.1). She was initially treated with intravenous immunoglobulin (IVIG) but was later changed to subcutaneous immunoglobulin (SCIG) treatment. She has had two episodes of meningitis while receiving immunoglobulin and has chronic diarrhea. Despite several functional endoscopic sinus surgical procedures, she continues to suffer recurrent upper respiratory tract infections. She is on thyroxine replacement for Hashimoto's thyroiditis and also meets the American College of Rheumatology (ACR) criteria for SLE. She has cytopenias, antinuclear antibodies, rashes, oral ulcers, nasal ulcers, and arthritis.

R. Ameratunga (✉)
Department of Clinical Immunology, Auckland City Hospital, Auckland, New Zealand

Department of Molecular Medicine and Pathology, Faculty of Medical and Health Sciences, University of Auckland, Auckland, New Zealand
e-mail: rohana@adhb.govt.nz

C. Allan
Department of Immunology, Auckland City Hospital, Auckland, New Zealand

S.-T. Woon
Department of Virology and Immunology, Auckland City Hospital, Auckland, New Zealand

Department of Molecular Medicine and Pathology, Faculty of Medical and Health Sciences, University of Auckland, Auckland, New Zealand

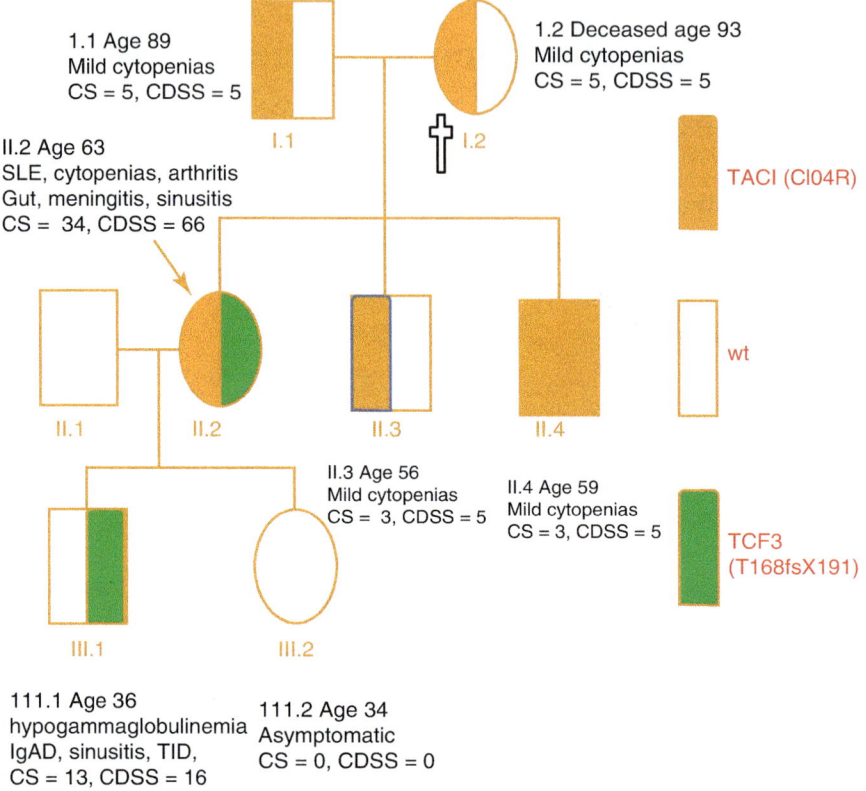

Fig. 7.1 Family with a digenic CVID-like disorder caused by epistatic interactions of *TNFRSF13B*/TACI and *TCF3* genes [1]. The proband (arrow) suffers from both a severe immunodeficiency and SLE. Other members are as described in our previous publications including a brother (II.3) with severe hypogammaglobulinemia caused by homozygous C104R mutations of the *TNFRSF13B*/TACI gene [2]. CDSS = CVID disease severity score [3]. CS = clinical score [4]. wt = wild type, SLE = systemic lupus erythematosus, TID = type 1 diabetes and IgAD = IgA deficiency. Male = square, Female = circle

Discordant Segregation of the **TNFRSF13B/TACI C104R** *Mutation in the Kindred and Subsequent Identification of the* **TCF3** *Mutation Causing a CVID-Like Disorder*

The proband was shown to be heterozygous for the C104R (c.310T>C) mutation of the *TNFRSF13B*/TACI gene in a previous study [2]. Her non-consanguineous parents (I.1 and I.2) were both heterozygous for the C104R mutation (see Fig. 7.1). Her mother recently passed away but both parents had mild asymptomatic hypogammaglobulinemia and thrombocytopenia.

The two male siblings carry the *TNFRSF13B*/TACI C104R mutation but are asymptomatic. One brother is heterozygous (II.3), and the other (II.4) is homozygous for the *TNFRSF13B*/TACI C104R mutation. Given his asymptomatic status, the proband's brother with the homozygous *TNFRSF13B*/TACI C104R mutation (II.4) does not meet our (Ameratunga et al. 2013) [5] criteria for probable CVID; he has normal albeit transient vaccine challenge responses despite being profoundly hypogammaglobulinemic (IgG 1.6 g/l, nr 7-14). He has declined immunoglobulin replacement and remains in excellent health.

Neither of the proband's children carry the *TNFRSF13B*/TACI C104R mutation (see Fig. 7.1). The proband's daughter (III.2) is in good health. The proband's son (III.1) has CVID-related phenotypes including symptomatic IgG deficiency, IgA deficiency, and type 1 diabetes and has recently developed seronegative arthritis. He has high titers of anti-parietal cell antibodies. His disorder may be in evolution, as he has an IgG of 6.5 g/l (nr 7-14). He suffers recurrent infections and had impaired responses to protein and carbohydrate vaccines. Both the proband and her son have reduced switched memory B cells, and the proband is lymphopenic.

Given the discordant segregation studies, we suspected a second, causative mutation in this family [2]. With the advent of next-generation sequencing (NGS), the proband and her symptomatic son were shown to have an additional causative nonsense mutation of the *TCF3* gene (T168fsX191), after which they were reclassified as having a CVID-like disorder (see Fig. 7.1) [1]. The proband, who had both mutations, was much more severely affected than her son or other relatives, indicating quantitative epistasis, as discussed below. Asymptomatic family members carrying the *TNFRSF13B*/TACI C104R mutation have possible CVID, while others have a CVID-like disorder caused by a mutation of *TCF3*.

Case Presentation 2: Sarcoidosis or the Granulomatous Variant of CVID (GVCVID) [6]

A 22-year-old male presented at age 14 years with epistaxis related to severe thrombocytopenia. Immune thrombocytopenic purpura (ITP) was diagnosed, and he was initially treated with high doses of prednisone. Prior to immunosuppression, his immunoglobulins were in the normal range (IgG 8.8 g/l, nr 7-14). Following 5 months of glucocorticoid therapy, he became hypogammaglobulinemic (IgG 4.3 g/l).

Once the severe hypogammaglobulinemia was identified, he was treated with monthly IVIG (2 g/kg), with the added expectation that the immunomodulatory doses of IVIG would reduce his risk of infections as well as potentially benefitting his ITP [7]. He then developed Evans syndrome with autoimmune hemolytic anemia while on IVIG, in addition to the ITP. He eventually responded to IVIG, and the prednisone dose was tapered to 10 mg daily and stopped.

He was well until 2013 when his ITP relapsed. On this occasion, he did not respond to high-dose prednisone, vincristine, cyclosporine, cyclophosphamide, or rituximab. Due to ongoing cytopenias, he underwent a splenectomy in 2014. Histology revealed the presence of splenic granulomas. Although the splenectomy was not successful, he remitted with eltrombopag, an activator of thrombopoietin receptors, in 2014.

He remained well until early 2017 when he developed diplopia due to impaired eye abduction secondary to bilateral cranial VI nerve palsies. He had headaches, fever, and signs of meningism. Lumbar puncture showed an elevated CSF opening pressure, but protein and other cellular parameters were normal. CSF bacterial culture, fungal antigen tests, and viral PCR studies excluded infection.

He had widespread lymphadenopathy including mediastinal and abdominal lymphadenopathy on MRI scanning. Excision biopsy of a left inguinal lymph node showed the presence of discrete non-caseating granulomas, reactive follicles, and overall normal lymph node architecture [6]. Plasma cells were present although slightly reduced compared to a normal control. His serum angiotensin-converting enzyme (ACE) level was normal.

The following week he developed increasing gait instability and was readmitted to the hospital. CSF examination again showed an increased opening pressure (23 cm, nr <20) and a raised protein level. The cell count and glucose levels were once more normal. A repeat MRI scan of the brain and spine revealed enhancing lesions in the cauda equina roots suggestive of granulomatous inflammation. Given the location of inflammation, a biopsy was not possible. Nerve conduction tests of the lower limbs were consistent with nerve root involvement. Several months after starting glucocorticoids, a gallium PET scan showed enhancing lesions of the lacrimal gland.

PCR studies of the CSF and blood were negative for toxoplasma and tuberculosis (TB), the two main infectious differential diagnoses for granulomatous infections in New Zealand. He had not recently travelled internationally. He had a good response to IV methylprednisolone (1 g) monthly, low-dose oral prednisone and mycophenolate with resolution of headaches, fever, and gait abnormalities. The improvement was reflected in the blood parameters, with the CRP decreasing from 69 to 7 mg/l within a week and improving cytopenias.

In mid-2018 when the immunosuppression was lifted, his IgG increased from 3.0 to 8.8 g/l, and the previously decreased IgA and IgM also normalized. This confirmed that sarcoidosis rather than the granulomatous variant of CVID (GVCVID) was the underlying diagnosis. Shortly afterward, he developed progressive renal impairment with a creatinine clearance of 36 ml/min (nr >120). Renal biopsy showed 18/42 sclerosed glomeruli. No granulomas were identified. He was restarted on mycophenolate and low-dose prednisone. There was insufficient time to undertake vaccine challenge responses or detailed immunophenotyping studies before the immunosuppression was urgently recommenced. Over the following 6 months, the creatinine clearance increased to 66 ml/min. The family has undergone whole exome sequencing for diagnosis and gene discovery, but no causative mutation was identified.

Introduction

Common variable immunodeficiency (CVID) disorders are a rare group of primary immunodeficiencies (PIDs) of unknown cause but presumably due to inborn errors of immunity (IEI). CVID is characterized by late-onset antibody failure (LOAF), which leads to immune system failure (ISF) [8]. For reasons that are unclear, onset of symptoms can occur from early childhood to the eighth decade or later [9]. There is increasing evidence of viral infections of the Herpes genus can alter the prognostic trajectory of patients with CVID and CVID-like disorders, triggering onset of symptoms.

Current estimates suggest a prevalence between 1:25,000 and 1:100,000 in Caucasians [10, 11]. CVID appears to be less frequent in Asian and African populations, although there may be ascertainment bias.

Most CVID patients experience severe bacterial infections. Delayed diagnosis can lead to chronic suppuration of the respiratory tract, frequently resulting in chronic rhinosinusitis and bronchiectasis. There is also an increased risk of malignancy [12]. Unexpectedly, 15–25% of CVID patients suffer autoimmune or inflammatory complications, presumably from defects in immune regulation [13].

A proportion of CVID patients also develop a granulomatous disorder resembling sarcoidosis (GVCVID) [13]. Similar to sarcoidosis, GVCVID typically involves the lung, liver, and lymph nodes. A variety of thoracic radiological features can be seen in GVCVID including lymphadenopathy and interstitial lung disease [14, 15]. The pulmonary changes are collectively referred to as granulomatous-lymphocytic interstitial lung disease (GLILD) [16, 17]. Histological correlates of GLILD include non-caseating granulomas, follicular bronchiolitis and lymphoid interstitial pneumonitis. In contrast to sarcoidosis, plasma cells are absent in GVCVID, and germinal centers are often poorly formed or disrupted [18].

Genetics of CVID

At this time, the molecular explanation for patients with CVID remains to be established [19]. Mutations of the inducible T-cell co-stimulator (*ICOS*) were discovered in 2003 [19]. All affected individuals in the Black Forest area of Germany carried the identical mutation indicating a founder population. Different mutations of *ICOS* were subsequently identified in other parts of the world, confirming allelic heterogeneity [20].

Mutations of the T-cell activator, calcium modulator, and cyclophilin ligand interactor (*TNFRSF13B*/TACI) were found soon after the discovery of *ICOS* mutations [21]. *TNFRSF13B*/TACI plays a critical role in in B-cell signaling and immunoglobulin isotype switching through the non-CD40 pathway. Mutations of *TNFRSF13B*/TACI were initially thought to be causative in CVID patients, but it soon became obvious that the same mutations were found in the general population at a far greater frequency than the lifetime incidence of CVID [22].

These variants including *TNFRSF13B*/TACI BAFFR (*TNFRSF13C*), TWEAK (*TNFSF12*), *MSH5*, and TRAIL (*TNFSF10*) are now thought to predispose to or modify disease severity and remain within the broad spectrum of CVID, as they do not cause the disorder. With our recent demonstration of the role of *TNFRSF13B*/TACI in epistatic interactions with *TCF3* (Case 1), there is now a clear argument that mutations linked to CVID should be categorized according to whether they cause or modify the condition (Fig. 7.2) [5, 24]. Epistasis is the nonlinear, synergistic interaction

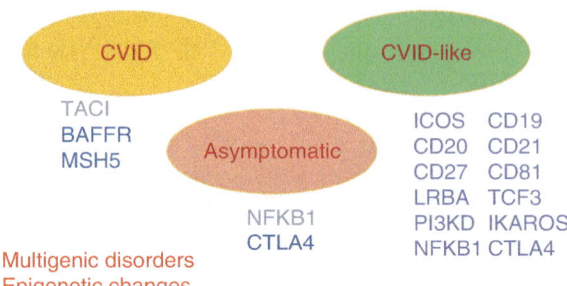

Fig. 7.2 The proposed relationship between CVID and CVID-like disorders and patients who are asymptomatic [23]. Digenic disorders should be considered CVID-like disorders as their cause is known

between two or more genetic loci leading either to a much more severe disorder or a different phenotype [1, 25]. The proband (Case 1), who carries both mutations, is much more severely affected than other members of the family (see Fig. 7.1).

In contrast, mutations of other genes including *NFKB1*, *NFKB2*, *CTLA4*, *TCF3*, etc. are causal [26, 27]. There is a high probability of symptomatic disease in individuals carrying these mutations. If a pathogenic mutation is identified, patients such as in Case 1 and her son are removed from the umbrella diagnosis of CVID and are reclassified as having a CVID-like disorder caused by a specific PID/IEI (see Fig. 7.2). All current diagnostic criteria exclude patients with known causes, which is the basis for removing such patients from the umbrella diagnosis of CVID [5, 28–30].

Locus heterogeneity (genocopy) is the most obvious feature of CVID-like disorders. Mutations of genes causing CVID-like disorders (*NFKB1*, *NFKB2*, *CTLA4*, *TCF3*, etc.) predominantly result in late-onset antibody failure leading to recurrent and severe infections as well as immune dysregulation causing autoimmunity [31]. This makes it very difficult to identify the mutated gene by clinical evaluation alone.

Occasionally, there may be clinical features such as alopecia and pituitary dysfunction, which suggest *NFKB2* mutations [31]. Severe autoimmunity might suggest *PIK3CD/PIK3R1* mutations (causing the activated protein kinase 3D syndrome, APDS) or *CTLA4/LRBA* mutations. Similarly, the presence of vasculitis in a patient with hypogammaglobulinemia could indicate *ADA2* deficiency [31]. Reduced numbers or absence of B cells may suggest *IKZF1/IKAROS* or some *TCF3* mutations [32].

CVID-like disorders are also characterized by phenotypic heterogeneity. This was illustrated in another NZ family where we co-discovered *NFKB1* mutations as a common cause for CVID-like disorders [23, 27]. All affected members of this kindred have heterozygous nonsense mutations of the *NFKB1* gene leading to haploinsufficiency. One affected brother was asymptomatic with normal immunoglobulins, while his sister recently passed away from late-onset combined immunodeficiency (LOCID) [23]. She had nodular regenerative hyperplasia of the liver, GLILD, cytopenias, and marginal zone non-Hodgkin's lymphoma. Our CVID disease severity score (CDSS) showed marked differences in clinical severity within the same family [3]. We speculated that the phenotypic heterogeneity could be a consequence of epigenetic influences, variable penetrance and expressivity, or, as we have shown in Case 1 [1], epistasis caused by gene-gene interactions.

In the last 15 years, approximately 40 genetic defects have been shown to predispose to CVID or to cause CVID-like disorders [31]. The marked genetic and phenotypic heterogeneity has precluded routine genetic analysis of CVID [33]. Serial

Sanger sequencing of this ever-increasing number of genes associated with CVID is an inefficient use of scarce resources [34].

Because of the poor yield, we have previously argued against routine Sanger sequencing of genes associated with CVID [28]. We believe there is now a good case for routine diagnostic genetic testing of patients with a CVID phenotype (Table 7.1) [35]. This change of strategy is both the result of identifying increasing

Table 7.1 Advantages of genetic diagnosis for patients with a CVID phenotype [35]

Establishing the diagnosis
Confirming the clinical diagnosis of a CVID-like disorder
Identifying novel presentations of other CVID-like disorders, e.g., LOCID
Identifying atypical presentations of other PIDs with hypogammaglobulinemia, e.g., XLP
Distinguishing genetic from acquired disorders, e.g., drug-induced hypogammaglobulinemia
Identifying digenic disorders
THA variability of IgG levels over time: some of these patients may have CVID-like disorders
Differences in diagnostic criteria for CVID: the presence of a CVID-like disorder will obviate the need to apply CVID diagnostic criteria
Identifying CVID-like disorders in patients who have already developed malignancy
Identifying CVID-like disorders in patients on SCIG/IVIG or immunosuppression
Treatment
Offering early SCIG/IVIG treatment for individuals carrying causative mutations
Identifying specific treatment options, e.g., abatacept for CTLA4/LRBA deficiency
Identifying patients who may benefit from gene-based therapy in the future
Prognosis
Asymptomatic patients with monogenic defects have a high probability of symptomatic disease, leading to long-term SCIG/IVIG treatment
May distinguish patients with THI, who may not recover till adulthood, and some have impaired vaccine responses
Presymptomatic testing
Where presymptomatic diagnosis (at any age) is not possible with protein-based tests, e.g., patients with CVID-like disorders who are asymptomatic with normal immunoglobulins
Diagnosis in infancy where conventional diagnostic tests are unreliable, e.g., because of transplacentally acquired IgG levels
Screening
Cascade screening of at-risk relatives with or without symptoms after genetic counseling
Identifying mutations from tissue samples from deceased relatives
Identifying mutations from Guthrie cards from deceased relatives
PID prevention
Prenatal diagnosis of chorionic villus sampling (CVS)
Preimplantation genetic diagnosis (PGD)
Research
Characterizing the role of molecules in cellular function
Assisting with the classification of primary immunodeficiency disorders
Identification of new genetic defects with trio analysis
Investigating animal models of CVID-like disorders
Identifying epistasis caused by digenic (or oligogenic) disorders

LOCID late-onset combined immunodeficiency, *SCIG/IVIG* subcutaneous of intravenous immunoglobulin treatment, *THA* transient hypogammaglobulinemia of adulthood, *THI* transient hypogammaglobulinemia of infancy, *XLP* X-linked lymphoproliferative disorder numbers of genetic defects and most importantly the advent of next-generation sequencing (NGS) technology [31]. In Table 7.1, the many overlapping advantages of identifying a causative mutation in patients with a CVID phenotype are summarized [36, 37].

Diagnostic Criteria in the Absence of a Causative Mutation

Case 2 illustrates the difficulty in making a diagnosis of CVID while on immunosuppression and IVIG treatment [13]. Standard diagnostic tests including vaccine responses were not possible, and he did not have a causative mutation. Given the presence of granulomas, the main differential diagnosis was sarcoidosis. GVCVID and sarcoidosis are both associated with organ dysfunction caused by multisystem granulomas [38]. There is a marked difference in long-term prognosis between the two conditions [39]. There are other important therapeutic advantages in determining the exact underlying condition. Patients without an underlying immunodeficiency may be better able to tolerate immunosuppression. Some drugs such as TNF inhibitors may be more effective for neurosarcoidosis than GVCVID.

Careful review of his lymph node histology and immunohistochemistry studies showed the presence of CD138+ staining plasma cells and intact germinal centers. Although plasma cells were reduced compared to the control, their presence is diagnostic of sarcoidosis, in the absence of other granulomatous disorders. The histological findings were strongly in favor of sarcoidosis during the period of IVIG treatment and immunosuppression [18]. The subsequent normalization of his immunoglobulins excluded GVCVID in Case 2, confirming the value of histology in making the correct diagnosis.

Because the etiology of CVID is unknown, there is no single clinical or laboratory feature which is pathognomonic for these disorders. In areas of uncertainty, diagnostic criteria can be very helpful. Diagnostic criteria for CVID continue to evolve [35]. The previous ESID/PAGID (1999) and the more recent ICON (2016) diagnostic criteria for CVID emphasize poor vaccine responses [28, 40]. Serological responses to vaccines can, however, be difficult to assess when patients are either being treated with subcutaneous or intravenous immunoglobulin (SCIG/IVIG) or when immunosuppressed for autoimmunity. Furthermore, our recent NZ hypogammaglobulinemia study (NZHS) has shown the variability of vaccine responses in such patients [36]. The ESID/PAGID (1999) and ICON (2016) criteria do not explicitly include any of the characteristic histological features of CVID. These vaccine-based CVID diagnostic criteria are thus difficult to apply to complex cases such as Case 2.

Prior to recovery of his IgG, Case 2 had many of the features of the revised ESID registry (2014) criteria for CVID as he had a granulomatous disorder, reduction in IgG and IgA, and absent switched memory B cells with an age of onset greater than 4 years. He did not, however, meet the revised ESID registry (2014) criteria for CVID because of the immunosuppression, where a secondary cause could not be excluded [30]. The absence of plasma cells is not part of the revised ESID registry (2014) criteria, which was probably the most important clue in allowing the correct diagnosis, prior to normalization of his immunoglobulins.

The second case illustrates the value of our CVID diagnostic criteria during the period of IVIG treatment and immunosuppression (Table 7.2). In 2013, we described new diagnostic criteria for CVID [5, 24]. These criteria include clinical, serological, and histological features of the disorder, which allows a more precise diagnosis. CVID was previously a diagnosis of exclusion but can now be made with greater certainty. To fulfill our CVID criteria, patients are required to have symptomatic hypogammaglobulinemia with no other explanation for the disorder. Supportive serological markers include poor or transient vaccine responses, absent

Table 7.2 New CVID diagnostic criteria [5] for CVID

A	Must meet all major criteria
	Hypogammaglobulinemia IgG <5 g/l [41] No other cause identified for immune defect [42] Age >4 years [43]
B	Sequelae directly attributable to immune system failure (ISF) (one or more)
	Recurrent, severe, or unusual infections Poor response to antibiotics Breakthrough infections in spite of prophylactic antibiotics Infections in spite of appropriate vaccination, e.g., HPV disease Bronchiectasis and/or chronic sinus disease Inflammatory disorders or autoimmunity [44]
C	Supportive laboratory evidence (three or more criteria)
	Concomitant reduction or deficiency of IgA (<0.8 g/l) and/or IgM (0.4 g/l) [45, 46] Presence of B cells but reduced memory B-cell subsets and/or increased CD21 low subsets by flow cytometry [47] IgG3 deficiency (<0.2 g/l) [48, 49] Impaired vaccine responses compared to age-matched controls [50] Transient vaccine responses compared with age-matched controls [2, 51] Absent isohemagglutinins (if not blood group AB) [52] Serological evidence of significant autoimmunity, e.g., Coombes test Sequence variations of genes predisposing to CVID, e.g., *TACI, BAFFR, MSH5*, etc. [22, 53]
D	Presence of relatively specific histological markers of CVID (not required for diagnosis but presence increases diagnostic certainty, in the context of Category A and B criteria)
	Lymphoid interstitial pneumonitis [54] Granulomatous disorder [13, 55] Nodular regenerative hyperplasia of the liver [56, 57] Nodular lymphoid hyperplasia of the gut [58] Absence of plasma cells on gut biopsy [59, 60]

Meeting criteria in categories ABC or ABD indicates probable CVID. Patients meeting criteria ABC and ABD should be treated with IVIG/SCIG (see Fig. 7.1). Patients meeting criteria A alone, AB or AC, or AD but not B are termed possible CVID. Some of these patients may need to be treated with IVIG/SCIG. Patients with levels of IgG >5 g/l, not meeting any other criteria, are termed hypogammaglobulinemia of uncertain significance (HGUS) [5]. These diagnostic criteria must be applied sequentially as none are specific individually isohemagglutinins, and IgG3, IgA, or IgM deficiency along with tests for significant autoimmunity.

Importantly, our CVID diagnostic criteria also include histological features of the disorder such as the absence of plasma cells (Category D of the Ameratunga et al. (2013) criteria). While these histological features can occur in other disorders, the primary symptomatic hypogammaglobulinemia confers specificity for CVID in our criteria [32].

Our reasoning was that histological features may be particularly useful, when SCIG/IVIG treatment or immunosuppression preclude assessing serological tests, as seen in Case 2. They can also be helpful in historical cases where the patient is deceased, if archived histological specimens are available from previous investigations. We have previously shown that histological features of our diagnostic criteria (see Table 7.2) were similarly helpful in another patient who had both CVID and drug-induced hypogammaglobulinemia [61].

Conclusion

We advise careful clinical and laboratory review of patients presenting with hypogammaglobulinemia to exclude secondary causes. We suggest early genetic testing in appropriate patients to determine if they have a CVID-like disorder, as seen in Case 1. If there is no obvious secondary cause or genetic explanation, we recommend application of our CVID diagnostic criteria to these patients. Given the limitations of protein-based tests, Case 2 highlights the value of histology in being able to make a firm diagnosis during IVIG treatment and immunosuppression, when protein-based tests cannot be applied. Patients with a diagnosis of CVID should also be periodically reviewed as it is possible that a causative mutation may be identified with the advent of new technology as seen in Case 1.

Clinical Pearls and Pitfalls
- At least 25% of patients with a CVID phenotype have a causative mutation. Therefore, all patients with a CVID phenotype should be offered genetic testing.
- The presence of a causative mutation excludes CVID, and patients are reclassified as having a CVID-like disorder.
- In the absence of a causative mutation, diagnostic criteria may be helpful in establishing the diagnosis of CVID with greater precision.
- Histology can provide helpful diagnostic information, particularly in patients on immunosuppression or those who have already commenced SCIG/IVIG, where protein-based studies are problematic.

Acknowledgments We thank our patients for participating in our studies for the benefit of others. We hope our studies will be of direct benefit to patients and their families. We thank the A+ Trust, AMRF, IDFNZ, and ASCIA for grant support.

The authors do not have any conflicts of interest.

References

1. Ameratunga R, Koopmans W, Woon ST, Leung E, Lehnert K, Slade CA, et al. Epistatic interactions between mutations of TACI (TNFRSF13B) and TCF3 result in a severe primary immunodeficiency disorder and systemic lupus erythematosus. Clin Transl Immunology. 2017;6:e159.
2. Koopmans W, Woon ST, Brooks AE, Dunbar PR, Browett P, Ameratunga R. Clinical variability of family members with the C104R mutation in transmembrane activator and calcium modulator and cyclophilin ligand interactor (TACI). J Clin Immunol. 2013;33:68–73.
3. Ameratunga R. Assessing disease severity in common variable immunodeficiency disorders (CVID) and CVID-like disorders. Front Immunol. 2018;9:2130.
4. Agarwal S, Cunningham-Rundles C. Treatment of hypogammaglobulinemia in adults: a scoring system to guide decisions on immunoglobulin replacement. J Allergy Clin Immunol. 2013;131:1699–701.
5. Ameratunga R, Woon ST, Gillis D, Koopmans W, Steele R. New diagnostic criteria for common variable immune deficiency (CVID), which may assist with decisions to treat with intravenous or subcutaneous immunoglobulin. Clin Exp Immunol. 2013;174:203–11.
6. Ameratunga R, Ahn Y, Tse D, Woon ST, Pereira J, McCarthy S, et al. The critical role of histology in distinguishing sarcoidosis from common variable immunodeficiency disorder (CVID) in a patient with hypogammaglobulinemia. Allergy Asthma Clin Immunol. 2019;15:78.
7. Ameratunga R. Initial intravenous immunoglobulin doses should be based on adjusted body weight in obese patients with primary immunodeficiency disorders. Allergy Asthma Clin Immunol. 2017;13:47.
8. Abbott JK, Gelfand EW. Common variable immunodeficiency: diagnosis, management, and treatment. Immunol Allergy Clin North Am. 2015;35:637–58.
9. Gathmann B, Mahlaoui N, CEREDIH, Gérard L, Oksenhendler E, Warnatz K, et al. Clinical picture and treatment of 2212 patients with common variable immunodeficiency. J Allergy Clin Immunol. 2014;134:116–26.
10. Selenius JS, Martelius T, Pikkarainen S, Siitonen S, Mattila E, Pietikäinen R, et al. Unexpectedly high prevalence of common variable immunodeficiency in Finland. Front Immunol. 2017;8:1190.
11. Westh L, Mogensen TH, Dalgaard LS, Bernth Jensen JM, Katzenstein T, Hansen AE, et al. Identification and characterization of a nationwide Danish adult common variable immunodeficiency cohort. Scand J Immunol. 2017;85:450–61.
12. Kralickova P, Milota T, Litzman J, Malkusova I, Jilek D, Petanova J, et al. CVID-Associated tumors: Czech Nationwide Study focused on epidemiology, immunology, and genetic background in a cohort of patients with CVID. Front Immunol. 2018;9:3135.
13. Ameratunga R, Becroft DM, Hunter W. The simultaneous presentation of sarcoidosis and common variable immune deficiency. Pathology. 2000;32:280–2.
14. de Boer S, Wilsher M. Review series: aspects of interstitial lung disease. Sarcoidosis. Chron Respir Dis. 2010;7:247–58.
15. Jolles S, Carne E, Brouns M, El-Shanawany T, Williams P, Marshall C, et al. FDG PET-CT imaging of therapeutic response in granulomatous lymphocytic interstitial lung disease (GLILD) in common variable immunodeficiency (CVID). Clin Exp Immunol. 2017;187:138–45.
16. Prasse A, Kayser G, Warnatz K. Common variable immunodeficiency-associated granulomatous and interstitial lung disease. Curr Opin Pulm Med. 2013;19:503–9.

17. Verbsky JW, Routes JM. Sarcoidosis and common variable immunodeficiency: similarities and differences. Semin Respir Crit Care Med. 2014;35:330–5.
18. Unger S, Seidl M, Schmitt-Graeff A, Böhm J, Schrenk K, Wehr C, et al. Ill-defined germinal centers and severely reduced plasma cells are histological hallmarks of lymphadenopathy in patients with common variable immunodeficiency. J Clin Immunol. 2014;34:615–26.
19. Grimbacher B, Hutloff A, Schlesier M, Glocker E, Warnatz K, Dräger R, et al. Homozygous loss of ICOS is associated with adult-onset common variable immunodeficiency. Nat Immunol. 2003;4:261–8.
20. Schepp J, Chou J, Skrabl-Baumgartner A, Arkwright PD, Engelhardt KR, Hambleton S, et al. 14 Years after discovery: clinical follow-up on 15 patients with inducible co-stimulator deficiency. Front Immunol. 2017;8:964.
21. Salzer U, Chapel HM, Webster AD, Pan-Hammarström Q, Schmitt-Graeff A, Schlesier M, et al. Mutations in TNFRSF13B encoding TACI are associated with common variable immunodeficiency in humans. Nat Genet. 2005;37:820–8.
22. Pan-Hammarstrom Q, Salzer U, Du L, Björkander J, Cunningham-Rundles C, Nelson DL, et al. Reexamining the role of TACI coding variants in common variable immunodeficiency and selective IgA deficiency. Nat Genet. 2007;39:429–30.
23. Ameratunga R, Ahn Y, Jordan A, Lehnert K, Brothers S, Woon ST. Keeping it in the family: the case for considering late onset combined immunodeficiency a subset of common variable immunodeficiency disorders. Expert Rev Clin Immunol. 2018;14:549–56.
24. Ameratunga R, Woon ST, Gillis D, Koopmans W, Steele R. New diagnostic criteria for CVID. Expert Rev Clin Immunol. 2014;10:183–6.
25. Ameratunga R, Woon ST, Bryant VL, Steele R, Slade C, Leung EY, et al. Clinical implications of digenic inheritance and epistasis in primary immunodeficiency disorders. Front Immunol. 2018;8:1965.
26. de Valles-Ibanez G, Esteve-Sole A, Piquer M, González-Navarro EA, Hernandez-Rodriguez J, Laayouni H, et al. Evaluating the genetics of common variable immunodeficiency: monogenetic model and beyond. Front Immunol. 2018;9:636.
27. Fliegauf M, Bryant VL, Frede N, Slade C, Woon ST, Lehnert K, et al. Haploinsufficiency of the NF-κB1 subunit p50 in common variable immunodeficiency. Am J Hum Genet. 2015;97:389–403.
28. Ameratunga R, Brewerton M, Slade C, Jordan A, Gillis D, Steele R, et al. Comparison of diagnostic criteria for common variable immunodeficiency disorder. Front Immunol. 2014;5:415.
29. Bonilla FA, Barlan I, Chapel H, Costa-Carvalho BT, Cunningham-Rundles C, de la Morena MT, et al. International Consensus Document (ICON): common variable immunodeficiency disorders. J Allergy Clin Immunol Pract. 2016;4:38–59.
30. Seidel MG, Kindle G, Gathmann B, Quinti I, Buckland M, van Montfrans J, et al. The European Society for Immunodeficiencies (ESID) Registry working definitions for the clinical diagnosis of inborn errors of immunity. J Allergy Clin Immunol Pract. 2019;7(6):1763–70.
31. Ameratunga R, Lehnert K, Woon ST, Gillis D, Bryant VL, Slade CA, et al. Review: diagnosing common variable immunodeficiency disorder in the era of genome sequencing. Clin Rev Allergy Immunol. 2018;54:261–8.
32. Ameratunga R, Woon ST. Perspective: evolving concepts in the diagnosis and understanding of common variable immunodeficiency disorders (CVID). Clin Rev Allergy Immunol. 2019;13:019–08765.
33. Ameratunga R, Steele R, Jordan A, Preece K, Barker R, Brewerton M, et al. The case for a national service for primary immune deficiency disorders in New Zealand. N Z Med J. 2016;129:75–90.
34. Woon ST, Ameratunga R. Comprehensive genetic testing for primary immunodeficiency disorders in a tertiary hospital: 10-year experience in Auckland, New Zealand. Allergy Asthma Clin Immunol. 2016;12:65.
35. Ameratunga R, Lehnert K, Woon S-T. All patients with common variable immunodeficiency disorders (CVID) should be routinely offered diagnostic genetic testing. Front Immunol. 2019;10:2678.

36. Ameratunga R, Ahn Y, Steele R, Woon S-T. The natural history of untreated primary hypogammaglobulinemia in adults: implications for the diagnosis and treatment of common variable immunodeficiency disorders (CVID). Front Immunol. 2019;10:1541.
37. Ameratunga R, Ahn Y, Steele R, Woon ST. Transient hypogammaglobulinemia of infancy: many patients recover in adolescence and adulthood. Clin Exp Immunol. 2019;198(2):224–32.
38. Shanks AM, Alluri R, Herriot R, Dempsey O. Misdiagnosis of common variable immune deficiency. BMJ Case Rep. 2014;2014:bcr2013202806. https://doi.org/10.1136/bcr-2013-202806.
39. Bouvry D, Mouthon L, Brillet PY, Kambouchner M, Ducroix JP, Cottin V, et al. Granulomatosis-associated common variable immunodeficiency disorder: a case-control study versus sarcoidosis. Eur Respir J. 2013;41:115–22.
40. Ameratunga R, Gillis D, Steele R. Diagnostic criteria for common variable immunodeficiency disorders. J Allergy Clin Immunol Pract. 2016;4:1017–8.
41. Oksenhendler E, Gerard L, Fieschi C, Malphettes M, Mouillot G, Jaussaud R, et al. Infections in 252 patients with common variable immunodeficiency. Clin Infect Dis. 2008;46:1547–54.
42. Agarwal S, Cunningham-Rundles C. Assessment and clinical interpretation of reduced IgG values. Ann Allergy Asthma Immunol. 2007;99:281–3.
43. Chapel H, Cunningham-Rundles C. Update in understanding common variable immunodeficiency disorders (CVIDs) and the management of patients with these conditions. Br J Haematol. 2009;145:709–27.
44. Knight AK, Cunningham-Rundles C. Inflammatory and autoimmune complications of common variable immune deficiency. Autoimmun Rev. 2006;5:156–9.
45. Cunningham-Rundles C, Bodian C. Common variable immunodeficiency: clinical and immunological features of 248 patients. Clin Immunol (Orlando, Fla). 1999;92:34–48.
46. Chapel H, Lucas M, Lee M, Bjorkander J, Webster D, Grimbacher B, et al. Common variable immunodeficiency disorders: division into distinct clinical phenotypes. Blood. 2008;112:277–86.
47. Wehr C, Kivioja T, Schmitt C, Ferry B, Witte T, Eren E, et al. The EUROclass trial: defining subgroups in common variable immunodeficiency. Blood. 2008;111:77–85.
48. Abrahamian F, Agrawal S, Gupta S. Immunological and clinical profile of adult patients with selective immunoglobulin subclass deficiency: response to intravenous immunoglobulin therapy. Clin Exp Immunol. 2010;159:344–50.
49. Olinder-Nielsen AM, Granert C, Forsberg P, Friman V, Vietorisz A, Bjorkander J. Immunoglobulin prophylaxis in 350 adults with IgG subclass deficiency and recurrent respiratory tract infections: a long-term follow-up. Scand J Infect Dis. 2007;39:44–50.
50. Musher DM, Manof SB, Liss C, McFetridge RD, Marchese RD, Bushnell B, et al. Safety and antibody response, including antibody persistence for 5 years, after primary vaccination or revaccination with pneumococcal polysaccharide vaccine in middle-aged and older adults. J Infect Dis. 2010;201:516–24.
51. Grabenstein JD, Manoff SB. Pneumococcal polysaccharide 23-valent vaccine: long-term persistence of circulating antibody and immunogenicity and safety after revaccination in adults. Vaccine. 2012;30:4435–44.
52. Tiller TL Jr, Buckley RH. Transient hypogammaglobulinemia of infancy: review of the literature, clinical and immunologic features of 11 new cases, and long-term follow-up. J Pediatr. 1978;92:347–53.
53. Salzer U, Bacchelli C, Buckridge S, Pan-Hammarström Q, Jennings S, Lougaris V, et al. Relevance of biallelic versus monoallelic TNFRSF13B mutations in distinguishing disease-causing from risk-increasing TNFRSF13B variants in antibody deficiency syndromes. Blood. 2009;113:1967–76.
54. Popa V. Lymphocytic interstitial pneumonia of common variable immunodeficiency. Ann Allergy. 1988;60:203–6.
55. Fasano MB, Sullivan KE, Sarpong SB, Wood RA, Jones SM, Johns CJ, et al. Sarcoidosis and common variable immunodeficiency. Report of 8 cases and review of the literature. Medicine (Baltimore). 1996;75:251–61.

56. Fuss IJ, Friend J, Yang Z, He JP, Hooda L, Boyer J, et al. Nodular regenerative hyperplasia in common variable immunodeficiency. J Clin Immunol. 2013;33:748–58.
57. Malamut G, Ziol M, Suarez F, Beaugrand M, Viallard JF, Lascaux AS, et al. Nodular regenerative hyperplasia: the main liver disease in patients with primary hypogammaglobulinemia and hepatic abnormalities. J Hepatol. 2008;48:74–82.
58. Luzi G, Zullo A, Iebba F, Rinaldi V, Sanchez Mete L, Muscaritoli M, et al. Duodenal pathology and clinical-immunological implications in common variable immunodeficiency patients. Am J Gastroenterol. 2003;98:118–21.
59. Malamut G, Verkarre V, Suarez F, Viallard JF, Lascaux AS, Cosnes J, et al. The enteropathy associated with common variable immunodeficiency: the delineated frontiers with celiac disease. Am J Gastroenterol. 2010;105:2262–75.
60. Agarwal S, Smereka P, Harpaz N, Cunningham-Rundles C, Mayer L. Characterization of immunologic defects in patients with common variable immunodeficiency (CVID) with intestinal disease. Inflamm Bowel Dis. 2011;17:251–9.
61. Ameratunga R, Lindsay K, Woon S-T, Jordan A, Anderson NE, Koopmans W. New diagnostic criteria could distinguish common variable immunodeficiency disorder from anticonvulsant-induced hypogammaglobulinemia. Clin Exp Neuroimmunol. 2015;6:83–8.

Part II
T-Cell Immunodeficiency

Chapter 8
Severe Combined Immunodeficiency

Jessica Galant-Swafford and Bob Geng

Introduction

Severe combined immunodeficiencies (SCID) are a heterogeneous group of rare, genetic diseases defined by significant lymphopenia resulting in complete lack of or profoundly impaired adaptive immune responses. If not diagnosed early, SCID can lead to life-threatening bacterial, fungal, and viral infections with both ordinary and opportunistic pathogens and is fatal without treatment. SCID was first reported in 1950 by Glanzmann and Rinker when they described Swiss infants with lymphopenia who died before 2 years of age [1]. SCID gained widespread attention in the 1980s when a movie described the life of David Vetter, the "bubble boy," a child with profound defects in cellular and humoral immunity who lived in isolation for over a decade because his brother had died of the disease. Unfortunately, David died from complications of an unsuccessful hematopoietic stem cell transplant (HSCT) in 1984.

Over the past 30 years, advances in molecular biology, genetics, and immunology have led to improved understanding of the pathophysiology of SCID and highlighted the importance of early treatment. Furthermore, the refinement of HSCT has revolutionized the care of these patients who likely would have died otherwise. Beginning in 2010, the incorporation of routine universal newborn screening (NBS) for SCID, now adopted by all 50 states, has greatly improved the detection and treatment of these patients with significantly reduced morbidity and mortality. Prior to NBS, retrospective data demonstrated a prevalence of SCID of 1/100,000 live births [2]; however,

J. Galant-Swafford
Department of Medicine, Division of Rheumatology, Allergy and Immunology, University of California, San Diego, San Diego, CA, USA

B. Geng (✉)
University of California, San Diego, and Rady Children's Hospital, Division of Allergy and Immunology, San Diego, CA, USA

© Springer Nature Switzerland AG 2021
J. A. Bernstein (ed.), *Primary and Secondary Immunodeficiency*,
https://doi.org/10.1007/978-3-030-57157-3_8

with the advent of screening and prospective analysis, the prevalence is understood to be about 1/58,000 live births [3]. Definitive management of SCID has traditionally required allogeneic HSCT; however, advanced therapies including gene therapy and gene editing have emerged as promising new therapeutic tools for particular subtypes of SCID. In this chapter, through the experiences of two real patient journeys, we will discuss basic principles in the diagnosis of SCID including interpreting newborn screening results and genetic sequencing, initial management considerations, and therapeutic options and challenges. Through the first case of a newborn infant, we will explore the initial clinical presentation as well as management of classic SCID, the value of the newborn screening, core concepts in immunophenotyping, utility of genotyping, and the basics of hematopoietic stem cell transplantation. From the second case of a teenager on chronic enzyme replacement for ADA deficiency, we will delve into nuances of this common subtype of SCID to illustrate the challenges of long-term clinical monitoring, benefits versus challenges of chronic enzyme replacement, and introduction to evolving and emerging curative treatments.

Case Presentation 1

We begin with the case of an abnormal newborn screening. A boy is born well at 39 weeks gestational age without perinatal complications. The newborn screening on his day of birth resulted in a TREC =1 (reference range >18). This result was confirmed with a repeat newborn screening, and subsequently flow cytometry testing was done (shown below). This is a representative report that one might expect to see from the Department of Public Health (Fig. 8.1). What conclusions can be drawn from these test results?

The most obvious initial finding is that the total white blood cell count is low, and, in particular, the absolute lymphocyte count is low for his age at 650 cells/μL. A low total lymphocyte count is often the first clue for detecting a cellular immune defect. The flow cytometry results show undetectable T cells for all T-cell subsets; there was notably absent naïve $CD4^+$ and $CD8^+$ T cells (CD3/CD45RA). T-lymphocyte differentiation and maturation can be further examined based on the expression of different isoforms of the common leukocyte antigen (CD45). Naïve cells express the high molecular weight isoform CD45RA; however, following stimulation, naive cells lose CD45RA and gain the low molecular weight isoform CD45RO, which is characteristic of the memory phenotype [4]. Therefore, the patient's flow cytometry results suggest absent naïve T cells (CD45RA). In patients with an absence of CD45RA cells, particularly an absence of recent thymic emigrants, naïve T cells expressing the surface marker CD31, the presence of CD45RO cells could represent T cells of maternal origin [5]. Returning to the laboratory results, we see that B cells are normal in number and expectedly higher in percentage, and NK cells are low normal in number and also higher in percentage. In summary, the results are consistent with a severe T-cell lymphopenia, in particular with a severe lack of naïve T cells. Is this SCID? What should we do next?

8 Severe Combined Immunodeficiency

Test	Result (* out of range)	Units
CBC (DIFF/PLT)		
WBC	7.7*	Thousand/μL
RBC	4.63	Million/μL
HGB	17.4	g/dL
HCT	48.0	%
MCV	103.7	fL
MCH	37.6*	pg
MCHC	36.3*	g/dL
PLT	370.0	Thousand/μL
MPV	11.2	fL
RDW	14.1	%
Absolute Neutrophils	3940	cells/μL
Absolute Lymphocytes	650*	cells/μL
Absolute Monocytes	2750*	cells/μL
Absolute Eosinophils	290	cells/μL
Absolute Basophils	40	cells/μL
Neutrophils	51.7	%
Lymphocytes	8.4	%
Monocytes	35.6	%
Eosinophils	3.8	%
Basophils	0.5	%
CD3+ T-Cells, Absolute	<20*	cells/μL
CD3+ T-Cells, Percent	1*	% of Lymphs
CD3+/CD4+ T-Helper, Abs	<20*	cells/μL
CD3+/CD4+ T-Helper, Percent	<1*	% of Lymphs
CD3+/CD8+ T-Cytotoxic, Abs	<20*	cells/μL
CD3+/CD8+ T-Cytotoxic, Percent	1*	% of Lymphs
CD19+ B-Cells, Absolute	433	cells/μL
CD19+ B-Cells, Percent	67*	% of Lymphs
CD16/CD56 NK-Cells, Abs	176	cells/μL
CD16/CD56 NK-Cells, Percent	27*	% of Lymphs
CD3/CD4/CD45RA, Absolute	<20*	cells/μL
CD3/CD4/CD45RA, Percent	<1	% of CD3/CD4
CD3/CD4/CD45RO, Absolute	<20*	cells/μL
CD3/CD4/CD45RO, Percent	<1*	% of CD3/CD4
CD3/CD8/CD45RA, Absolute	<20*	cells/μL
CD3/CD8/CD45RA, Percent	<1	% of CD3/CD8
CD3/CD8/CD45RO, Absolute	<20*	cells/μL
CD3/CD8/CD45RO, Percent	<1*	% of CD3/CD8

Fig. 8.1 Sample flow cytometry from a newborn screen

Diagnosis of SCID

The Primary Immune Deficiency Treatment Consortium (PIDTC) has established diagnostic criteria to distinguish between the two main subtypes of SCID: typical or atypical ("leaky") SCID (Table 8.1). Infants with typical SCID have <300 autologous T cells per μL, have very low T-cell function as measured by proliferative responses to the mitogen phytohemagglutinin (PHA) <10%, and may demonstrate the presence of T cells of maternal origin. Atypical SCID involves patients with reduced numbers of CD3 T cells defined by age, <30% of the lower limit of T-cell

Table 8.1 SCID definition according to the PIDTC

Type of SCID	CD3+ T-cell count	CD3+ T cell function	T cells of maternal origin
Typical SCID	<300/μL	<10% (lower limit of normal by response to PHA)	May be present
Atypical or "leaky" SCID	<1000/μL (up to age 2 years) <800/μL (up to age 4 years) <600/μL (>4 years)	<30%	Absent

Adapted from [110]

function, and an absence of maternal engraftment. Atypical SCID is usually the result of hypomorphic mutations that lead to a reduced, but not completely absent, T-cell compartment that is sufficient to prevent maternal engraftment, but not protective against infections.

An important distinguishing feature between typical and atypical SCID is the presence or absence of maternal T-cell engraftment. T cells of maternal origin that have crossed the placenta are present in approximately 40% of patients with SCID [6]. As discussed earlier, CD45RO cells in a patient with absent naive T cells can suggest T cells of maternal origin. While the immunocompetent fetus can reject the histocompatibility leukocyte antigen (HLA)-mismatched maternal lymphocytes, the SCID fetus fails to reject these. These maternally engrafted T cells express a restricted TCR repertoire and respond poorly to mitogens, explaining how they do not adequately protect the newborn from infections [7, 8]. These maternally engrafted cells can lead to multiorgan inflammation similar to GVHD and can interfere with the engraftment donor cells post-HSCT [9]. Typical SCID with maternal engraftment can look similar to leaky SCID with oligoclonal, but endogenous, T-cell populations. Therefore, it is important to evaluate for the presence of maternal engraftment in any newborn with SCID, which is done by using non inherited HLAs and variable-number tandem repeat analysis or fluorescent in situ hybridization (FISH). The absence of such cells is a diagnostic criterion for atypical SCID.

Omenn syndrome is a subset of atypical SCID in which CD3+ T cells are present; however, an oligoclonal proliferation of autoreactive memory T cells invades peripheral tissues and causes widespread inflammation, leading to a phenotype that is similar to graft-versus-host disease (GVHD). As a subset of atypical SCID, patients with Omenn syndrome must demonstrate detectable CD3 T cells ≥300/μL, <30% T-cell proliferation to PHA, and an absence of maternal engraftment. However, specifically, patients with Omenn syndrome must have other clinical features. Most commonly patients present with a generalized skin rash but may also have hepatosplenomegaly, lymphadenopathy, elevated IgE, and elevated absolute eosinophil counts. The presence of oligoclonal T cells, to be discussed later, can further support the diagnosis.

Case 1 Continued

Functional studies were completed to evaluate T-cell proliferation in our newborn boy. His report is seen in Fig. 8.2. The first step is to check the viability of the lymphocytes obtained by the laboratory. If the viability is low, then the sample may not be adequate to test proliferation. One common reason for low viability is that the sample is left unrefrigerated or unfrozen for a prolonged period of time. This is especially relevant when blood samples are being shipped to other institutions for processing. However, low viability can also be present in patients with T-cell lymphopenia. The next step is to evaluate nonspecific T-cell proliferation through stimulation with pokeweed mitogen (PWM) and phytohemagglutinin (PHA). Antigen-specific T-cell proliferation is usually not done as the newborn has not been exposed to a wide range of antigens and has not been vaccinated. The results indicate that he has nearly absent proliferation to stimulation with both PWM and PHA. PWM is a potent stimulator of B cells and is thus reported as a percentage of CD19 cells, whereas PHA is a potent stimulator of T cells and is reported as a percentage of CD3. Therefore, taken together with the flow cytometry results, our patient meets criteria for typical SCID.

Fig. 8.2 Laboratory test results during the initial workup of a patient with SCID

Viab of Lymphs at Day 0		MCR
⚠ 27.1 % [Low]		Reference Value ≥75.0
Max Prolif of PWM as % CD45		MCR
⚠ 0.7 % [Low]		Reference Value ≥4.5
Max Prolif of PWM as % CD3		MCR
⚠ 1.4 % [Low]		Reference Value ≥3.5
Max Prolif of PWM as % CD19		MCR
⚠ 0.0% [Low]		Reference Value ≥3.9
Max Prolif of PHA as % CD45		MCR
⚠ 0.1 % [Low]		Reference Value ≥49.9
Max Prolif of PHA as % CD3		MCR
⚠ 0.1 % [Low]		Reference Value ≥58.5

Newborn Screening for SCID

As SCID is a potentially life-threatening genetic disease for which pre-symptomatic detection and treatment is critical to survival, this condition is an ideal candidate for newborn screening (NBS). In August 2010, California instituted a state-wide screening program for SCID based on successful pilot programs, and it was added to the Recommended Uniform Screening Panel for all newborns. Using dried blood spots obtained routinely from newborns by heel stick, the SCID NBS test is a polymerase chain reaction (PCR) test that measures T-cell receptor excision circles (TRECs), which are DNA biomarkers of normal T-cell lymphopoiesis. Newborns with SCID have undetectable or low numbers of TRECs, though the cutoff between normal and abnormal is not standardized across locations. In the state in which the patient in our first case was diagnosed, the cutoff at the time was 18 TRECs/microliter.

In order to produce T cells with diverse antigen specificities, normal thymic maturation of T cells requires cutting and splicing of the DNA sequence encoding the T-cell antigen receptor (TCR) in a process called recombination. As a byproduct of this process, excised DNA forms T-cell receptor excision circles (TRECs) (Fig. 8.3). PCR amplification of the dRec-uJa TREC, which is one species of TRECs produced in late maturation by 70% of human T cells that express αβ TCRs, reflects the amount of newly formed T cells [10–12].

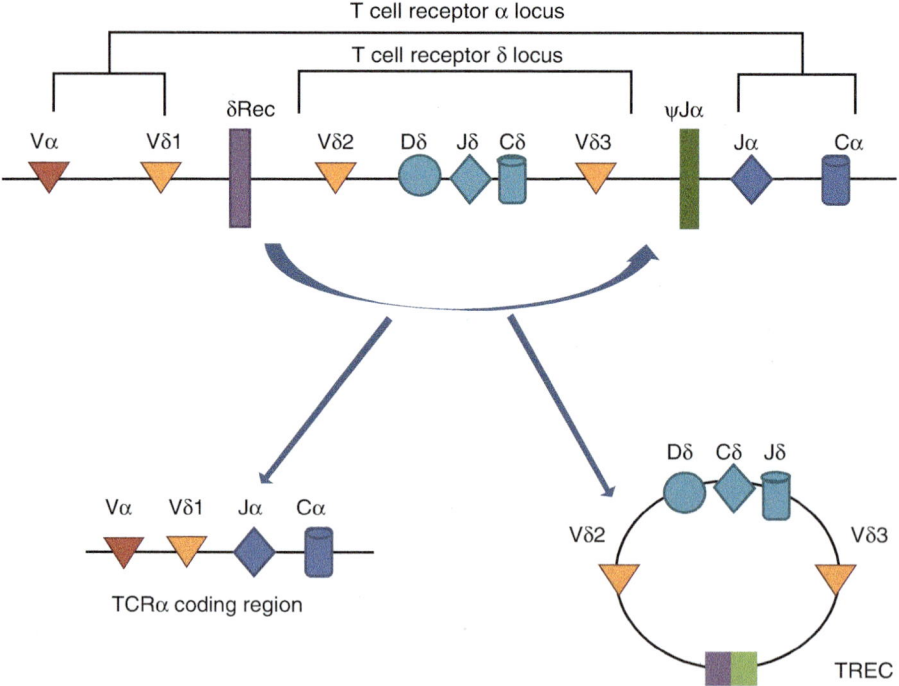

Fig. 8.3 Formation of T-cell receptor excision circles (TRECs). (Adapted from [112, 113])

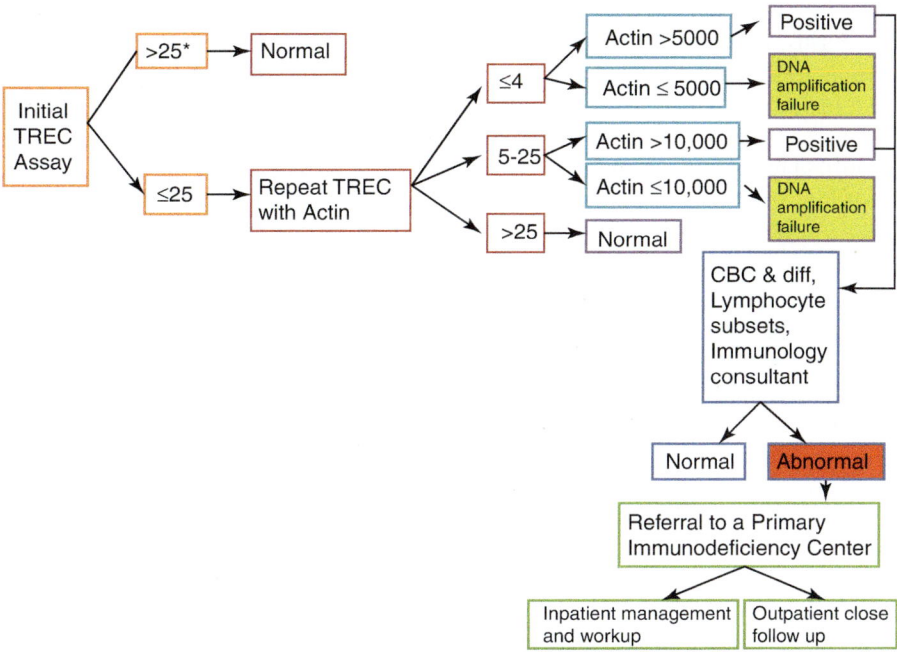

Fig. 8.4 Sample algorithm for newborn screening for SCID. (Adapted from [114]). *Threshold of 25 adapted from lower threshold seen in [16]

If the initial TREC assay is abnormal, an algorithm designed by the founders of the SCID NBS can help guide the next steps (Fig. 8.4). If initially abnormal, the PCR must be repeated with a ß-actin control which serves as a marker of DNA that is suitable for PCR. Once an abnormal TREC level is confirmed, the blood is sent for flow cytometry and T-cell subset characterization.

While SCID is defined by T-cell lymphopenia (TCL), not all TCL is SCID. For this reason, NBS for SCID can result in false positives. Abnormal TREC screens are readily seen in premature infants (<37 weeks of age). Genetic syndromes associated with T-cell lymphopenia, including DiGeorge syndrome (22q11 deletion), CHARGE syndrome (CHD7 mutation), ataxia telangiectasia, trisomy 21, and others, need to be distinguished from SCID as they have very different treatments such as thymus transplants for the complete DiGeorge syndrome patients. False negatives can also occur with NBS. For instance, patients with MHC II deficiency (bare lymphocyte syndrome) and ZAP70 mutations can have normal TRECs but will inevitably develop severe or recurrent infections [13, 14]. Therefore, patients with a high index of clinical suspicion for SCID should be referred for further testing even with a normal newborn screening.

By the end of 2018, SCID NBS was adopted population-wide in all 50 states including the District of Columbia, Puerto Rico, and also in many countries including Israel, Norway, and New Zealand. In examining the SCID NBS from 2010 to

2017 in California, clinically significant TCL was detected at a rate of 1 in 15,300 live births. Of these, 50 cases of SCID or (1 in 65,000 births) were identified and prompt treatment led to 94% survival. Infants with non-SCID TCL were also identified, including four patients with complete DiGeorge who underwent thymic transplants. Two infants with leaky SCID had normal TREC screens, but were clinically identified before age 2 of life [15].

While it is evident that screening has been critically effective in identifying cases of SCID, there is a lack of consensus in screening algorithms. Specifically, TREC cut-off values differ across states and countries and naturally affect the sensitivity and positive predictive value of the NBS for SCID. In the US, TREC cut-off values range from 25 to 252 [16]. One analysis found that the sensitivity of NBS for typical SCID across geographic locations was 100%; however, the positive predictive value was highly variable ranging from 0.8% to 11.2% for SCID and 18.3–81.0% for TCL. In this review, the individual TREC contents among all the patients with SCID was <25 TRECs/μL. In summary, a lower cut-off reduces the need for retesting and the number of false positives without necessarily compromising sensitivity.

Case 1 Continued

Upon referral to a pediatric hospital, a full history and physical examination was obtained. During the first 2 weeks of life, he had been well. He had not had fevers, cough, rash, vomiting, or diarrhea. He had been strictly breastfed since birth and had not had significant weight loss. Parents denied consanguinity, and he was their first child; mom had two miscarriages previously, both at 9–10 weeks of gestation. There was no family history of immunodeficiency, autoimmunity, or early childhood death. He received his routine hepatitis B vaccine at birth. He had not had any illnesses, had never been prescribed antibiotics, and was not taking any other medications.

Physical examination was notable for a 1.35% BMI with otherwise normal vital signs. The remainder of his examination was otherwise normal.

Clinical Presentation of SCID

The clinical presentation of SCID can vary widely. Typically, patients are asymptomatic at birth; however, within a few weeks or months, they may present with severe, recurrent, and atypical infections and failure to thrive. Infections with opportunistic and fungal organisms (*Pneumocystis jirovecii*, *Cryptococcus*, *Candida*) are commonly observed in SCID reflective of the defect in cellular immunity. Pulmonary infections due to common viral organisms (*respiratory syncytial virus* (RSV), *Myxovirus*, *Adenovirus*, *Influenza*) can lead to severe pneumonia requiring mechanical ventilation. Sepsis is common; bacterial infections with *Pseudomonas*, *Streptococcus*, and *Staphylococcus* species can quickly become diffuse and systemic. Intestinal infections with *Rotavirus*, *Norovirus*, and *Adenovirus* can cause chronic diarrhea leading to severe malnutrition and weight loss. Live vaccines such as *Rotavirus* or *Bacille Calmette-Guérin* (BCG) can lead to atypical infections. *Cytomegalovirus* (CMV) infection can lead to diffuse cardiac, liver, gastrointestinal, ocular, and even central nervous system involvement and is one of the most feared infections among SCID patients. In addition to infections, patients with Omenn syndrome can present with signs of diffuse autoimmunity that reflect widespread inflammation involving nearly every organ system.

A detailed history should be followed by a careful physical examination. History should focus on infections and hospitalizations. Family history should include investigating for family members with recurrent infections, known immunodeficiency diseases, autoimmune conditions, early childhood deaths, and consanguinity. The physical examination, particularly in those diagnosed via NBS, can seem normal; however, one should be on high alert for subtle findings and rapid changes in clinical status. Vital signs may show persistent or high fever, hypotension due to sepsis or dehydration, tachycardia or arrhythmia due to volume loss or myocardial infection, and tachypnea with hypoxemia in the setting of pulmonary infection. Patients with SCID are often underweight and may appear listless or cachectic on initial impression. Head and neck examination may reveal microcephaly or facial dysmorphia depending on the specific mutation. Oropharyngeal examination may demonstrate thrush secondary to candidiasis, and lymphadenopathy may be present. Lungs may be clear or may demonstrate wheezing or crackling in the setting of infection. The abdomen can be distended, and hepatosplenomegaly may be present. Extremities may demonstrate pitting edema, in the setting of protein loss from chronic diarrhea. Skin may appear normal, but generalized rash (specifically in Omenn syndrome), skin abscesses, and urticaria can be present. Non-SCID syndromes associated with T-cell lymphopenia can result in particular physical features. For example, patients with DiGeorge and CHARGE syndrome (coloboma, heart defects, choanal atresia, growth retardation, and genital and ear abnormalities) may demonstrate particular abnormal facies and cardiac abnormalities on examination.

Case 1 Continued

The newborn underwent extensive diagnostic testing while in the hospital. Results of some of this testing are detailed in Table 8.2.

Table 8.2 Additional laboratory test results for a patient with SCID

Complete blood count			Day of birth	Day 7 of life
	WBC (thousand/µL)		7.7	10.9
	HGB (million/µL)		17.4	18.5
	PLT (thousand/µL)		370	274
	ANC (cells/µL)		3940	7957
	ALC (cells/µL)		650	436
	AEC (cells/µL)		290	218
Complete metabolic panel	Normal			
Respiratory viral panel	Negative			
Blood, urine, stool culture	No growth			
HIV PCR	Negative			
CMV PCR	Negative			
Quantitative immunoglobulins	IgG 630 IgM 6 IgA <5 IgE <2			
Chest radiograph	Normal cardiothymic silhouette. Low lung volumes. No focal opacity. Mild ground glass opacities suggest atelectasis			
Echocardiogram	Patent foramen ovale with bidirectional atrial shunting, otherwise normal			
Chromosomal microarray	Normal			

WBC white blood count, *HGB* hemoglobin, *PLT* platelets, *ANC* absolute neutrophil count, *ALC* absolute lymphocyte count, *AEC* absolute eosinophil count

Laboratory Testing for SCID

If NBS is not available, SCID should be suspected in the presence of severe lymphopenia; however, a normal lymphocyte count can be due to maternal engraftment of T cells or autoreactive oligoclonal T-cell populations. Therefore, if a CBC is not available, SCID should be considered with a history of severe or recurrent infections or failure to thrive. The most important next diagnostic test is flow cytometry to analyze lymphocyte subpopulations and functional analysis. Thymic dysfunction is suggested by a lack of naïve T lymphocytes (CD3+CD4+CD45RA+CCR7+) or recent thymic emigrants (CD4+CD45RA+CD31+). Reduced proliferation to PHA can confirm the diagnosis of SCID; however, it can be difficult to interpret when T-lymphocyte counts are low. Antigen-specific simulation of T-cell proliferation, typically done with *Candida* or *Tetanus*, is often not useful for infants as they have not been exposed to these organisms or the tetanus vaccine. If diagnosed by NBS, CBC with differential and lymphocyte proliferation assays should be repeated in the hospital to confirm the results reported by the screening program and to evaluate for changes including the development of anemia or thrombocytopenia, worsening lymphopenia, or any recovery of T or B numbers or function.

If symptoms are suggestive of atypical SCID or Omenn syndrome, T-cell repertoire analysis can be important for evaluating oligoclonal maternal or autologous autoreactive T-lymphocyte populations. Diversity of the T-cell receptor is elemental to responding to a wide variety of different antigens. As discussed previously, T-cell receptor (TCR) precursors undergo gene rearrangements in the thymus, the same process that generates TRECs. During VDJ recombination, one allele in each gene segment is recombined with others to form a variable region, which is then combined with a constant gene segment to form a functional TCR transcript. The variable region of TCRα and TCRδ chains are encoded by variable (V) and joining (J) genes, while the TCRß and TCRγ chains are encoded by diversity (D) genes. As well, random nucleotides are added or deleted at junction sites. The combinatorial variation from VDJ recombination in addition to the junctional diversity of nucleotide addition and deletion creates a highly variable TCR repertoire [17, 18]. Then, the rearranged TCRα and TCRß chains pair to yield the TCR heterodimers, which determines the antigen specificity for new T cells. The structure of each TCR contains three complementarity determining regions (CDR1-3). CDR3 is most essential for the interaction of TCR with the peptide-MHC complex and accounts for the majority of the variability of a TCR [19]. CDR3 is encoded in the junctional region between the V and J or D and J genes. In particular, the Vß-Jß region is associated with the greatest variability. Analysis of the CDR3 in a population of T cells, using polymerase chain reaction of the individual Vß family genes, can thus provide a measure of TCR diversity [20]. Skewing of the TCR repertoire, or reduced variability such that one or more Vß CDR3 transcripts is disproportionately represented, is often seen in atypical SCID and predisposes to the autoinflammatory phenotype seen in these patients [21, 22].

An infectious workup is critically important in the evaluation of SCID and T-cell lymphopenia, as these patients will not mount a normal immune response to infections and can show evidence of infection even with a normal examination. Obtaining blood, urine, sputum, and CSF cultures is guided by clinical history and physical examination. HIV status must be assessed due to its association with CD4+ T-cell lymphopenia. PCR or antigen testing for HSV, EBV, hepatitis B, parvovirus B19, respiratory viruses, and rotavirus should also be done keeping in mind that serologic testing is insufficient and can be misleading since humoral immunity is likely impaired and IgG is mostly maternal during the first 4–6 months of life. CMV PCR shells should be checked weekly for the first 4 weeks and then at routine intervals. A metabolic panel can be especially useful to evaluate calcium levels (which can be abnormal in DiGeorge syndrome), albumin levels (which could suggest protein-calorie malnutrition), and bilirubin levels and test renal and liver function for autoimmune or infectious inflammation which is also helpful for establishing a baseline for administering prophylactic antibiotics.

Immunoglobulin levels may be difficult to interpret as IgG levels are of mostly of maternal origin for the first few months of life, and IgA can be absent in the normally functioning infant immune system. Hypogammaglobulinemia in a newborn may relate more to a protein-losing process such as nephropathy or enteropathy. However, increased IgE is a usual component of Omenn syndrome and can be present even in the setting of significant B-cell lymphopenia.

It is important to rule out DiGeorge syndrome or other thymic disorders for which the therapeutic strategy would involve thymic transplantation. Unless concern for radiosensitive SCID exists, chest radiograph should be completed to look for absence of a thymic shadow, which can be present in SCID and DiGeorge syndrome. Echocardiography to evaluate for cardiac abnormalities seen in DiGeorge or CHARGE syndrome is also an important imaging tool. Adenosine deaminase (ADA) and purine nucleoside phosphorylase (PNP) enzyme and purine metabolite testing should be completed to evaluate for particular phenotypes of SCID especially if genetic testing is delayed. HLA typing should be done on the infant, parents, and full siblings, to evaluate the latter as potential HCT donors. Chromosomal microarray to evaluate for DiGeorge syndrome (22q11 deletion) should be done if available.

Case 1 Continued

For our representative case, his examination and results are consistent with a diagnosis of typical SCID, specifically T-B+NK- SCID. His results do not suggest DiGeorge syndrome or other non-SCID T cell lymphopenia. While his NK cell count is on the cusp of the lower limit of normal, these cells are likely also dysfunctional.

Immunophenotypic Classification of SCID

Prior to the widespread availability of genetic sequencing, immunophenotyping of SCID based on the prevalence of T, B, and NK cells helped to predict which stage of immune cell development or function was affected [23]. In typical SCID, the immunophenotype is characterized by an absence or profound decrease in T cells, while the effect on the B-cell and NK-cell compartment depends on the underlying defect. Patients with T-B+NK+ SCID are those who have defects specific to T-cell development but leave other cells spared; these include defects in the TCR (CD3 complex) or T-cell survival signaling (IL-7R defects). Those with T-B-NK+ SCID have defects that affect developmental pathways which T and B cells have in common, such as the formation of the TCR and BCR. Recombination-activating gene 1 (*RAG1*) and recombination-activating gene 2 (*RAG2*) encode proteins expressed early in T- and B-cell development and initiate the process of V(D)J recombination by introducing DNA double-strand breaks (DSB) [24, 25]. The result is the formation of a sealed hairpin coding end and a blunt signal end, which are joined by means of non-homologous end joining (NHEJ) pathway, a process that depends on genes such as Artemis nuclease (*DCLRE1C*), which, in complex with DNA-dependent protein kinase (*PRKDC*), binds to and cleaves the DNA hairpin exposing the 3′ termini to the deletion and addition of nucleotides that contribute ultimately to TCR diversity. DSB are ultimately joined by DNA ligase 4 (*LIG4*) [26, 27]. Therefore, defects in *RAG1*, *RAG2*, *DCLRE1C*, *PRKDC*, and *LIG4* can all lead to T-B-NK+ SCID. Patients with T-B+NK- SCID are those in which pathways affecting only T and NK cells are affected but B cells are spared. These include defects in the common gamma chain (γ_c chain), which forms part of the receptor for multiple cytokines including T-cell survival signals IL-2 and IL-7, signals promoting T-cell differentiation including IL-4 and IL-9, and NK-cell survival signals IL-15 and IL-21 [28–32]. A key signaling molecule in this pathway is the Janus kinase 3 (*JAK3*), a tyrosine-protein kinase that binds to the γ_c chain and helps initiate signaling [33]. Therefore, defects in the γ_c chain [29, 34] and *JAK3* [35] are associated with T-B+NK- SCID. Lastly, processes that affect all three cell lines leading to T-B-NK- SCID are those characterized by defects in the hematopoietic lymphoid progenitor or the accumulation of toxic metabolites. For example, adenosine deaminase (ADA) deficiency results in the accumulation of toxic metabolites of the purine salvage pathway which cause widespread damage to multiple cell types and organ systems. Similarly, mutations in the *AK2* gene, which codes for a protein that is a key regulator of mitochondrial metabolism, lead to defective differentiation and proliferation of hematopoietic stem cells, which affects all lymphocyte lineages [36].

Case 1 Continued

Our newborn boy subsequently underwent whole genome sequencing (Fig. 8.5). He was found to have a pathogenic mutation in the gene *IL2RG*. This mutation is associated with X-linked SCID, and, expectedly, sequencing of the patient's mother confirmed the presence of this variant.

Genetic Classification of SCID

Over 90% of patients with SCID can be genetically characterized (Table 8.3) [37]. The advent of widespread genetic sequencing has revolutionized the identification and stratification SCID patients; however, understanding the immunophenotype is

> **TEST RESULT:** A pathogenic, hemizygous c.676C>T. p.Arg226Cys variant in the IL2RG gene was detected in this individual. Pathogenic variation in IL2RG is associated with X-linked combined immunodeficiency (OMIM: 300400). This variant was confirmed by Sanger sequencing. Analysis of the maternal sample was positive for the variant. Analysis of the paternal sample was not applicable to this variant due to the X-linked inheritance.

Patient phenotype

Combined immunodeficiency

Primary findings - Variants in genes associated with patient's reported phenotype

Confirmation status	Gene & transcript	Condition	Chromosome: genomic coordinates	Variant	Zygosity	Inheritance	Classifaction
Confirmed	IL2RG ENST00000374202	Combined immun odeficiency, X-Linked	x70329159	c.676C>T pArg226Cys	Hemizygous		Pathogenic

Fig. 8.5 Sample genetic test result for X-linked SCID

Table 8.3 Classification of SCID

Immunophenotype	Disease	Genetic defect	Inheritance	Distinguishing clinical features
T-B+NK+	IL7Rα	*IL7R*	AR	Failure to thrive, chronic diarrhea, recurrent pneumonia
	CD45 deficiency	*PTPRC*	AR	Same as above
	CD3δ deficiency	*CD3D*	AR	Same as above
	CD3ε deficiency	*CD3E*	AR	Same as above
	CD3ξ deficiency	*CD247*	AR	Same as above
	Coronin-1A deficiency	*CORO1A*	AR	Same as above
	LAT deficiency	*LAT*	AR	Same as above
T-B+NK-	γc deficiency (common gamma chain SCID, CD132 deficiency, X-linked SCID)	*IL2RG*	XL	Infant males, chronic diarrhea candidiasis, dermatitis
	CD25 deficiency	*IL2RA*	AR	IPEX-like: chronic diarrhea, endocrinopathy, dermatitis
	JAK3 deficiency	*JAK3*	AR	Chronic diarrhea, candidiasis, pneumonia, dermatitis, warts
T-B-NK+	RAG 1 deficiency	*RAG1*	AR	Failure to thrive, chronic diarrhea, candidiasis *Pneumocystis jirovecii* pneumonia
	RAG 2 deficiency	*RAG2*	AR	Same as above
	DCLRE1C (Artemis) deficiency	*DCLRE1C*	AR	Same as above
	DNA PKcs deficiency	*PRKDC*	AR	Same as above
	Cernunnos/XLF	*NHEJ1*	AR	Radiosensitivity, growth retardation, microcephaly/bird-like facies, malignancy
	DNA Ligase IV deficiency	*LIG4*	AR	Same as above
T-B-NK-	Reticular dysgenesis	*AK2*	AR	Neutropenia, anemia, chronic diarrhea, hearing impairment
	Adenosine deaminase (ADA) deficiency	*ADA*	AR	Neutropenia, anemia, developmental delay, bone abnormalities, pulmonary alveolar proteinosis, autoimmunity

Adapted from [41, 111]

not only critically important to predicting the clinical manifestations of the various subtypes of SCID but, most importantly, can affect the outcomes of HSCT and the type of conditioning necessary. This will be discussed in greater detail later in this chapter.

There are approximately 20 known SCID-causing mutations with novel culprits being described more readily since the advent of newborn screening. The most common mutations include defects in *IL2RG* (46%), ADA (16.1%), IL-7Rα (10.3%), JAK3 (6.9%), and RAG1/2 (3.4%) [38].

Case 1 Continued

Following immunologic consultation and preliminary diagnostic evaluation, the newborn was monitored carefully in the neonatal intensive care unit for the development of infectious or inflammatory symptoms. He was isolated in the hospital with strict droplet and contact precautions with no sick visitors permitted. He was immediately treated with acyclovir and fluconazole prophylaxis and was given palivizumab for RSV prophylaxis. Breastfeeding was halted pending evaluation of mother's CMV status. IVIG was initiated at 1 month of age as his IgG dropped to <500 mg/dL. Trimethoprim-sulfamethoxazole was also initiated at 1 month of age for PJP prophylaxis as there were no contraindications. Live vaccinations were held and discouraged for any family members. The immunology, infectious diseases, hematology-oncology, and social work services were consulted. Per hematology-oncology recommendations, he, his parents, and his siblings underwent HLA typing, and arrangements were made to select the correct medical institution in preparation for an eventual HSCT.

Initial Management of SCID

A diagnosis or high clinical suspicion for SCID should be considered an urgent medical condition because life-threatening infections can develop at any time. Therefore, patients with a high clinical suspicion for SCID should be admitted to a pediatric hospital with experience in managing SCID. However, not all patients with a positive newborn screening need admission to the hospital. It is important to remember that patients with idiopathic T-cell lymphopenia may be monitored carefully as outpatients because there is a significant likelihood of T-cell recovery. However, patients with abnormal TRECS and abnormal lymphocyte flow cytometry suggesting SCID do warrant inpatient admission for further workup and management. The initial management of SCID patients is focused on infection prophylaxis and preparing for HSCT or other definitive therapies. The goal is initially supportive to prevent, monitor for, and quickly treat any infections and to involve rapid consultation support from an interdisciplinary team that includes an immunologist, hematology/oncologist, infectious disease specialist, genetic counselor, nutritionist, and social worker.

Antibiotic prophylaxis and isolation are required to prevent infection with opportunistic and common viral, fungal, and bacterial organisms. History of or active infection at time of HSCT has been shown to decrease the likelihood of 5-year survival and increased risk of graft failure [39]. Approximately 42% of infants diagnosed by NBS develop infections before HSCT [40]. Acyclovir should be provided to prevent herpes zoster infections, and fluconazole or itraconazole should be given for fungal prophylaxis with monitoring of liver and renal function. Palivizumab (Synagis), a monoclonal antibody directed against an epitope in the antigenic site of the F protein of RSV, should also be given. *Pneumocystis jirovecii* pneumonia is a common complication in SCID patients due to defective cellular immunity, and prophylaxis should be initiated. Trimethoprim/sulfamethoxazole (5 mg/kg/day trimethoprim by mouth 3 times per week) is the preferred regimen and should be started no sooner than day 30 of life to avoid the risk of kernicterus and bone marrow suppression. If trimethoprim/sulfamethoxazole is not tolerated or contraindicated, alternative regimens include pentamidine isethionate (5 mg/kg every 4 weeks), dapsone (1 mg/kg/day), or atovaquone (30 mg/kg/day) [41]. Blood products, if needed, should be CMV-negative, irradiated, and leukoreduced [41].

Breastfeeding should be halted until the CMV status of mothers is confirmed. CMV is highly prevalent in the general population and is readily found in the breast milk of CMV-positive mothers [42]. CMV can cause devastating infectious consequences in infants with SCID including cytopenias, hepatitis, enteritis, and neurologic dysfunction. Importantly, CMV infection has been associated with poorer HSCT outcomes [43]. CMV-negative mothers can potentially resume breastfeeding; however, infant blood CMV PCR should be routinely evaluated because there is still a possible risk of seroconversion of the mother even if initially negative. While general consensus is that CMV-positive mothers should not breastfeed a CMV-negative infant, there is considerable debate as breastfeeding offers other significant emotional, immunologic, and nutritional benefits to the infant. Approaches including breastfeeding with milk from seronegative mothers and novel methods to remove or inactivate CMV from breast milk have been considered, but further research is required to further illuminate its benefits and risks [44].

Immunoglobulin replacement should be initiated in all patients diagnosed with SCID. In SCID newborns, while the IgG level may be normal due to the transfer of maternal immunoglobulin, these levels can quickly decline in the setting of B-cell dysfunction particularly around 4–6 months of age when immunocompetent infants will begin to make their own IgG. More importantly, endogenous immunoglobulin production is generally assumed to be insufficient and ineffective in SCID patients in the absence of functional T-cell help. SCID patients should not receive live vaccines and will have dysfunctional responses to inactivated vaccines. Generally, Ig replacement should be given to maintain an IgG level that is normal for age (>500 mg/dL for newborn, >800 mg/dL for older children and adults particularly those with pulmonary manifestations of disease [45]) and should be continued throughout definitive therapy with either HSCT or GT [46]. A significant number of transplanted SCID patients continue to require Ig replacement after transplant due to failed or delayed B-cell engraftment [47]. Therefore, Ig replacement should be continued until there is concrete evidence of humoral immune reconstitution. In patients with atypical SCID and Omenn syndrome who may have aggressive autoreactive oligoclonal T cells, immunosuppression with glucocorticoids, calcineurin-inhibitors, anti-thymocyte globulin, or anti-CD52 monoclonal antibody is usually required as a bridge to HSCT [46].

Best isolation practices to reduce infectious exposures to SCID patients are less well-defined and are often met with social challenges. In general, SCID patients should be isolated from others with no sick contacts permitted in the same room, and individuals should wear gloves, gown, and mask when interacting with the patient. Patients and family members should not receive live vaccinations. Discharging patients is challenging, particularly if there are siblings in the home who may readily carry viruses they have acquired from daycare or school. If this is the case, patients might be safer staying in the hospital.

Case 1 Continued

Our patient underwent HLA typing, and no matched related donor was identified. He was ultimately transferred directly to a transplanting institution. He underwent HSCT with a 10/10 matched unrelated donor on day 88 of life. Prior to transplant, he underwent conditioning with anti-thymocyte globulin and busulfan with TCR α/ß/CD19+ depleted PBSCs. T-cell engraftment was noted at day 24 post-transplant. He has received inactivated vaccinations, and live vaccinations are continuing to be held. He continues on intravenous immunoglobulin due to delayed B-cell engraftment, but he has overall done well without serious complications or infections.

HSCT in SCID

Hematopoietic stem cell transplant (HSCT) is the definitive therapy for SCID. Prospective cohorts have shown overall survival to be between 85% and 90% [48]. While the most important factor predicting survival is using a matched related donor, other variables contributing to survival include younger age, fewer ongoing and past infections at time of HSCT, and genotype [39, 49, 50]. For instance, despite both being T-B-NK+ phenotypes, survival in patients with *RAG* mutations is superior to that of *DCLRE1C* mutations [49]. Uniquely, HSCT in patients with SCID, compared to HSCT for other disorders, can be performed without a conditioning regimen (CR) for matched-related, matched-unrelated, or haploidentical donors with maternal chimerism. However, as HLA mismatch percentage increases, conditioning may be required for B-cell engraftment [51].

Conditioning practices vary across health centers. Conditioning can lead to immediate and prolonged toxicity in patients with SCID, especially in the setting of DNA-repair defects and active infection. In fact, immunosuppression-only regimens without conditioning have been associated with lower acuity of GVHD [49]. However, reduced-intensity myeloablative conditioning (RIC/MAC) has been associated with improved T- and B-cell reconstitution. Patients with dysfunctional but present B cells (*IGR2G*, *JAK3*) typically require some degree of conditioning in order for B cells to reconstitute and function well post-transplant [52–54]. Delayed B-cell engraftment can explain why a sizable proportion of patients require long-term Ig replacement therapy post-HSCT. In one cohort study of 124 patients with SCID post-HSCT without pre-transplant conditioning, 53% of children required long-term Ig replacement; however, over half of these children had IL-2RG- and JAK3-deficient SCID [55].

Careful monitoring and demonstration of B-cell reconstitution are therefore required prior to stopping Ig replacement. In general, naïve and memory T-cell, NK-cell, and B-cell subsets should be measured every 4 weeks until normal and then every 3 months for the first year of life. B-cell reconstitution can be defined as CD19+ B-cell counts >150 cells/mL with normal age-adjusted IgA and IgM levels [46]. Baseline IgG titers specific to tetanus toxoid, diphtheria toxoid, *Haemophilus influenzae type B*, and *Streptococcus pneumoniae* should be obtained 3 months after the last IgG infusion and 4–6 weeks following the inactivated vaccine series. If T- and B-cell reconstitution is demonstrated, protective titers to inactivated vaccines are present, and lymphocyte proliferation to tetanus toxoid is normal, then live attenuated vaccines should be given.

When a matched related or matched unrelated donor is unavailable, a haploidentical donor can be considered. Haploidentical donors are mismatched related or unrelated donors, typically a parent, in which half of the HLAs are matched between the donor and the recipient. Mother-to-child HSCTs are typically superior to father-to-child HSCTs. This is thought to be due to fetal microchimerism, the presence of fetal cells in the donor HSCs of the mother that persist in some mothers even years after the birth of their child [56–58]. The reason why only some mothers display fetal microchimerism is currently unknown. Regardless, because the HLAs are incompletely matched, in order to prevent GVHD, HSCTs from haploidentical must undergo additional processing to deplete T-cell receptor (TCR) α/β cells prior to transplant [59, 60]. Additional considerations need to be taken for unrelated donors and SCID patients with evidence of maternal T cell engraftment, which has been associated with an increased risk of GVHD [9]. In these cases, pre-HSCT serotherapy with rabbit anti-thymocyte globulin has been successful [61].

More recent efforts have been focused on designing reduced toxicity conditioning regimens including those that move away from alkylating agents and purine analogs (fludarabine) and more toward novel antibody-based protocols including anti-CD45 or anti-CD117 (anti-c-Kit receptor) therapy [62]. One of the major challenges is that because of the rarity of SCID it is difficult to create genotype-specific guidelines. In particular, for radiosensitive SCID (deficiencies in Artemis, DNA ligase IV, DNA-dependent protein catalytic subunit, Cernunnos-XLF, and nibrin, which causes Nijmegen breakage syndrome), increased sensitivity to alkylating agents requires careful selection of both donor and conditioning regimen. In addition, for atypical SCID and Omenn syndrome, a conditioning regimen is required. Another challenge is determining the biomarkers that suggest the need for re-transplantation. Low CD4+ and CD4+CD45RA+ cells at 6 months post-HSCT are associated with reduced survival and increased length of time to immune reconstitution [49]; however, these biomarkers fall short of predicting precisely which patients will require a repeat HSCT. Patients with IL-2RG and JAK3-SCID and those with poor NK-cell engraftment post-HSCT can still be at risk of developing HPV-related warts and HPV-related cancers due to defective anti-viral immunity as a sequela of profoundly reduced or dysfunctional NK cells [63].

Treatment of SCID for patients who do not have access to a matched related donor (MRD)/matched unrelated donor (MUD) or HSC-GT (discussed later) is challenging. Many centers abandoned haplo-HSCT altogether as survival rates were not promising early on (around 43% in the 1980s) [64]. Advances including sequence-based HLA typing, newer graft engineering techniques to deplete donor T cells, as well as post-transplant chemotherapies have improved possibilities for these patients [65]. Psychosocial stressors for patients and families, including post-traumatic stress disorder and postpartum depression, are also important in mediating long-term survival and deserve further study. Genetic manipulation, as we will discuss, may offer a solution to many of these challenges.

Case Presentation 2

A 13-year-old patient presents with ADA SCID, and a history of autoimmune thyroiditis has been treated with PEG-ADA infusions since her diagnosis. Newborn screening was not available in the state where she was born at the time. As an infant, she developed failure to thrive and recurrent pneumonia as well as persistent diarrhea. She was diagnosed based on clinical presentation along with flow cytometry findings of severe lymphopenia across all three subsets. Fortunately, she did not develop any of the neurologic, skeletal, or other extra-immune complications of ADA deficiency.

Adenosine Deaminase Deficiency SCID

Adenosine deaminase (ADA) deficiency is a subtype of T-B-NK- SCID. We discuss it in this chapter because it is one of the most common genotypes of SCID, has a well-described phenotype, and has been the focus of advanced therapeutics that are paving the way for targeted therapies in other types of SCID. It is also the only form of SCID where the defective protein, or enzyme, in this case, can be given in a replacement product. This has made it possible for some patients with ADA SCID to survive into adulthood even without HSCT.

ADA is one of the key enzymes involved in purine metabolism. Deficiency in ADA leads to accumulation of its substrates adenosine (Ado) and 2′-deoxyadenosine (dAdo) as well as their phosphorylated derivatives (dATPs). Increased concentrations of dATPs can block DNA synthesis by inhibiting ribonucleotide reductase and can affect processes dependent on transmethylation via inhibition of S-adenosylhomocysteine hydrolase [66]. Because ADA deficiency leads to a buildup of toxic metabolites throughout the body, it affects all three immune cell lines leading to a T-B-NK- SCID immunophenotype. ADA deficiency is considered a systemic metabolic disorder because, in addition to reduced lymphocyte number and function, it is associated with neutropenia, skeletal abnormalities [67], neurologic abnormalities and behavioral impairments [68], lung complications specifically pulmonary alveolar proteinosis [69], as well as liver [70] and renal impairment [71]. Patients with ADA SCID are also at increased risk of malignancy due to defects in tumor surveillance [72].

Therefore, history and physical examination may reveal clues to this particular SCID genotype and phenotype, and high suspicion can inform directed testing. Diagnosis of ADA SCID is established by demonstrating <1% normal ADA activity accompanied by elevated levels of dATP. Genetic testing as discussed previously should be done to confirm the diagnosis. While ADA SCID is usually diagnosed via NBS, patients with hypomorphic ADA mutations may have TRECs above threshold values resulting in a false-negative screening test. As these hypomorphic mutations often lead to a delayed onset, older children should be considered if clinical presentation is consistent with SCID [73].

Case 2 Continued

On enzyme replacement therapy, our patient had overall been doing well without severe infections or other manifestations of ADA deficiency. Lymphocyte analysis showed normal proliferation of T cells to PHA; however she had persistent chronic moderate lymphopenia with CD4 T cells consistently below 200 requiring prophylaxis with trimethoprim/sulfamethoxazole as well as hypogammaglobulinemia requiring Ig replacement. Her dose of PEG-ADA required careful monitoring. Figure 8.6 illustrates the patient's ADA enzyme and dAXP levels every 6 months since starting therapy with PEG-ADA at approximately 6 months of age.

Initial Management of ADA SCID: Enzyme Replacement Therapy

The history and management advancements of ADA SCID reflect the general principles and challenges of evaluating immunodeficiency patients as well as promising future treatments.

Weeks of Therapy	Normal weekly dose PEG-ADA U/kg/inj	Plasma ADA nmol/h/ml <0.5*	Erythrocyte AXP µmol/ml RBC < .465 ± 0.38*	Nucleotides dAXP µmol/ml RBC < 0.002*	% dAXP < 0.2*
0			1.954	0.127	6.1
-2	-2	-	2.461	0.222	8.3
3	30/30	50.93	1.670	0.022	1.3
9	30/30	46.49	1.602	0.011	0.7
37	30/30	46.93	2.469	0.012	0.5
56	30/30	51.07	1.519	0.005	0.4
71	30/30	96.02	0.800	0.000	0.0
101	30/30	60.02	1.198	0.000	0.0
123	30/30	104.08	0.000	0.000	0.0
172	30/30	131.02	0.000	0.000	0.0
175	30/30	105.47	1.323	0.004	0.3
222	30/30	63.51	1.730	0.015	0.9
230	30/30	72.74	1.550	0.010	0.7
279	?	26.43	1.665	0.000	0.0
349	?	52.29	1.931	0.000	0.0
411	?	38.93	1.472	0.000	0.0
440	?	52.48	1.469	0.000	0.0
451	?	38.15	1.407	0.030	2.1
464	?	40.12	2.015	0.007	0.3
512	?	24.34	1.824	0.012	0.7
524	?	29.15	2.037	0.026	1.2
553	?	32.15	2.238	0.014	0.6
622	?	20.88	2.308	0.029	1.2
639	?	34.63	1.878	0.019	1.0
667	?	32.30	1.854	0.020	1.1
699	?	26.22	2.139	0.021	1.0
752	?	16.43	2.145	0.021	1.0
800	?	24.81	1.571	0.000	0.0

Fig. 8.6 Sample of ADA and ATP level monitoring chart in a patient with ADA SCID

The advent of newborn screening has changed the treatment of ADA SCID dramatically, as these patients previously presented with life-threatening infections and multiorgan dysfunction. Initial management is similar to that in the previous case, with certain special considerations. For instance, alternatives to trimethoprim/sulfamethoxazole are often used for PJP prophylaxis in ADA SCID patients due to the common presence of severe neutropenia. In addition to hematologic parameters, monitoring of the ADA SCID patient requires specific attention to neurologic [68] and hepatorenal function [70] as well as respiratory status, given that pulmonary alveolar proteinosis can be a rapid cause of decompensation [74].

In 1990, a significant advancement in the treatment of ADA SCID became available when PEGylated bovine ADA (Adagen) was approved for ADA

SCID. Enzyme replacement therapy (ERT) with PEG-ADA rapidly normalizes dATP levels and improves T- and B-lymphocyte counts, reducing the metabolic toxicity that leads to hepatic, pulmonary, and skeletal abnormalities. However, ERT has not been shown to mitigate all of the defects associated with ADA SCID, particularly existing neurologic sequelae. It is now standard of care to start patients with ADA SCID on ERT soon after diagnosis. It is estimated that the overall survival of patients on ERT is approximately 78%; however, if patients are alive at 6 months after starting ERT, their survival is 90% [75]. Patients treated with PEG-ADA require regular monitoring of plasma ADA activity (trough levels), dATP content (red cell dATP content), and parameters of immune function in order to determine the optimal dose and for monitoring continued effectiveness. A decline in plasma ADA activity and increase in dATP content suggest the formation of anti-ADA antibodies.

Data of the past 30 years have illuminated many challenges associated with ERT. Multiple treatment centers have reported a progressive decline in lymphocyte counts and function with long-term ERT [76–78]. The mechanism may be related to change in the pharmacokinetics of the ERT product or the presence of anti-ADA neutralizing antibodies which develop in approximately 10% of patients during the first year of treatment [79]. With such decline, complications begin to appear including a decline in antiviral immunity and tumor surveillance [80]. Recently, the use of bovine tissue to purify ADA has raised safety concerns and poses challenges to consistent production of Adagen. Therefore, a recombinant version of bovine ADA conjugated to PEG, elapegademase-lvlr (Revcovi), has replaced Adagen as the standard of care. Thus, the general consensus for ADA SCID diagnosed in infancy is that ERT should be a bridge to definitive therapy with either HSCT or HSC-GT (discussed later) unless these therapies are not available and carry significant risk or a suitable donor for HSCT cannot be found. However, this concept is controversial since there are a number of older teenagers and adults who are doing well on long-term ERT.

Case 2 Continued

At age 13, our patient presented to the hospital with petechiae, bruising, and bleeding shortly after an upper respiratory infection. Pertinent laboratory values at the time included the following: WBC 3.7 TH/μL (4.0–10.5 Th/μL), ANC 2997 cells/μL (1800–8000 cells/μL), ALC 266 cells/μL (1200–5200 cells/μL), hemoglobin 11.6 g/dL (12.5–15.0 g/dL), platelets 4 TH/μL (140–440 TH/μL), PT 15 seconds (11.5–14.3 seconds), PTT 23 seconds (24–37 seconds), INR 1.2 (0.9–1.2), reticulocytes 3.3% (0.5–1.5%), IgG 1179 mg/dL (749–1640 mg/dL), IgM 119 mg/dL (34–225 mg.dL), and IgA 47 mg/dL (62–241 mg/dL). Direct Coombs IgG was positive. No splenomegaly was present, and she did not undergo evaluation for pulmonary embolism. She was initially treated with IVIG at immunomodulatory dosing of

1 mg/kg (total 65 g), compared to her replacement dosing at baseline (4 g every 7 days for a total of 28 g per month). Though the immunomodulatory IVIG helped initially, she had a relapse of her thrombocytopenia. She was subsequently treated with dexamethasone, after which time her platelets returned to normal. Her clinical course and laboratory findings were consistent with a diagnosis of Evans syndrome, a rare disease characterized by both autoimmune hemolytic anemia (AIHA) and immune thrombocytopenia (ITP), and sometimes accompanying neutropenia, and often associated with rheumatologic diseases such as systemic lupus erythematosus (SLE) in addition to both SCID and non-SCID primary immunodeficiency diseases [81–84].

Autoimmunity in ADA SCID

Autoimmune complications are often seen in SCID, particularly in patients with oligoclonal autoreactive T-cell populations. This compromised immune tolerance is thought to occur via multiple mechanisms. Patients with ADA SCID demonstrate a loss of B-cell tolerance checkpoints [85] and defective regulatory T cells (Treg) [84]. Under normal circumstances, regulatory T cells suppress T-cell responses by maintaining homeostasis and self-tolerance and preventing autoimmunity. Mouse and human models have demonstrated that ADA-deficient Tregs have decreased suppressive ability and are exquisitely sensitive to extracellular adenosine concentrations [84].

As described in our patient, autoimmune complications are not only associated with the clinical presentation of SCID but can also occur as a consequence of the SCID treatment due to different degrees of immune reconstitution achieved by the various treatment options. This breakdown in immune tolerance can present in multiple organ systems. Treatment of ADA SCID with PEG-ADA has been associated with autoimmune hypothyroidism, diabetes mellitus, and hemolytic anemia and autoimmune thrombocytopenia as was seen in this case [84, 86, 87]. Therefore, increased vigilance in monitoring for autoimmunity in patients with SCID is warranted regardless of the treatment. As mentioned, monitoring ADA enzyme and dAXP levels is necessary to track response to therapy and evaluate for neutralizing antibodies.

Because of the limitations of ERT, if MSD/MFD is available, HSCT should be performed as soon as possible and can be undertaken without cytoreductive conditioning. One multicenter study found an overall survival rate of 85.2% with 100% donor engraftment in patients who did not receive conditioning, and only 3.7% of patients required continuing Ig replacement therapy. 5.6% of patients died from treatment-related causes [64]. Subsequent studies have found that a sizable proportion of these patients require a repeat HSCT procedure [88], the mechanism of which may relate to the restoration of immune function that occurs with pre-HSCT ERT. Therefore, some centers choose to discontinue ERT prior to HSCT or perform reduced-intensity conditioning [75].

Novel Therapeutic Approaches to SCID: HSCT-GT and Gene Editing

HSCT-GT

ADA deficiency was the first disease to be treated with autologous HSCT gene therapy (HSC-GT). Results have demonstrated excellent safety and efficacy [89–91] and are paving the way for HSC-GT for other types of SCID including X-SCID, Artemis-deficient SCID, and other primary immunodeficiency diseases (PIDD) including chronic granulomatous disease (CGD), Wiskott-Aldrich syndrome (WAS), and leukocyte adhesion deficiency-1 (LAD-1) [88, 92–95]. The process of HSC-GT involves removing bone marrow (BM) HSCs from patients, introducing a retroviral or lentiviral vector containing the desired gene and then transplanting those cells back into the patient. Compared to HSCT, as an autologous procedure, HSC-GT avoids the risk of GVHD and can be done with less conditioning. In a landmark trial conducted by the San Raffaele Telethon Institute for Gene Therapy (SR-TIGET) in Milan, Italy, a low-dose busulfan conditioning regimen proved efficacious for engraftment and expansion of ADA-corrected cells [96]. Following these results, in 2016, HSC-GT for ADA deficiency, Strimvelis, was approved for use in the European Union in patients for whom matched sibling donor (MSD) is not available.

There are a number of limitations and challenges to HSC-GT to discuss. First, there must be a sufficient amount of bone marrow hematopoietic stem cells (HSCs), which can be challenging to acquire in older patients. Second, active infections with viral pathogens, such as CMV and HCV, can affect the processing of HSCs in manufacturing facilities, though newer antivirals can effectively clear these infections prior to HSC-GT [97]. Third, Strimvelis is a fresh cell product; therefore, the cells must be infused shortly after they are transduced to allow for the maximum likelihood of successful engraftment. This creates the challenge of patients potentially needing to travel distantly to be treated. Newer ADA-HSC-GT products, including those being designed in the US, can be cryopreserved, allowing for greater convenience to patients. Studies are ongoing to characterize how cryopreservation affects the cells prior to infusion. Importantly, concerns about safety of HSC-GT arose when one trial for gamma retroviral vector HSC-GT for CGD showed good initial results but later was associated with the development of leukemia [98]. These results led to the development of newer self-inactivating (SIN) lentiviral vectors that are now being employed widely in other disease types and reduce the potential for leukoproliferation.

Gene Editing

A novel approach to gene therapy for SCID involves gene editing, in which the endogenous gene is modified rather than added exogenously with a viral vector. Gene editing involves the use of site-specific endonucleases to induce double-stranded DNA breaks near the sequences to be edited. These endonucleases include zinc finger nucleases (ZNF) [99], transcription activator-like effector nucleases (TALEN) [100], and the clustered regularly interspaced short palindromic repeats (CRISPR)-associated protein 9 (Cas 9) [101, 102]. Gene editing is being developed for many forms of SCID including X-SCID [101, 103] and ADA SCID [104] as well as other primary immunodeficiency diseases such as X-CGD [105, 106] and hyper-IgM syndrome [96, 107, 108]. One of the challenges of gene editing is to obtain high enough frequencies of gene edits while preserving the ability of the HSCs to engraft and support blood cell production. Clinical trials are ongoing for these novel therapies [96].

Conclusion

Since the 1980s, advances in HSCT, molecular biology, and genetics as well as the initiation of newborn screening have dramatically improved the care of patients with SCID by allowing for early diagnosis and treatment. Outcomes in SCID, particularly following MRD/MUD HSCT, are overall excellent; however, regular monitoring is important. Long-term sequelae can develop as a consequence of therapy or as a result of the underlying genetic defect. For example, as discussed in Case 2, patients with not only ADA SCID but also DNA ligase IV and Cernunnos defects are associated with neurologic impairment and reticular dysgenesis with sensorineural defects [109], neither of which are corrected with HSCT. As well, SCID patients carry a predisposition to malignancy and autoimmunity, such as autoimmune cytopenias, warranting close monitoring for the life of the patient. Importantly, conditioning regimens can have lasting toxic consequences including endocrine and growth abnormalities particularly in radiosensitive SCID patients. Varying degrees of B-cell engraftment post-transplant often lead to potential need for long-term Ig replacement therapy even following HSCT. As SCID patients are now surviving past childhood into young adulthood and beyond, psychosocial and quality-of-life concerns require increasing attention and rigorous study. While there are many challenges ahead, the treatment of SCID has been one of the earliest models of the possibilities of personalized and precision medicine and continues to serve as an example for innovation in the treatment of primary immunodeficiencies and other rare genetic diseases.

> **Clinical Pearls and Pitfalls**
> - Severe combined immunodeficiencies (SCID) are a heterogeneous group of rare, genetic diseases that lead to profoundly impaired adaptive immune responses characterized by severe, recurrent infections and failure to thrive and are fatal without treatment.
> - The advent of universal newborn screening, measuring T-cell receptor excision circles in the peripheral blood, has led to improved early detection of SCID.
> - SCID is classified as either typical or atypical, depending on the quantity and function of CD3 T cells and is further classified by immunophenotype and genotype.

- Initial management of SCID usually involves isolation, infectious workup, antibiotic prophylaxis, immune globulin replacement therapy, HLA typing, evaluation for maternal T-cell engraftment, and the involvement of a multidisciplinary team.
- Factors that improve survival following HSCT for SCID include matched related donor, younger age at transplant, fewer ongoing and past infections at time of HSCT, as well as particular genotypes.
- Adenosine deaminase (ADA) deficiency is one of the most common causes of SCID and results in immunodeficiency and multiorgan dysfunction due to the accumulation of toxic metabolites of purine metabolism.
- First-line therapy for ADA SCID involves immediate treatment with adenosine deaminase enzyme replacement therapy, either the PEGylated bovine form (Adagen) or the newer recombinant product (elapegademase-lvlr, Recvovi).
- Gene replacement therapy and gene editing are novel strategies that have shown promising results in treating SCID and have addressed some of the challenges with HSCT.
- A normal newborn screening does not necessarily rule out SCID as TREC thresholds vary across states and countries, and patients with hypomorphic mutations can present later in childhood; therefore, high clinical suspicion for SCID should prompt investigation.
- False-positive newborn screens can be due to non-SCID forms of T-cell lymphopenia including DiGeorge syndrome and CHARGE syndrome or can be idiopathic.
- Conditioning is associated with improved lymphocyte engraftment in many cases of SCID; however it is often associated with toxicity; guidelines for choosing an appropriate conditioning regimen are not well defined.
- SCID, in particular ADA SCID, is often associated with autoimmune complications and a susceptibility to malignancy, a risk that is reduced but not entirely eliminated by successful HSCT. Therefore, post-HSCT monitoring is critical.
- Continued immune globulin replacement therapy is required in the post-transplant period until B-cell reconstitution has been demonstrated, and avoidance of live attenuated vaccinations is recommended until both T- and B-cell reconstitution is established.
- While enzyme replacement (ERT) has dramatically improved the survival of ADA SCID patients, regular monitoring of ADA enzyme and dAXP levels is required as the development of antibodies to the enzyme replacement product is common over time.
- Self-inactivating lentiviral vectors have reduced the risk of leukoproliferation due to off-target gene insertion when using gene therapy for SCID.
- Mutation-specific guidelines are difficult to establish given the rare nature of SCID and because therapeutic and monitoring strategies often vary widely across centers.

References

1. Glanzmann E. Essetielle Lymphocytophthise. Ein neues Krankheitsbild aus der Sauglingspathologie. Ann Paediatr (Basel). 1950;175:1–32.
2. Buckley RH, Schiff RI, Schiff SE, Louise Markert M, Williams LW, Harville TO, et al. Human severe combined immunodeficiency: genetic, phenotypic, and functional diversity in one hundred eight infants. J Pediatr. 1997:378–87. https://doi.org/10.1016/s0022-3476(97)70199-9.
3. Kwan A, Abraham RS, Currier R, Brower A, Andruszewski K, Abbott JK, et al. Newborn screening for severe combined immunodeficiency in 11 screening programs in the United States. JAMA. 2014;312:729–38.
4. Summers KL, O'Donnell JL, Hart DN. Co-expression of the CD45RA and CD45RO antigens on T lymphocytes in chronic arthritis. Clin Exp Immunol. 1994;97:39–44.
5. Liu C, Duffy B, Bednarski JJ, Calhoun C, Lay L, Rundblad B, et al. Maternal T-cell engraftment interferes with human leukocyte antigen typing in severe combined immunodeficiency. Am J Clin Pathol. 2016;145:251–7.
6. Denianke KS, Frieden IJ, Cowan MJ, Williams ML, McCalmont TH. Cutaneous manifestations of maternal engraftment in patients with severe combined immunodeficiency: a clinicopathologic study. Bone Marrow Transplant. 2001;28:227–33.
7. Lev A, Simon AJ, Ben-Ari J, Takagi D, Stauber T, Trakhtenbrot L, et al. Co-existence of clonal expanded autologous and transplacental-acquired maternal T cells in recombination activating gene-deficient severe combined immunodeficiency. Clin Exp Immunol. 2014;176:380–6.
8. Knobloch C, Goldmann SF, Friedrich W. Limited T cell receptor diversity of transplacentally acquired maternal T cells in severe combined immunodeficiency. J Immunol. 1991;146:4157–64.
9. Wahlstrom J, Patel K, Eckhert E, Kong D, Horn B, Cowan MJ, et al. Transplacental maternal engraftment and posttransplantation graft-versus-host disease in children with severe combined immunodeficiency. J Allergy Clin Immunol. 2017;139:628–633.e10.
10. Verschuren MC, Wolvers-Tettero IL, Breit TM, Noordzij J, van Wering ER, van Dongen JJ. Preferential rearrangements of the T cell receptor-delta-deleting elements in human T cells. J Immunol. 1997;158:1208–16.
11. Hazenberg MD, Verschuren MC, Hamann D, Miedema F, van Dongen JJ. T cell receptor excision circles as markers for recent thymic emigrants: basic aspects, technical approach, and guidelines for interpretation. J Mol Med. 2001;79:631–40.
12. Chan K, Puck JM. Development of population-based newborn screening for severe combined immunodeficiency. J Allergy Clin Immunol. 2005;115:391–8.
13. Kuo CY, Chase J, Garcia Lloret M, Stiehm ER, Moore T, Aguilera MJM, et al. Newborn screening for severe combined immunodeficiency does not identify bare lymphocyte syndrome. J Allergy Clin Immunol. 2013;131:1693–5.
14. Buckley RH. The long quest for neonatal screening for severe combined immunodeficiency. J Allergy Clin Immunol. 2012;129:597–604; quiz 605–6.
15. Amatuni GS, Currier RJ, Church JA, Bishop T, Grimbacher E, Nguyen AA-C, et al. Newborn screening for severe combined immunodeficiency and T-cell lymphopenia in California, 2010–2017. Pediatrics. 2019;143 https://doi.org/10.1542/peds.2018-2300.
16. van der Spek J, Groenwold RHH, van der Burg M, van Montfrans JM. TREC Based newborn screening for severe combined immunodeficiency disease: a systematic review. J Clin Immunol. 2015;35:416–30.
17. Rosati E, Marie Dowds C, Liaskou E, Henriksen EKK, Karlsen TH, Franke A. Overview of methodologies for T-cell receptor repertoire analysis. BMC Biotechnol. 2017. https://doi.org/10.1186/s12896-017-0379-9
18. Schatz DG, Ji Y. Recombination centres and the orchestration of V (D) J recombination. Nat Rev Immunol. 2011;11:251–63.
19. Bassing CH, Swat W, Alt FW. The mechanism and regulation of chromosomal V (D) J recombination. Cell. 2002;109:S45–55.

20. Pannetier C, Even J, Kourilsky P. T-cell repertoire diversity and clonal expansions in normal and clinical samples. Immunol Today. 1995;16:176–81.
21. Sarzotti M, Patel DD, Li X, Ozaki DA, Cao S, Langdon S, et al. T cell repertoire development in humans with SCID after nonablative allogeneic marrow transplantation. J Immunol. 2003;170:2711–8.
22. Lev A, Simon AJ, Amariglio N, Rechavi G, Somech R. Thymic functions and gene expression profile distinct double-negative cells from single positive cells in the autoimmune lymphoproliferative syndrome. Autoimmun Rev. 2012;11:723–30.
23. Al-Herz W, Bousfiha A, Casanova J-L, Chatila T, Conley ME, Cunningham-Rundles C, et al. Primary immunodeficiency diseases: an update on the classification from the International Union of Immunological Societies Expert Committee for primary immunodeficiency. Front Immunol. 2014;5:162.
24. Kalman L, Lindegren ML, Kobrynski L, Vogt R, Hannon H, Howard JT, et al. Mutations in selected genes required for T cell development: IL7R, CD45, IL2R gamma chain, JAK3, RAG1, RAG2, ARTEMIS and ADA and severe combined immunodeficiency. Genet Med. 2004;6:16–26.
25. Villa A, Sobacchi C, Notarangelo LD, Bozzi F, Abinun M, Abrahamsen TG, et al. V (D) J recombination defects in lymphocytes due to RAG mutations: severe immunodeficiency with a spectrum of clinical presentations. Blood J Am Soc Hematol. 2001;97:81–8.
26. Lieber MR, Ma Y, Pannicke U, Schwarz K. The mechanism of vertebrate nonhomologous DNA end joining and its role in V(D)J recombination. DNA Repair. 2004;3:817–26.
27. Felgentreff K, Baxi SN, Lee YN, Dobbs K, Henderson LA, Csomos K, et al. Ligase-4 deficiency causes distinctive immune abnormalities in asymptomatic individuals. J Clin Immunol. 2016;36:341–53.
28. Takeshita T, Asao H, Ohtani K, Ishii N, Kumaki S, Tanaka N, et al. Cloning of the gamma chain of the human IL-2 receptor. Science. 1992;257:379–82.
29. Noguchi M, Nakamura Y, Russell SM, Ziegler SF, Tsang M, Cao X, et al. Interleukin-2 receptor gamma chain: a functional component of the interleukin-7 receptor. Science. 1993;262:1877–80.
30. Russell SM, Keegan AD, Harada N, Nakamura Y, Noguchi M, Leland P, et al. Interleukin-2 receptor gamma chain: a functional component of the interleukin-4 receptor. Science. 1993;262:1880–3.
31. Asao H, Okuyama C, Kumaki S, Ishii N, Tsuchiya S, Foster D, et al. Cutting edge: the common γ-chain is an indispensable subunit of the IL-21 receptor complex. J Immunol. 2001;167:1–5.
32. Giri JG, Ahdieh M, Eisenman J, Shanebeck K, Grabstein K, Kumaki S, et al. Utilization of the beta and gamma chains of the IL-2 receptor by the novel cytokine IL-15. EMBO J. 1994;13:2822–30.
33. O'Shea JJ. Jaks, STATs, cytokine signal transduction, and immunoregulation: are we there yet? Immunity. 1997;7:1–11.
34. Puck JM, Deschênes SM, Porter JC, Dutra AS, Brown CJ, Willard HF, et al. The interleukin-2 receptor gamma chain maps to Xq13.1 and is mutated in X-linked severe combined immunodeficiency, SCIDX1. Hum Mol Genet. 1993;2:1099–104.
35. Roberts JL, Lengi A, Brown SM, Chen M, Zhou Y-J, O'Shea JJ, et al. Janus kinase 3 (JAK3) deficiency: clinical, immunologic, and molecular analyses of 10 patients and outcomes of stem cell transplantation. Blood. 2004;103:2009–18.
36. Lagresle-Peyrou C, Six EM, Picard C, Rieux-Laucat F, Michel V, Ditadi A, et al. Human adenylate kinase 2 deficiency causes a profound hematopoietic defect associated with sensorineural deafness. Nat Genet. 2009;41:106–11.
37. Dvorak CC, Haddad E, Buckley RH, Cowan MJ, Logan B, Griffith LM, et al. The genetic landscape of severe combined immunodeficiency in the United States and Canada in the current era (2010–2018). J Allergy Clin Immunol. 2019;143:405–7.
38. Buckley RH. The multiple causes of human SCID. J Clin Invest. 2004;114:1409–11.

39. Antoine C, Müller S, Cant A, Cavazzana-Calvo M, Veys P, Vossen J, et al. Long-term survival and transplantation of haemopoietic stem cells for immunodeficiencies: report of the European experience 1968–99. Lancet. 2003;361:553–60.
40. Heimall J, Logan BR, Cowan MJ, Notarangelo LD, Griffith LM, Puck JM, et al. Immune reconstitution and survival of 100 SCID patients post-hematopoietic cell transplant: a PIDTC natural history study. Blood. 2017;130:2718–27.
41. Bonilla FA, Khan DA, Ballas ZK, Chinen J, Frank MM, Hsu JT, et al. Practice parameter for the diagnosis and management of primary immunodeficiency. J Allergy Clin Immunol. 2015;136:1186–205.e1–78.
42. Peckham CS, Johnson C, Ades A, Pearl K, Chin KS. Early acquisition of cytomegalovirus infection. Arch Dis Child. 1987;62:780–5.
43. Maschmann J, Hamprecht K, Dietz K, Jahn G, Speer CP. Cytomegalovirus infection of extremely low-birth weight infants via breast milk. Clin Infect Dis. 2001;33:1998–2003.
44. Bryant P, Morley C, Garland S, Curtis N. Cytomegalovirus transmission from breast milk in premature babies: does it matter? Arch Dis Child Fetal Neonatal Ed. 2002;87:F75–7.
45. Orange JS, Hossny EM, Weiler CR, Ballow M, Berger M, Bonilla FA, et al. Use of intravenous immunoglobulin in human disease: a review of evidence by members of the Primary Immunodeficiency Committee of the American Academy of Allergy, Asthma and Immunology. J Allergy Clin Immunol. 2006;117:S525–53.
46. Dorsey MJ, Dvorak CC, Cowan MJ, Puck JM. Treatment of infants identified as having severe combined immunodeficiency by means of newborn screening. J Allergy Clin Immunol. 2017;139:733–42.
47. Buckley RH. Advances in the understanding and treatment of human severe combined immunodeficiency. Immunol Res. 2000;22:237–51.
48. Dvorak CC, Cowan MJ, Logan BR, Notarangelo LD, Griffith LM, Puck JM, et al. The natural history of children with severe combined immunodeficiency: baseline features of the first fifty patients of the primary immune deficiency treatment consortium prospective study 6901. J Clin Immunol. 2013;33:1156–64.
49. Haddad E, Logan BR, Griffith LM, Buckley RH, Parrott RE, Prockop SE, et al. SCID genotype and 6-month posttransplant CD4 count predict survival and immune recovery. Blood. 2018;132:1737–49.
50. Pai S-Y, Logan BR, Griffith LM, Buckley RH, Parrott RE, Dvorak CC, et al. Transplantation outcomes for severe combined immunodeficiency, 2000–2009. N Engl J Med. 2014;371:434–46.
51. Haddad E, Hoenig M. Hematopoietic stem cell transplantation for severe combined immunodeficiency (SCID). Front Pediatr. 2019;7:481.
52. Buckley RH, Win CM, Moser BK, Parrott RE, Sajaroff E, Sarzotti-Kelsoe M. Post-transplantation B cell function in different molecular types of SCID. J Clin Immunol. 2013;33:96–110.
53. Haddad E, Leroy S, Buckley RH. B-cell reconstitution for SCID: should a conditioning regimen be used in SCID treatment? J Allergy Clin Immunol. 2013;131:994–1000.
54. Abd Hamid IJ, Slatter MA, McKendrick F, Pearce MS, Gennery AR. Long-term outcome of hematopoietic stem cell transplantation for IL2RG/JAK3 SCID: a cohort report. Blood. 2017;129:2198–201.
55. Railey MD, Lokhnygina Y, Buckley RH. Long-term clinical outcome of patients with severe combined immunodeficiency who received related donor bone marrow transplants without pretransplant chemotherapy or post-transplant GVHD prophylaxis. J Pediatr. 2009;155:834–840.e1.
56. Stern M, Ruggeri L, Mancusi A, Bernardo ME, de Angelis C, Bucher C, et al. Survival after T cell-depleted haploidentical stem cell transplantation is improved using the mother as donor. Blood. 2008;112:2990–5.
57. Kruchen A, Stahl T, Gieseke F, Binder TMC, Özcan Z, Meisel R, et al. Donor choice in haploidentical stem cell transplantation: fetal microchimerism is associated with better outcome in pediatric leukemia patients. Bone Marrow Transplant. 2015;50:1367–70.

58. Wang Y, Chang Y-J, Xu L-P, Liu K-Y, Liu D-H, Zhang X-H, et al. Who is the best donor for a related HLA haplotype-mismatched transplant? Blood. 2014;124:843–50.
59. Dvorak CC, Hassan A, Slatter MA, Hönig M, Lankester AC, Buckley RH, et al. Comparison of outcomes of hematopoietic stem cell transplantation without chemotherapy conditioning by using matched sibling and unrelated donors for treatment of severe combined immunodeficiency. J Allergy Clin Immunol. 2014;134:935–943.e15.
60. Brodszki N, Turkiewicz D, Toporski J, Truedsson L, Dykes J. Novel treatment of severe combined immunodeficiency utilizing ex-vivo T-cell depleted haploidentical hematopoietic stem cell transplantation and CD45RA+ depleted donor lymphocyte infusions. Orphanet J Rare Dis. 2016;11:5.
61. Dvorak CC, Hung G-Y, Horn B, Dunn E, Oon C-Y, Cowan MJ. Megadose CD34(+) cell grafts improve recovery of T cell engraftment but not B cell immunity in patients with severe combined immunodeficiency disease undergoing haplocompatible nonmyeloablative transplantation. Biol Blood Marrow Transplant. 2008;14:1125–33.
62. Lum SH, Hoenig M, Gennery AR, Slatter MA. Conditioning regimens for hematopoietic cell transplantation in primary immunodeficiency. Curr Allergy Asthma Rep. 2019;19:52.
63. Kamili QUA, Seeborg FO, Saxena K, Nicholas SK, Banerjee PP, Angelo LS, et al. Severe cutaneous human papillomavirus infection associated with natural killer cell deficiency following stem cell transplantation for severe combined immunodeficiency. J Allergy Clin Immunol. 2014;134:1451–1453.e1.
64. Hassan A, Booth C, Brightwell A, Allwood Z, Veys P, Rao K, et al. Outcome of hematopoietic stem cell transplantation for adenosine deaminase-deficient severe combined immunodeficiency. Blood. 2012;120:3615–24; quiz 3626.
65. Carapito R, Jung N, Kwemou M, Untrau M, Michel S, Pichot A, et al. Matching for the nonconventional MHC-I MICA gene significantly reduces the incidence of acute and chronic GVHD. Blood. 2016;128:1979–86.
66. Flinn AM, Gennery AR. Adenosine deaminase deficiency: a review. Orphanet J Rare Dis. 2018;13:65.
67. Sauer AV, Mrak E, Hernandez RJ, Zacchi E, Cavani F, Casiraghi M, et al. ADA-deficient SCID is associated with a specific microenvironment and bone phenotype characterized by RANKL/OPG imbalance and osteoblast insufficiency. Blood. 2009;114:3216–26.
68. Sauer AV, Hernandez RJ, Fumagalli F, Bianchi V, Poliani PL, Dallatomasina C, et al. Alterations in the brain adenosine metabolism cause behavioral and neurological impairment in ADA-deficient mice and patients. Sci Rep. 2017;7:40136.
69. Booth C, Algar VE, Xu-Bayford J, Fairbanks L, Owens C, Gaspar HB. Non-infectious lung disease in patients with adenosine deaminase deficient severe combined immunodeficiency. J Clin Immunol. 2012;32:449–53.
70. Bollinger ME, Arredondo-Vega FX, Santisteban I, Schwarz K, Hershfield MS, Lederman HM. Brief report: hepatic dysfunction as a complication of adenosine deaminase deficiency. N Engl J Med. 1996;334:1367–71.
71. Ratech H, Greco MA, Gallo G, Rimoin DL, Kamino H, Hirschhorn R. Pathologic findings in adenosine deaminase-deficient severe combined immunodeficiency. I. Kidney, adrenal, and chondro-osseous tissue alterations. Am J Pathol. 1985;120:157–69.
72. Migliavacca M, Assanelli A, Ponzoni M, Pajno R, Barzaghi F, Giglio F, et al. First occurrence of plasmablastic lymphoma in adenosine deaminase-deficient severe combined immunodeficiency disease patient and review of the literature. Front Immunol. 2018;9:113.
73. Hershfield M. Adenosine deaminase deficiency. In: Adam MP, Ardinger HH, Pagon RA, Wallace SE, Bean LJH, Stephens K, et al., editors. GeneReviews®. Seattle: University of Washington, Seattle; 2006.
74. Grunebaum E, Cutz E, Roifman CM. Pulmonary alveolar proteinosis in patients with adenosine deaminase deficiency. J Allergy Clin Immunol. 2012;129:1588–93.
75. Gaspar HB, Aiuti A, Porta F, Candotti F, Hershfield MS, Notarangelo LD. How I treat ADA deficiency. Blood. 2009;114:3524–32.

76. Scott O, Kim VH-D, Reid B, Pham-Huy A, Atkinson AR, Aiuti A, et al. Long-term outcome of adenosine deaminase-deficient patients-a single-center experience. J Clin Immunol. 2017;37:582–91.
77. Baffelli R, Notarangelo LD, Imberti L, Hershfield MS, Serana F, Santisteban I, et al. Diagnosis, treatment and long-term follow up of patients with ADA deficiency: a single-center experience. J Clin Immunol. 2015;35:624–37.
78. Chan B, Wara D, Bastian J, Hershfield MS, Bohnsack J, Azen CG, et al. Long-term efficacy of enzyme replacement therapy for adenosine deaminase (ADA)-deficient severe combined immunodeficiency (SCID). Clin Immunol. 2005;117:133–43.
79. Chaffee S, Mary A, Stiehm ER, Girault D, Fischer A, Hershfield MS. IgG antibody response to polyethylene glycol-modified adenosine deaminase in patients with adenosine deaminase deficiency. J Clin Invest. 1992;89:1643–51.
80. Kapoor N, Jung LK, Engelhard D, Filler J, Shalit I, Landreth KS, et al. Lymphoma in a patient with severe combined immunodeficiency with adenosine deaminase deficiency, following unsustained engraftment of histoincompatible T cell-depleted bone marrow. J Pediatr. 1986;108:435–8.
81. Aladjidi N, Fernandes H, Leblanc T, Vareliette A, Rieux-Laucat F, Bertrand Y, et al. Evans syndrome in children: long-term outcome in a prospective French national observational cohort. Front Pediatr. 2015;3:79.
82. Hadjadj J, Aladjidi N, Fernandes H, Leverger G, Magérus-Chatinet A, Mazerolles F, et al. Pediatric Evans syndrome is associated with a high frequency of potentially damaging variants in immune genes. Blood. 2019;134:9–21.
83. Grimbacher B, Warnatz K, Yong PFK, Korganow A-S, Peter H-H. The crossroads of autoimmunity and immunodeficiency: lessons from polygenic traits and monogenic defects. J Allergy Clin Immunol. 2016;137:3–17.
84. Sauer AV, Brigida I, Carriglio N, Aiuti A. Autoimmune dysregulation and purine metabolism in adenosine deaminase deficiency. Front Immunol. 2012;3:265.
85. Sauer AV, Morbach H, Brigida I, Ng Y-S, Aiuti A, Meffre E. Defective B cell tolerance in adenosine deaminase deficiency is corrected by gene therapy. J Clin Invest. 2012;122:2141–52.
86. Notarangelo LD, Stoppoloni G, Toraldo R, Mazzolari E, Coletta A, Airò P, et al. Insulin-dependent diabetes mellitus and severe atopic dermatitis in a child with adenosine deaminase deficiency. Eur J Pediatr. 1992;151:811–4.
87. Ozsahin H, Arredondo-Vega FX, Santisteban I, Fuhrer H, Tuchschmid P, Jochum W, et al. Adenosine deaminase deficiency in adults. Blood. 1997;89:2849–55.
88. Kohn DB, Hershfield MS, Puck JM, Aiuti A, Blincoe A, Gaspar HB, et al. Consensus approach for the management of severe combined immune deficiency caused by adenosine deaminase deficiency. J Allergy Clin Immunol. 2019;143:852–63.
89. Cicalese MP, Ferrua F, Castagnaro L, Rolfe K, De Boever E, Reinhardt RR, et al. Gene therapy for adenosine deaminase deficiency: a comprehensive evaluation of short- and medium-term safety. Mol Ther. 2018;26:917–31.
90. Aiuti A, Roncarolo MG, Naldini L. Gene therapy for ADA-SCID, the first marketing approval of an ex vivo gene therapy in Europe: paving the road for the next generation of advanced therapy medicinal products. EMBO Mol Med. 2017;9:737–40.
91. Candotti F, Shaw KL, Muul L, Carbonaro D, Sokolic R, Choi C, et al. Gene therapy for adenosine deaminase-deficient severe combined immune deficiency: clinical comparison of retroviral vectors and treatment plans. Blood. 2012;120:3635–46.
92. Mamcarz E, Zhou S, Lockey T, Abdelsamed H, Cross SJ, Kang G, et al. Lentiviral gene therapy combined with low-dose busulfan in infants with SCID-X1. N Engl J Med. 2019;380:1525–34.
93. Punwani D, Kawahara M, Yu J, Sanford U, Roy S, Patel K, et al. Lentivirus mediated correction of Artemis-deficient severe combined immunodeficiency. Hum Gene Ther. 2017;28:112–24.
94. Hacein-Bey Abina S, Gaspar HB, Blondeau J, Caccavelli L, Charrier S, Buckland K, et al. Outcomes following gene therapy in patients with severe Wiskott-Aldrich syndrome. JAMA. 2015;313:1550–63.

95. Ferrua F, Cicalese MP, Galimberti S, Giannelli S, Dionisio F, Barzaghi F, et al. Lentiviral haemopoietic stem/progenitor cell gene therapy for treatment of Wiskott-Aldrich syndrome: interim results of a non-randomised, open-label, phase 1/2 clinical study. Lancet Haematol. 2019;6:e239–53.
96. Kohn DB, Kuo CY. New frontiers in the therapy of primary immunodeficiency: from gene addition to gene editing. J Allergy Clin Immunol. 2017;139:726–32.
97. Tucci F, Calbi V, Barzaghi F, Migliavacca M, Ferrua F, Bernardo ME, et al. Successful treatment with ledipasvir/sofosbuvir in an infant with severe combined immunodeficiency caused by adenosine deaminase deficiency with HCV allowed gene therapy with strimvelis. Hepatology. 2018;68:2434–7.
98. Stein S, Ott MG, Schultze-Strasser S, Jauch A, Burwinkel B, Kinner A, et al. Genomic instability and myelodysplasia with monosomy 7 consequent to EVI1 activation after gene therapy for chronic granulomatous disease. Nat Med. 2010;16:198–204.
99. Urnov FD, Rebar EJ, Holmes MC, Zhang HS, Gregory PD. Genome editing with engineered zinc finger nucleases. Nat Rev Genet. 2010;11:636–46.
100. Miller JC, Tan S, Qiao G, Barlow KA, Wang J, Xia DF, et al. A TALE nuclease architecture for efficient genome editing. Nat Biotechnol. 2011;29:143–8.
101. Schiroli G, Ferrari S, Conway A, Jacob A, Capo V, Albano L, et al. Preclinical modeling highlights the therapeutic potential of hematopoietic stem cell gene editing for correction of SCID-X1. Sci Transl Med. 2017;9 https://doi.org/10.1126/scitranslmed.aan0820.
102. Biffi A. Clinical translation of TALENS: treating SCID-X1 by gene editing in iPSCs. Cell Stem Cell. 2015;16:348–9.
103. Pavel-Dinu M, Wiebking V, Dejene BT, Srifa W, Mantri S, Nicolas CE, et al. Gene correction for SCID-X1 in long-term hematopoietic stem cells. Nat Commun. 2019;10:1634.
104. Calero-Garcia M, Carmo M, Thrasher A, Bobby GH. 140. Point mutation correction for ADA SCID. Mol Ther. 2016;24:S57.
105. De Ravin SS, Reik A, Liu P-Q, Li L, Wu X, Su L, et al. Targeted gene addition in human CD34(+) hematopoietic cells for correction of X-linked chronic granulomatous disease. Nat Biotechnol. 2016;34:424–9.
106. De Ravin SS, Li L, Wu X, Choi U, Allen C, Koontz S, et al. CRISPR-Cas9 gene repair of hematopoietic stem cells from patients with X-linked chronic granulomatous disease. Sci Transl Med. 2017;9(372). Epub 2017/01/13. https://doi.org/10.1126/scitranslmed.aah3480. PMID: 28077679.
107. Kuo CY, Long JD, Campo-Fernandez B, de Oliveira S, Cooper AR, Romero Z, et al. Site-specific gene editing of human hematopoietic stem cells for X-Linked Hyper-IgM syndrome. Cell Rep. 2018;23:2606–16.
108. Hubbard N, Hagin D, Sommer K, Song Y, Khan I, Clough C, et al. Targeted gene editing restores regulated CD40L function in X-linked hyper-IgM syndrome. Blood. 2016;127:2513–22.
109. Pannicke U, Hönig M, Hess I, Friesen C, Holzmann K, Rump E-M, et al. Reticular dysgenesis (aleukocytosis) is caused by mutations in the gene encoding mitochondrial adenylate kinase 2. Nat Genet. 2009;41:101–5.
110. Shearer WT, Dunn E, Notarangelo LD, Dvorak CC, Puck JM, Logan BR, et al. Establishing diagnostic criteria for severe combined immunodeficiency disease (SCID), leaky SCID, and Omenn syndrome: the Primary Immune Deficiency Treatment Consortium experience. J Allergy Clin Immunol. 2014;133:1092–8.
111. Picard C, Bobby Gaspar H, Al-Herz W, Bousfiha A, Casanova J-L, Chatila T, et al. International Union of Immunological Societies: 2017 Primary Immunodeficiency Diseases Committee report on inborn errors of immunity. J Clin Immunol. 2018;38:96–128.
112. Chiarini M, Zanotti C, Serana F, Sottini A, Bertoli D, Caimi L, et al. T-cell receptor and K-deleting recombination excision circles in newborn screening of T- and B-cell defects: review of the literature and future challenges. J Public Health Res. 2013;2:9–16.
113. Somech R, Etzioni A. A call to include severe combined immunodeficiency in newborn screening program. Rambam Maimonides Med J. 2014;5:e0001.
114. Puck JM. Neonatal screening for severe combined immunodeficiency. Curr Opin Pediatr. 2011;23:667–73.

Chapter 9
Idiopathic CD4 Lymphopenia

Yuliya Afinogenova and Joel P. Brooks

Case Presentation 1

A 40-year-old woman with no significant past medical history who was not on any medications presented with a 1-month history of progressive headaches suffering from confusion, dizziness, nausea, and vomiting. She was afebrile. She did not have any focal neurological deficits on exam. Brain MRI revealed leptomeningeal enhancement. Lumbar puncture was performed and was positive for *Cryptococcus neoformans*. Her immunologic profile revealed absolute CD4 count of 90 cells/microL and a CD8 count of 80 cells/microL. She was initiated on treatment with amphotericin B and flucytosine and had a full recovery. She remained on maintenance treatment with oral fluconazole and prophylactic trimethoprim/sulfamethoxazole (TMP/SMX).

As an outpatient, her repeat CD4 count remained low. Over the course of investigating the source of her CD4 lymphopenia, she was tested for HIV and was found to be negative. She had not traveled recently nor was she exposed to any sick contacts. Testing for other infectious etiologies, including tuberculosis, was unremarkable. To exclude an autoimmune basis for her CD4 lymphopenia, her rheumatologic review of systems was unremarkable, and all laboratory workup returned negative. She was up to date with age-appropriate cancer screening and did not have any signs or symptoms that would suggest a malignancy. She did not have lymphadenopathy or hepatosplenomegaly. Flow cytometry obtained for quantification of T, B, and NK cells did not show clonality. There was no family or personal history of

Y. Afinogenova
Department of Rheumatology, Allergy & Immunology, Yale New Haven Hospital and Yale School of Medicine, New Haven, CT, USA

J. P. Brooks (✉)
Department of Allergy and Immunology, George Washington University School of Medicine and Health Sciences, Children's National Health System, Washington, DC, USA
e-mail: jpbrooks@childrensnational.org

immunodeficiency or frequent or severe infections except for this episode. Her B and NK cells as well as immunoglobulin levels were within normal limits. Ultimately, she was diagnosed with idiopathic CD4 lymphopenia.

Background

Idiopathic CD4 lymphopenia was formally described in the literature published by the American Centers for Disease Control and Prevention (CDC) in 1992 [1]. It is defined as persistent CD4 lymphopenia <300 cells/microL or <20% of the total T cells on more than one cell count at least 6 weeks apart, without evidence of HIV infection or any other secondary causes of depressed CD4 cell counts. To arrive at this diagnosis, all secondary causes of CD4 lymphopenia must be excluded. HIV is the most recognized infection leading to CD4 lymphopenia. Severe CD4 lymphopenia is a hallmark of HIV and is the main underlying etiology of serious opportunistic infections and malignancies. Other secondary causes for CD4 lymphopenia include mycobacterial infections, viral infections in addition to HIV, malignancies, autoimmune disorders, drugs such as corticosteroids, chemotherapy, and cytotoxic agents (Table 9.1). Other

Table 9.1 Differential diagnosis of CD4 lymphopenia

Infections	HIV
	Hepatitis B and C
	Mycobacterium tuberculosis
	Nontuberculous mycobacterium
	EBV
	CMV
	HTLV
Malignancies	Lymphoma
	Myelodysplastic syndrome
	Aplastic anemia
Autoimmune diseases	Systemic lupus erythematous
	Sjogren's syndrome
	Sarcoidosis
	Multiple sclerosis
Medications	Corticosteroids
	Cytotoxic immunosuppressants
	Chemotherapy
Immunodeficiency syndromes	Severe combined immunodeficiencies
	Combined immunodeficiencies
	Common variable immunodeficiency
Genetic syndromes	IL-2-inducible T-cell kinase deficiency
	Uncoordinated 119 (UNC119) mutation
	Warts, hypogammaglobulinemia, infections, and myelokathexis (WHIM)
	X-linked magnesium deficiency with EBV infection and neoplasia (XMEN)
Miscellaneous	OKT4 epitope deficiency

This is not an all-inclusive list

immunodeficiency conditions, such as common variable immunodeficiency, must be excluded. Genetic etiologies for immunodeficiencies must also be excluded based on the standard definition of idiopathic CD4 lymphopenia.

Diagnosis/Management

The diagnosis of idiopathic CD4 lymphopenia can be difficult to make as it is a diagnosis of exclusion. It is important to note that, initially, it is often difficult to understand the cause of CD4 lymphopenia. For instance, in patients presenting with severe infection, it is hard to determine whether the infection is the result of or the cause of CD4 lymphopenia. It is important to monitor CD4 counts over a time period and assess for improvement with the resolution of infection. Similarly, the association of CD4 lymphopenia with autoimmune diseases is complex. Patients with autoimmune diseases such as systemic lupus erythematosus and Sjogren's syndrome can present with lymphopenia secondary to their autoimmune disease; however, autoimmune disease can also stem from primary lymphopenia possibly due to a compensatory T-cell proliferation and break in tolerance. Immunosuppressive medications, such as azathioprine, corticosteroids, cyclosporine, cyclophosphamide, methotrexate, and mycophenolate, also lead to CD4 T-cell lymphopenia. The medication list needs to be carefully reviewed to identify possible causative agents.

To make the diagnosis of idiopathic CD4 lymphopenia, a detailed history followed by a thorough physical exam should be performed to assess for signs and symptoms of other infectious, immunologic, rheumatologic, or hematologic conditions. Some authors recommend initial investigations with lymphocyte flow cytometry to assess CD4, CD8, B cell, and natural killer subsets and function, quantitative immunoglobulin levels, infectious workup, and an autoantibody panel to screen for rheumatologic conditions. Further disease-specific workup should be pursued if clinically indicated based on the patient's history and physical exam [2].

Most patients with idiopathic CD4 lymphopenia have normal B cells and CD8 T cells. It is important to note that some patients have depressed CD4 and CD8 numbers, and these patients should not be excluded based on the 1992 CDC definition. There is data supporting the fact that depressed CD8 counts may represent a separate disease subset, possibly increasing the risk of infections [3]. In idiopathic CD4 lymphopenia, CD4 levels typically remain stable, in contrast to an HIV infection, where a natural decline in CD4 counts is expected without treatment. A minority of patients with idiopathic CD4 lymphopenia spontaneously restore to normal CD4 levels.

Some patients with idiopathic CD4 lymphopenia remain asymptomatic for many years, and CD4 lymphopenia may be discovered incidentally. However, in the majority of cases, idiopathic CD4 lymphopenia is diagnosed due to a presentation with an opportunistic infection, such as in our patient. Many different opportunistic infections have been reported in patients with idiopathic CD4 lymphopenia. These include infections caused by *Mycobacterium tuberculosis*, *Mycobacterium avium-intracellulare* (MAC), unusual types of *Salmonella*, *Cytomegalovirus*, *human polyomavirus 2*, *human papilloma virus* (HPV), *varicella-zoster virus*, *herpes simplex virus*, *human herpesvirus-8*, *Aspergillus*, *Histoplasma capsulatum*, *Leishmania*, *Candida albicans*, *Cryptococcus neoformans*, *Pneumocystis jirovecii* (PJP) and *Toxoplasma gondii*, among others. Many case reports of such opportunistic infections may be found in the literature. Most common opportunistic infections in one study were reported to be with *Cryptococcus*, HPV, and nontuberculous mycobacterium, such as MAC [3]. It is of interest to note that although both idiopathic CD4 lymphopenia and HIV/AIDS have low CD4 counts, the opportunistic infection profiles in both diseases differ in regard to frequencies of different opportunistic pathogens. For instance, cryptococcal infections appear to be the most common infections among opportunistic pathogens in idiopathic CD4 lymphopenia. In contrast, PJP infections are at the top of the list of the most common opportunistic pathogens occurring in HIV/AIDS [4, 5].

It is important to consider that patients with CD4 lymphopenia can be otherwise healthy. Therefore, the immunodeficiency is typically not suspected resulting in a long delay before diagnosis is made. In particular, many cases of cryptococcal meningitis present without fevers, which further complicates the diagnosis [6]. Some patients may also present with malignancy secondary to idiopathic CD4 lymphopenia. These malignancies may include disseminated Kaposi sarcoma, HPV-associated malignancies, and Epstein-Barr virus-related lymphoproliferative disease leading to B-cell lymphoma. Some of these patients also appear to be more prone to autoimmune disease [4].

It is hard to determine the true prevalence of idiopathic CD4 lymphopenia as some patients are likely asymptomatic and do not present for medical care. There is no sex predilection. Cases have been reported in both pediatric and adult populations, although the disorder is thought to be a disease of adulthood.

The pathogenesis of idiopathic CD4 lymphopenia is not clearly understood and may stem from decreased CD4 cell production or increased destruction or sequestration within the spleen and lymph nodes. It is conceivable that patients with CD4 lymphopenia have different etiologies leading to the same common manifestation of depressed CD4 counts. This could possibly contribute to different disease phenotypes. Decreased T-cell production has been attributed to decreased bone marrow precursors, abnormal cell signaling that is important for maintenance of peripheral T cells, and disrupted thymic T-cell maturation [7–9]. There is evidence that CD4 T cells in patients with idiopathic CD4 lymphopenia undergo accelerated programmed cell death [10, 11]. CD4 T cells also seem to have blunted response to IL-7 [2]. Increased activation and turnover of the CD4 T cells have also been observed. CD4 T cells have been shown to exhibit higher proportions of memory-activated CD4 T cells, suggesting restriction of pathogen recognition, which may also contribute to infections [12]. Functional T-cell defects may also be present [13]. T-cell trafficking and tissue distribution have not been fully explored in idiopathic CD4 T-cell lymphopenia, but there is suggestion that CD4 T cells may have abnormal expression of CXCR4 resulting in abnormal chemotactic responses [14].

The presentation of idiopathic CD4 lymphopenia in our case is, to a degree, typical. An otherwise healthy host presents with opportunistic infection. Her infection was likely not suspected given that she had no prior history of an immunodeficiency. As in our case, approximately 50% of patients with cryptococcal meningitis present without a fever. Fortunately, the diagnosis was confirmed based on the lumbar puncture results, and the patient was appropriately treated, resulting in a full recovery. Her CD4 levels remained persistently low, requiring further workup. Infectious, rheumatic, immunologic, and oncologic causes were all negative, allowing for the diagnosis of exclusion of idiopathic CD4 lymphopenia. It was further noteworthy that the patient's CD8 levels were also low. This may portend a worse prognosis and can be seen in patients with more severe opportunistic infections.

Case Presentation 2

A 60-year-old otherwise healthy man with no history of smoking was admitted to the hospital in fulminant respiratory failure after developing high-grade fevers and a dry cough. Chest X-ray showed diffuse bilateral infiltrates. A lactate dehydrogenase was elevated. Bronchoscopy with alveolar lavage was eventually performed, and the patient was diagnosed with PJP pneumonia. He was started on oral trimethoprim/sulfamethoxazole (TMP/SMX) therapy with good response.

Given a diagnosis of PJP pneumonia in an otherwise healthy man, further diagnostic workup was performed. He was found to have a CD4 count of 160 cells/microL. No underlying hematologic, rheumatologic, malignancy, or immunodeficiency causes were identified.

CD4 count was repeated on outpatient basis after resolution of PJP pneumonia and was persistently <200 cells/microL. After excluding all other causes for a low CD4 count, a diagnosis of idiopathic CD4 T-cell lymphopenia was made. The patient was started on TMP/SMX prophylaxis with close outpatient monitoring by specialists.

Treatment of idiopathic CD4 lymphopenia primarily targets treating and preventing opportunistic infections. Although most experts agree on the need for secondary prophylaxis in cases of opportunistic infections, the guidelines for primary prophylaxis are less clear. Current recommendations are to follow prophylaxis guidelines extrapolated from established guidelines in HIV/AIDS literature. However, it is important to note that infectious profiles in idiopathic CD4 lymphopenia and HIV/AIDS are likely distinct. There is data to suggest that at least some opportunistic infections are less common in patients with idiopathic CD4 lymphopenia compared to HIV/AIDS. In particular, patients with idiopathic CD4 lymphopenia appear to be less susceptible to Pneumocystis jirovecii pneumonia (PJP) and Mycobacterium avium complex (MAC).

Based on HIV/AIDS data, PJP prophylaxis is recommended with CD4 count <200 cells/microL. Prophylaxis is typically continued until the CD4 count rises above 200 cells/microL. Toxoplasmosis prophylaxis is recommended with CD4 count <100 and a positive serology. Toxoplasmosis prophylaxis can be achieved with trimethoprim/sulfamethoxazole (TMP/SMX) or other combination therapies, if the patient is intolerant to TMP/SMX. TMP/SMX is the preferred agent for PJP prophylaxis for patients who can tolerate a sulfa drug. The specific dose strength and frequency are dependent on factors that include the additional need for toxoplasmosis prophylaxis and renal function. Patients with good renal function being treated for PJP alone can be treated with one single-strength tablet (trimethoprim 80 mg–sulfamethoxazole 400 mg) daily or one double-strength tablet (trimethoprim 160 mg–sulfamethoxazole 800 mg) three times per week. If PJP and toxoplasmosis prophylaxis are necessary, then both can be treated with one double-strength tablet (trimethoprim 160 mg–sulfamethoxazole 800 mg) daily or three times per week. When patients are intolerant to sulfa, alternative agents, such as dapsone or atovaquone, can be substituted and used for PJP and, if necessary, toxoplasmosis prophylaxis.

Preventative therapy for cryptococcal disease is generally not recommended in HIV cases. However, cryptococcal disease appears to affect a higher percentage of patients with idiopathic CD4 lymphopenia compared to patients with HIV/AIDS. Therefore, prophylaxis with an anti-fungal agent against *Cryptococcus*, such as fluconazole, may be considered. This is particularly true in patients with a worse prognosis, such as those with low CD8 in addition to low CD4 [15]. Azithromycin prophylaxis may be considered with CD4 <100 based on HIV data. When necessary, one preferred dosing regimen is 1200 mg once weekly. Alternatively, 600 mg twice weekly has been utilized as well.

Live vaccines should be avoided in patients with CD4 lymphopenia. The efficacy of protective effects of non-live vaccines is unknown, but these vaccines appear to be safe and should be recommended.

Patients with idiopathic CD4 lymphopenia are at a higher risk of lymphoma as well as HPV-related cancers. Patients should undergo age-appropriate cancer screening. Additional cancer screening recommendations are less clear, but it is important to have frequent follow-up with routine histories and physicals, close monitoring for development of any suspicious symptoms, and prompt evaluations.

The treatment experiences aimed at augmenting CD4 numbers are very limited and based on case report data. These treatments are reserved for patients with a history of life-threatening infections or persistent opportunistic infections. More data is needed to support their widespread use. Some treatments that have been investigated target IL-2, IFN-gamma, and IL-7 [16–21]. The use of hematopoietic stem cell transplantation in idiopathic CD4 lymphopenia has also been reported [22, 23]. It is important to note that there is a possibility of publication bias toward positive results.

Pneumocystis jirovecii pneumonia was present in our case. It is a rare, opportunistic infection in patients with idiopathic CD4 lymphopenia. Our current guidelines extrapolate from HIV/AIDS data on opportunistic infections, and prophylaxis with TMP/SMX or an alternative agent is recommended for patients with CD4 <200 cells/microL. However, the overall risk of PJP infection is possibly lower in patients with idiopathic CD4 lymphopenia compared to HIV/AIDS.

Conclusion

Idiopathic CD4 lymphopenia is a rare condition resulting in low CD4 lymphocyte counts. It is a diagnosis of exclusion, once other causes of primary and secondary lymphopenia are ruled out. It is a heterogeneous disorder, with patient presentation's ranging from asymptomatic to severe opportunistic infections. Cryptococcal meningitis remains the most common opportunistic infection. There are a number of other diseases associated with ICL, including several malignancies and autoimmune disorders. There are no standard guidelines for this condition. Attention should be focused on rapid treatment of opportunistic infections, management of any associated conditions, and supportive care. Infection prophylaxis should be implemented based on HIV guidelines and include therapies for PJP, toxoplasmosis, and MAC prevention. While there is no clear consensus on monitoring, it would be reasonable to check CD4 counts twice yearly in most stable patients. The overall prognosis is variable and depends on the degree and duration of immune suppression, as well as the presence of any comorbidities and associated infections. Patients with low CD8 cell counts in addition to low CD4 counts have a worse overall prognosis and should be followed more closely.

Clinical Pearls and Pitfalls

- Consider idiopathic CD4 lymphopenia in patients with persistent CD4 lymphopenia <300 cells/microL or <20% of the total T cells on more than one cell count at least 6 weeks apart.
- It is important to exclude any alternative diagnoses leading to CD4 lymphopenia, such as infections, malignancy, autoimmunity, drugs, and other immunodeficiency syndromes.
- Some patients present with severe opportunistic infections, while a minority may be asymptomatic.
- For some patients with idiopathic CD4 lymphopenia, CD4 counts may improve spontaneously without treatment.
- The mainstay of treatment is aggressive care of any opportunistic infections, initiation of prophylaxis, and general health care maintenance.
- Data on prophylaxis is extrapolated from HIV/AIDS data, although the opportunistic infection profile is distinct in idiopathic CD4 lymphopenia as compared to HIV/AIDS.
- Vigilant monitoring for infections, malignancy, and autoimmunity at routine follow-up visits is imperative in patients with idiopathic CD4 lymphopenia.
- Patients should be up to date with vaccines. Live vaccines are contraindicated in patients with low CD4 counts.
- Stable patients with ICL should have their CD4 counts checked at least twice per year.
- Additional treatments to augment CD4 T-cell numbers may be considered, but more research is needed to support their use.

References

1. Smith DK, Neal JJ, Holmberg SD. Unexplained opportunistic infections and CD4+ T-lymphocytopenia without HIV infection. An investigation of cases in the United States. The Centers for Disease Control Idiopathic CD4+ T-lymphocytopenia Task Force. N Engl J Med. 1993;328(6):373–9.
2. Zonios D, Sheikh V, Sereti I. Idiopathic CD4 lymphocytopenia: a case of missing, wandering or ineffective T cells. Arthritis Res Ther. 2012;14(4):222.
3. Zonios DI, Falloon J, Bennett JE, Shaw PA, Chaitt D, Baseler MW, et al. Idiopathic CD4+ lymphocytopenia: natural history and prognostic factors. Blood. 2008;112(2):287–94.
4. Ahmad DS, Esmadi M, Steinmann WC. Idiopathic CD4 Lymphocytopenia: spectrum of opportunistic infections, malignancies, and autoimmune diseases. Avicenna J Med. 2013;3(2):37–47.
5. Buchacz K, Baker RK, Palella FJ Jr, Chmiel JS, Lichtenstein KA, Novak RM, et al. AIDS-defining opportunistic illnesses in US patients, 1994–2007: a cohort study. AIDS. 2010;24(10):1549–59.
6. Shribman S, Noyce A, Gnanapavan S, Lambourne J, Harrison T, Schon F. Cryptococcal meningitis in apparently immunocompetent patients: association with idiopathic CD4+ lymphopenia. Pract Neurol. 2018;18(2):166–9.
7. Isgro A, Sirianni MC, Gramiccioni C, Mezzaroma I, Fantauzzi A, Aiuti F. Idiopathic CD4+ lymphocytopenia may be due to decreased bone marrow clonogenic capability. Int Arch Allergy Immunol. 2005;136(4):379–84.
8. Hubert P, Bergeron F, Ferreira V, Seligmann M, Oksenhendler E, Debre P, et al. Defective p56Lck activity in T cells from an adult patient with idiopathic CD4+ lymphocytopenia. Int Immunol. 2000;12(4):449–57.
9. Fruhwirth M, Clodi K, Heitger A, Neu N. Lymphocyte diversity in a 9-year-old boy with idiopathic CD4+ T cell lymphocytopenia. Int Arch Allergy Immunol. 2001;125(1):80–5.
10. Laurence J, Mitra D, Steiner M, Lynch DH, Siegal FP, Staiano-Coico L. Apoptotic depletion of CD4+ T cells in idiopathic CD4+ T lymphocytopenia. J Clin Invest. 1996;97(3):672–80.
11. Roger PM, Bernard-Pomier G, Counillon E, Breittmayer JP, Bernard A, Dellamonica P. Overexpression of Fas/CD95 and Fas-induced apoptosis in a patient with idiopathic CD4+ T lymphocytopenia. Clin Infect Dis. 1999;28(5):1012–6.
12. Signorini S, Pirovano S, Fiorentini S, Stellini R, Bianchi V, Albertini A, Imberti L. Restriction of T-cell receptor repertoires in idiopathic CD4+ lymphocytopenia. Br J Haematol. 2000;110(2):434–7.
13. Netea MG, Brouwer AE, Hoogendoorn EH, Van der Meer JW, Koolen M, Verweij PE, et al. Two patients with cryptococcal meningitis and idiopathic CD4 lymphopenia: defective cytokine production and reversal by recombinant interferon- gamma therapy. Clin Infect Dis. 2004;39(9):e83–7.
14. Scott-Algara D, Balabanian K, Chakrabarti LA, Mouthon L, Dromer F, Didier C, et al. Idiopathic CD4+ T-cell lymphocytopenia is associated with impaired membrane expression of the chemokine receptor CXCR4. Blood. 2010;115(18):3708–17.
15. Yarmohammadi H, Cunningham-Rundles C. Idiopathic CD4 lymphocytopenia: pathogenesis, etiologies, clinical presentations and treatment strategies. Ann Allergy Asthma Immunol. 2017;119(4):374–8.
16. Cunningham-Rundles C, Murray HW, Smith JP. Treatment of idiopathic CD4 T lymphocytopenia with IL-2. Clin Exp Immunol. 1999;116(2):322–5.
17. Yilmaz-Demirdag Y, Wilson B, Lowery-Nordberg M, Bocchini JA Jr, Bahna SL. Interleukin-2 treatment for persistent cryptococcal meningitis in a child with idiopathic CD4(+) T lymphocytopenia. Allergy Asthma Proc. 2008;29(4):421–4.
18. Warnatz K, Draeger R, Schlesier M, Peter HH. Successful IL-2 therapy for relapsing herpes zoster infection in a patient with idiopathic CD4+ T lymphocytopenia. Immunobiology. 2000;202(2):204–11.

19. Moniuszko M, Fry T, Tsai WP, Morre M, Assouline B, Cortez P, et al. Recombinant interleukin-7 induces proliferation of naive macaque CD4+ and CD8+ T cells in vivo. J Virol. 2004;78(18):9740–9.
20. Holland SM, Eisenstein EM, Kuhns DB, Turner ML, Fleisher TA, Strober W, et al. Treatment of refractory disseminated nontuberculous mycobacterial infection with interferon gamma. A preliminary report. N Engl J Med. 1994;330(19):1348–55.
21. Sheikh V, Porter BO, DerSimonian R, Kovacs SB, Thompson WL, Perez-Diez A, et al. Administration of interleukin-7 increases CD4 T cells in idiopathic CD4 lymphocytopenia. Blood. 2016;127(8):977–88.
22. Petersen EJ, Rozenberg-Arska M, Dekker AW, Clevers HC, Verdonck LF. Allogeneic bone marrow transplantation can restore CD4+ T-lymphocyte count and immune function in idiopathic CD4+ T-lymphocytopenia. Bone Marrow Transplant. 1996;18(4):813–5.
23. Cervera C, Fernández-Avilés F, de la Calle-Martin O, Bosch X, Rovira M, Plana M, et al. Nonmyeloablative hematopoietic stem cell transplantation in the treatment of severe idiopathic CD4+ lymphocytopenia. Eur J Haematol. 2011;87(1):87–91.

Chapter 10
Hyper IgE Syndrome

Taha Al-Shaikhly

Case Presentation 1

A 7-year-old boy presented for evaluation of recurrent infections. A detailed infectious history revealed that he had recurrent otitis media starting by 8 months of age which necessitated the placement of bilateral tympanostomy tubes by age 3. Tympanostomy tubes helped in reducing the frequency of his ear infections. He had a history of three episodes of staphylococcal neck abscess requiring incision and drainage at ages 1.5, 2, and 4 years and a history of paronychia at 3 years of age. His abscesses were notable for lack of erythema and fever. He was hospitalized at 10 months of age with a *respiratory syncytial virus* bronchiolitis. He had two episodes of pneumonia, at age 3 and 6 years, both of which required hospitalization and treatment with parenteral antibiotics. The latter episode of pneumonia was complicated by pleural effusion and *Streptococcus pneumoniae* bacteremia. Further review of his hospitalization course revealed that, despite the severity of his pneumonia, he only developed low-grade fever (up to 100.4° F), and his C-reactive protein (CRP) remained normal (highest recorded, 2.2 mg/L). Early in his life, he had recurrent episodes of oral thrush, but he had no history of recurrent or difficult-to-treat skin warts and no history of recurrent infections with herpes viruses. His mother states that, after the last episode of pneumonia, he had persistent respiratory symptoms and was eventually diagnosed with asthma. In addition to asthma and recurrent infections, his past medical history was also significant for eczema, which was diagnosed by 3 months of age. He was using daily moisturizer and topical triamcinolone. Bleach baths were especially helpful per his mother. Physical examination was notable for high-arched palate, a broad nasal bridge, and crowded teeth. He had eczema on his cheeks, the flexural surfaces of his elbows, the posterior aspects

---

T. Al-Shaikhly (✉)
Department of Medicine, Penn State College of Medicine, Hershey, PA, USA
e-mail: talshaikhly@pennstatehealth.psu.edu

© Springer Nature Switzerland AG 2021
J. A. Bernstein (ed.), *Primary and Secondary Immunodeficiency*,
https://doi.org/10.1007/978-3-030-57157-3_10

of his neck, and upper back. The big toenails were brittle with yellowish discoloration. He had bilateral rhonchi on lung auscultation. Hypermobility of his elbow, wrist, and finger joints was also noted. Computerized tomography of his chest revealed bronchiectatic changes affecting multiple lung lobes and a pneumatocele in the left upper lobe. Because of the unusual frequency and severity of his infections, an immunological evaluation was pursued. His complete blood count showed anemia (hemoglobin, 10.9 g/dL; normal, 12–15 g/dL) and leukocytosis (WBC, 12,100 cells/μL; normal, 4000–11,000 cells//μL), with an absolute eosinophil count (AEC) of 2800 cells/μL (normal, 0–350 cells/μL). He had normal neutrophil oxidative burst as assessed by dihydrorhodamine (DHR) flow cytometry. His total complement hemolytic activity (CH50) was 73 U/mL (normal. 42–95 U/mL). Quantitative immunoglobulin levels were measured, and his serum IgG level was 915 mg/dL (normal, 463–1236 mg/dL), IgM level was 110 (normal 48–207 mg/dL), and IgA level was 90 mg/dL (normal, 33–202 mg/dL). However, his serum IgE level was 53,323 IU/mL (normal, 1.03–161.3 IU/mL). He had protective antibody titer to tetanus vaccine (0.3 IU/L; normal, >0.1 IU/L). Four weeks after the administration of pneumococcal polysaccharide vaccine-23 booster, he mounted protective antibody titers to 7 out of the 23 tested pneumococcal serotypes. Fluorescence-activated cell sorting (FACS) analysis of the patient's peripheral blood mononuclear cells (PBMCs) showed a $CD3^+$ count of 1750 cells/μL (normal, 1200–2600 cells/μL), with a normal CD4:CD8 ratio. His $CD19^+$ B-cell number was also normal at 460 cells/μL (normal, 270–860 cells/μL), but he had decreased proportion of $CD27^+$ memory B cells. In vitro stimulation of his PBMCs with mitogen phytohemagglutinin (PHA) as well as with anti-CD3 was normal. Further subset analysis of his PBMCs revealed decreased percentage of IL-17-producing $CD4^+$ T cells (Th17). Sequencing of the *STAT3* gene revealed a heterozygous missense mutation in the highly conserved DNA-binding domain (c.1396 A>G, p.N466D). The patient was started on intravenous immunoglobulin replacement therapy at 400 mg/kg/month and trimethoprim/sulfamethoxazole prophylaxis. Further radiographic evaluation confirmed the presence of three retained primary teeth which were surgically removed. At 10 years of age, he had a left radioulnar fracture after minor trauma which was successfully treated with immobilization.

Diagnosis/Assessment

Clinical Features

Autosomal dominant (AD)-HIES, formerly known as Job syndrome, is a rare disease with an estimated incidence of 1/1,000,000 [1]. AD-HIES is caused by a heterozygous dominant negative mutation in the *signal transducer and activator of transcription-3 (STAT3)* gene [2–4]. The majority of the reported mutations affect either the DNA-binding domain as observed in the case presented or the Src homology 2 (SH2) domain of the STAT3 protein [2–7]. STAT3 is a transcription factor essential for signal transduction of multiple key cytokines including interleukin (IL)-6, IL-10, IL-11, IL-27, IL-21, and IL-23, explaining the broad clinical manifestations of the disease consisting of both immune and nonimmune manifestations [1, 4, 5, 8, 9].

The immunological manifestations include both recurrent infections and atopic diseases. Early-onset neonatal rash followed by the eventual development of eczematoid dermatitis occurs in almost all patients (90% of patients). The eczematoid rash often has a predilection for the scalp and face, as with our patient, and appears to be driven at least in part by frequent skin infections or colonization with *Staphylococcus aureus* [10]. Other atopic features include both food (20% of patients) and environmental (12%) allergies [1, 6]. A good proportion of patients (~28%) also suffer from asthma [1, 6]. A predominant role for the impaired IL-6 signaling pathway in the development of these atopic features is conjectured by (1) a recent identification of biallelic loss-of-function mutations in *IL6R* gene as a novel cause for HIES in two patients presenting predominantly with atopy and recurrent infections [11] and (2) by genome-wide association study linking *IL6R* gene polymorphism with asthma and poor lung function in the Han Chinese population [12]. Alternatively, STAT3 deficiency causes defective mast cell degranulation which may explain the relatively lower prevalence of atopy when compared to DOCK8-deficient patients [13].

In addition to humoral immunodeficiency (discussed below), Th17 deficiency secondary to impaired signal transduction of IL-6, a cytokine critical for the development of these cells [14], is thought to mainly account for the infectious susceptibility seen in patients with AD-HIES. Recurrent skin and lung infections are hallmarks of the disease and are most commonly caused by *Staphylococcus aureus* [1, 6, 7, 15]. Skin infections, most often in the form of skin abscesses and less frequently cellulitis, occur in virtually all patients [1, 6, 7, 15]. Recurrent pneumonias occur in 90–95% of patients and are most often caused by *Staphylococcus aureus*. Pneumonias are often associated with pleural effusion and less frequently pneumothorax [6]. Recurrent pneumonias can be complicated by bronchiectasis as well as by the formation of pneumatoceles (lung cysts) which can be seen in almost half of these patients [1, 6, 7, 15]. Pneumatocele infections are most often caused by *Aspergillus fumigatus* or by *Pseudomonas aeruginosa,* reminiscent of cystic fibrosis patients, and represent a major cause of morbidity [1, 6]. In addition to recurrent skin and lung infections, half of the patients with STAT3 deficiency suffer from recurrent otitis and sinusitis [1, 6]. Although patients with AD-HIES may present with bacterial infections without cardinal signs of inflammation (aka cold abscesses), they more often do [1]. In addition to bacterial infections, over half of the patients suffer from mucocutaneous candidiasis (oral thrush and onychomycosis). Disseminated endemic mycosis such as with *Histoplasma, Cryptococcus, and Coccidioides* has also been reported in patients with AD-HIES and has predilection for gastrointestinal involvement [16]. Viral infections are uncommon among STAT3-deficient patients (~10%) [1, 6] and are most often caused by *herpes simplex virus*. The virtual absence of viral infection distinguishes patients with AD-HIES from those with autosomal recessive-HIES (AR-HIES) secondary to DOCK8 deficiency who often present with recurrent cutaneous viral infections (discussed below) [17]. Beyond atopy and recurrent infections, lymphoma has been reported in ~5% of patients [1, 6, 18]. The molecular basis for the predisposition to lymphoma in STAT3-deficient patients remains unknown.

The non-immunological manifestations distinguish STAT3-deficient patients from other causes of HIES (Table 10.1). These features include (1) facial dysmorphism observed in 90–95% of patients [6, 7, 15] which includes prominent forehead, broad nasal bridge, prognathism, retrognathism, increased interalar distance, and high-arched palate; (2) skeletal malformations (30–40% of patients) such as pathological

Table 10.1 Selected disorders presenting with recurrent infections and elevated IgE levels

Disorder	Inheritance/gene affected	Key clinical and laboratory features
Job syndrome (AD-HIES or STAT3 deficiency)	AD[a]/*STAT3*	Recurrent pneumonias, skin abscesses (cold abscesses), mucocutaneous candidiasis, pneumatocele, skeletal and dental abnormalities, no susceptibility to cutaneous viral infections. Normal Ig levels, T- and B-lymphocyte counts, and mitogen studies, but decreased percentage of Th17 and memory B cells
ZNF431 deficiency [21, 22]	AR/*ZNF431*	Phenocopy of Job syndrome but with *lower prevalence of skeletal and dental abnormalities*. Normal Ig levels, T-cell count, and mitogen studies, but decreased percentage of Th17 and memory B cells
GP130 deficiency [23, 24]	AR/*IL6ST*	Phenocopy of Job syndrome, also *keratitis*, limited skeletal abnormalities (scoliosis and craniosynostosis), less susceptibility to fungal infections. Normal Ig levels, T-cell count, and mitogen studies, but decreased percentage of memory B cells, with *normal or reduced percentage of Th17*
IL6 receptor deficiency [11]	AR/*IL6R*	Phenocopy of Job syndrome *without skeletal or dental abnormalities and no susceptibly to fungal infections*. Normal Ig levels, normal T-lymphocyte count and function, normal percentage of Th17
DOCK8 deficiency	AR/*DOCK8*	Combined immunodeficiency with *cutaneous viral infections*, autoimmunity, malignancy, and neurological complications. Low T-lymphocyte count and poor responses to mitogens, *low IgM levels*, normal or high IgA and IgG levels
Wiskott-Aldrich syndrome	X-linked/*WAS*	Similar to DOCK8 deficiency, also *colitis*, and bleeding tendency with small platelets (*microthrombocytopenia*-pathognomonic)
PGM3 deficiency [67, 68, 74]	AR/*PGM3*	A congenital disorder of glycosylation disorder, presenting with a combined immunodeficiency phenotype, *developmental delay, and motor symptoms* (ataxia, hypotonia), neutropenia, hypergammaglobulinemia, low T lymphocytes, and poor responses to mitogens
CARD11 deficiency [75, 76]	AD[a] / *CARD11*	Similar to DOCK8 but milder phenotype and with less susceptibility to cutaneous viral infections

Table 10.1 (continued)

Disorder	Inheritance/gene affected	Key clinical and laboratory features
Comel-Netherton syndrome [77, 78]	AR/SPINK5	Ichthyosis and *bamboo hair*, poor vaccine responses including to bacteriophage and NK cell dysfunction
Omenn Syndrome [79]	Variable	Opportunistic infections, *diarrhea and erythroderma, lymphadenopathy, and hepatosplenomegaly*. Oligoclonal T-cell lymphocytosis, with poor or absent response to mitogens
IPEX [80, 81]	X-linked/*FOXP3*	Early-onset *enteropathy, diabetes,* and failure to thrive. Decreased FOXP3$^+$ CD25$^+$ T cells
Atopic dermatitis [15]	Polygenic	Infections, if any, are limited to the skin with *absence of deep infections* such as pneumonia. Normal immunological evaluation and *low NIH HIES score* (<20)

Abbreviations: *Ig* Immunoglobulin, *ZNF431* zinc finger protein 431, *GP130* glycoprotein 130, *PGM3* phosphoglucomutase-3, *CARD11* caspase activation and recruitment domain-11, *IPEX* immunodysregulation polyendocrinopathy enteropathy X-linked
[a]Heterozygous mutation with dominant negative effect

fractures, craniosynostosis, scoliosis, and joint hypermobility; (3) retention of deciduous teeth observed in ~40–70% of patients; (4) pneumatocele present in ~50% of patients; and (5) vascular malformation such as cardiovascular and brain aneurysms [19]. While there is no considerable genotype-phenotype correlation, patients with mutations affecting the SH2 domain of STAT3 are more likely to develop severe scoliosis, high-arched palate, and increased interalar distance [20]. These non-immunological manifestations are not unique to STAT3 deficiency (Fig. 10.1) and are observed with (1) ZNF431 deficiency, which is a newly recognized autosomal recessive cause of HIES associated with a functional STAT3 deficiency state [21, 22] and with (2) biallelic mutations in the *IL6ST* gene which result in deficiency of gp130, a receptor subunit necessary for the signal transduction of IL-6, IL-27, and IL-11 cytokines to STAT3 [23, 24]. The skeletal malformations may be explained by impaired signal transduction of both IL-11 [25] and leukemia inhibitory factor (LIF), the latter of which is involved in regulation of osteoclastogenesis [26]. On the other hand, dysregulated metalloproteases may account for the rare occurrence of vascular malformation among STAT3-deficient patients [27–29]. Counterintuitive to the fact that suppression of STAT3 prevents platelet aggregation [30] and lower extremity thrombosis [31], a rare and under-recognized complication of STAT3 deficiency is venous thrombophlebitis [6] which may be attributed to vascular abnormalities.

Laboratory Features

While complete blood count in patients with AD-HIES often reveals eosinophilia, a recent review of the STAT3-deficient patients collected at the US Immunodeficiency Network (USIDNET) registry also highlights anemia as an under-recognized

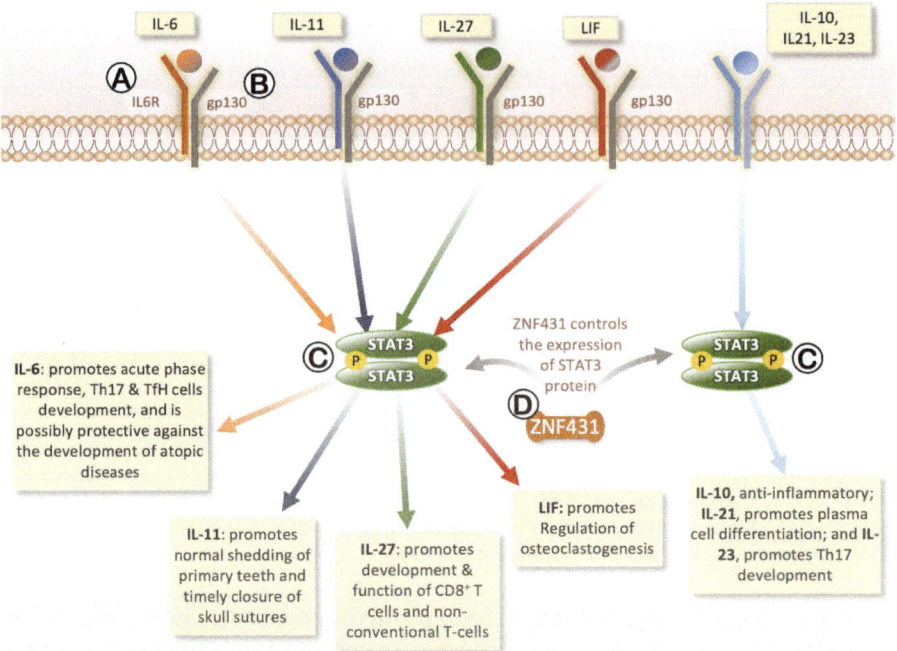

Fig. 10.1 ZNF431 is a transcription factor that controls the expression of STAT3 protein especially in hematopoietic cells. STAT3, another transcription factor, is activated by several cytokines including IL-6, IL-11, IL-21, IL-23, IL-27, IL-10, and LIF. The key functions of these cytokines are illustrated. Glycoprotein 130 (gp130) is a receptor subunit utilized by some of these cytokines. Deficiency of IL6R subunit (A) results in atopy, elevated IgE level, and recurrent staphylococcal skin and lung infections with impaired inflammatory response. Deficiency of gp130 receptor subunit (B) can additionally result in craniosynostosis, scoliosis, and delayed shedding of primary teeth secondary to defective IL-11 signal transduction. Deficiency of the downstream molecules such as STAT3 or ZNF431 transcription factors (C and D) results in a broader clinical phenotype with additional features of mucocutaneous candidiasis, pathological fractures, and vascular malformations. Th17, T-helper 17; TfH, T follicular helper cell; LIF, leukemia inhibitory factor; ZNF431, zinc finger protein 431

finding occurring in 41% of patients [1] as was observed in this case presentation. Finding of anemia may be explained by an autoimmune phenomenon or direct effects of STAT3 deficiency which can accelerate the destruction of erythrocytes by splenic macrophages [32]. Marked elevation in serum IgE levels (up to 93,000 IU/mL) [1, 6] is observed in almost all patients [1, 6, 7, 15], and those with mutations affecting the DNA-binding domain of STAT3 tend to have relatively higher serum IgE levels [20]. However, the level of serum IgE only begins to rise after birth and decreases or even normalizes during adulthood [1, 33]. In fact, 4% of patients reported in the literature had a normal serum level of IgE [6, 15]. In addition to increased IgE levels, serum IgD levels can also be elevated [6, 34]. The underlying molecular basis for the elevated IgE levels and eosinophil count is not completely understood but may be related to an unopposed IL-4 signal secondary to impaired

10 Hyper IgE Syndrome

IL-10 and IL-21 signal transduction [35] and/or to impaired IL-6 signal transduction [11, 21–24]. Neither IgE level nor eosinophilia correlates with disease activity.

Serum levels of other immunoglobulin isotypes, including IgG, IgA, and IgM, are often normal. However, antibody responses to vaccines or to bacteriophage can be impaired [1, 6, 36] as illustrated in the patient presented. Impaired IL-6 signal transduction, which is important for early stages of T follicular helper cell (TfH) development [37], and impaired IL-21 signal transduction in B cells, which is important for plasma cell maturation [38], are thought to underlie the impairment in antibody responses. This is further supported by a recent study demonstrating a critical role for STAT3 signaling in affinity maturation and B-cell differentiation [39]. The numbers of T, B, and NK cells are often normal. However, almost all STAT3-deficient patients have decreased percentages of Th17 and of CD27$^+$CD19$^+$ memory B cells [6, 36], and these two findings are useful diagnostic clues [6, 15].

Diagnosis

Suspicion for AD-HIES is based on the clinical and laboratory findings, but sequencing of the *STAT3* gene is ultimately required to establish a definitive diagnosis [7]. Figure 10.2 provides a suggested stepwise approach to patients presenting with the HIES triad. Because STAT3 deficiency is an autosomal dominant disorder, the

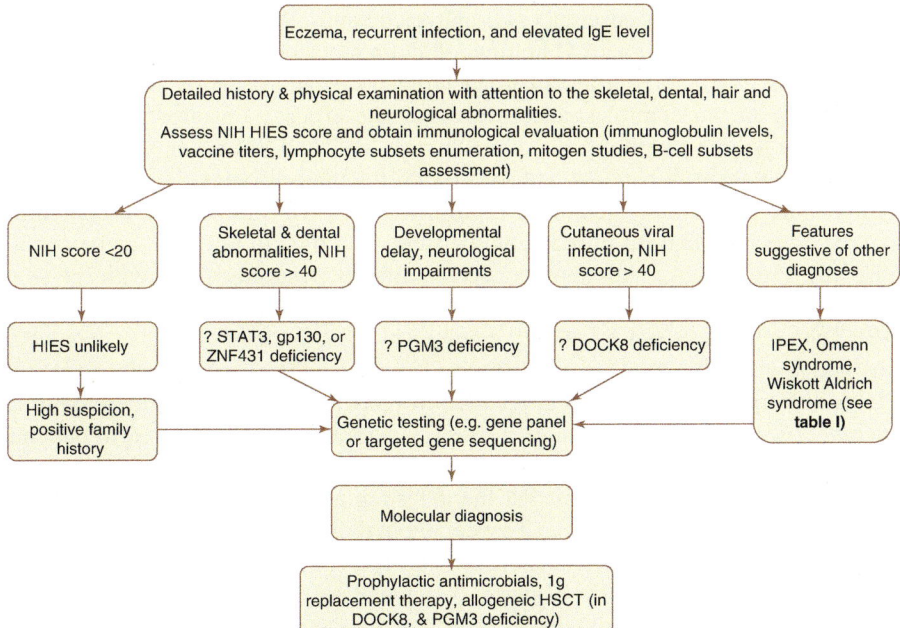

Fig. 10.2 A stepwise approach to patients presenting with eczema, recurrent infections, and elevated serum IgE levels

presence of a positive family history can be another useful diagnostic clue. However, almost half of the patients registered by the USIDNET had no other affected family members. Based on aggregate data from five large cohorts [6–9, 15] describing the clinical characteristics of patients with AD-HIES, a scoring system was developed by the National Institute of Health (NIH HIES score). The NIH HIES score accounts for the presence and severity of 21 clinical and laboratory findings [40] and has proven useful in identifying patients who are candidates for further genetic testing. It is estimated that 76–96% of patients with STAT3 deficiency would have a score equal or greater than 40, indicating a high probability for this diagnosis [6, 7, 15]. The NIH HIES scoring system should, however, not replace the physician's judgment or preclude genetic testing if the clinical suspicion is high and especially in the presence of a compatible family history [7]. It is important to recognize that the clinical phenotype of AD-HIES remains variable even among those with the same genetic defect [6] and that the non-immunological features accrue over time and may be absent early in life explaining the delay in diagnosis of these patients [1, 6] with an average age at diagnosis being about 10 years old.

Management/Outcome

While there are no established treatment guidelines for AD-HIES, observational studies describing patients with AD-HIES suggest five mainstays for treatment: (1) meticulous skin care for eczema, (2) prophylactic antimicrobials, (3) vigilance and early treatment of infections, (4) immunoglobulin replacement therapy, and (5) special attention to the nonimmune manifestations (skeletal and dental abnormalities). While there are no control studies evaluating the efficacy of anti-staphylococcal prophylaxis with trimethoprim-sulfamethoxazole (TMP-SMX) or an equivalent antimicrobial agent in patients with AD-HIES, the majority of patients reported in the literature were maintained on such prophylaxis [1, 6]. Antibacterial prophylaxis may be especially helpful in reducing the frequency of skin infection and external otitis [6]. Prophylactic anti-staphylococcal antibiotics can also help with the skin disease because bacterial colonization of the skin contributes to eczema severity [10]. The prevalence of drug allergy among AD-HIES patients is higher than what was initially thought (24% of patients) and can pose a therapeutic challenge [1, 6]. Cloxacillin offers an attractive alternative in patients with sulfonamide antibiotic allergy; however it is not available in the US market [6]. As compared to patients with DOCK8 deficiency, a relatively less proportion of patients (~50%) would require antimycotic prophylaxis, but the latter remains a consideration in patients with recurrent fungal infections and especially in those with structural lung diseases [1, 6]. Itraconazole and voriconazole are the most frequently utilized antifungal agents in that regard [1, 6]. Because skin and lung infections in patients with AD-HIES may lack the cardinal signs of inflammation, vigilance for infections and low threshold for antibiotic initiation should be maintained. It is also important to recognize that the synthesis of CRP, a commonly used inflammatory marker to indicate the presence of bacterial infections, is also dependent on an intact STAT3 signaling pathway (see Fig. 10.1), and hence CRP may not be a reliable biomarker for infections [11, 23, 24, 41]. Furthermore, the lack of inflammatory response or the appropriate rise in CRP is not a unique feature of STAT3-HIES, as it has been observed with newly recognized genetic causes of HIES, all of which interfere with the IL-6 signaling pathway including biallelic loss-of-function mutations in *IL6R* [11], *ZNF431* [21, 22], or *IL6ST* [23, 24] (see Fig. 10.1).

As discussed above, STAT3-HIES patients have reduced memory B cells and may fail to mount a protective antibody response to T-cell-dependent antigens. However, irrespective of the presence of such qualitative antibody deficiency, immunoglobulin replacement therapy may be beneficial and can reduce the risk of pneumonia [1, 6]. The impact of IgG replacement therapy on the incidence of pneumonia has been evaluated in the French cohort of AD-HIES and was proven to significantly reduce the incidence of pneumonia from 27.8 to 9.3 per 100 patients [6]. Eczematous dermatitis should be treated per established guidelines, and as seen in the patient presented, bleach baths can be especially helpful [42]. Although theoretically tempting, a role for using biologics such as mepolizumab to target the IL-5 cytokine pathway or dupilumab to target the IL4 receptor-alpha (IL4Ra) is yet to be elucidated. However, three patients with a clinical diagnosis of HIES and refractory eczematous dermatitis were reported to have a favorable response to omalizumab (a humanized monoclonal antibody to IgE), albeit having significantly elevated IgE levels (>3000 IU/mL) [43–45].

Nonimmune manifestations require special attention. For example, retained primary teeth should be surgically removed, and a lower threshold should be maintained for bone fracture evaluation, even after a minor trauma. In addition, patients should also be monitored for the development of scoliosis [8]. Therapy with bisphosphonates can improve bone mineral density in patients with AD-HIES, but its role in reducing the frequency of pathological fractures remains unclear [42, 46]. Because of the high prevalence of vascular malformations in these patients [19], clinicians should ensure proper blood pressure control and maintain a lower threshold for considering vascular events. Lastly, the psychological burden of the disease should not be overlooked. Depression has been reported in ~20% of patients with STAT3 deficiency and especially among those with pneumatocele [1]. Therefore, screening for the presence of depression, as recommended by the US Preventive Services Task Force (USPSTF), is also advocated.

In the search for a definitive treatment for AD-HIES, conflicting results were obtained from allogeneic hematopoietic stem cell transplantation (HSCT) probably owing to the presence of extra-immunological manifestations. After two initial reports demonstrating poor outcome [47, 48], subsequent reports were more encouraging at least for correcting the underlying immunological defects [49–51]. Surprisingly, HSCT also corrected the osteoporosis and halted further development of the non-immunological manifestations in one patient [49]. Compared to patients with DOCK8 deficiency (see below), the prognosis of patients with AD-HIES is relatively good provided that multiple prophylactic measures, including immunoglobulin replacement therapy, are employed [6]. Patients with AD-HIES are reported to live into their sixth decades [1, 6], and the majority of these patients (>85%) enjoyed no or only minor impairment in their quality of life [1]. However, those with pneumatocele, such as the patient described in the case presentation, tend to have a worse prognosis [52]. Severe infections, including pneumatocele fungal and pseudomonal infections, remain the number one cause of death [6, 52].

Case Presentation 2

A 6-year-old boy presented for evaluation of recurrent infections and hypereosinophilia with an absolute eosinophil count of 45,130 cells/μL. He was born to a consanguineous family from Iran and was diagnosed with eczema early in his infancy. His eczema affected his face, and extremities, and he was being treated with daily moisturizer and topical anti-inflammatory agents including triamcinolone and tacrolimus. Despite proper skin care, his eczema was complicated by multiple episodes of skin abscesses including a recent episode of a skin abscess in his left arm that required incision and drainage. Bleach baths provided partial improvement of his eczema and reduced the frequency of skin abscesses per his mother. In addition to skin abscesses, he also suffered from recurrent otitis media starting early in his life, and by 3 years of age he had bilateral tympanostomy tube placement. His mother states that he often gets "viral colds" and that he had difficult time getting over his cold symptoms frequently leading to bronchitis. By 3.5 years of age, he was hospitalized for necrotizing staphylococcal pneumonia which was complicated by empyema. In addition to recurrent ear infections and upper and lower respiratory tract infections, he had multiple skin warts which were difficult to treat and a history of recurrent herpes simplex stomatitis. His past medical history was also notable for asthma diagnosed by 5 years of age and multiple food allergy including anaphylactic reaction to peanut. Because of his eczema, he had food allergy testing at age 1 which revealed IgE sensitization to soy, wheat, peanut and tree nuts. At 2 years of age, he developed autoimmune hemolytic anemia which was successfully treated with prednisone and high-dose intravenous immunoglobulin. He had no family history of immunodeficiency or autoimmune disorders. In addition to topical triamcinolone and tacrolimus, his home medications included as needed albuterol and twice daily budesonide-formoterol (80/4.5 mcg) inhaler. Physical examination revealed eczematous changes on his face, upper arms, and thighs. Multiple umbilicated warty lesions (aka Mollusca) were noted on his back. He also had three skin warts on his left hand and two warts on his right hand. Dystrophic changes affecting several of his toenails were noted. He had no dysmorphic facial features. A white patch was also noted in his oropharynx, and bilateral rhonchi were appreciated on lung auscultation.

Because of the patient's unusual history of recurrent infections and eczema, a primary immunodeficiency disorder was suspected, and an in-depth evaluation of his immune system was performed. His quantitative immunoglobulin levels revealed a serum IgG level of 1354 mg/dL (normal, 633–1280 mg/dL), IgA of 102 mg/dL (normal, 33–202 mg/dL), and IgM of 40 mg/dL (normal, 48–207 mg/dL). His serum IgE level was 3492 IU/mL (normal, 1.03–161.3 IU/mL). He had protective antibody titers to tetanus (0.24 IU/L; normal, >0.1 IU/L), and diphtheria (0.4 IU/L; normal, >0.1 IU/L), but 4 weeks after a booster dose of pneumococcal polysaccharide vaccine-23 (PPSV-23), he mounted a protective response to only 3 out of the 23 tested pneumococcal serotypes. Lymphocyte subset analysis by flow cytometry showed decreased number of $CD3^+$ T cells (762 cells/μL; normal, 1200–2600 cells/μL) affecting both the $CD4^+$ (500 cells/μL; normal, 650–1500 cells/μL) and $CD8^+$ (250 cells/μL; normal 370–1100 cells/μL) T-cell populations. His $CD19^+$ B cells were also slightly reduced (220 cells/μL; normal, 270–860 cells/μL). His $CD16^+CD56^+$ NK-cell number was normal. In vitro stimulation of his PBMCs with PHA was adequate at 65% of control (normal ≥30%), but his T cells failed to respond adequately to anti-CD3 or to specific antigens such as candida and tetanus. The patient was started on intravenous immunoglobulin at a dose of 400 mg/kg/month. Because of the observed combined cellular and humoral immune defects, a monogenic cause was speculated, and a gene panel which analyzes four genes associated with HIES (*STAT3*, *DOCK8*, *PGM3*, and *SPINK5*) by next-generation sequencing was ordered revealing biallelic large 5′ deletion extending to exon 27 in the *DOCK8* gene. The patient was started on TMP-SMX and eventually underwent allogenic stem cell transplantation from a matched related donor. He received a reduced busulfan-based conditioning regimen, and his post-transplantation course was largely uneventful. By 2 years post-transplantation, he had appropriate B- and T-cell reconstitutions, his eczema had largely resolved, and his asthma had improved, but he continues to require daily controller therapy although he is no longer experiencing recurrent infections.

Diagnosis/Assessment

Clinical Features

The second patient illustrates the same classic triad observed in STAT3 deficiency, namely, an elevated IgE level with eosinophilia, recurrent sinopulmonary infections, and eczema. However, there are several distinguishing features. This patient lacked the connective tissue and skeletal abnormalities seen in the first patient and distinctively exhibited a more pronounced history of atopic diseases including asthma and IgE-mediated food allergy. Furthermore, he had an unusual susceptibility to cutaneous viral infections, which was not observed in the first patient. Dedicator of cytokinesis 8 (DOCK8) deficiency is now recognized as the number one cause for the autosomal recessive variant of HIES [53, 54]. The majority of pathogenic mutations in the *DOCK8* gene are due to deletions ranging from a few base pairs to large segments [53–56]. The prevalence of DOCK8 deficiency is not defined, but it is more prevalent among populations with higher rates of consanguineous marriages such as those of Turkish and Arabic descents [17]. DOCK8 is a guanine nucleotide exchange factor that functions upstream of Wiskott-Aldrich Syndrome protein (WASp) promoting actin polymerization and cytoskeleton rearrangement which is critical for vast arrays of immune function including migration of immune cells, such as dendritic cells, and immune synapse formation between the various players of the immune system, such as B- and T-cell interaction. Therefore, DOCK8 deficiency is best viewed as an example of an actin-related combined immunodeficiency disorder [57].

The clinical features of DOCK8 deficiency are largely confined to the immune system and consist of atopy, recurrent infections, autoimmunity, and malignancy [17, 53, 54, 56]. Atopic features include early-onset atopic dermatitis (seen in 99% of patients), IgE-mediated food allergies (85% of patients), and asthma (54% of patients) [17, 56]. Patients with DOCK8 deficiency have impaired suppressive function of regulatory T cells [58] and an expanded population of T-helper 2 (Th2) cells which may explain the atopic diathesis seen in these patients [59].

Similar to STAT3 deficiency, infectious complications include recurrent sinopulmonary infections (91% of patients), staphylococcal skin infections (84% of patients), and mucocutaneous candidiasis (60–90% of patients) [17, 56]. The phenotypic overlap between DOCK8 deficiency and STAT3 deficiency may be rationalized by DOCK8 being necessary for STAT3 translocation to the nucleus [60]. Recurrent pneumonias, however, can lead to the development of bronchiectasis and rarely to pneumatocele [17, 56]. Distinctively, patients with DOCK8 are especially susceptible to cutaneous viral infections, such as infections with *herpes simplex virus*, *varicella-zoster virus*, *human papillomavirus* (HPV), and *Molluscum contagiosum* virus. These cutaneous viral infections can occur in up to 60–80% of patients [17, 56]. Additionally, progressive multifocal leukoencephalopathy secondary to John Cunningham (JC) virus and viral encephalitis have also been reported [17, 56]. There are several postulated reasons for such heightened vulnerability to viral infection in DOCK8-deficient patients including (1) deficiency of plasmacytoid dendritic cells [61, 62] which is a major source of antiviral interferon-alpha, (2) impaired cytolytic granule release from NK cells [63] and cytotoxic $CD8^+$ T lymphocytes [62], and (3) cytothripsis (aka cell death by shattering) of DOCK8-deficient $CD8^+T$ cells which prevents the generation of long-lived skin-resident memory CD8 T cells [64], another important effector cell for fighting cutaneous viral infections.

Reminiscent to Wiskott-Aldrich syndrome [65] (see Table 10.1), autoimmunity and malignancy complement the combined immunodeficiency phenotype of DOCK8 deficiency. Susceptibility to viral infections such as to HPV and Epstein-Barr virus and defective tumor surveillance are likely contributors to the high prevalence of lymphomas and squamous cell carcinomas seen in these patients [17, 56]. Autoimmunity, such as autoimmune hemolytic anemia and vasculitis, is observed in up to 13% of patients [17]. DOCK8 deficiency impairs peripheral B-cell tolerance [66] and the suppressive function of regulatory T cell [58] which may contribute to the pathogenesis of autoimmune diseases in these patients. Other diverging points from STAT3-HIES are the virtual absence of skeletal, dental, and connective tissue abnormalities [17, 56], as well as the high prevalence of neurologic manifestations, including infectious and non-infectious manifestations (vasculitis, vascular aneurysms, and brain infarcts) [17]. The mechanisms for these non-infectious neurologic manifestations remain to be elucidated [33].

Laboratory Features

Laboratory evaluation in patients with DOCK8 deficiency almost always reveals eosinophilia (96% of patients) and elevated IgE levels (98% of patients) [17]. Unlike in AD-HIES, immunological evaluation in DOCK8-deficient patients can reveal lymphopenia, especially T-cell lymphopenia, which can be observed in ~20–40% of patients [17, 56]. T-cell lymphopenia can affect both the $CD4^+$ and $CD8^+$ populations. This is an important distinction from phosphoglucomutase-3 (PGM3) deficiency, which is another cause of AR-HIES that can preferentially affect the $CD4^+$ population of T cells [67, 68]. Less frequently, patients with DOCK8 deficiency can develop NK-cell cytopenia (28% of patients) or B-cell lymphopenia (12% of patients) [17, 56]. Additionally, patients with DOCK8 deficiency often demonstrate diminished lymphocyte proliferation in response to mitogens, as was illustrated in this second patient. Quantitative immunoglobulin levels are variable [17, 56]. Serum IgM level appears to decline with age, and almost all patients older than 12 years of age will have low serum IgM levels [17], whereas IgG and IgA levels are usually normal or elevated [17, 56]. Qualitative antibody deficiency with poor vaccine responses, especially to polysaccharide antigens, is a common finding [17]. By virtue of its effect on actin polymerization, DOCK8 deficiency can disrupt B-cell receptor signaling by regulating the expression of CD19 resulting in an ineffective activation of memory B cells [69]. This can partly explain the humoral immunodeficiency observed in these patients.

Diagnosis

The presence of HIES triad in a patient with cutaneous viral infections, autoimmunity, and/or malignancy should alert the treating providers to the possibility of DOCK8 deficiency (Fig. 10.2). Given the considerable clinical overlap between STAT3 deficiency and DOCK8 deficiency, patients with DOCK8 deficiency can have an NIH HIES score of ≥40, but this remains less frequently observed compared to patients with STAT3 deficiency (67% of patients) [56]. To assist in differentiating between these two disorders, Engelhardt and colleagues proposed a modified weighted NIH HIES scoring system (aka DOCK8 score) based on 5 out of the 20 clinical and laboratory findings used in the original NIH HIES. These five features include parenchymal lung abnormalities, eosinophilia, otitis/sinusitis, retained primary teeth, and fracture with minor trauma [56]. A DOCK8 score greater than 30 predicts a DOCK8 mutation [56]. The second patient had an NIH HIES score of 34 and a DOCK8 score of 64.58. Definitive diagnosis of DOCK8 deficiency requires molecular confirmation of absent DOCK8 expression by flow cytometry or targeted gene sequencing demonstrating biallelic mutations in the

DOCK8 gene. Flow cytometric analysis for DOCK8 protein expression is a reliable diagnostic tool since most patients have mutations that interfere with normal protein expression [70]. However, a subset of patients, however, can have somatic reversions leading to normal protein expression, and hence genetic testing remains the gold standard [71].

Management/Outcome

Akin to STAT3 deficiency, TMP-SMX and an azole-based antifungal are often utilized in hope of reducing the frequency of bacterial and fungal infections and may prove useful in some patients [17]. Further, antiviral prophylaxis with valacyclovir may offer additional benefit in these patients [17]. Because of the well-characterized humoral immune defect seen in patients with DOCK8 deficiency, immunoglobulin replacement therapy represents a cornerstone of treatment and is reported to be effective in 60% of patients [17]. Despite these aforementioned prophylactic measures and IgG replacement therapy, survival without allogeneic HSCT remains poor [17]. In a retrospective review of 136 patients with DOCK8 deficiency, the median survival was only 20 years. Furthermore, the disease course of these patients was often complicated by significant life-threatening complications [17]. Infections and malignancy were the most common causes of death accounting for 75% of mortalities in these patients [17]. Contrary to STAT3 deficiency, and since DOCK8 deficiency predominantly affects the immune system, allogeneic HSCT can provide a potential cure for these patients. Indeed, in a recent retrospective analysis of 81 patients with DOCK8 deficiency who underwent allogeneic HSCT, survival was 84% at 2 years post-transplantation and was associated with improvement or resolution of most of the disease-related features including reduction in the frequency of infections, eczema, and food allergies [72]. Reduced intensity conditioning regimens and early transplantation prior to 8 years of age were associated with better survival outcomes [72]. Another study examined the clinical and immunological impacts of allogenic HSCT in 18 patients with DOCK8 deficiency, documenting restoration of both T- and B-cell functions in parallel with an observed clinical improvement [73].

Clinical Pearls and Pitfalls
- Recurrent infections in a patient with an elevated serum IgE level should alert the clinician to the possibility of HIES.
- Normal IgE level in the setting of a compatible clinical phenotype should not preclude further evaluation including genetic testing for a possible HIES diagnosis.
- In addition to DOCK8 and STAT3 deficiency, HIES is an umbrella diagnosis for a growing number of monogenic immunodeficiencies including

IL6R, *IL6ST*, *PGM3*, *ZNF431*, *CARD11*, and *SPINK*. Careful attention to both the clinical and the immunological phenotypes may be useful in identifying these disorders, but molecular diagnosis remains indispensable to establish a definitive diagnosis and guide further management.
- Recurrent cutaneous viral infections, a hallmark of DOCK8 deficiency, are virtually absent in STAT3 deficiency. Conversely, extra-immune manifestations, characteristics of STAT3, ZNF431, and gp130 deficiencies, are nearly absent in DOCK8 deficiency.
- Deficiency of IL-17-producing helper T cells underlies many of the infectious susceptibilities seen in both AD-HIES and DOCK8 deficiency and signifies a critical role for DOCK8 in proper STAT3 activation.
- The multisystem nature of AD-HIES (or Job syndrome) warrants a multidisciplinary approach to prevent and treat infections as well as to identify and, when possible, correct the non-immunological manifestations.
- Similar to Wiskott-Aldrich syndrome, the exclusive and deleterious effect of DOCK8 deficiency on the immune system results in a combined immunodeficiency phenotype which can be corrected with early allogeneic HSCT.

References

1. Gernez Y, Freeman AF, Holland SM, Garabedian E, Patel NC, Puck JM, et al. Autosomal dominant hyper-IgE syndrome in the USIDNET registry. J Allergy Clin Immunol. 2018;6(3):996–1001.
2. Renner ED, Torgerson TR, Rylaarsdam S, Añover-Sombke S, Golob K, LaFlam T, et al. STAT3 mutation in the original patient with job's syndrome. N Engl J Med. 2007;357(16):1667–8.
3. Minegishi Y, Saito M, Tsuchiya S, Tsuge I, Takada H, Hara T, et al. Dominant-negative mutations in the DNA-binding domain of STAT3 cause hyper-IgE syndrome. Nature. 2007;448:1058.
4. Holland SM, DeLeo FR, Elloumi HZ, Hsu AP, Uzel G, Brodsky N, et al. STAT3 mutations in the hyper-IgE syndrome. N Engl J Med. 2007;357(16):1608–19.
5. Renner ED, Rylaarsdam S, Anover-Sombke S, Rack AL, Reichenbach J, Carey JC, et al. Novel signal transducer and activator of transcription 3 (STAT3) mutations, reduced T(H)17 cell numbers, and variably defective STAT3 phosphorylation in hyper-IgE syndrome. J Allergy Clin Immunol. 2008;122(1):181–7.
6. Chandesris MO, Melki I, Natividad A, Puel A, Fieschi C, Yun L, et al. Autosomal dominant STAT3 deficiency and hyper-IgE syndrome: molecular, cellular, and clinical features from a French national survey. Medicine (Baltimore). 2012;91(4):e1–19.
7. Woellner C, Gertz EM, Schäffer AA, Lagos M, Perro M, Glocker EO, et al. Mutations in STAT3 and diagnostic guidelines for hyper-IgE syndrome. J Allergy Clin Immunol. 2010;125(2):424–32.e8.
8. Grimbacher B, Holland SM, Gallin JI, Greenberg F, Hill SC, Malech HL, et al. Hyper-IgE syndrome with recurrent infections — an autosomal dominant multisystem disorder. N Engl J Med. 1999;340(9):692–702.
9. Jiao H, Tóth B, Erdos M, Fransson I, Rákóczi E, Balogh I, et al. Novel and recurrent STAT3 mutations in hyper-IgE syndrome patients from different ethnic groups. Mol Immunol. 2008;46(1):202–6.

10. Eberting CL, Davis J, Puck JM, Holland SM, Turner ML. Dermatitis and the newborn rash of hyper-IgE syndrome. Arch Dermatol. 2004;140(9):1119–25.
11. Spencer S, Köstel Bal S, Egner W, Lango Allen H, Raza SI, Ma CA, et al. Loss of the interleukin-6 receptor causes immunodeficiency, atopy, and abnormal inflammatory responses. J Exp Med. 2019;216(9):1986–98.
12. Wang Y, Hu H, Wu J, Zhao X, Zhen Y, Wang S, et al. The IL6R gene polymorphisms are associated with sIL-6R, IgE and lung function in Chinese patients with asthma. Gene. 2016;585(1):51–7.
13. Siegel AM, Stone KD, Cruse G, Lawrence MG, Olivera A, Jung MY, et al. Diminished allergic disease in patients with STAT3 mutations reveals a role for STAT3 signaling in mast cell degranulation. J Allergy Clin Immunol. 2013;132(6):1388–96.
14. Foley JF. STAT3 regulates the generation of Th17 cells. Sci STKE. 2007;2007(380):tw113.
15. Schimke LF, Sawalle-Belohradsky J, Roesler J, Wollenberg A, Rack A, Borte M, et al. Diagnostic approach to the hyper-IgE syndromes: immunologic and clinical key findings to differentiate hyper-IgE syndromes from atopic dermatitis. J Allergy Clin Immunol. 2010;126(3):611–7.e1.
16. Odio CD, Milligan KL, McGowan K, Rudman Spergel AK, Bishop R, Boris L, et al. Endemic mycoses in patients with STAT3-mutated hyper-IgE (Job) syndrome. J Allergy Clin Immunol. 2015;136(5):1411–3.e1–2.
17. Aydin SE, Kilic SS, Aytekin C, Kumar A, Porras O, Kainulainen L, et al. DOCK8 deficiency: clinical and immunological phenotype and treatment options – a review of 136 patients. J Clin Immunol. 2015;35(2):189–98.
18. Leonard GD, Posadas E, Herrmann PC, Anderson VL, Jaffe ES, Holland SM, et al. Non-Hodgkin's lymphoma in Job's syndrome: a case report and literature review. Leuk Lymphoma. 2004;45(12):2521–5.
19. Chandesris MO, Azarine A, Ong KT, Taleb S, Boutouyrie P, Mousseaux E, et al. Frequent and widespread vascular abnormalities in human signal transducer and activator of transcription 3 deficiency. Circ Cardiovasc Genet. 2012;5(1):25–34.
20. Heimall J, Davis J, Shaw PA, Hsu AP, Gu W, Welch P, et al. Paucity of genotype-phenotype correlations in STAT3 mutation positive hyper IgE syndrome (HIES). Clin Immunol. 2011;139(1):75–84.
21. Frey-Jakobs S, Hartberger JM, Fliegauf M, Bossen C, Wehmeyer ML, Neubauer JC, et al. ZNF341 controls STAT3 expression and thereby immunocompetence. Sci Immunol. 2018;3(24):eaat4941.
22. Beziat V, Li J, Lin JX, Ma CS, Li P, Bousfiha A, et al. A recessive form of hyper-IgE syndrome by disruption of ZNF341-dependent STAT3 transcription and activity. Sci Immunol. 2018;3(24):eaat4956.
23. Shahin T, Aschenbrenner D, Cagdas D, Bal SK, Conde CD, Garncarz W, et al. Selective loss of function variants in IL6ST cause Hyper-IgE syndrome with distinct impairments of T-cell phenotype and function. Haematologica. 2019;104(3):609–21.
24. Nieminen T, Twigg SRF, Aschenbrenner D, Manrique S, Miller KA, Taylor IB, et al. A biallelic mutation in IL6ST encoding the GP130 co-receptor causes immunodeficiency and craniosynostosis. J Exp Med. 2017;214(9):2547–62.
25. Nieminen P, Morgan NV, Fenwick AL, Parmanen S, Veistinen L, Mikkola ML, et al. Inactivation of IL11 signaling causes craniosynostosis, delayed tooth eruption, and supernumerary teeth. Am J Hum Genet. 2011;89(1):67–81.
26. Sims NA, Johnson RW. Leukemia inhibitory factor: a paracrine mediator of bone metabolism. Growth Factors. 2012;30(2):76–87.
27. Pyo R, Lee JK, Shipley JM, Curci JA, Mao D, Ziporin SJ, et al. Targeted gene disruption of matrix metalloproteinase-9 (gelatinase B) suppresses development of experimental abdominal aortic aneurysms. J Clin Invest. 2000;105(11):1641–9.
28. Pradhan-Palikhe P, Vikatmaa P, Lajunen T, Palikhe A, Lepantalo M, Tervahartiala T, et al. Elevated MMP-8 and decreased myeloperoxidase concentrations associate significantly

with the risk for peripheral atherosclerosis disease and abdominal aortic aneurysm. Scand J Immunol. 2010;72(2):150–7.
29. Sekhsaria V, Dodd LE, Hsu AP, Heimall JR, Freeman AF, Ding L, et al. Plasma metalloproteinase levels are dysregulated in signal transducer and activator of transcription 3 mutated hyper-IgE syndrome. J Allergy Clin Immunol. 2011;128(5):1124–7.
30. Xu Z, Xu Y-J, Hao Y-N, Ren L-J, Zhang Z-B, Xu X, et al. A novel STAT3 inhibitor negatively modulates platelet activation and aggregation. Acta Pharmacol Sin. 2017;38(5):651–9.
31. Li NX, Sun JW, Yu LM. Evaluation of the circulating MicroRNA-495 and Stat3 as prognostic and predictive biomarkers for lower extremity deep venous thrombosis. J Cell Biochem. 2018;119(7):5262–73.
32. Ohkubo N, Suzuki Y, Aoto M, Yamanouchi J, Hirakawa S, Yasukawa M, et al. Accelerated destruction of erythrocytes in Tie2 promoter-driven STAT3 conditional knockout mice. Life Sci. 2013;93(9–11):380–7.
33. Al-Shaikhly T, Ochs HD. Hyper IgE syndromes: clinical and molecular characteristics. Immunol Cell Biol. 2019;97(4):368–79.
34. Josephs SH, Buckley RH. Serum IgD concentrations in normal infants, children, and adults and in patients with elevated IgE. J Pediatr. 1980;96(3 Pt 1):417–20.
35. Avery DT, Ma CS, Bryant VL, Santner-Nanan B, Nanan R, Wong M, et al. STAT3 is required for IL-21–induced secretion of IgE from human naive B cells. Blood. 2008;112(5):1784–93.
36. Meyer-Bahlburg A, Renner ED, Rylaarsdam S, Reichenbach J, Schimke LF, Marks A, et al. Heterozygous signal transducer and activator of transcription 3 mutations in hyper-IgE syndrome result in altered B-cell maturation. J Allergy Clin Immunol. 2012;129(2):559–62, 62.e1-2.
37. Crotty S. T follicular helper cell differentiation, function, and roles in disease. Immunity. 2014;41(4):529–42.
38. Kuchen S, Robbins R, Sims GP, Sheng C, Phillips TM, Lipsky PE, et al. Essential role of IL-21 in B cell activation, expansion, and plasma cell generation during CD4+ T cell-B cell collaboration. J Immunol. 2007;179(9):5886–96.
39. van de Veen W, Krätz CE, McKenzie CI, Aui PM, Neumann J, van Noesel CJM, et al. Impaired memory B-cell development and antibody maturation with a skewing toward IgE in patients with STAT3 hyper-IgE syndrome. Allergy. 2019;74(12):2394-2405.
40. Grimbacher B, Schäffer AA, Holland SM, Davis J, Gallin JI, Malech HL, et al. Genetic linkage of hyper-IgE syndrome to chromosome 4. Am J Hum Genet. 1999;65(3):735–44.
41. Zhang D, Sun M, Samols D, Kushner I. STAT3 participates in transcriptional activation of the C-reactive protein gene by interleukin-6. J Biol Chem. 1996;271(16):9503–9.
42. Freeman AF, Holland SM. The hyper-IgE syndromes. Immunol Allergy Clin N Am. 2008;28(2):277. –viii.
43. Alonso-Bello CD, Jimenez-Martinez MDC, Vargas-Camano ME, Hierro-Orozco S, Ynga-Durand MA, Berron-Ruiz L, et al. Partial and transient clinical response to Omalizumab in IL-21-induced low STAT3-phosphorylation on hyper-IgE syndrome. Case Reports Immunol. 2019;2019:6357256.
44. Etikan P, Kocatürk E, Tüzün B, Sahillioğlu N, Yazıcı A, Oguz Topal I. Omalizumab for the treatment of hyperimmunoglobulin E syndrome: a 12-year-old case. Dermatol Sin. 2016;35:48–49.
45. Chularojanamontri L, Wimoolchart S, Tuchinda P, Kulthanan K, Kiewjoy N. Role of omalizumab in a patient with hyper-IgE syndrome and review dermatologic manifestations. Asian Pac J Allergy Immunol. 2009;27(4):233–6.
46. Sowerwine KJ, Shaw PA, Gu W, Ling JC, Collins MT, Darnell DN, et al. Bone density and fractures in autosomal dominant hyper IgE syndrome. J Clin Immunol. 2014;34(2):260–4.
47. Gennery AR, Flood TJ, Abinun M, Cant AJ. Bone marrow transplantation does not correct the hyper IgE syndrome. Bone Marrow Transplant. 2000;25(12):1303–5.
48. Nester TA, Wagnon AH, Reilly WF, Spitzer G, Kjeldsberg CR, Hill HR. Effects of allogeneic peripheral stem cell transplantation in a patient with Job syndrome of hyperimmunoglobulinemia E and recurrent infections. Am J Med. 1998;105(2):162–4.

49. Goussetis E, Peristeri I, Kitra V, Traeger-Synodinos J, Theodosaki M, Psarra K, et al. Successful long-term immunologic reconstitution by allogeneic hematopoietic stem cell transplantation cures patients with autosomal dominant hyper-IgE syndrome. J Allergy Clin Immunol. 2010;126(2):392–4.
50. Patel NC, Gallagher JL, Torgerson TR, Gilman AL. Successful haploidentical donor hematopoietic stem cell transplant and restoration of STAT3 function in an adolescent with autosomal dominant hyper-IgE syndrome. J Clin Immunol. 2015;35(5):479–85.
51. Yanagimachi M, Ohya T, Yokosuka T, Kajiwara R, Tanaka F, Goto H, et al. The potential and limits of hematopoietic stem cell transplantation for the treatment of autosomal dominant hyper-IgE syndrome. J Clin Immunol. 2016;36(5):511–6.
52. Freeman AF, Kleiner DE, Nadiminti H, Davis J, Quezado M, Anderson V, et al. Causes of death in hyper-IgE syndrome. J Allergy Clin Immunol. 2007;119(5):1234–40.
53. Zhang Q, Davis JC, Lamborn IT, Freeman AF, Jing H, Favreau AJ, et al. Combined immunodeficiency associated with DOCK8 mutations. N Engl J Med. 2009;361(21):2046–55.
54. Engelhardt KR, McGhee S, Winkler S, Sassi A, Woellner C, Lopez-Herrera G, et al. Large deletions and point mutations involving the dedicator of cytokinesis 8 (DOCK8) in the autosomal-recessive form of hyper-IgE syndrome. J Allergy Clin Immunol. 2009;124(6):1289–302.e4.
55. Biggs CM, Keles S, Chatila TA. DOCK8 deficiency: insights into pathophysiology, clinical features and management. Clin Immunol. 2017;181:75–82.
56. Engelhardt KR, Gertz EM, Keles S, Schäffer AA, Sigmund EC, Glocker C, et al. The extended clinical phenotype of 64 patients with DOCK8 deficiency. J Allergy Clin Immunol. 2015;136(2):402–12.
57. Burns SO, Zarafov A, Thrasher AJ. Primary immunodeficiencies due to abnormalities of the actin cytoskeleton. Curr Opin Hematol. 2017;24(1):16–22.
58. Singh AK, Eken A, Hagin D, Komal K, Bhise G, Shaji A, et al. DOCK8 regulates fitness and function of regulatory T cells through modulation of IL-2 signaling. JCI Insight. 2017;2(19):e94275.
59. Boos AC, Hagl B, Schlesinger A, Halm BE, Ballenberger N, Pinarci M, et al. Atopic dermatitis, STAT3- and DOCK8-hyper-IgE syndromes differ in IgE-based sensitization pattern. Allergy. 2014;69(7):943–53.
60. Keles S, Charbonnier LM, Kabaleeswaran V, Reisli I, Genel F, Gulez N, et al. DOCK8 regulates STAT3 activation and promotes Th17 cell differentiation. J Allergy Clin Immunol. 2016;138(5):1384–94.e2.
61. Keles S, Jabara HH, Reisli I, McDonald DR, Barlan I, Hanna-Wakim R, et al. Plasmacytoid dendritic cell depletion in DOCK8 deficiency: rescue of severe herpetic infections with IFN-α 2b therapy. J Allergy Clin Immunol. 2014;133(6):1753–5.e3.
62. Randall KL, Chan SSY, Ma CS, Fung I, Mei Y, Yabas M, et al. DOCK8 deficiency impairs CD8 T cell survival and function in humans and mice. J Exp Med. 2011;208(11):2305–20.
63. Ham H, Guerrier S, Kim J, Schoon RA, Anderson EL, Hamann MJ, et al. DOCK8 interacts with Talin and WASP to regulate natural killer cell cytotoxicity. J Immunol (Baltimore, Md: 1950). 2013;190(7). https://doi.org/10.4049/jimmunol.1202792.
64. Zhang Q, Dove CG, Hor JL, Murdock HM, Strauss-Albee DM, Garcia JA, et al. DOCK8 regulates lymphocyte shape integrity for skin antiviral immunity. J Exp Med. 2014;211(13):2549–66.
65. Ochs HD, Thrasher AJ. The Wiskott-Aldrich syndrome. J Allergy Clin Immunol. 2006;117(4):725–38.
66. Janssen E, Morbach H, Ullas S, Bannock JM, Massad C, Menard L, et al. Dedicator of cytokinesis 8-deficient patients have a breakdown in peripheral B-cell tolerance and defective regulatory T cells. J Allergy Clin Immunol. 2014;134(6):1365–74.
67. Sassi A, Lazaroski S, Wu G, Haslam SM, Fliegauf M, Mellouli F, et al. Hypomorphic homozygous mutations in phosphoglucomutase 3 (PGM3) impair immunity and increase serum IgE levels. J Allergy Clin Immunol. 2014;133(5):1410–9.e13.
68. Zhang Y, Yu X, Ichikawa M, Lyons JJ, Datta S, Lamborn IT, et al. Autosomal recessive phosphoglucomutase 3 (PGM3) mutations link glycosylation defects to atopy, immune

deficiency, autoimmunity, and neurocognitive impairment. J Allergy Clin Immunol. 2014;133(5):1400–9, 9.e1–5.
69. Sun X, Wang J, Qin T, Zhang Y, Huang L, Niu L, et al. Dock8 regulates BCR signaling and activation of memory B cells via WASP and CD19. Blood Adv. 2018;2(4):401–13.
70. Pai SY, de Boer H, Massaad MJ, Chatila TA, Keles S, Jabara HH, et al. Flow cytometry diagnosis of dedicator of cytokinesis 8 (DOCK8) deficiency. J Allergy Clin Immunol. 2014;134(1):221–3.
71. Jing H, Zhang Q, Zhang Y, Hill BJ, Dove CG, Gelfand EW, et al. Somatic reversion in dedicator of cytokinesis 8 immunodeficiency modulates disease phenotype. J Allergy Clin Immunol. 2014;133(6):1667–75.
72. Aydin SE, Freeman AF, Al-Herz W, Al-Mousa HA, Arnaout RK, Aydin RC, et al. Hematopoietic stem cell transplantation as treatment for patients with DOCK8 deficiency. J Allergy Clin Immunol Pract. 2019;7(3):848–55.
73. Pillay BA, Avery DT, Smart JM, Cole T, Choo S, Chan D, et al. Hematopoietic stem cell transplant effectively rescues lymphocyte differentiation and function in DOCK8-deficient patients. JCI Insight. 2019;4(11):e127527.
74. Stray-Pedersen A, Backe Paul H, Sorte Hanne S, Mørkrid L, Chokshi Niti Y, Erichsen Hans C, et al. PGM3 mutations cause a congenital disorder of glycosylation with severe immunodeficiency and skeletal dysplasia. Am J Hum Genet. 2014;95(1):96–107.
75. Dadi H, Jones TA, Merico D, Sharfe N, Ovadia A, Schejter Y, et al. Combined immunodeficiency and atopy caused by a dominant negative mutation in caspase activation and recruitment domain family member 11 (CARD11). J Allergy Clin Immunol. 2018;141(5):1818–30.e2.
76. Ma CA, Stinson JR, Zhang Y, Abbott JK, Weinreich MA, Hauk PJ, et al. Germline hypomorphic CARD11 mutations in severe atopic disease. Nat Genet. 2017;49(8):1192–201.
77. Renner ED, Hartl D, Rylaarsdam S, Young ML, Monaco-Shawver L, Kleiner G, et al. Comel-Netherton syndrome defined as primary immunodeficiency. J Allergy Clin Immunol. 2009;124(3):536–43.
78. Smith DL, Smith JG, Wong SW, deShazo RD. Netherton's syndrome: a syndrome of elevated IgE and characteristic skin and hair findings. J Allergy Clin Immunol. 1995;95(1):116–23.
79. Villa A, Notarangelo LD, Roifman CM. Omenn syndrome: inflammation in leaky severe combined immunodeficiency. J Allergy Clin Immunol. 2008;122(6):1082–6.
80. Barzaghi F, Amaya Hernandez LC, Neven B, Ricci S, Kucuk ZY, Bleesing JJ, et al. Long-term follow-up of IPEX syndrome patients after different therapeutic strategies: an international multicenter retrospective study. J Allergy Clin Immunol. 2018;141(3):1036–49.e5.
81. Barzaghi F, Passerini L, Bacchetta R. Immune dysregulation, polyendocrinopathy, enteropathy, X-linked syndrome: a paradigm of immunodeficiency with autoimmunity. Front Immunol. 2012;3:211.

Chapter 11
Genetic Syndromes with Associated Immunodeficiencies

Rebecca A. Marsh and Andrew W. Lindsley

Introduction

There are a variety of genetic syndromes that are associated with defects in the immune system. They are sometimes collectively referred to as "syndromic primary immunodeficiencies" (PIDs) or "syndromic immunodeficiencies" [1, 2]. Syndromic PIDs are usually considered to encompass diseases which feature *prominent* non-immune system problems that form a recognizable syndrome. The immunodeficiencies associated with these syndromes can be highly variable, and not all patients may have immunodeficiency.

The International Union of Immunological Societies (IUIS) primary immunodeficiency expert committee regularly publishes a classification of inborn errors of immunity. The 2019 update on the classification included over 400 inborn errors of immunity [3]. More than 60 genetic diseases with associated immunodeficiencies are classified as "combined immunodeficiencies with associated or syndromic features," and additional inborn errors of immunity with syndromic features can be found elsewhere in the IUIS Classification. For instance, DNA ligase IV deficiency due to mutations in *LIG4*, which is characterized by microcephaly, is classified with the severe combined immune deficiencies, and several pigmentary syndromes are classified with the diseases of immune dysregulation because they also cause hemophagocytic lymphohistiocytosis (HLH).

Genetic syndromes with associated immunodeficiencies can be caused by known single-gene defects or complex chromosomal abnormalities, or the cause of disease

R. A. Marsh (✉)
Bone Marrow Transplantation and Immune Deficiency, University of Cincinnati, Cincinnati Children's Hospital Medical Center, Cincinnati, OH, USA
e-mail: Rebecca.Marsh@cchmc.org

A. W. Lindsley
Department of Allergy and Immunology, University of Cincinnati, Cincinnati Children's Hospital Medical Center, Cincinnati, OH, USA

may be unknown. The spectrum of immunologic defects varies from severe and life-threatening to relatively mild. Even within the same disorder the clinical spectrum of immunologic disease may be wide. A good example of this clinical heterogeneity is DiGeorge syndrome. A patient with DiGeorge syndrome may have a complete athymia and absence of T cells (complete DiGeorge syndrome) which will result in life-threatening infections and a high likelihood of death without correction, or may manifest with only very mild/subtle immune abnormalities which can be asymptomatic [4]. While a complete review of all genetic syndromes associated with syndromic immunodeficiency is outside the scope of this chapter, we present two representative cases to illustrate their complexity and discuss additional generalities.

Case Presentation 1

A 10-year-old female was referred to immunology clinic for a history of recurrent upper respiratory infections, otitis media, and two episodes of pneumonia. She had a history of developmental delay and dysmorphism. The patient did not walk until 2.5 years of age, and speech development was also delayed. She is below grade level at school and has been in special reading and math classes. She wears hearing aids. She has not been fully vaccinated due to parental concern for association with developmental delay.

Physical examination revealed a well-nourished but short pre-pubertal female whose height and weight were <3rd percentile and 40th percentile, respectively. Facial abnormalities were noted and included long palpebral fissures, eversion of the lower lateral eyelids, long eyelashes, arched eyebrows, flattened tip of nose, and large ears (Fig. 11.1). A close inspection of the hands revealed that the fifth fingers bilaterally appeared abnormally shorter than the other digits.

Given the characteristic facial features and developmental delay, Kabuki syndrome, an autosomal dominant congenital epigenetic disease, was suspected. Laboratory evaluations were notable for low levels of IgG (240 mg/dL), IgA (13 mg/dL), and IgM (24 mg/dL). Lymphocyte subset analysis was normal. Mitogen-stimulated proliferation studies were normal. Complete blood count revealed a mildly low platelet count of 97×10^3/mcL. Genetic testing revealed a de novo heterozygous pathologic variant in the *KMT2D* gene, which is the most common cause of Kabuki syndrome (also known as type 1 Kabuki syndrome). *KMT2D* encodes lysine-specific methyltransferase 2D, part of a family of proteins that function as histone methyltransferases [5]. In contrast, type 2 Kabuki syndrome is caused by pathologic variants in *KDM6A* which encodes lysine-specific demethylase 6A, a histone demethylase located in the pseudoautosomal region of the X chromosome [5]. Defects in either enzyme lead to abnormal histone methylation and are thought to disrupt normal regulation of genes important in developmental and other processes [5].

11 Genetic Syndromes with Associated Immunodeficiencies

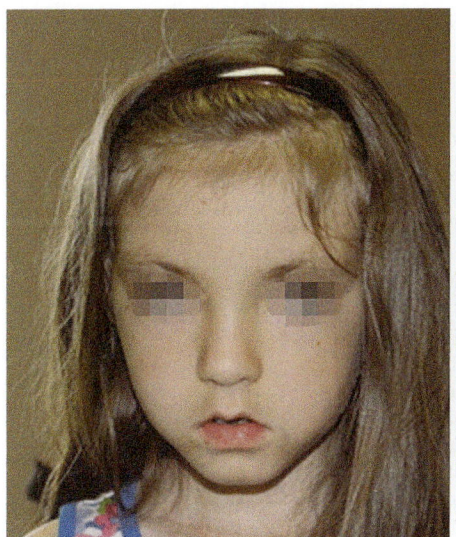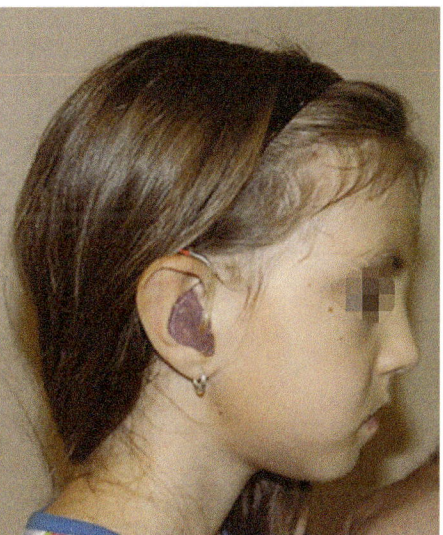

Fig. 11.1 Typical facial features of a patient with Kabuki syndrome

Following the diagnosis, the patient was started on immunoglobulin replacement for treatment of humoral deficiency [6]. Additional screening evaluations were undertaken to look for clinical abnormalities associated with Kabuki syndrome (Table 11.1) such as renal/urinary tract and cardiac malformations which can be observed in approximately 30–40% and 40–50% of patients, respectively [7]. An abdominal ultrasound was normal. A cardiac echo revealed an atrial septal defect, and the patient was referred to cardiology. Skeletal X-rays were normal. An endocrinology referral was made for evaluation of short stature, and the patient was found to be growth hormone deficient, another complication of Kabuki syndrome [7]. A hematology referral was made and a diagnosis of immune thrombocytopenia was made after testing for platelet autoantibodies. The patient was also referred to genetics and developmental clinics.

Case Presentation 2

A 15-month-old female was referred to immunology clinic for a history of recurrent severe infections. At 3 months of age, she required hospitalization for diarrhea and respiratory distress requiring oxygen. She was found to have enterovirus and rhinovirus infections. At 4 months of age, she was hospitalized with enterovirus meningitis. At that time, she was noted to have a low IgG and was started on intravenous immunoglobulin replacement. At 6 months of age, she developed *Pneumocystis jirovecii* pneumonia. She also had a history of failure to thrive.

Table 11.1 Selected non-immune features that may be present in a number of genetic syndromes with associated immunodeficiencies

Disease	Molecular defect	Selected non-immune features which may be present	OMIM	Reference(s)
3-Methylglutaconic aciduria type VII	CLPB	Progressive encephalopathy, movement abnormalities, microcephaly, developmental delay, cataracts, seizures	616254	[17]
Ataxia telangiectasia	ATM	Radiation sensitivity; cerebellar ataxia, telangiectasia, dysarthric speech, oculomotor apraxia, predisposition to malignancy	607585	[18]
Ataxia telangiectasia-like disease	MRE11	Radiation sensitivity; cerebellar degeneration, ataxia	600814	[19–21]
Barth syndrome (3-methylglutaconic aciduria type II)	TAZ	Cardiomyopathy, dysmorphism, growth retardation, cognitive impairment	300394	[22]
BCL11B deficiency	BCL11B	Developmental delays, intellectual disability, dysmorphism	606558	[23, 24]
Bloom syndrome	BLM	Microcephaly, intrauterine and postnatal growth retardation, telangiectatic erythema, cancer predisposition, endocrine abnormalities	604610	[25]
Ca2+ channel deficiency	STIM1, ORAI1	Hypotonia, abnormal dental enamel, anhidrotic ectodermal dysplasia	605921, 610277	[26]
Cartilage-hair hypoplasia	RMRP	Sparse hair, short-limbed dwarfism, ligamentous laxity, anemia, Hirschsprung's disease, cancer predisposition	157660	[27]
Cernunnos deficiency	NHEJ1	Radiation sensitivity; microcephaly, intrauterine and postnatal growth retardation	611290	[28]

Table 11.1 (continued)

Disease	Molecular defect	Selected non-immune features which may be present	OMIM	Reference(s)
CHARGE syndrome	*CHD7*	Colobomas, congenital heart malformations, choanal atresia, growth retardation, genital anomalies, ear anomalies, tracheoesophageal fistula, dysmorphism	608892	[29]
Chediak-Higashi syndrome	*LYST*	Partial albinism, neurologic problems	606897	[30]
Cohen syndrome	*VPS13B*	Developmental delay, microcephaly, facial dysmorphism, truncal obesity, joint hypermobility, neutropenia	607817	[31, 32]
Netherton syndrome	*SPINK5*	Congenital ichthyosiform erythroderma, trichorrhexis invaginata, atopy	605010	[33, 34]
DiGeorge syndrome	*22q11.2 deletion*	Congenital heart malformations, hypocalcemia, palatal abnormalities, developmental delay, behavioral problems, learning disabilities, renal abnormalities	602054	[35]
DNA ligase IV deficiency	*LIG4*	Radiation sensitivity; microcephaly, dysmorphism, bone abnormalities, growth retardation	601837	[36]
Dyskeratosis congenita	*DKC1, TERC, TERT, TINF2, RTEL1, ACD, NOP10, NHP2, WRAP53, PARN*	Short telomeres, marrow failure, pulmonary fibrosis, nail dystrophy, oral leukoplakia	300126, 602322, 187270, 604319, 608833, 609377, 606471, 606470, 612661, 604212	[37]
ERCC6L2 deficiency	*ERCC6L2*	Marrow failure, learning disabilities, microcephaly	615667	[38, 39]

(continued)

Table 11.1 (continued)

Disease	Molecular defect	Selected non-immune features which may be present	OMIM	Reference(s)
EXTL3 deficiency	*EXTL3*	Platyspondyly, cervical malformations, short stature, developmental delay, intellectual disabilities	605744	[40, 41]
G6PC3 deficiency (SCN4)	*G6PC3*	Congenital heart malformations, prominent superficial venous pattern, uro-genital anomalies	611045	[42]
GINS1 deficiency	*GINS1*	Prenatal and postnatal growth retardation, facial dysmorphism	610608	[43]
Griscelli syndrome	*RAB27A*	Partial albinism	603868	[44]
Hennekam-lymphangiectasia-lymphedema syndrome	*CCBE1*	Lymphedema, lymphangiectasia, dysmorphism, developmental delay	612753	[45]
Hepatic veno-occlusive disease with immunodeficiency	*SP110*	Hepatic veno-occlusive disease	604457	[46]
Hyper IgE syndrome AD	*STAT3*	Distinctive/coarse facial features, eczema, retained primary teeth, joint hyperflexibility, scoliosis, bone fractures	102582	[47]
ICF syndrome	*DNMT3B, ZBTB24, CDCA7, HELLS*	Dysmorphism, centromeric instability	602900, 614064, 609937, 603946	[9, 48–50]
Immune deficiency with multiple intestinal atresias	*TTC7A*	Intestinal atresia	609332	[51, 52]
IκBα (ectodermal dysplasia and immunodeficiency 2)	*IκBα*	Anhidrotic ectodermal dysplasia	164008	[53]
JAGN1 deficiency	*JAGN1*	Bone and dental abnormalities	616012	[54]

Table 11.1 (continued)

Disease	Molecular defect	Selected non-immune features which may be present	OMIM	Reference(s)
Kabuki syndrome	*KMT2D, KDM6A*	Distinctive facial features, growth delay, intellectual disability, skeletal abnormalities, short stature, cardiac abnormalities, renal abnormalities, autoimmunity	602113, 300128	[5, 7]
Leukocyte adhesion deficiency type II	*SLC35C1*	Dysmorphism, developmental delay, short stature	605881	[55]
Leukocyte adhesion deficiency type III	*FERMT3*	Bleeding tendency	607901	[56, 57]
MCM4 deficiency	*MCM4*	Glucocorticoid deficiency/adrenal failure, failure to thrive, short stature	602638	[58]
MOPD1 deficiency (Roifman syndrome)	*RNU4ATAC*	Dysmorphism, growth retardation, cognitive delay, spondyloepiphyseal dysplasia	601428	[59]
NEMO	*NEMO*	Ectodermal dysplasia, conical or missing teeth, hypohydrosis	300248	[60]
Nijmegen breakage syndrome	*NBS1*	Radiation sensitivity; microcephaly, bird-like facies, growth retardation, intellectual disability	602667	[61]
NSMCE3 deficiency	*NSMCE3*	Dysmorphism, failure to thrive, psychomotor retardation	608243	[62]
PNP (purine nucleoside phosphorylase) deficiency	*PNP*	Neurologic problems such as spasticity, ataxia, developmental delay, intellectual disability	164050	[63]
RAD50 deficiency	*RAD50*	Radiation sensitivity; dysmorphism, microcephaly, growth retardation	604040	[64]
Schimke immuno-osseous dysplasia	*SMARCAL1*	Spondyloepiphyseal dysplasia, short stature, nephropathy, dysmorphism, cerebral infarcts	606622	[65]

(continued)

Table 11.1 (continued)

Disease	Molecular defect	Selected non-immune features which may be present	OMIM	Reference(s)
Shwachman-Diamond syndrome	SBDS, DNAJC21, EFL1	Marrow failure, exocrine pancreatic insufficiency, skeletal abnormalities, intellectual disability	607444, 617052, 617941	[66]
SMARCD2 deficiency	SMARCD2	Dysmorphism, developmental delay, bone marrow fibrosis, dysplasia	601736	[67]
STAT5b deficiency	STAT5b	Poor growth due to growth hormone insensitivity	604260	[68]
Vici syndrome	EPG5	Agenesis of the corpus callosum, cataracts, pigmentary defects, cardiomyopathy	615068	[69]
VPS45 deficiency (SCN5)	VPS45	Bone marrow fibrosis	610035	[70, 71]
WHIM	CXCR4	Warts (though related to the immune deficiency), myelokathexis	162643	[72]
Wiskott-Aldrich syndrome	WAS	Small platelets, eczema, predisposition to malignancy	300392	[73]

On examination, the patient was noted to be thin with a protuberant abdomen. Facial features were notable for mild hypertelorism and low-set ears. Immunologic evaluations were notable for undetectable IgA and IgM, normal lymphocyte subset analysis, lack of class-switched memory B cells, normal distribution of naïve and memory T cells, and normal mitogen-stimulated proliferation studies.

A syndromic immune deficiency was suspected based on the facial features. A large commercially available genetic panel for primary immunodeficiencies was ordered and resulted with one likely pathologic and one variant of uncertain clinical significance in the *DNMT3B* gene which is associated with immunodeficiency, centromeric instability, and facial dysmorphism (ICF) syndrome [1]. ICF syndrome is caused by defective chromosomal methylation. Metaphase chromosomes from phytohemagglutinin-stimulated blood cultures that are performed during routine clinical chromosome analysis can exhibit several anomalies such as whole-arm deletions and pericentromeric breaks of chromosomes 1, 9 and 16, and multiradial configurations containing three or more arms of these chromosomes are striking [8–12]. A routine chromosome analysis was performed and revealed the typical multi-radial configurations involving chromosome 1, which confirmed the clinical diagnosis (Fig. 11.2) [13]. Due to the severity of the primary immunodeficiency, the patient ultimately underwent successful allogeneic hematopoietic cell transplantation.

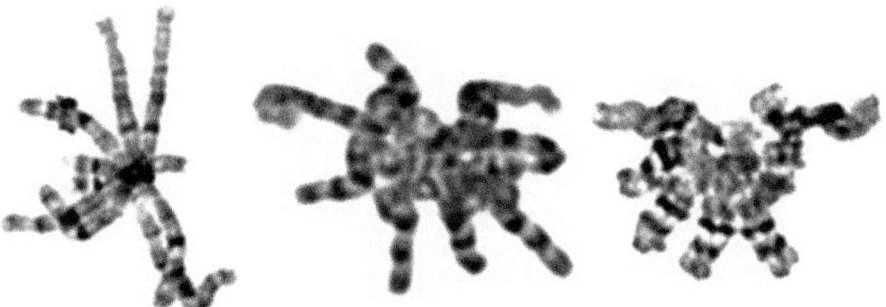

Fig. 11.2 Radial figures identified for chromosome 1 after phytohemagglutinin stimulation of a blood sample collected from a patient with ICF syndrome. (Image courtesy of Teresa Smolarek, PhD)

General Considerations in Genetic Syndromes with Associated Immunodeficiencies

The immune evaluation for patients suspected to have a primary immunodeficiency component of their syndromic disease is essentially the same as for other patients suspected to have primary immunodeficiencies. Evaluations can be tailored or emphasized depending on the underlying disorder if it is known. For example, a patient with Barth syndrome should have a complete blood count to screen for neutropenia, and a patient with GINS1 deficiency should be screened for neutropenia as well as NK-cell deficiency. A known Kabuki syndrome patient should have careful humoral deficiency evaluations [14, 15]. A patient with DiGeorge syndrome should have careful T-cell deficiency evaluations since the syndrome is associated with athymia and partial athymia but should also have humoral deficiency evaluations since a small percentage of patients have evidence of humoral deficiency [16]. Beyond disease-specific evaluations, most patients should have broad immunologic screening tests performed as suggested in Table 11.2.

In patients who lack a known genetic syndrome diagnosis, immunologic testing and genetic testing should be performed in tandem when appropriate. Routine chromosome analysis and microarray should be considered in patients who lack a known underlying genetic diagnosis. Additionally, targeted sequencing of any genes linked to suspected genetic disorders should be performed. Alternatively, a primary immunodeficiency panel or whole-exome sequencing should be pursued in appropriate patients with a clear immune phenotype, syndromic features, but no obvious unifying genetic diagnosis. Collaboration with a clinical geneticist should be considered during the evaluation of complex patients so that newly described, emerging, or very rare genetic syndromes that are not common to the immunologist are not overlooked.

After a thorough immune evaluation, any needed interventions can be instigated as appropriate. Treatment is highly variable depending on the underlying disorder

Table 11.2 Suggested initial screening immunologic evaluations to consider in patients suspected of having a genetic syndrome with associated immunodeficiency

Clinical test	To evaluate
Complete blood count	Neutrophil, lymphocyte, eosinophil, and monocyte percentages and numbers, hemoglobin/hematocrit, platelet count
Lymphocyte subset enumeration	CD4+ T-cell, CD8+ T-cell, NK-cell, and B-cell percentages and numbers
T-cell phenotyping and/or TREC testing	Presence of naive and memory T-cell subsets, recent thymic emigrants
Mitogen and/or antigen-stimulated proliferation assays	Proliferative responses
B-cell phenotyping	Presence of memory B cells and class-switched memory B cells
Vaccine titers (if appropriately vaccinated)	Antibody responses to vaccinations
Vaccine challenge (if indicated)	Antibody responses to vaccinations

More limited, expanded, or alternative testing may be indicated based on clinical scenario

and the extent of immune deficiency, as observed in the two example cases above. Patients with humoral deficiency should be started on immunoglobulin replacement. Patients with significant T-cell deficiencies may require prophylaxis against *Pneumocystis jirovecii* and other pathogens. Patients with severe neutropenia may need antifungal and other appropriate antimicrobial prophylaxis or treatment with granulocyte-colony stimulating factor. These interventions can significantly improve the quality of life for patients and prevent life-threatening infections. Some patients with severe disorders are optimally treated with allogeneic hematopoietic cell transplantation.

Importantly, many patients will require multi-specialty evaluations and care. Obvious problems such as a cleft lip or palate will be easy to recognize and more straightforward to treat. Some syndromic complications are not obvious, and thoughtful consideration should be given to screening evaluations when appropriate if they have not been performed prior to referral to immunology clinic. For example, patients with CHARGE syndrome should be examined/evaluated for many associated problems such as colobomas, heart malformations, kidney malformations, choanal atresia, cleft lip, cleft palate, tracheoesophageal fistula, growth problems, ear malformations, hearing problems, genital abnormalities, problems with the digits or limbs, cognitive abnormalities or learning disabilities, and other problems. Selected associated complications of other syndromic PID disorders are listed in Table 11.2. Patients may need consultation and/or care with specialists in clinical genetics, neurology, cardiology, developmental pediatrics, gastroenterology, nutrition, nephrology, urology, pulmonology, otolaryngology, orthopedics, general and specialty surgery, and psychiatry and other specialists along with a variety of physical, occupational, and speech therapy services. Appropriate placements in schools and individualized education program (IEP) development may be needed as children progress through school. Multi-subspecialty care clinics can be helpful when available.

Conclusion

The evaluation and treatment of patients with genetic syndromes with associated immunodeficiencies can be complex. There are a large number of phenotypically heterogeneous disorders, many with overlapping non-immune features and a wide spectrum of immunologic defects. Some disorders are common in the primary immunodeficiency clinic and are simple to manage. For syndromes that are ill-defined or complex, evaluations and treatments can be undertaken in collaboration with clinical geneticists and multi-disciplinary specialists as appropriate. Immunologists are often able to have a significant positive impact on the quality of life of patients with syndromic PIDs through the recognition and treatment of the associated immunodeficiencies in these patients.

Clinical Pearls and Pitfalls
- Genetic syndromes with associated immunodeficiencies are diverse.
- Most patients suspected to have a syndromic immunodeficiency should have broad immunologic and genetic testing performed to quantify the degree of immunodeficiency and determine the underlying genetic disorder.
- Patients may need multi-subspecialty evaluations and care.
- Treatment interventions for immunodeficiency depend on the underlying disorder and extent of immunodeficiency.

References

1. Kersseboom R, Brooks A, Weemaes C. Educational paper: syndromic forms of primary immunodeficiency. Eur J Pediatr. 2011;170(3):295–308.
2. Ming JE, Stiehm ER. Genetic syndromic immunodeficiencies with antibody defects. Immunol Allergy Clin N Am. 2008;28(4):715–36, vii.
3. Tangye SG, Al-Herz W, Bousfiha A, Chatila T, Cunningham-Rundles C, Etzioni A, et al. Human inborn errors of immunity: 2019 update on the classification from the international union of immunological societies expert committee. J Clin Immunol. 2020;40(1):24–64.
4. Davies EG. Immunodeficiency in DiGeorge syndrome and options for treating cases with complete athymia. Front Immunol. 2013;4:322.
5. Lavery WJ, Barski A, Wiley S, Schorry EK, Lindsley AW. KMT2C/D COMPASS complex-associated diseases [KCDCOM-ADs]: an emerging class of congenital regulopathies. Clin Epigenetics. 2020;12(1):10.
6. Lindsley AW, Saal HM, Burrow TA, Hopkin RJ, Shchelochkov O, Khandelwal P, et al. Defects of B-cell terminal differentiation in patients with type-1 Kabuki syndrome. J Allergy Clin Immunol. 2016;137(1):179–87. e110.
7. Bogershausen N, Wollnik B. Unmasking Kabuki syndrome. Clin Genet. 2013;83(3):201–11.
8. Ehrlich M, Jackson K, Weemaes C. Immunodeficiency, centromeric region instability, facial anomalies syndrome (ICF). Orphanet J Rare Dis. 2006;1:2.
9. Maraschio P, Zuffardi O, Dalla Fior T, Tiepolo L. Immunodeficiency, centromeric heterochromatin instability of chromosomes 1, 9, and 16, and facial anomalies: the ICF syndrome. J Med Genet. 1988;25(3):173–80.

10. Tiepolo L, Maraschio P, Gimelli G, Cuoco C, Gargani GF, Romano C. Multibranched chromosomes 1, 9, and 16 in a patient with combined IgA and IgE deficiency. Hum Genet. 1979;51(2):127–37.
11. Carpenter NJ, Filipovich A, Blaese RM, Carey TL, Berkel AI. Variable immunodeficiency with abnormal condensation of the heterochromatin of chromosomes 1, 9, and 16. J Pediatr. 1988;112(5):757–60.
12. Tuck-Muller CM, Narayan A, Tsien F, Smeets DF, Sawyer J, Fiala ES, et al. DNA hypomethylation and unusual chromosome instability in cell lines from ICF syndrome patients. Cytogenet Cell Genet. 2000;89(1–2):121–8.
13. Kellner ES, Rathbun PA, Marshall GS, Tolusso LK, Smolarek TA, Sun M, et al. The value of chromosome analysis to interrogate variants in DNMT3B causing immunodeficiency, centromeric instability, and facial anomaly syndrome type I (ICF1). J Clin Immunol. 2019;39(8):857–9.
14. Hoffman JD, Ciprero KL, Sullivan KE, Kaplan PB, McDonald-McGinn DM, Zackai EH, et al. Immune abnormalities are a frequent manifestation of Kabuki syndrome. Am J Med Genet A. 2005;135(3):278–81.
15. Adam MP, Banka S, Bjornsson HT, Bodamer O, Chudley AE, Harris J, et al. Kabuki syndrome: international consensus diagnostic criteria. J Med Genet. 2019;56(2):89–95.
16. Patel K, Akhter J, Kobrynski L, Benjamin Gathmann MA, Davis O, Sullivan KE, et al. Immunoglobulin deficiencies: the B-lymphocyte side of DiGeorge Syndrome. J Pediatr. 2012;161(5):950–3.
17. Wortmann SB, Zietkiewicz S, Kousi M, Szklarczyk R, Haack TB, Gersting SW, et al. CLPB mutations cause 3-methylglutaconic aciduria, progressive brain atrophy, intellectual disability, congenital neutropenia, cataracts, movement disorder. Am J Hum Genet. 2015;96(2):245–57.
18. Chun HH, Gatti RA. Ataxia-telangiectasia, an evolving phenotype. DNA Repair (Amst). 2004;3(8–9):1187–96.
19. Stewart GS, Maser RS, Stankovic T, Bressan DA, Kaplan MI, Jaspers NG, et al. The DNA double-strand break repair gene hMRE11 is mutated in individuals with an ataxia-telangiectasia-like disorder. Cell. 1999;99(6):577–87.
20. Delia D, Piane M, Buscemi G, Savio C, Palmeri S, Lulli P, et al. MRE11 mutations and impaired ATM-dependent responses in an Italian family with ataxia-telangiectasia-like disorder. Hum Mol Genet. 2004;13(18):2155–63.
21. Fernet M, Gribaa M, Salih MA, Seidahmed MZ, Hall J, Koenig M. Identification and functional consequences of a novel MRE11 mutation affecting 10 Saudi Arabian patients with the ataxia telangiectasia-like disorder. Hum Mol Genet. 2005;14(2):307–18.
22. Finsterer J. Barth syndrome: mechanisms and management. Appl Clin Genet. 2019;12:95–106.
23. Lessel D, Gehbauer C, Bramswig NC, Schluth-Bolard C, Venkataramanappa S, van Gassen KLI, et al. BCL11B mutations in patients affected by a neurodevelopmental disorder with reduced type 2 innate lymphoid cells. Brain. 2018;141(8):2299–311.
24. Punwani D, Zhang Y, Yu J, Cowan MJ, Rana S, Kwan A, et al. Multisystem anomalies in severe combined immunodeficiency with mutant BCL11B. N Engl J Med. 2016;375(22):2165–76.
25. Cunniff C, Bassetti JA, Ellis NA. Bloom's syndrome: clinical spectrum, molecular pathogenesis, and cancer predisposition. Mol Syndromol. 2017;8(1):4–23.
26. Feske S, Picard C, Fischer A. Immunodeficiency due to mutations in ORAI1 and STIM1. Clin Immunol. 2010;135(2):169–82.
27. Ridanpaa M, van Eenennaam H, Pelin K, Chadwick R, Johnson C, Yuan B, et al. Mutations in the RNA component of RNase MRP cause a pleiotropic human disease, cartilage-hair hypoplasia. Cell. 2001;104(2):195–203.
28. Buck D, Malivert L, de Chasseval R, Barraud A, Fondanèche M-C, Sanal O, et al. Cernunnos, a novel nonhomologous end-joining factor, is mutated in human immunodeficiency with microcephaly. Cell. 2006;124(2):287–99.
29. Hsu P, Ma A, Wilson M, Williams G, Curotta J, Munns CF, et al. CHARGE syndrome: a review. J Paediatr Child Health. 2014;50(7):504–11.

30. Kaplan J, De Domenico I, Ward DM. Chediak-Higashi syndrome. Curr Opin Hematol. 2008;15(1):22–9.
31. Kolehmainen J, Black GC, Saarinen A, Chandler K, Clayton-Smith J, Träskelin A-L, et al. Cohen syndrome is caused by mutations in a novel gene, COH1, encoding a transmembrane protein with a presumed role in vesicle-mediated sorting and intracellular protein transport. Am J Hum Genet. 2003;72(6):1359–69.
32. Chandler KE, Kidd A, Al-Gazali L, Kolehmainen J, Lehesjoki A-E, Black GCM, et al. Diagnostic criteria, clinical characteristics, and natural history of Cohen syndrome. J Med Genet. 2003;40(4):233–41.
33. Chavanas S, Bodemer C, Rochat A, Hamel-Teillac D, Ali M, Irvine AD, et al. Mutations in SPINK5, encoding a serine protease inhibitor, cause Netherton syndrome. Nat Genet. 2000;25(2):141–2.
34. Bitoun E, Chavanas S, Irvine AD, Lonie L, Bodemer C, Paradisi M, et al. Netherton syndrome: disease expression and spectrum of SPINK5 mutations in 21 families. J Invest Dermatol. 2002;118(2):352–61.
35. Sullivan KE. Chromosome 22q11.2 deletion syndrome and DiGeorge syndrome. Immunol Rev. 2019;287(1):186–201.
36. Altmann T, Gennery AR. DNA ligase IV syndrome; a review. Orphanet J Rare Dis. 2016;11(1):137.
37. Niewisch MR, Savage SA. An update on the biology and management of dyskeratosis congenita and related telomere biology disorders. Expert Rev Hematol. 2019;12(12):1037–52.
38. Tummala H, Kirwan M, Walne AJ, Hossain U, Jackson N, Pondarre C, et al. ERCC6L2 mutations link a distinct bone-marrow-failure syndrome to DNA repair and mitochondrial function. Am J Hum Genet. 2014;94(2):246–56.
39. Zhang S, Pondarre C, Pennarun G, Labussiere-Wallet H, Vera G, France B, et al. A nonsense mutation in the DNA repair factor Hebo causes mild bone marrow failure and microcephaly. J Exp Med. 2016;213(6):1011–28.
40. Oud MM, Tuijnenburg P, Hempel M, van Vlies N, Ren Z, Ferdinandusse S, et al. Mutations in EXTL3 cause Neuro-immuno-skeletal dysplasia syndrome. Am J Hum Genet. 2017;100(2):281–96.
41. Volpi S, Yamazaki Y, Brauer PM, van Rooijen E, Hayashida A, Slavotinek A, et al. EXTL3 mutations cause skeletal dysplasia, immune deficiency, and developmental delay. J Exp Med. 2017;214(3):623–37.
42. Banka S, Newman WG. A clinical and molecular review of ubiquitous glucose-6-phosphatase deficiency caused by G6PC3 mutations. Orphanet J Rare Dis. 2013;8:84.
43. Cottineau J, Kottemann MC, Lach FP, Kang Y-H, Vély F, Deenick EK, et al. Inherited GINS1 deficiency underlies growth retardation along with neutropenia and NK cell deficiency. J Clin Invest. 2017;127(5):1991–2006.
44. Ménasché G, Pastural E, Feldmann J, Certain S, Ersoy F, Dupuis S, et al. Mutations in RAB27A cause Griscelli syndrome associated with hemophagocytic syndrome. Nat Genet. 2000;25:173–6.
45. Alders M, Hogan BM, Gjini E, Salehi F, Al-Gazali L, Hennekam EA, et al. Mutations in CCBE1 cause generalized lymph vessel dysplasia in humans. Nat Genet. 2009;41(12):1272–4.
46. Roscioli T, Cliffe ST, Bloch DB, Bell CG, Mullan G, Taylor PJ, et al. Mutations in the gene encoding the PML nuclear body protein Sp110 are associated with immunodeficiency and hepatic veno-occlusive disease. Nat Genet. 2006;38(6):620–2.
47. Yong PF, Freeman AF, Engelhardt KR, Holland S, Puck JM, Grimbacher B. An update on the hyper-IgE syndromes. Arthritis Res Ther. 2012;14(6):228.
48. Sterlin D, Velasco G, Moshous D, Touzot F, Mahlaoui N, Fischer A, et al. Genetic, cellular and clinical features of ICF syndrome: a French National Survey. J Clin Immunol. 2016;36(2):149–59.
49. de Greef JC, Wang J, Balog J, den Dunnen JT, Frants RR, Straasheijm KR, et al. Mutations in ZBTB24 are associated with immunodeficiency, centromeric instability, and facial anomalies syndrome type 2. Am J Hum Genet. 2011;88(6):796–804.

50. Thijssen PE, Ito Y, Grillo G, Wang J, Velasco G, Nitta H, et al. Mutations in CDCA7 and HELLS cause immunodeficiency-centromeric instability-facial anomalies syndrome. Nat Commun. 2015;6:7870.
51. Chen R, Giliani S, Lanzi G, Mias GI, Lonardi S, Dobbs K, et al. Whole-exome sequencing identifies tetratricopeptide repeat domain 7A (TTC7A) mutations for combined immunodeficiency with intestinal atresias. J Allergy Clin Immunol. 2013;132(3):656–64. e617.
52. Samuels ME, Majewski J, Alirezaie N, Fernandez I, Casals F, Patey N, et al. Exome sequencing identifies mutations in the gene TTC7A in French-Canadian cases with hereditary multiple intestinal atresia. J Med Genet. 2013;50(5):324–9.
53. Boisson B, Puel A, Picard C, Casanova JL. Human IκBα gain of function: a severe and syndromic immunodeficiency. J Clin Immunol. 2017;37(5):397–412.
54. Boztug K, Jarvinen PM, Salzer E, Racek T, Mönch S, Garncarz W, et al. JAGN1 deficiency causes aberrant myeloid cell homeostasis and congenital neutropenia. Nat Genet. 2014;46(9):1021–7.
55. Etzioni A, Frydman M, Pollack S, Avidor I, Phillips ML, Paulson JC, et al. Brief report: recurrent severe infections caused by a novel leukocyte adhesion deficiency. N Engl J Med. 1992;327(25):1789–92.
56. Kuijpers TW, van Bruggen R, Kamerbeek N, Tool ATJ, Hicsonmez G, Gurgey A, et al. Natural history and early diagnosis of LAD-1/variant syndrome. Blood. 2007;109(8):3529–37.
57. Svensson L, Howarth K, McDowall A, Patzak I, Evans R, Ussar S, et al. Leukocyte adhesion deficiency-III is caused by mutations in KINDLIN3 affecting integrin activation. Nat Med. 2009;15(3):306–12.
58. Hughes CR, Guasti L, Meimaridou E, Chuang C-H, Schimenti JC, King PJ, et al. MCM4 mutation causes adrenal failure, short stature, and natural killer cell deficiency in humans. J Clin Invest. 2012;122(3):814–20.
59. Merico D, Roifman M, Braunschweig U, Yuen RKC, Alexandrova R, Bates A, et al. Compound heterozygous mutations in the noncoding RNU4ATAC cause Roifman Syndrome by disrupting minor intron splicing. Nat Commun. 2015;6:8718.
60. Orange JS, Jain A, Ballas ZK, Schneider LC, Geha RS, Bonilla FA. The presentation and natural history of immunodeficiency caused by nuclear factor kappaB essential modulator mutation. J Allergy Clin Immunol. 2004;113(4):725–33.
61. Chrzanowska KH, Gregorek H, Dembowska-Baginska B, Kalina MA, Digweed M. Nijmegen breakage syndrome (NBS). Orphanet J Rare Dis. 2012;7:13.
62. van der Crabben SN, Hennus MP, McGregor GA, Ritter DI, Nagamani SCS, Wells OS, et al. Destabilized SMC5/6 complex leads to chromosome breakage syndrome with severe lung disease. J Clin Invest. 2016;126(8):2881–92.
63. Markert ML. Purine nucleoside phosphorylase deficiency. Immunodefic Rev. 1991;3(1):45–81.
64. Waltes R, Kalb R, Gatei M, Kijas AW, Stumm M, Sobeck A, et al. Human RAD50 deficiency in a Nijmegen breakage syndrome-like disorder. Am J Hum Genet. 2009;84(5):605–16.
65. Boerkoel CF, O'Neill S, Andre JL, Benke PJ, Bogdanović R, Bulla M, et al. Manifestations and treatment of Schimke immuno-osseous dysplasia: 14 new cases and a review of the literature. Eur J Pediatr. 2000;159(1–2):1–7.
66. Nelson AS, Myers KC. Diagnosis, treatment, and molecular pathology of Shwachman-Diamond syndrome. Hematol Oncol Clin North Am. 2018;32(4):687–700.
67. Witzel M, Petersheim D, Fan Y, Bahrami E, Racek T, Rohlfs M, et al. Chromatin-remodeling factor SMARCD2 regulates transcriptional networks controlling differentiation of neutrophil granulocytes. Nat Genet. 2017;49(5):742–52.
68. Kofoed EM, Hwa V, Little B, Woods KA, Buckway CK, Tsubaki J, et al. Growth hormone insensitivity associated with a STAT5b mutation. N Engl J Med. 2003;349(12):1139–47.
69. Finocchi A, Angelino G, Cantarutti N, Corbari M, Bevivino E, Cascioli S, et al. Immunodeficiency in Vici syndrome: a heterogeneous phenotype. Am J Med Genet A. 2012;158A(2):434–9.
70. Stepensky P, Saada A, Cowan M, Tabib A, Fischer U, Berkun Y, et al. The Thr224Asn mutation in the VPS45 gene is associated with the congenital neutropenia and primary myelofibrosis of infancy. Blood. 2013;121(25):5078–87.

71. Vilboux T, Lev A, Malicdan MC, Simon AJ, Järvinen P, Racek T, et al. A congenital neutrophil defect syndrome associated with mutations in VPS45. N Engl J Med. 2013;369(1):54–65.
72. McDermott DH, Murphy PM. WHIM syndrome: immunopathogenesis, treatment and cure strategies. Immunol Rev. 2019;287(1):91–102.
73. Massaad MJ, Ramesh N, Geha RS. Wiskott-Aldrich syndrome: a comprehensive review. Ann N Y Acad Sci. 2013;1285:26–43.

Part III
Immune Dysregulation Syndromes

Chapter 12
Autoimmune Lymphoproliferative Syndrome

David T. Yang

Case Presentation 1

A 5-year-old male with a history of idiopathic thrombocytopenic purpura (ITP) presents for evaluation of posterior auricular lymphadenopathy. His mother reports that she has noted swelling behind his left ear for 1–2 years but feels it has recently enlarged. The patient has not had any fevers, night sweats, or weight loss nor has he had any skin rashes, bruising, joint pains, diarrhea, abdominal pain, cough, shortness of breath, pain with urination, visual disturbances, or trouble with gait. He was diagnosed with ITP at age 2, and his thrombocytopenia responded to treatment with intravenous immunoglobulin G. There is no family history of autoimmune disorders, lymphoproliferation, or malignancy. Physical exam reveals a soft, mobile, 3 cm left posterior auricular lymph node and multiple smaller palpable nodes along the bilateral anterior and posterior cervical chains. Abdominal exam reveals a palpable spleen 4 cm below the costal margin without a palpable liver edge. Initial laboratory testing (Table 12.1) showed a normal leukocyte and platelet count with mild normocytic anemia, elevated erythrocyte sedimentation rate and vitamin B12 levels, abnormal immunoglobulin levels with elevated IgA and IgG with decreased IgM, and negative serologies for a panel of viral and fungal infections. CT scan showed extensive diffuse cervical and upper mediastinal lymphadenopathy up to 21 mm in greatest dimension and numerous bilateral axillary, hilar, mesenteric, and inguinal lymph nodes that were increased in number, but did not meet CT size criteria for lymphadenopathy. The patient subsequently underwent a lymph node biopsy and further evaluation for suspected autoimmune lymphoproliferative syndrome (ALPS).

D. T. Yang (✉)
Department of Pathology and Laboratory Medicine, University of Wisconsin, Madison, WI, USA
e-mail: dtyang@wisc.edu

Table 12.1 Case 1 laboratory results

				Reference range
Complete blood count				
	WBC	6.8	K/uL	(4.0–12.0 K/uL)
	Hgb	10.9	g/dL	(11.5–14.5 g/dL)
	Hct	31	%	(33–43 %)
	MCV	78	fL	(76–90 fL)
	Plts	267	K/uL	(160–370 K/uL)
LDH		218	U/L	(192–321 U/L)
Direct Coombs			Negative	
ESR		40	mm/hr	(0–15 mm/hr)
IgA		264	mg/dL	(27–195 mg/dL)
IgG		2248	mg/dL	(540–1822 mg/dL)
IgM		27	mg/dL	(41–183 mg/dL)
Ferritin		87	ng/mL	(7–142 ng/mL)
Vitamin B12		>2000	pg/mL	(200–900 pg/mL)
Monospot		Negative		
Parvovirus B19			Negative	
HIV		Negative		
Blastomyces serology		Negative		
Histoplasma serology		Negative		
CMV serology		Negative		
EBV serology		Negative		
B. henselae serology		Negative		
Mycoplasma serology		Negative		

Results out of the reference range are highlighted in red.

The lymph node biopsy showed an expansion of interfollicular T cells that lacked expression of CD4 and CD8 with additional histologic features of sinus histiocytosis with massive lymphadenopathy (Rosai-Dorfman disease) that together were suggestive of ALPS. Flow cytometry performed on the peripheral blood showed an expanded population of alpha-beta T cells that lacked CD4 and CD8 expression (double-negative T cells) and comprised 12% of the CD3-positive T cells. Next-generation sequencing of *CASP8, CASP10, FADD, FAS, FASLG, NRAS*, and *KRAS* showed a pathogenic *FAS* c.676 + 1G > A mutation.

Diagnosis/Assessment

Pathogenesis

Autoimmune lymphoproliferative syndrome (ALPS) was first described by Canale and Smith in 1967 [1] and then recognized as an autoimmune syndrome in 1992 when Sneller et al. [2] documented the similarities between strains of mice with FAS pathway mutations and children suffering from a progressive lymphoproliferative disorder associated with autoimmunity. The clinical manifestations of ALPS are due to a disruption in FAS pathway-mediated apoptosis in T cells that alters normal development of the immune system.

In quiescent T cells, FAS and FAS ligand (FASL) are sequestered in the cytoplasm (Fig. 12.1a). Upon activation, FAS and FASL are expressed on the surface of T cells where FASL can bind FAS receptors on neighboring T cells and cause clustering of FAS receptors (Fig. 12.1b, c). Clustering of FAS receptors allows binding of FAS-associated protein with death domain (FADD) and recruitment of caspase 8 and caspase 10 to form the death-inducing signaling complex (DISC), which in turn propagates a signal leading to terminal caspase activation and cellular apoptosis. This process of activation-induced cell death (AICD) is vital in eliminating T cells that recognize self-antigens, thereby preventing the expansion of these auto reactive T cells that can lead to autoimmune disease [3]. Because patients with ALPS have mutations that impede AICD, they accumulate atypical T cells that include a characteristic population of alpha-beta T cells that lack CD4 and CD8 expression. These are referred to as double-negative T cells and are a hallmark of ALPS.

Clinical Manifestations

Case 1 illustrates the typical clinical manifestations of ALPS with early-onset chronic lymphadenopathy and splenomegaly often associated with immune cytopenias. The median age of diagnosis is 3 years, but some patients are diagnosed later in life. The spectrum of presenting clinical symptoms and signs are all related to the

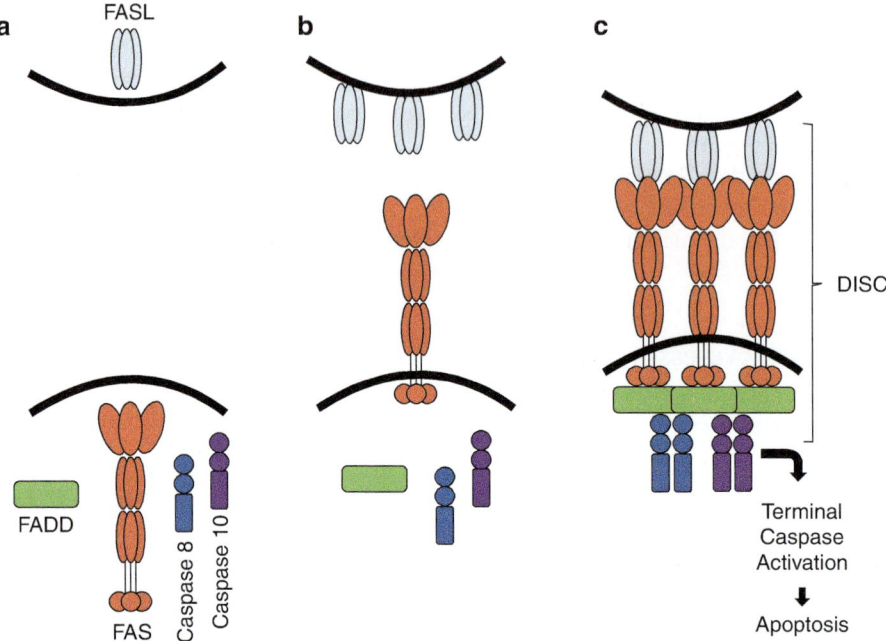

Fig. 12.1 Depiction of the FAS signaling pathway in T cells. (**a**) In resting T cells, FAS ligand (FASL) and FAS protein are not expressed on the cell surface. (**b**) Membrane-bound FASL and FAS appear on the surface of T cells shortly after activation. (**c**) Membrane-bound FASL binds FAS, causing clustering of FAS, which in turn leads to recruitment of the adaptor FAS-associated protein with death domain (FADD), caspase 8, and caspase 10. Together, this complex is referred to as the death-inducing signaling complex (DISC), which propagates a pro-apoptotic signal via the activation of terminal caspases

progressive accumulation of autoreactive B and T cells [4, 5]. Diagnostic criteria for ALPS were initially established in 1999 and subsequently revised in 2009 to reflect unifying clinical manifestations and laboratory findings of approximately 500 patients diagnosed with the disorder in the 10-year interim (Table 12.2) [6].

Lymphadenopathy and splenomegaly in ALPS are the consequence of non-infectious, non-malignant polyclonal lymphoproliferation. Their presence for at least a 6-month duration is part of the required diagnostic criteria (see Table 12.2). While not part of the diagnostic criteria, lymphoproliferation can also lead to hepatomegaly, which is found in approximately 50% of patients with ALPS [7].

Autoimmunity is the second most common manifestation of ALPS and is included as an accessory diagnostic criteria (see Table 12.2) when patients present with documented autoimmune cytopenias associated with elevated immunoglobulin G levels (polyclonal hypergammaglobulinemia). Immune-mediated cytopenias associated with polyclonal hypergammaglobulinemia are the most frequent clinical manifestation of autoimmunity, with autoimmune hemolytic anemia, immune thrombocytopenia, and autoimmune neutropenia found in 29%, 23%, and 19% of

Table 12.2 Autoimmune lymphoproliferative syndrome (ALPS) diagnostic criteria from the 2009 NIH International Workshop [6]

Definitive diagnosis = both required criteria plus one primary accessory criterion
Probable diagnosis = both required criteria plus one secondary accessory criterion
Required criteria
1. Chronic (>6 months), non-malignant, non-infectious lymphadenopathy or splenomegaly or both
2. Elevated CD3+, TCRαβ+, CD4-, CD8- double-negative T cells (>1.5% of total lymphocytes or 2.5% of CD3+ lymphocytes) in the setting of normal or elevated lymphocyte counts
Accessory criteria
Primary
1. Defective lymphocyte apoptosis (in 2 separate assays)
2. Somatic or germline pathogenic mutations in *FAS, FASLG,* or *CASP10*
Secondary
1. Elevated plasma sFASL levels (>200 pg/mL) *or*
Elevated plasma IL-10 levels (>20 pg/mL) *or*
Serum or plasma B12 levels (>1500 ng/L) *or*
Elevated plasma IL-18 levels (>500 pg/mL)
2. Typical immunohistological findings as reviewed by an experienced hematopathologist
3. Autoimmune cytopenias (hemolytic anemia, thrombocytopenia, or neutropenia) *and*
Elevated immunoglobulin G levels (polyclonal hypergammaglobulinemia)
4. Family history of a non-malignant/non-infectious lymphoproliferation with or without autoimmunity

patients, respectively [8]. Patients with significant cytopenias may present with fatigue, pallor, icterus, mucocutaneous hemorrhage, or recurrent infections. Autoimmune syndromes involving the solid organs are less common, but uveitis, glomerulonephritis, hepatitis, thyroiditis, dermatitis, encephalitis, and myelitis have been reported [4, 9–11].

Laboratory Findings

As noted above, no single finding is diagnostic of ALPS, but instead, a definitive or probable diagnosis can be made based on fulfillment of required and accessory criteria (see Table 12.2) [6]. The two required diagnostic criteria are documentation of chronic lymphadenopathy or splenomegaly and evidence of an expanded population of double-negative T cells (alpha-beta T cells that lack CD4 and CD8). Thus, performing flow cytometric evaluation of circulating T cells to quantify double-negative T cells is an essential part of the laboratory evaluation for suspected ALPS patients (Fig. 12.2). For diagnosis, double-negative T cells must comprise a minimum of 1.5% of the total lymphocytes or 2.5% of the CD3-positive T cells. Quantification of double-negative T cells must be based on expression of T-cell receptor alpha-beta, as normal gamma-delta T cells lack CD4 and CD8 and need to

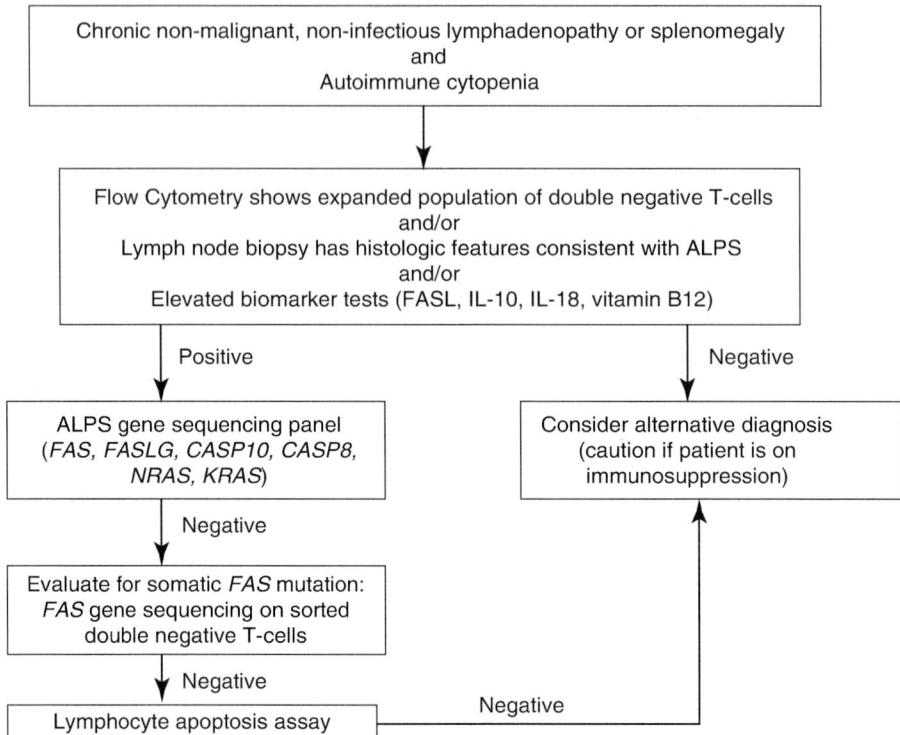

Fig. 12.2 Diagnostic algorithm for autoimmune lymphoproliferative syndrome (ALPS). In patients with clinical features of ALPS, pursuing more specific laboratory testing is the next step. Flow cytometric evaluation for circulating double-negative T cells and enzyme immunoassays for plasma FASL, IL-10, IL18, and vitamin B12 is typically available through a combination of local laboratories and reference laboratories. Biopsies should be evaluated by an experienced hematopathologist who is familiar with the histologic features of ALPS. If any combination of these tests is positive, gene sequencing of a panel of ALPS-related genes should be considered. If gene sequencing is negative, there is a possibility that the patient is harboring a somatic *FAS* mutation in the double-negative T cells that is being obscured by the predominance of normal lymphocytes. Gene sequencing of isolated double-negative T cells can be performed to diagnose ALPS with somatic FAS mutations (ALPS-sFAS). If negative, a diagnosis of ALPS with unknown genetic cause (ALPS-U) should be considered and can be confirmed by a positive lymphocyte apoptosis assay

be excluded from the quantification. Also of note, while the necessary diagnostic number of double-negative T cells appears to be low, it is important to recognize that double-negative T cells comprising >3% of total lymphocytes is seldom seen in any condition other than ALPS [12]. The double-negative T cells in ALPS are believed to be a subset of effector memory T cells that are typically eliminated through the FAS apoptosis pathway, and their persistence likely drives abnormal B-cell activity and autoimmunity [13, 14]. A reflection of the B-cell activation is polyclonal hypergammaglobulinemia that often has a characteristic pattern, demonstrated in Case 1 (see Table 12.1), of elevated immunoglobulin G and immunoglobulin A with decreased immunoglobulin M due to exacerbated class switching [15].

For a probable diagnosis of ALPS, one secondary accessory criterion must be fulfilled in addition to the two required criteria (see Table 12.2). The secondary criteria include a set of plasma biomarkers that are frequently elevated in patients with pathogenic *FAS* mutations. Soluble FAS ligand (sFASL) may be the most sensitive biomarker to rule out a *FAS* mutation with 97% of patients harboring germline *FAS* mutations demonstrating levels greater than 200 pg/mL [12]. Likewise, elevated levels of the cytokines IL-10 and IL-18 greater than 20 pg/mL and 500 pg/mL, respectively, are associated with a high probability of *FAS* mutation [12]. Interestingly, patients with ALPS have also been noted to have elevated plasma vitamin B12 levels, and levels above 1500 ng/L have been deemed high enough to fulfill secondary accessory criteria for ALPS diagnosis [6]. The etiology of elevated vitamin B12 in ALPS may be related to increased expression of haptocorrin (also known as transcobalamin-1 (TC-1) or cobalophilin), a plasma B12-binding protein, on lymphocytes of ALPS patients [16].

Other secondary accessory diagnostic criteria include histologic findings, presence of autoimmune cytopenias (described in the Clinical Manifestations section above), and a family history of non-malignant, non-infectious lymphoproliferation. Patients presenting with chronic lymphadenopathy frequently undergo lymph node biopsy as part of their evaluation for malignant or infectious etiologies. The enlarged lymph nodes in ALPS patients have characteristic histologic features that include follicular hyperplasia and a florid paracortical expansion comprised of a polymorphous population of small proliferative lymphocytes, immunoblasts, and plasma cells. Mitotic figures are frequent; however, the overall architecture of the lymph node is intact, differentiating this polyclonal T-cell proliferation from T-cell lymphoma [17]. In some cases, like Case 1, features of sinus histiocytosis with massive lymphadenopathy (Rosai-Dorfman disease) are present characterized by a marked expansion of sinus histiocytes that demonstrate the unique feature of emperipolesis with lymphocytes transiting through the histiocyte cytoplasm [18]. Immunohistochemical staining of the lymph node biopsy shows increased numbers of CD3-positive, CD4-negative, and CD8-negative double-negative T cells, but no aberrant loss of other pan-T-cell antigens such as CD2, CD5, and CD7, which would be more typical of T-cell lymphoma.

Fulfillment of the two required diagnostic criteria and either of the two primary accessory diagnostic criteria is sufficient for a definitive diagnosis of ALPS. The two primary accessory criteria are demonstration of defective lymphocyte apoptosis and demonstration of somatic or germline mutations in *FAS*, *FASLG*, or *CASP10* (see Table 12.2). Lymphocyte apoptotic assays assess the percentage of in vitro activated T cells that undergo apoptosis after FAS activation by agonist antibodies, recombinant FAS ligand, or cytokine starvation compared to control T cells [19, 20]. While apoptotic assays were once held as the gold standard for the diagnosis of ALPS, they have fallen out of favor as a frontline diagnostic test because very few laboratories offer this labor-intensive and difficult-to-standardize test. In addition, patients with somatic mutations of *FAS* and germline mutations of *FASLG* will have

Table 12.3 Classification of autoimmune lymphoproliferative syndrome (ALPS) [6]

ALPS-FAS	Patients fulfill ALPS diagnostic criteria and have a germline *FAS* mutation
ALPS-sFAS	Patients fulfill ALPS diagnostic criteria and have a somatic *FAS* mutation
ALPS-FASLG	Patients fulfill ALPS diagnostic criteria and have a germline *FASL* mutation
ALPS-CASP10	Patients fulfill ALPS diagnostic criteria and have a germline *CASP10* mutation
ALPS-U	Patients fulfill ALPS diagnostic criteria, but no genetic defect in *FAS, FASL,* or *CASP10* is detected

normal apoptotic assays [21]. Accordingly, to make a definitive diagnosis of ALPS, most diagnostic algorithms recommend pursuing gene sequencing of *FAS, FASLG,* and *CASP10* before pursuing apoptosis assays [22, 23]. A practical diagnostic algorithm would be to first pursue flow cytometry, lymph node biopsy, and biomarker testing in patients who present with chronic lymphadenopathy and autoimmune cytopenia suspected of having ALPS (see Fig. 12.2). If any of these tests are positive, the suspicion for ALPS is further heightened, and an ALPS gene sequencing panel should be pursued (see Fig. 12.2).

Mutations in *FAS, FASLG,* or *CASP10* are found in approximately 70% of patients with ALPS, and these patients can be further subclassified based on mutation type (Table 12.3) [6, 24]. Many mutation testing panels also include gene sequencing for *CASP8, NRAS,* and *KRAS* as patients with germline mutations in *CASP8* and somatic mutations in *NRAS* and *KRAS* can have similar clinical and laboratory features as ALPS patients. However, patients with mutations in these alternative genes typically lack the characteristic double-negative T cells found in ALPS and those with *RAS* pathway mutations frequently have associated myeloid abnormalities resembling juvenile myelomonocytic leukemia [25–27]. Accordingly, patients with *CASP8, NRAS,* or *KRAS* mutations are classified as having ALPS-related apoptosis disorders. Similarly, patients who otherwise meet diagnostic criteria for ALPS, but lack a recognized genetic cause (unknown), are classified as ALPS-U, denoting a yet to be defined category (see Table 12.3). These patients are typically diagnosed via a positive lymphocyte apoptosis assay (see Fig. 12.2).

The majority of patients with ALPS have germline heterozygous missense *FAS* mutations that lead to an amino acid substitution in the intracellular protein domain that in turn imparts a dominant negative effect on the wild type protein, likely by inhibiting FAS trimerization (see Fig. 12.1) [28]. While these more common *FAS* mutations have high clinical penetrance, 20–30% of germline heterozygous *FAS* mutations are nonsense, splice site, or frameshift mutations found in the extracellular domain that lead to decreased FAS expression and haploinsufficiency with low clinical penetrance [29]. In contrast to germline *FAS* mutations, 10–15% of patients with *FAS* mutations harbor somatic mutations. These sporadically acquired mutations appear in hematopoietic stem cells and tend to be restricted to double-negative T cells thereby often requiring sequencing analysis to be performed on enriched samples of sorted double-negative T cells to facilitate detection (see Fig. 12.2) [21, 30]. Patients with somatic *FAS* mutations are segregated from those with germline mutations and are classified as ALPS-sFAS rather than ALPS-FAS, respectively (see Table 12.3). ALPS patients with *FASLG* or *CASP10* mutations are also separately classified as ALPS-FASLG and ALPS-CASP10, respectively (see Table 12.3). These are uncommon ALPS mutations with only a small number of cases described in the literature [31–33].

Differential Diagnosis

The differential diagnosis for chronic lymphadenopathy and splenomegaly combined with immune mediated cytopenias is broad and includes numerous infectious and malignant possibilities. Among these, self-limited viral infections are especially common in the pediatric population. Epstein-Barr virus (EBV) infection has similar clinical manifestations as ALPS, with patients frequently presenting with lethargy, fatigue, lymphadenopathy, and splenomegaly. Serologic and viral nucleic acid testing are typically the most efficient methods to differentiate EBV-related illness from ALPS. If a lymph node biopsy is obtained, the histologic features of EBV-related lymphadenopathy have some overlap with ALPS with a marked paracortical expansion of polymorphous lymphocytes, but immunohistochemistry demonstrates the lymphocytes are predominantly CD8 positive T cells as opposed to double-negative T cells in ALPS [17]. Of note, EBV infection elicits an expansion of gamma-delta T cells, and because gamma-delta T cells lack CD4 and CD8 expression, they can be mistaken for the double-negative alpha-beta T cells characteristic of ALPS unless alpha-beta and gamma-delta markers are assessed simultaneously [34].

Immune-mediated cytopenias occur in many settings other than ALPS and are classified as primary autoimmune cytopenias (previously referred to as idiopathic) and secondary autoimmune cytopenias that are a result of another cause such as rheumatologic disorders, medications, or malignancy. In adults, secondary autoimmune cytopenias are more common than the primary, but the opposite is true in children. Primary autoimmune cytopenias usually only affects a single lineage but will occasionally cause multi-lineage cytopenias, typically involving red cells and platelets, and is referred to as Evans syndrome [35]. Evans syndrome appears to overlap with ALPS where, in a subset of patients, double-negative T cells are similarly increased and persistent lymphoproliferation has been noted, but lymphadenopathy is typically absent [36].

Common variable immune deficiency (CVID) is an immunodeficiency disorder of unknown cause that, similar to ALPS, typically manifests in children with lymphadenopathy and autoimmunity. CVID is associated with recurrent infections and low levels of circulating immunoglobulin with diminished memory B cells. Patients with CVID can be differentiated from ALPS patients by lack of ALPS-associated mutations, no increase of double-negative T cells, and intact FAS-mediated lymphocyte apoptosis. However, a subset of ALPS patients has been described that appear to have co-morbid CVID, often appearing years after initial diagnosis, with decreased immunoglobulin A or immunoglobulin M and susceptibility to infection

[15, 37]. Additional inherited conditions that should be considered in the differential diagnosis include X-linked lymphoproliferative syndrome, Wiskott-Aldrich syndrome, hyperimmunoglobulin M syndrome, gray platelet syndrome, and RAS-associated autoimmune leukoproliferative disorder [26].

Finally, malignant lymphoma should be considered in the differential diagnosis of any patient presenting with lymphadenopathy and cytopenias. On lymph node biopsies, the histologic features of ALPS can mimic malignant T-cell lymphoma due to architectural distortion from the proliferation of double-negative T cells and, coupled with splenic and bone marrow involvement by T cells, can make a compelling picture for T-cell lymphoma. In such cases, demonstration of polyclonal T-cell receptor rearrangements is helpful in ruling out a clonal T-cell neoplasm.

Management/Outcome

Treatment

Not all ALPS patients require treatment although a majority require immunosuppression to manage autoimmune manifestations, primarily autoimmune cytopenias. The goal of managing cytopenias is to prevent life-threatening cytopenias while avoiding splenectomy [24]. Short bursts of glucocorticoids are usually successful for treating cytopenias in the acute setting, and patients are then transitioned to glucocorticoid-sparing immunosuppressive regimens such as mycophenolate mofetil to avoid the complications associated with long-term glucocorticoid therapy [38]. Of note, unlike non-ALPS patients with autoimmune cytopenias, those with ALPS typically do not respond to intravenous immunoglobulin G [39]. Rituximab, an anti-CD20 monoclonal antibody, has been reported to be effective in treating ALPS patients with chronic refractory thrombocytopenia but not autoimmune hemolytic anemia [24]. Caution should be exercised with using rituximab though, due to the risk of prolonged hypogammaglobulinemia in ALPS patients, likely associated with reduced proportions of marginal zone and memory B cells in patients with ALPS [24, 40]. Recombinant granulocyte-colony-stimulating factor is useful in patients suffering from recurrent infections due to autoimmune neutropenia. Sirolimus, a mammalian target of rapamycin (mTOR) inhibitor, has been shown to be remarkably effective in treating autoimmune cytopenias in ALPS patients [41]. Upregulation of mTOR occurs in abnormal lymphocytes, including double-negative T cells, and mTOR inhibitors are effective in inducing cell death and apoptosis in these cells [42]. By reducing lymphoproliferation, patients on sirolimus also show reduction in lymphadenopathy and splenomegaly. Like other glucocorticoid-sparing immunosuppressive regimens, patients need to be maintained on sirolimus long term with careful monitoring of drug levels, dose adjustment, and regular evaluation for toxicities that include T-cell immunosuppression, hypercholesterolemia, and stomatitis.

Splenectomy should be avoided in patients with ALPS as it is associated with a high rate of recurrence of cytopenias (56%), sepsis (29%), and overall worse outcomes compared to ALPS patients managed without splenectomy [43]. ALPS patients are particularly prone to post-splenectomy sepsis because they have defective anti-polysaccharide IgM antibody production due to a deficit of memory B cells. Accordingly, post-splenectomy ALPS patients are unable to mount or sustain protective levels of antibodies against pneumococcal polysaccharide antigens after vaccination [40]. ALPS patients should only undergo splenectomy if it is the only remaining option to treat refractory life-threatening cytopenias. ALPS patients who have undergone splenectomy should take daily antibiotic prophylaxis, be regularly re-vaccinated using a combination of both 13-valent conjugate and 23-valent polysaccharide vaccines every 4 to 5 years, and wear Medic alert bracelets that convey their risk for life-threatening sepsis [24].

As noted above, splenomegaly should be treated conservatively. Use of molded thermoplastic spleen guards has been reported to be protective in active children to prevent splenic rupture [24]. Sirolimus may be considered for patients with symptomatic splenomegaly as it has demonstrated efficacy in reducing spleen size [41].

Counseling

Autosomal dominant transmission of germline heterozygous *FAS* mutations comprises the majority of ALPS cases [7]. Accordingly, assessment of relatives of ALPS probands frequently identifies first-degree relatives who harbor the same mutation, although their clinical manifestations may differ from the proband, dependent upon the variable penetrance of the specific mutation. Genetic counseling should be a part of the diagnostic process where patients and family members are educated regarding inheritance patterns, disease manifestations, and the necessity of close follow-up of affected patients for emerging complications.

Case Presentation 2

A 25-year-old male presents with complaints of increasing cervical adenopathy and night sweats. He has a history of ALPS diagnosed at age 3 years when he presented with thrombocytopenia and splenomegaly. His cytopenias have responded to several short courses of glucocorticoids, and he is currently taking mycophenolate mofetil. He has regular follow-ups, and review of his chart notes that while his adenopathy and splenomegaly have periodically waxed and waned, both have overall been diminishing over the past 10 years. He denies any fevers, chills, cough, or weight loss. Physical exam reveals prominent non-tender bilateral cervical adenopathy that has doubled in size since the previous recorded examination performed 6 months ago. A lymph node biopsy is performed and shows effacement of normal architecture by a predominance of small lymphocytes with scattered eosinophils, plasma cells, and rare large atypical Hodgkin and Reed-Sternberg cells, diagnostic for classic Hodgkin lymphoma.

Management

Next to post-splenectomy sepsis, lymphoma is the second most common cause of death in ALPS patients [43]. The risk for malignant lymphoma in ALPS patients is estimated to be 50-fold that of the general public for developing Hodgkin lymphoma and 14-fold for non-Hodgkin lymphoma, with the risk extending across mutation types and not diminishing with age [44]. Biologically, *FAS* is a tumor suppressor gene and is frequently found to be mutated in cancer, including up to 20% of Hodgkin lymphomas, and loss of tumor suppressor function likely contributes to the risk of patients harboring germline inactivating *FAS* mutations to develop lymphoma [45]. These observations underscore both the importance of cancer surveillance in patients diagnosed with ALPS and the importance of awareness of the possibility of underlying ALPS in young lymphoma patients who have an unusual history of chronic lymphadenopathy and idiopathic cytopenias.

Case 2 illustrates the typical fluctuation in lymphadenopathy experienced by ALPS patients that complicates lymphoma surveillance. Careful examination and documentation of changes in site-specific lymph node groups at regular intervals with a standardized grading system can be helpful in determining when lymphoma transformation should be suspected. Similarly, splenomegaly should be regularly documented as the palpable distance below the costal margin at the midclavicular line by physical exam [24]. Imaging by serial computed tomography (CT) and positron emission tomography (PET) can provide more accurate assessment of interval changes in lymph node and spleen size, but cost and radiation exposure limit the surveillance frequency of these modalities compared to physical examination. Clinical suspicion and focal exacerbation of lymphadenopathy require follow-up with a biopsy to rule out lymphoma, and in some cases, ALPS patients are subjected to multiple repeated biopsies. Whole-body PET with 2-deoxy-2-[fluorine-18]fluoro-D-glucose uptake (FDG-PET) may be able to discriminate between ALPS-associated lymphadenopathy and ALPS-associated lymphoma based on FDG distribution and is currently being investigated as a noninvasive surveillance modality.

Outcomes

The major determinants of morbidity and mortality for patients with ALPS are the severity of their autoimmune disease and the development of lymphoma. Autoimmune disease can lead to life-threatening cytopenias and immune-related organ failure, necessitating management by immunosuppression or splenectomy, but long-term follow-up studies show that post-splenectomy sepsis is the leading cause of mortality in ALPS patients [7, 43]. Accordingly, avoiding splenectomy is a critical part of the management plan which can be bolstered by the idea of bridging pediatric patients through autoimmune cytopenias without resorting to splenectomy predicated on the observation that autoimmunity appears to improve with age as 44% of patients showed remission in autoimmune cytopenias over a median follow-up of 28 years [7]. Likewise, lymphoproliferation (lymphadenopathy and splenomegaly) also improved in patients in the same study with complete remission in 66% and significant improvement in 34% [7]. In contrast, the risk for developing lymphoma does not diminish with age, and the cumulative risk of developing lymphoma before age 30 is 15% [7]. Current investigations are focused on correlating specific ALPS-related mutations with prognosis to guide more personalized management decisions, but the rarity of this disorder combined with its relative genetic heterogeneity poses a significant challenge.

Clinical Pearls and Pitfalls
- ALPS is caused by a deficient FAS-mediated apoptosis pathway in T cells and typically manifests in children as lymphadenopathy, splenomegaly, and autoimmune cytopenias.
- An expanded population of atypical CD4- and CD8-negative alpha-beta T cells is a hallmark of ALPS.
- Gene sequencing of a panel of ALPS-related genes is an efficient way to definitively diagnose ALPS in patients who fulfill criteria for a probable diagnosis.
- Management of ALPS is based on treating autoimmune cytopenias, avoiding splenectomy, and surveillance for lymphoma, keeping in mind that lymphoproliferative and autoimmune manifestations typically improve with age.

References

1. Canale VC, Smith CH. Chronic lymphadenopathy simulating malignant lymphoma. J Pediatr. 1967;70(6):891–9.
2. Sneller MC, Straus SE, Jaffe ES, Jaffe JS, Fleisher TA, Stetler-Stevenson M, et al. A novel lymphoproliferative/autoimmune syndrome resembling murine lpr/gld disease. J Clin Invest. 1992;90(2):334–41.
3. Green DR, Droin N, Pinkoski M. Activation-induced cell death in T cells. Immunol Rev. 2003;193:70–81.
4. Sneller MC, Wang J, Dale JK, Strober W, Middelton LA, Choi Y, et al. Clinical, immunologic, and genetic features of an autoimmune lymphoproliferative syndrome associated with abnormal lymphocyte apoptosis. Blood. 1997;89(4):1341–8.

5. Lambotte O, Neven B, Galicier L, Magerus-Chatinet A, Schleinitz N, Hermine O, et al. Diagnosis of autoimmune lymphoproliferative syndrome caused by FAS deficiency in adults. Haematologica. 2013;98(3):389–92.
6. Oliveira JB, Bleesing JJ, Dianzani U, Fleisher TA, Jaffe ES, Lenardo MJ, et al. Revised diagnostic criteria and classification for the autoimmune lymphoproliferative syndrome (ALPS): report from the 2009 NIH International Workshop. Blood. 2010;116(14):e35–40.
7. Neven B, Magerus-Chatinet A, Florkin B, Gobert D, Lambotte O, De Somer L, et al. A survey of 90 patients with autoimmune lymphoproliferative syndrome related to TNFRSF6 mutation. Blood. 2011;118(18):4798–807.
8. Sneller MC, Dale JK, Straus SE. Autoimmune lymphoproliferative syndrome. Curr Opin Rheumatol. 2003;15(4):417–21.
9. Kanegane H, Vilela MM, Wang Y, Futatani T, Matsukura H, Miyawaki T. Autoimmune lymphoproliferative syndrome presenting with glomerulonephritis. Pediatr Nephrol. 2003;18(5):454–6.
10. Pensati L, Costanzo A, Ianni A, Accapezzato D, Iorio R, Natoli G, et al. Fas/Apo1 mutations and autoimmune lymphoproliferative syndrome in a patient with type 2 autoimmune hepatitis. Gastroenterology. 1997;113(4):1384–9.
11. Lim WK, Ursea R, Rao K, Buggage RR, Suhler EB, Dugan F, et al. Bilateral uveitis in a patient with autoimmune lymphoproliferative syndrome. Am J Ophthalmol. 2005;139(3):562–3.
12. Caminha I, Fleisher TA, Hornung RL, Dale JK, Niemela JE, Price S, et al. Using biomarkers to predict the presence of FAS mutations in patients with features of the autoimmune lymphoproliferative syndrome. J Allergy Clin Immunol. 2010;125(4):946–9.e6.
13. Rensing-Ehl A, Völkl S, Speckmann C, Lorenz MR, Ritter J, Janda A, et al. Abnormally differentiated CD4+ or CD8+ T cells with phenotypic and genetic features of double-negative T cells in human Fas deficiency. Blood. 2014;124(6):851–60.
14. Ohga S, Nomura A, Takahata Y, Ihara K, Takada H, Wakiguchi H, et al. Dominant expression of interleukin 10 but not interferon gamma in CD4(−)CD8(−)alphabetaT cells of autoimmune lymphoproliferative syndrome. Br J Haematol. 2002;119(2):535–8.
15. Campagnoli MF, Garbarini L, Quarello P, Garelli E, Carando A, Baravalle V, et al. The broad spectrum of autoimmune lymphoproliferative disease: molecular bases, clinical features and long-term follow-up in 31 patients. Haematologica. 2006;91(4):538–41.
16. Bowen RA, Dowdell KC, Dale JK, Drake SK, Fleisher TA, Hortin GL, et al. Elevated vitamin B_{12} levels in autoimmune lymphoproliferative syndrome attributable to elevated haptocorrin in lymphocytes. Clin Biochem. 2012;45(6):490–2.
17. Lim MS, Straus SE, Dale JK, Fleisher TA, Stetler-Stevenson M, Strober W, et al. Pathological findings in human autoimmune lymphoproliferative syndrome. Am J Pathol. 1998;153(5):1541–50.
18. Maric I, Pittaluga S, Dale JK, Niemela JE, Delsol G, Diment J, et al. Histologic features of sinus histiocytosis with massive lymphadenopathy in patients with autoimmune lymphoproliferative syndrome. Am J Surg Pathol. 2005;29(7):903–11.
19. Teachey DT, Manno CS, Axsom KM, Andrews T, Choi JK, Greenbaum BH, et al. Unmasking Evans syndrome: T-cell phenotype and apoptotic response reveal autoimmune lymphoproliferative syndrome (ALPS). Blood. 2005;105(6):2443–8.
20. Muppidi JR, Siegel RM. Ligand-independent redistribution of Fas (CD95) into lipid rafts mediates clonotypic T cell death. Nat Immunol. 2004;5(2):182–9.
21. Holzelova E, Vonarbourg C, Stolzenberg MC, Arkwright PD, Selz F, Prieur AM, et al. Autoimmune lymphoproliferative syndrome with somatic Fas mutations. N Engl J Med. 2004;351(14):1409–18.
22. Teachey DT, Seif AE, Grupp SA. Advances in the management and understanding of autoimmune lymphoproliferative syndrome (ALPS). Br J Haematol. 2010;148(2):205–16.
23. Matson DR, Yang DT. Autoimmune lymphoproliferative syndrome: an overview. Arch Pathol Lab Med. 2020;144(2):245–51.

24. Rao VK, Oliveira JB. How I treat autoimmune lymphoproliferative syndrome. Blood. 2011;118(22):5741–51.
25. Chun HJ, Zheng L, Ahmad M, Wang J, Speirs CK, Siegel RM, et al. Pleiotropic defects in lymphocyte activation caused by caspase-8 mutations lead to human immunodeficiency. Nature. 2002;419(6905):395–9.
26. Niemela JE, Lu L, Fleisher TA, Davis J, Caminha I, Natter M, et al. Somatic KRAS mutations associated with a human nonmalignant syndrome of autoimmunity and abnormal leukocyte homeostasis. Blood. 2011;117(10):2883–6.
27. Oliveira JB, Bidère N, Niemela JE, Zheng L, Sakai K, Nix CP, et al. NRAS mutation causes a human autoimmune lymphoproliferative syndrome. Proc Natl Acad Sci U S A. 2007;104(21):8953–8.
28. Fisher GH, Rosenberg FJ, Straus SE, Dale JK, Middleton LA, Lin AY, et al. Dominant interfering Fas gene mutations impair apoptosis in a human autoimmune lymphoproliferative syndrome. Cell. 1995;81(6):935–46.
29. Kuehn HS, Caminha I, Niemela JE, Rao VK, Davis J, Fleisher TA, et al. FAS haploinsufficiency is a common disease mechanism in the human autoimmune lymphoproliferative syndrome. J Immunol. 2011;186(10):6035–43.
30. Dowdell KC, Niemela JE, Price S, Davis J, Hornung RL, Oliveira JB, et al. Somatic FAS mutations are common in patients with genetically undefined autoimmune lymphoproliferative syndrome. Blood. 2010;115(25):5164–9.
31. Del-Rey M, Ruiz-Contreras J, Bosque A, Calleja S, Gomez-Rial J, Roldan E, et al. A homozygous Fas ligand gene mutation in a patient causes a new type of autoimmune lymphoproliferative syndrome. Blood. 2006;108(4):1306–12.
32. Sobh A, Crestani E, Cangemi B, Kane J, Chou J, Pai SY, et al. Autoimmune lymphoproliferative syndrome caused by a homozygous FasL mutation that disrupts FasL assembly. J Allergy Clin Immunol. 2016;137(1):324–7.e2.
33. Miano M, Cappelli E, Pezzulla A, Venè R, Grossi A, Terranova P, et al. FAS-mediated apoptosis impairment in patients with ALPS/ALPS-like phenotype carrying variants on CASP10 gene. Br J Haematol. 2019;187(4):502–8.
34. Long HM, Meckiff BJ, Taylor GS. The T-cell response to Epstein-Barr Virus-new tricks from an old dog. Front Immunol. 2019;10:2193.
35. Norton A, Roberts I. Management of Evans syndrome. Br J Haematol. 2006;132(2):125–37.
36. Seif AE, Manno CS, Sheen C, Grupp SA, Teachey DT. Identifying autoimmune lymphoproliferative syndrome in children with Evans syndrome: a multi-institutional study. Blood. 2010;115(11):2142–5.
37. Rensing-Ehl A, Warnatz K, Fuchs S, Schlesier M, Salzer U, Draeger R, et al. Clinical and immunological overlap between autoimmune lymphoproliferative syndrome and common variable immunodeficiency. Clin Immunol. 2010;137(3):357–65.
38. Kossiva L, Theodoridou M, Mostrou G, Vrachnou E, Le Deist F, Rieux-Laucat F, et al. Mycophenolate mofetil as an alternate immunosuppressor for autoimmune lymphoproliferative syndrome. J Pediatr Hematol Oncol. 2006;28(12):824–6.
39. Bleesing JJ, Straus SE, Fleisher TA. Autoimmune lymphoproliferative syndrome. A human disorder of abnormal lymphocyte survival. Pediatr Clin N Am. 2000;47(6):1291–310.
40. Neven B, Bruneau J, Stolzenberg MC, Meyts I, Magerus-Chatinet A, Moens L, et al. Defective anti-polysaccharide response and splenic marginal zone disorganization in ALPS patients. Blood. 2014;124(10):1597–609.
41. Teachey DT, Greiner R, Seif A, Attiyeh E, Bleesing J, Choi J, et al. Treatment with sirolimus results in complete responses in patients with autoimmune lymphoproliferative syndrome. Br J Haematol. 2009;145(1):101–6.
42. Völkl S, Rensing-Ehl A, Allgäuer A, Schreiner E, Lorenz MR, Rohr J, et al. Hyperactive mTOR pathway promotes lymphoproliferation and abnormal differentiation in autoimmune lymphoproliferative syndrome. Blood. 2016;128(2):227–38.

43. Price S, Shaw PA, Seitz A, Joshi G, Davis J, Niemela JE, et al. Natural history of autoimmune lymphoproliferative syndrome associated with FAS gene mutations. Blood. 2014;123(13):1989–99.
44. Straus SE, Jaffe ES, Puck JM, Dale JK, Elkon KB, Rösen-Wolff A, et al. The development of lymphomas in families with autoimmune lymphoproliferative syndrome with germline Fas mutations and defective lymphocyte apoptosis. Blood. 2001;98(1):194–200.
45. Poppema S, Maggio E, van den Berg A. Development of lymphoma in Autoimmune Lymphoproliferative Syndrome (ALPS) and its relationship to Fas gene mutations. Leuk Lymphoma. 2004;45(3):423–31.

Chapter 13
Autoinflammatory Syndromes

James M. Fernandez, John McDonnell, and Christine A. Royer

Introduction

Autoinflammatory diseases consist of a wide variety of immunologically mediated syndromes most frequently characterized by abnormalities in innate immunity that result in a secondary loss of antigenic tolerance to self. These diseases have vast variety of symptoms that may be organ-specific or systemic. The innate immune response exists to protect an organism from potential dangers or threats. The goal of the immune response is to eliminate the danger and restore homeostasis. Autoinflammatory syndromes are caused by a dysregulation in this innate process [1]. Primary immunodeficiency diseases include several diseases that affect different components of the adaptive [acquired] but also this innate immunity. At its core, it would seem that primary immunodeficiencies and autoinflammatory diseases are independent or even opposing entities. However, after uncovering knowledge into the pathophysiological processes involving T-cell development, immune tolerance, T-cell signaling, complement pathway, and inflammation, they are now accepted as interconnected processes, sharing some common mechanisms [2]. In fact, some primary immunodeficiencies such as immune dysregulation, polyendocrinopathy, enteropathy, X-linked (IPEX) syndrome and autoimmune lymphoproliferative syndrome (ALPS) are defined by their autoimmune component with nearly 100% of the affected patients having an autoinflammatory component. The high prevalence of autoinflammatory syndromes in primary immunodeficiency demonstrates the close relationships between the mechanisms of these two conditions. Defects in central and peripheral tolerance of T regulatory cells appear to be integral in the

J. M. Fernandez (✉) · J. McDonnell · C.A. Royer
Department of Allergy and Clinical Immunology,
Cleveland Clinic Foundation, Cleveland, OH, USA
e-mail: fernanj2@ccf.org

development of autoimmunity in this susceptible population. Diagnosis, monitoring, and treating these conditions can be challenging and require a fine balance between immune replacement and immunosuppression. Balancing immunosuppressive therapy in patients with susceptibility to infection is highly dependent on correcting the underlying immune dysregulation while minimizing nonspecific immune suppression [3].

Case Presentation 1

A 20-year-old male with a history of psoriasis presents to the office for evaluation of chronic infections. He reports a history of waxing and waning fevers, diarrhea, tender lymphadenopathy, and recurrent sinusitis and pneumonias starting around age 11, requiring on average six to seven rounds of antibiotics a year. He states that the sinus infections are usually diagnosed clinically based on his presentation with headaches and fevers, and these do seem to respond to one round of oral antibiotics. He had a sinus CT at one point which showed pansinusitis and even had sinus surgery at the age of 17. His fevers have been occurring since childhood and are marked by occasional high spiking fevers of 101°F. These bouts of fever last a few days and then can resolve for months at a time. He does not feel the episodes of diarrhea are associated with the fevers, but his tender cervical lymphadenopathy seems to occur around the fevers. He has had chest X-ray-diagnosed pneumonia on three occasions affecting different anatomical locations. During one of his episodes of pneumonia, he was admitted to the hospital and required IV antibiotics to clear the infection. He has been seen by a local rheumatologist in the past where he was noted to be ANA positive (1:80) with homogenous pattern, and his ESR and CRP were slightly elevated at the time. On examination, he had a small amount of bleeding from his nose, tender hepatosplenomegaly, and a blanching petechial rash on his bilateral lower legs. His immunologic testing post visit revealed thrombocytopenia with a platelet count of 5000/uL. He was diagnosed with immune thrombocytopenic purpura and started on prednisone at 1 mg/kg daily. In addition, given his recurrent infections, further immunologic testing was ordered which showed an IgG of 444 mg/dL, 23 mg/dL, 10 mg/dL, and only 2 of 23 pneumococcal titers above 1.3 ug/dL post vaccine. He was also noted to have low titers of diphtheria and tetanus antibodies despite having had these routine vaccinations at appropriate times in the past. His cellular immune testing showed a slightly low CD4 count of 455 cells/uL but a normal CD4/CD8 ratio. B cells were low at 2% and 55 cells/uL. He was diagnosed with CVID and started on IVIG at 400 mg/kg. His infections improved, but he continued to suffer from severe diarrhea, abdominal cramping and pain, as well as almost daily fevers of 101°F. A chest/abdomen/pelvis CT revealed pulmonary nodules and an enlarged spleen. A colonoscopy and EGD with biopsy were unrevealing. Further B-cell phenotyping showed an enhanced population of CD21 (lo) B cells, and whole-exome sequencing (WES) revealed a nonsense mutation in CTLA4 at position c.105 (C35*) – a known pathogenic variant. He was started on abatacept – a protein composed of the Fc region of the immunoglobulin IgG1 fused to the extracellular domain of CTLA-4.

Diagnosis/Assessment

Symptoms/Clinical Presentation

As demonstrated in this case, the symptoms in various primary immunodeficiency and autoinflammatory syndromes can be diverse (Table 13.1). The most frequent clinical presentation in patients with primary immunodeficiency is recurrent (and in many instances) severe infections. The most common infections are sinopulmonary but can be highly varied depending on the immunologic deficit. In this case, the patient's recurrence of pneumonia and sinus infections tends to point toward a

Table 13.1 Autoimmune and immune disease differential by symptom

Symptoms	Autoimmune differential (major)	Immune deficiency differential (major)
Digestive (abdominal pain, vomiting, diarrhea)	FMF, TRAPS, MKD	XLA, CVID, CTLA4, LRBA, IPEX, STAT3-GOF,CGD
Cutaneous	CAPS (urticaria)	CVID (alopecia, vitiligo), LRBA (eczema, alopecia, scleroderma), STAT1-GOF (eczema, alopecia, vitiligo, psoriasis), WAS (eczema)
Joint	DADA2	CVID, XLA, CTLA4, LRBA, STAT3-GOF, WAS
Neurologic	HA20 (meningitis), DADA2 (stroke)	ALPS (Guillain-Barre syndrome), DiGeorge syndrome (hypocalcemic seizures)
Ocular	Still disease, TRAPS, CAPS	ALPS (uveitis), LRBA (uveitis), CGD
ENT (lymphadenopathy)	CAPS (hearing loss)	CVID, ALPS, LRBA, IPEX, STAT3-GOF
Hematologic (cancers, cytopenias, hepatosplenomegaly)	MKD, DADA2	CVID, XLA, ALPS, CTLA4, LRBA, IPEX, STAT3-GOF, WAS
Pulmonary	FMF (chest pain)	CVID, CTLA4, LRBA, STAT3-GOF, CGD

Abbreviations: *ALPS* autoimmune lymphoproliferative syndrome, *CAPS* cryopyrin-associated periodic syndrome, *CGD* chronic granulomatous disease, *CTLA4* cytotoxic T-lymphocyte-associated protein 4, *CVID* common variable immunodeficiency, *DADA2* deficiency of adenosine deaminase 2, *FMF* familial Mediterranean fever, *HA20* A20 haploinsufficiency, *IPEX* immunodysregulation polyendocrinopathy enteropathy X-linked, *LRBA* LPS-responsive and beige-like anchor protein, *MKD* mevalonate kinase deficiency, *STAT1-GOF* STAT1 gain-of-function, *STAT3-GOF* STAT3 gain-of-function, *TRAPS* tumor necrosis factor receptor-associated periodic system, *WAS* Wiskott-Aldrich syndrome, *XLA* X-linked agammaglobulinemia potential humoral deficit while opportunistic, viral, or fungal infections would make cellular deficits more likely. Beyond infections, patients with autoinflammatory syndromes frequently suffer from vague and nonspecific symptoms. As in this case, fevers, diarrhea, and lymphadenopathy are present in a number of diseases. Recurrent (or periodic) fevers are generally characterized by flares with short to even prolonged intervals of feeling asymptomatic. Many of these conditions are genetic and encompass a family of hereditary recurrent fever syndromes (HRF). In certain cases, a specific gene mutation is known to result in disease. For example, Familial Mediterranean Fever (FMF) is caused by mutations of *MEFV*, mevalonate kinase deficiency (MKD) by mutations of the mevalonate kinase gene (*MVK*), tumor necrosis factor (TNF) receptor-associated periodic fever syndrome (TRAPS) by mutations of type I TNF receptor (*TNFSRF1A*), and cryopyrin-associated periodic syndromes (CAPS) by mutations of *NLRP3*. Other fever syndromes such as periodic fever, aphthosis, pharyngitis, and adenitis (PFAPA) syndrome represent a multifactorial process but still result from a single genetic defect [4]. Although the criteria to diagnose these diseases can be difficult without genetic assessment, the current major criteria (Tel-Hashomer clinical criteria) consist of ≥3 attacks of the same type, with rectal temperature ≥38 °C, lasting 12 h to 3 days, as well as peritonitis, pleuritis or pericarditis, monoarthritis (hip, knee, ankle), or an isolated fever [3, 4]. However, as highlighted in our case, merely meeting these criteria in the absence of other supportive factors is insufficient as many other types of PID and AIS also present with similar symptoms.

Lymphadenopathy and splenomegaly are two other nonspecific features typically seen with these syndromes, as highlighted in this case. Splenomegaly is frequently noted as a noninfectious complication in CVID and other PIDs but is also found in autoinflammatory diseases such as PAMI syndrome (PSTPiP1-associated myeloid-related-proteinemia inflammatory syndrome), MAI with immune deficiency, H syndrome (a rare autosomal recessive disease characterized by cutaneous hyperpigmentation, hypertrichosis, hepatosplenomegaly, hearing loss, heart anomalies, hypogonadism, hyperglycemia, low height, and hallux valgus), and adult-onset Still's disease [1].

Many immunodysregulatory diseases present with lymphadenopathy, either localized or systemic. Chief among these are MKD, PFAPA [5], CVID, ALPS, CTLA4, LRBA, IPEX, and STAT3-GOF [4] (see Table 13.1). Although lymphadenopathy can be an isolated finding in some of these processes, particularly with the primary immune deficiencies, it often occurs in complex with other lymphoproliferative pathology such as hepatosplenomegaly, granulomatous and lymphocytic interstitial lung disease, leukemia, or lymphoma [6]. In CVID, for example, splenomegaly is found in about 25–30% [7]. Similarly, lymphadenopathy is seen in about 25% of CVID [8]. As mentioned earlier, these complications of splenomegaly, autoimmunity, and lymphadenopathy frequently occur together and may be a consequence of impaired B-cell maturation or selection [9].

Diarrhea and GI manifestations are common in PID and AIS, particularly patients with CVID, chronic granulomatous disease (CGD), IPEX and IPEX-like disorders, XIAP deficiency, IL-10 and IL-10 receptor deficiency, Omenn syndrome, NEMO deficiency, Wiskott-Aldrich syndrome (WAS), X-linked agammaglobulinemia (XLA), and others (see Table 13.1). The most common clinical symptoms of enteropathy are diarrhea and weight loss or failure to thrive. In this case, vague abdominal pain and diarrhea played a significant clinical role. PIDs have been associated with a broad clinical spectrum of autoimmune GI disorders including pernicious anemia, autoimmune enteropathy (AIE), inflammatory bowel disease, and celiac disease. Multiple autoinflammatory diseases also result in gastrointestinal complications. One review noted that of 180 patients with autoinflammatory syndromes (AIS), 58% had some form of gastrointestinal symptoms with abdominal pain (49%), vomiting (25%), and diarrhea (17%) being the most common [10]. In this patient, as in many CTLA4-deficient patients, diarrhea and GI complications are also found [11].

Diagnostic Testing

Diagnostic tools associated with defining PID and AIS are advancing at a fast pace. As in our case, initial diagnostic studies including serologic evaluation of white blood cell counts, platelets, autoantibodies, and inflammatory markers can help further guide more sophisticated testing. An extremely common finding is autoimmune cytopenia (Table 13.2). The diagnosis of autoimmune cytopenias is suspected in the setting of a persistently abnormal complete blood count. A positive direct Coombs test is helpful for confirming a diagnosis of autoimmune hemolytic anemia (AIHA). In the case of suspected ITP with persistent disease or with more than one cell lineage affected, a bone marrow biopsy is typically recommended to address the question of whether sufficient cells are being produced and to rule out the possibility of a malignancy or bone marrow failure syndrome [12].

The fact that this patient had recurrent infections pointed to the need to test his humoral and cellular immunity. Initial tests for these include immunoglobulin test; flow cytometry for T, B, and NK cells; and pre- and post-vaccine titers to assess humoral function. One characteristic feature of CTLA4 haploinsufficiency, not always found in other PID/AIS disorders, is hypogammaglobulinemia. The etiology of hypogammaglobulinemia in this disorder is unknown, but it has been suggested that the immune dysregulation observed in LPS-responsive beige-like anchor protein (LRBA) deficiency is also related to a decreased level of CTLA4 on T cells. This occurs because LRBA, a constituent of the innate immune system, plays an important role in recycling CTLA4 to the cell surface which is important for regulating immune responses [12].

As mentioned before, lymphadenopathy is often noted in the evaluation of patients with immunodysregulatory disorders. Here it is critical for the clinician to rely heavily on the history and physical exam in order to interpret this otherwise nonspecific physical finding in the proper context. Particularly in cases where the lymphadenopathy is persistent, refractory to antibiotic treatments, or associated with other signs of lymphoproliferative pathology, it is worth considering further diagnostic workup. Reasonable next steps include neck ultrasound (for pediatric

Table 13.2 Association between primary immunodeficiencies and autoimmune diseases

Primary immunodeficiency	Frequency of autoimmunity (%)	Associated autoimmune diseases
IPEX	100	AIE, T1D, autoimmune cytopenias, Hashimoto's thyroiditis, eczema
Omenn syndrome (OS)	100	Hashimoto's thyroiditis, IBD, ITP
APECED	Almost 100	Autoimmune hypoparathyroidism, Hashimoto's thyroiditis, Graves' disease, primary biliary cholangitis, T1D, AIH, vitiligo psoriasis
ALPS	>80	AIHA, ITP, autoimmune neutropenia [41]
C1q deficiency	93	SLE, AIHA, cryoglobulinemia [42]
C4, C1r/ C1s and C2 deficiencies	75, 65, and 10–25	
Wiskott-Aldrich syndrome	40–72	AIHA, autoimmune neutropenia, both small and large vessel vasculitis, IBD, renal diseases [43]
Selective IgA deficiency	7–38	AIH, RA, ITP, AIHA, IBD, SLE, celiac disease, vitiligo, T1D
CVID	26	AIHA, ITP, pernicious anemia, SLE, JIA, RA, T1D, Hashimoto's thyroiditis, IBD, vitiligo
Hyper-IgM type 2 (AID deficiency)	21–25	
X-linked Hyper-IgM (CD4OL deficiency)	20	
NEMO deficiencies (XL-EDA-ID))	23	
C3 and C5–9 deficiencies X-linked agammaglobulinemia	<20	
Incomplete DiGeorge syndrome	5–10	ITP, AIHA, Hashimoto's thyroiditis, Graves' disease, IBD, uveitis, JIA
X-linked agammaglobulinemia		JIA, RA, IBD, T1D, autoimmune cytopenias
LRBA deficiency		GLILD, autoimmune cytopenias, Hashimoto's thyroiditis, T1D, IBD, SLE, autoimmune thyroid disease, JIA
Chronic granulomatous disease		SLE, IBD, ITP, T1D, JIA, RA
XLP		HLH

Adapted from [44]

Abbreviations: *AIE* autoimmune enteropathy, *AIH* autoimmune hepatitis, *AIHA* autoimmune hemolytic anemia, *ALPS* autoimmune lymphoproliferative syndrome, *APECED* autoimmune polyendocrinopathy-candidiasis-ectodermal dystrophy, *CVID* common variable autoimmunodeficiency, *GLILD* granulomatous-lymphocytic interstitial lung disease, *HLH* hemophagocytic lymphohistiocytosis, *IBD* inflammatory bowel disease, *IPEX* immunodysregulation polyendocrinopathy enteropathy X-linked syndrome, *ITP* immune thrombocytopenic purpura, *JIA* juvenile idiopathic arthritis, *RA* rheumatoid arthritis, *SLE* systemic lupus erythematosus, *T1D* type 1 diabetes patients) or computed tomography with fine-needle aspiration or biopsy if the clinical picture mandates a more intensive approach [13]. The findings on lymph node biopsy can vary by patient and disease process. CVID patients, for example, may range from having totally normal lymph node biopsy findings to showing abnormal and distorted germinal center architecture lacking well-defined lymphoid cuffs [14]. In most instances, biopsies show benign lymphoid hyperplasia, but there appears to be a strong inflammatory process linked to this finding as well [15]. In one study of CVID patients, granulomatous inflammation was seen in 2 of 10 biopsies of hyperplastic lymph nodes [15], while a study in non-CVID patients showed an even greater association of lymphoid hyperplasia with granulomatous inflammation, as 20 of 38 biopsies demonstrated granulomas [16]. The concern in many instances is the potential of transformation to lymphoid malignancy. For example, CVID patients with benign lymphoproliferation have a higher risk of developing lymphoid malignancy than other CVID patients, with non-Hodgkin's B-cell lymphomas being most common [17]. Despite the increased risk, in most cases, lymphoid hyperplasia does not transform to malignancy, and repetitive biopsies in the same patient frequently show benign pathology [18].

The diagnosis of the GI manifestations can be extremely difficult. A broad net is usually cast with a comprehensive approach that includes physical examination; laboratory tests such as complete blood count, acute phase reactants (CRP and ESR), albumin, and pre-albumin; and liver function tests such as AST/ALT and bilirubin levels. Fecal calprotectin is a marker of bowel inflammation that can rise as much as 40 times the normal values during inflammatory processes, although this finding is nonspecific and can also be seen in irritable bowel syndrome. In the interest of maintaining an appropriate differential, clinicians would do well to consider the possibility of gastrointestinal infection and perform appropriate, targeted evaluations to rule this out such as stool culture, specific immunofluorescent stains, and PCR to common pathogens [12]. For those patients in whom inflammatory bowel disease (IBD) is suspected, a colonoscopy with biopsies is performed. The most common histological findings include granulomas, atrophy of the villi of the small intestine, nodular lymphoid hyperplasia, and lymphocytic and eosinophilic infiltrates, markers suggestive of an autoimmune rather than infectious process [12, 19].

Genetic testing is becoming more of a mainstay in the diagnosis of PID and AIS. As mentioned previously, various PIDs and many AIS (including the periodic fever syndromes) are associated with single gene defects. To date, more than 350 gene mutations associated with primary immunodeficiency and autoinflammatory syndromes have been discovered [20]. The explosion of genetic knowledge in this field is startling when one considers that in the early 1990s there were less than 20 genes identified [20]. Although whole-exome sequencing (WES) may seem like a costly measure, it can ultimately lead to specific disease phenotyping that would change clinical management. In a study of 278 families with PID of unknown genetic cause, whole-exome sequencing identified a candidate molecular cause in 110 (40%) cases, leading to a clear change and targeted change in management in 60 cases (>20% of cases tested) [21]. Genetic counseling should be provided before and after genetic testing with an immunologist or genetic counselor with expertise in primary immunodeficiency. Case 1 highlights the potential benefit of establishing a genetic diagnosis as in many instances, such as CTLA4 deficiency; such a diagnosis can change management and even drive a decision to pursue hematopoietic stem cell transplantation. The use of disease-specific panels versus whole-genome sequencing can be considered on a case-by-case basis with certain factors such as patient preference and insurance reimbursement requiring consideration. The use and application of individual Sanger sequencing tests, gene panels, and broader genomic approaches have varying costs and turn-around-time considerations that should be discussed with the patient, family, and genetic counselors [22].

Management and Outcomes

Treatment of autoimmune and immunologic manifestations varies depending on the specific disease, genetic mutation, and immunologic breach (Table 13.3). In this case, where poor humoral function was obviously at play, replacement with regular immunoglobulin infusions seems like a reasonable initial option which would not only protect from infections but also possibly aid in other secondary clinical symptoms such as diarrhea or fevers. Immunoglobulin replacement with either intravenous or subcutaneous routes between 400 and 800 mg/kg per month is typically initiated. Dose, frequency, and route adjustments are then usually made clinically or per the patient preference and tolerance. In many cases, the noninfectious

Table 13.3 Treatment of autoimmunity in patients with primary immunodeficiency

Category	Specific autoimmune diseases	Treatments of choice
Autoimmune hematologic syndromes	ITP, AIHA	Steroids, immunosuppression (AZA, Vcr, Vbl, cyclophosphamide, MTX, MMF, sirolimus), immunoglobulin G replacement
Autoimmune GI disorders	IBD, celiac disease, autoimmune enteropathy, pernicious anemia	Systemic steroids, NSAIDS, antibiotics, immunosuppression (6-MP, AZA, cyclosporine), infliximab, adalimumab, etanercept, vedolizumab, microbiota
Rheumatic disease		Hydroxychloroquine, cyclophosphamide, AZA, MMF, DMARDs, etanercept, adalimumab, infliximab, abatacept, rituximab, belimumab
Autoimmune lung disease		Steroids, immunosuppression (AZA, CY), infliximab, rituximab
Autoimmune skin disorders		Moisturizing lotions, steroid ointments, rituximab, tofacitinib

Adapted from [6]
Abbreviations: *AIHA* autoimmune hemolytic anemia, *AZA* azathioprine, *DMARDs* disease-modifying antirheumatic drugs, *GI* gastrointestinal disorder, *GLILD* granulomatous-lymphocytic interstitial lung disease, *MMF* mycophenolate mofetil, *MTX* methotrexate, *NSAIDs* nonsteroidal anti-inflammatory drugs, *RA* rheumatoid arthritis, *SLE* systemic lupus erythematosus, *Vcr* vincristine, *Vbl* vinblastine

complications themselves require specific treatment modalities beyond immunoglobulin replacement. Autoimmune cytopenias are commonly treated with corticosteroids and/or IVIG (see Case 2). Fevers and lymphadenopathy associated with these syndromes usually are a secondary manifestation, and treating the underlying problem will generally aid in symptom improvement. Treatment of AIS frequently entails some form of immunosuppression. For the classic periodic fever syndromes, daily colchicine and treatment targeting specific inflammatory pathways such as TNFa, anti-IL1, and anti-IL-6 inhibitors are generally considered first-line [1]. Similarly, GI manifestations are generally treated with TNF-a inhibitors as well as the anti-a4b7 integrin monoclonal, vedolizumab, an inhibitor of Treg-cell trafficking to the GI mucosa, which has been anecdotally reported to be effective [23]. Fortunately, in this case presented, a genetic diagnosis of CTLA4 haploinsufficiency was made which provided a more specific treatment option. As abatacept is a soluble version of CTLA-4 itself, it was initiated as a CTLA-4 replacement therapy with the hope for improvement in the patient's GI symptoms as well as joint pains and fever. Further investigations are needed to fully assess the efficacy of abatacept in similar settings as well as other PID/AIS syndromes.

If specific molecular treatments are not available or are ineffective, the next step is consideration of a hematopoietic stem cell transplant (HSCT). Classically, HSCT has been used in the treatment of severe combined immunodeficiency and Wiskott-Aldrich syndrome with cure rates of 90% for the former and 95% for the latter [2]. This therapy is also considered the treatment of choice for hemophagocytic lymphohistiocytosis (HLH) and X-linked lymphoproliferative disease (XLP) and is being increasingly used for chronic granulomatous disease (CGD) as well. In addition to the possibility of life-threatening infections in the peri-transplant period, clinicians need to be mindful of the need to monitor for graft-versus-host rejection disease, long-term autoimmune cytopenias, and thyroid disease [2].

Case Presentation 2

A 25-year-old female presents to the clinic for immune evaluation due to recurrent infections, eczema, fevers, and joint pains. She has a past medical history of type I diabetes diagnosed at age 5 and autoimmune hemolytic anemia (AIHA) based on fatigue and significant pancytopenia as a child. She was treated with a regimen of corticosteroids and cyclosporine. She has had no recurrences of anemia since the initial treatment to her knowledge. She had been evaluated by an allergist/immunologist years ago and was diagnosed with eczema. Skin prick testing showed a positive result to dust mites and multiple grasses. She was treated with oral H1-antihistamines and nasal corticosteroids but not allergen immunotherapy. She suffers from two to four sinus infections per year requiring oral antibiotics, and these episodes were deemed clinically consistent with allergies. A sinus CT showed only mild inflammation in the maxillary sinuses bilaterally. She is short in stature at 4 feet 9 inches tall and over the past few years has been complaining of knee and wrist pain with swelling and daily fevers of 100 °F. These episodes occur daily during "flares," but the flares come and go periodically, usually lasting 1–3 weeks and then spontaneously resolving. She received a Medrol dose pack during one episode that seemed to aid the severity and length of the symptoms. She saw a rheumatologist the previous year and had a negative ANA, with a normal ESR and CRP. She was prescribed NSAIDs which helped her pain but had no impact on her fevers. She also complained of hair loss and previously was told by a dermatologist that she had autoimmune alopecia. At age 24, she had been suffering from recurrent tender cervical lymphadenopathy with shortness of breath and was eventually diagnosed as having pneumonia confirmed by chest X-ray. Due to difficulty clearing her infection with antibiotics, she had a chest CT which showed suspected granulomas and lymphadenopathy. Immunologic tests at the time revealed an IgG of 566 mg/dL with a slightly decreased but not absent IgA and an elevated IgM. Flow cytometry showed mildly decreased numbers of CD4, CD8, and NK cells but normal NK cell cytotoxicity. She was challenged with Pneumovax 23 and tetanus vaccine but showed no response in titers 6 weeks post vaccination. Due to continued fevers and SOB, she underwent an open lung biopsy which revealed granulomatous-lymphocytic interstitial lung disease (GLILD). She was diagnosed with CVID and placed on IVIG therapy. Over the next year, she had no infections but continued to suffer from bouts of fevers, shortness of breath, and joint pains. A deeper analysis of her T cells showed an increased population of double-negative T cells. Given her clinical picture, a STAT3 gain of function mutation was suspected and eventually confirmed on genetic testing. She was started on tocilizumab (an anti-IL-6 receptor mAb) with significant clinical improvement in joint pains and fevers at 6 months post initiation.

Symptoms/Clinical Presentation

This case highlights the complexity and diversity of clinical aspects related to immune dysfunction. The initial picture of a pancytopenia and eventual diagnosis of AIHA at a young age was apparently the first clinical consequence of her autoinflammatory syndrome. Although the diagnosis of AIHA in this case did not prompt a suspicion for an associated PID, warning signs beyond recurrent infections may have included multilineage cytopenias, no response to first-line therapy, persistent/chronic ITP, and autoimmune neutropenia in a patient older than 2 years and/or that was persistent for more than 24 months [24]. Neutropenia is a rare complication in most primary immunodeficiencies and has been reported in less than 10% of the cases. When it is present, the most common complications usually do include autoimmunity and lymphoproliferative disease [25]. Her early diagnosis of type I diabetes also may have been a consequence of overall immune dysfunction. STAT3 gain-of-function mutation is one of several immunodeficiency syndromes that can manifest with endocrinopathies including loss of function mutations of STAT5, IPEX, APECED, NFkB2 LOF, MALT1, and NEMO as well as STAT1 gain-of-function mutations [26]. The endocrinopathy in IPEX syndrome commonly presents as diabetes and thyroiditis [27], whereas in autoimmune polyendocrinopathy-candidiasis-ectodermal dystrophy (APECED), primary adrenocortical insufficiency and hypoparathyroidism make up part of the classic triad of signs and symptoms [28].

Her short stature and development of fevers and joint pains with swelling raised a concern for some type of inflammatory process. Given her age, various forms of AIS would need to be considered in this setting including the interferonopathies. These are frequently a pediatric-onset heterogeneous group of diseases characterized by increased expression of interferon (IFN) type 1 that can lead to the secretion of proinflammatory cytokines by innate immune cells resulting in fevers, joint pains, and various other ailments. One such interferonopathy that frequently manifests with pulmonary involvement, such as in this case, is stimulator of interferon gene (STING)-associated vasculopathy with onset in infancy (SAVI), which is frequently associated with gain-of-function gain mutations of TMEM173, encoding a protein called STING. Musculoskeletal complaints and fevers are the hallmark of many autoinflammatory syndromes. The musculoskeletal abnormalities range from arthralgias, myalgias, bone erosions, fasciitis, and bone deformities [29]. A review of a large population of patients with confirmed autoinflammatory syndromes showed a high instance of arthralgias (59%), myalgias (44%), and oligoarthritis (18%) [10]. Daily fever is not typically a sign of primary immunodeficiency but is consistent with many different autoinflammatory syndromes including chronic infantile neurologic cutaneous and articular syndrome (CINCA), familial cold autoinflammatory syndrome (FCAS), familial Mediterranean fever (FMF), mevalonate kinase deficiency (MKD), Muckle-Wells syndrome (MWS), neonatal-onset multisystem inflammatory disease (NOMID), and tumor necrosis factor receptor-associated periodic syndrome (TRAPS). As our patient progressed, her infectious history became more significant in adulthood with continuation of the fevers and joint pains. A diagnosis of CVID was made, and despite typical therapies, her noninfectious symptoms did not resolve. A major clinical symptom in this case that ultimately drove further testing was shortness of breath and pulmonary-related issues. Pulmonary disease is one of the most common clinical features in patients with PID. There are multiple causes for pulmonary disease including infection, malignancy, and autoimmunity. Granulomatous-lymphocytic interstitial lung disease (GLILD) is one of these causes and is likely the consequence of chronic and recurrent infections combined with inflammatory/autoimmune-mediated disease resulting from the underlying immune dysregulation associated with the disorder [30]. If left untreated or undiagnosed, this can lead to chronic lung disease including bronchiectasis, pulmonary fibrosis resulting in decreased exercise tolerance, increased fatigue, chronic cough, and oxygen dependence late in disease [12].

Among AIS, FMF is the most prevalent condition and is characterized by self-limiting recurrent episodes of fever, frequently associated with polyserositis but predominantly manifesting as acute abdominal and chest pain [29]. The pain is often subacute and generally disappears within 2 weeks, though flexion contractures of involved joints may occur infrequently [31]. In contrast to the positive outcome of acute and subacute forms, chronic arthritis can affect knees and hips with destructive sequelae, often leading to early prosthetic joint replacement [32]. To avoid severe hip deterioration, Sohar et al. recommended repeated arthrocentesis of the hip in order to prevent compression-related ischemia [33].

Diagnosis/Assessment

The initial evaluation in this case is similar to Case 1. Evaluation of cell counts and inflammatory markers is generally performed as screening tests in these diseases. A close physical exam and in many cases joint imaging are required to evaluate the etiology and severity of the musculoskeletal disease. Later in the course, immunologic tests to help explain the infections including difficult-to-treat pneumonia were ultimately helpful. This led to the CT scan of the chest and eventual discovery of granulomas. In any patient with continued shortness of breath, further evaluation with pulmonary function tests and DLCO are reasonable first options in the assessment. If the patient demonstrates a clinical decline or has declining lung function on PFTs, a chest CT scan should be considered. The findings of lung nodules, ground glass opacities, and adenopathy on high-resolution chest CT are common and useful in the diagnosis of an inflammatory-related pulmonary manifestation. In order to assess the cellular infiltrates in tissue, a biopsy is usually needed. This is usually performed as a video-assisted thoracoscopic (VATS) wedge biopsy from an affected region of lung that should be stained for CD3+ T cells as well as CD19+/CD20+ B cells [34].

In our case, the patient was not initially suffering from frequent infections. In fact, her infectious history was quite unremarkable, notable only for one to two sinus infections per year. In contrast, autoimmune consequences dominated her clinical symptoms. Therefore, a pursuit of a genetic or molecular diagnosis was deemed the best option for unifying her symptoms and personalizing her management. Medical research has now elucidated several genetically defined immunodeficiency disorders that are associated with an increased risk of autoimmunity (see Table 13.2). One such defect is a STAT3 gain-of-function mutation, which results in STAT3 phosphorylation in follicular helper T cells and increased secretion of IL-21 causing decreased programmed cell death and decreased inducible co-stimulator (ICOS) on T cells. Ultimately, the patient is left with a paucity of follicular helper T cells with resultant interruption of normal B-cell terminal differentiation into plasma and memory cells. In contrast, STAT3 loss-of-function mutations are associated with impaired differentiation of follicular helper T cells. Whole-exome sequencing and individualized or disease-specific panels for these various conditions such as primary immunodeficiency, CVID, periodic fever syndromes, or autoinflammatory diseases are now available commercially. Use of these options should be made on a case-by-case basis.

Management/Outcomes

In our case, the patient developed autoimmune hemolytic anemia at an early age, one of the more common autoimmune cytopenias in primary immunodeficiency. There is growing clinical evidence for treatment of autoimmune cytopenias with a variety of approaches. As was the case with this patient, first-line therapy for most autoimmune cytopenias is corticosteroids. A typical dose may be 1–2 mg/kg/day in one or more divided doses. In more severe cases, higher doses of corticosteroids up to 30 mg/kg of methylprednisolone have been administered intravenously. IVIG is also used periodically for treatment of ITP and autoimmune neutropenia. In these instances, IVIG is often administered concurrently with corticosteroids at immunomodulatory doses of 1–2 g/kg. A good treatment response can also serve as confirmation of the correct diagnosis for this case as it is generally considered evidence of an autoimmune-mediated mechanism if there is an increase in cell counts after administration of IVIG, even if a specific autoantibody has not been identified [35]. Of note, IVIG for treatment of autoimmune hemolytic anemia has been less successful than treatment for ITP [36]. With the explosion of biologics, anti-CD20 antibody (rituximab) is now considered an effective second-line therapy for the treatment of ITP, although randomized clinical trials are lacking. In general, rituximab has been demonstrated to have a durable treatment response rate of 59% for treatment-resistant cases such as for patients who are corticosteroid dependent (56%), on immunomodulatory therapy (44%), or who had a previous splenectomy (21%). It has been proposed that rituximab be considered a standard second-line therapy, before splenectomy and/or other immunomodulatory therapy, in CVID-associated autoimmune cytopenias. Although 24% of patients developed severe bacterial infections after rituximab treatment, half of these cases were off immunoglobulin replacement therapy and/or had undergone splenectomy [37]. Splenectomy now is usually considered a last resort therapy for autoimmune cytopenias, particularly for AIHA in which response rates are reportedly between 20% and 65%.

Given the patient's pneumonia, hypogammaglobulinemia, and poor vaccine response, immunoglobulin replacement was initiated. But as in many cases, this did not help curtail the noninfectious comorbidities. As previously mentioned, the diagnosis of GLILD or other pulmonary diseases is not an uncommon manifestation of immune dysfunction. Regardless of the histologic analysis, corticosteroids have traditionally been used as a first-line therapy in many acute patients if necessary, although long-term use is not a viable option for most patients. In GLILD and other diseases such as follicular bronchiolitis, a lung biopsy typically shows both B- and T-cell infiltrates. In these instances, B-cell depletion with rituximab along with a T-cell inhibitor such as azathioprine has shown efficacy and can be highly effective at improving symptoms and pulmonary function. If the lung biopsy is highly enriched in only T cells, cyclosporine and rapamycin have shown efficacy [34].

Finally, this case once again emphasizes the importance of a genetic diagnosis. Uncovering a STAT3 GOF mutation allows for a better understanding of her disease and will hopefully aid in a better therapeutic plan. STAT3 GOF syndrome affects many organ systems resulting in endocrine and gastrointestinal disease which appears early in the course of illness as in our case. Polyautoimmunity with greater than or equal to two autoimmune diseases was frequent (29 of 42), and greater than three autoimmune diseases were reported in 16 of 42 patients. Single-organ autoimmune disease was reported in ten patients, and three patients had no obvious autoimmunity [38].

Most of the symptomatic patients with STAT3 GOF syndrome (as well as other autoinflammatory syndromes) require significant immunosuppressive therapy (see Table 13.3). In most instances, corticosteroids are offered as acute management but transitioning to a corticosteroid sparing agent such as azathioprine, hydroxychloroquine, rituximab, infliximab, or another appropriate agent needs to be considered sooner rather than later [39]. In our case, tocilizumab was initiated and appeared to have a positive impact. It is thought that the use of tocilizumab, an anti-IL6R antibody, is beneficial by blocking upstream IL-6-induced STAT3 activation [40].

Conclusion

As demonstrated by these cases, the presence of autoinflammatory disease in the setting of a primary immunodeficiency can have diverse clinical impacts that are difficult to manage. Autoinflammatory disease is common and can even predefine patients with primary immunodeficiency. In many instances, symptoms related to inflammation are the first manifestation suggesting a clinical problem. Regulatory T cells and dysfunction in the innate immune system appear to be the main factors associated with the presence of autoimmunity in PID. The presence of autoimmune and inflammatory diseases frequently complicates the diagnosis and management of patients with primary immunodeficiency. As suggested by Walter et al., treatment strategies in PID should be targeted not only to the clinical spectrum of autoimmunity (cytopenias, rheumatologic disease, and/or GI disease) but also to the underlying molecular cause of immune dysregulation (B-cell, T-cell, and/or innate immune pathology). Achieving this level of diagnostic and prognostic clarity often requires thorough genetic evaluation with the hopes of identifying a specific mutation. As we advance our understanding of mechanisms involved in the link between autoimmunity in PID, we hope to improve our ability to diagnose and treat the patients at the intersection of primary immunodeficiency and autoimmune and inflammatory disease [3].

Clinical Pearls and Pitfalls
- Autoinflammatory disorders are diverse and remain a diagnostic challenge especially in the setting of a primary immunodeficiency.
- In many instances, the autoinflammatory manifestations predate any signs of a primary immunodeficiency.

- Although it seems contradictory, autoinflammatory syndromes and primary immunodeficiency frequently coexist. The fine balance between protecting and suppressing the immune system remains a challenge.
- Advances in understanding the genetics involved in these syndromes have dramatically improved diagnostic and treatment strategies in this patient population.
- Although many of the monogenic autoinflammatory and immunodeficiency disorders begin in childhood, adults may also be affected with new-onset or continued inflammatory disease.

References

1. Georgin-Lavialle S, Fayand A, Rodrigues F, Bachmeyer C, Savey L, Grateau G. Autoinflammatory diseases: state of the art. Presse Med. 2019;48(1 Pt 2):e25–48. PubMed PMID: 30686513. Epub 2019/01/24. eng.
2. Amaya-Uribe L, Rojas M, Azizi G, Anaya JM, Gershwin ME. Primary immunodeficiency and autoimmunity: a comprehensive review. J Autoimmun. 2019;99:52–72. PubMed PMID: 30795880. Epub 2019/02/20. eng.
3. Walter JE, Farmer JR, Foldvari Z, Torgerson TR, Cooper MA. Mechanism-based strategies for the management of autoimmunity and immune dysregulation in primary immunodeficiencies. J Allergy Clin Immunol Pract. 2016;4(6):1089–100. PubMed PMID: 27836058. PMCID: PMC5289744. eng.
4. Gattorno M, Hofer M, Federici S, Vanoni F, Bovis F, Aksentijevich I, et al. Classification criteria for autoinflammatory recurrent fevers. Ann Rheum Dis. 2019;78(8):1025–32. PubMed PMID: 31018962. Epub 2019/04/24. eng.
5. Westwell-Roper C, Niemietz I, Tucker LB, Brown KL. Periodic fever syndromes: beyond the single gene paradigm. Pediatr Rheumatol Online J. 2019;17(1):22. PMCID: PMC6515597. Epub 2019/05/14. eng. PubMed PMID: 31088470.
6. Azizi G, Bagheri Y, Tavakol M, Askarimoghaddam F, Porrostami K, Rafiemanesh H, et al. The clinical and immunological features of patients with primary antibody deficiencies. Endocr Metab Immune Disord Drug Targets. 2018;18(5):537–45. PubMed PMID: 29651973. Epub 2018/04/14.
7. Chapel H, Lucas M, Lee M, Bjorkander J, Webster D, Grimbacher B, et al. Common variable immunodeficiency disorders: division into distinct clinical phenotypes. Blood. 2008;112(2):277–86. PubMed PMID: 18319398. Epub 2008/03/06.
8. Wehr C, Kivioja T, Schmitt C, Ferry B, Witte T, Eren E, et al. The EUROclass trial: defining subgroups in common variable immunodeficiency. Blood. 2008;111(1):77–85. PubMed PMID: 17898316. Epub 2007/09/28.
9. Roskin KM, Simchoni N, Liu Y, Lee JY, Seo K, Hoh RA, et al. IgH sequences in common variable immune deficiency reveal altered B cell development and selection. Sci Transl Med. 2015;7(302):302ra135. PubMed PMID: 26311730. PMCID: PMC4584259. Epub 2015/08/28.
10. Ter Haar NM, Eijkelboom C, Cantarini L, Papa R, Brogan PA, Kone-Paut I, et al. Clinical characteristics and genetic analyses of 187 patients with undefined autoinflammatory diseases. Ann Rheum Dis. 2019;78(10):1405–11. PubMed PMID: 31278138. Epub 2019/07/07.
11. Verma N, Burns SO, Walker LSK, Sansom DM. Immune deficiency and autoimmunity in patients with CTLA-4 (CD152) mutations. Clin Exp Immunol. 2017;190(1):1–7. PMCID: PMC5588810. Epub 2017/06/11. PubMed PMID: 28600865.

12. Allenspach E, Torgerson TR. Autoimmunity and primary immunodeficiency disorders. J Clin Immunol. 2016;36(Suppl 1):57–67. PubMed PMID: 27210535. Epub 2016/05/24. eng.
13. Gaddey HL, Riegel AM. Unexplained lymphadenopathy: evaluation and differential diagnosis. Am Fam Physician. 2016;94(11):896–903. PubMed PMID: 27929264. Epub 2016/12/09.
14. da Silva SP, Resnick E, Lucas M, Lortan J, Patel S, Cunningham-Rundles C, et al. Lymphoid proliferations of indeterminate malignant potential arising in adults with common variable immunodeficiency disorders: unusual case studies and immunohistological review in the light of possible causative events. J Clin Immunol. 2011;31(5):784–91. PubMed PMID: 21744182. PMCID: PMC3428024. Epub 2011/07/12. eng.
15. Unger S, Seidl M, Schmitt-Graeff A, Bohm J, Schrenk K, Wehr C, et al. Ill-defined germinal centers and severely reduced plasma cells are histological hallmarks of lymphadenopathy in patients with common variable immunodeficiency. J Clin Immunol. 2014;34(6):615–26. PubMed PMID: 247897. Epub 2014/05/03.
16. Ko HM, da Cunha SG, Darling G, Pierre A, Yasufuku K, Boerner SL, et al. Diagnosis and subclassification of lymphomas and non-neoplastic lesions involving mediastinal lymph nodes using endobronchial ultrasound-guided transbronchial needle aspiration. Diagn Cytopathol. 2013;41(12):1023–30. PubMed PMID: 2163048. Epub 2011/06/02.
17. Maglione PJ. Autoimmune and lymphoproliferative complications of common variable immunodeficiency. Curr Allergy Asthma Rep. 2016;16(3):19. PubMed PMID: 2685701. Epub 2016/02/10.
18. Piquer Gibert M, Alsina L, Giner Munoz MT, Cruz Martinez O, Ruiz Echevarria K, Dominguez O, et al. Non-Hodgkin lymphoma in pediatric patients with common variable immunodeficiency. Eur J Pediatr. 2015;174(8):1069–76. PubMed PMID: 25749928. Epub 2015/03/10.
19. Chatzikonstantinou M, Konstantopoulos P, Stergiopoulos S, Kontzoglou K, Verikokos C, Perrea D, et al. Calprotectin as a diagnostic tool for inflammatory bowel diseases. Biomed Rep. 2016;5(4):403–7. PubMed PMID: 27699005. PMCID: PMC5038578. Epub 2016/10/05.
20. Ziegler JB, Ballow M. Primary immunodeficiency: new approaches in genetic diagnosis, and constructing targeted therapies. J Allergy Clin Immunol Pract. 2019;7(3):839–41. PubMed PMID: 30832894. eng.
21. Stray-Pedersen A, Sorte HS, Samarakoon P, Gambin T, Chinn IK, Coban Akdemir ZH, et al. Primary immunodeficiency diseases: genomic approaches delineate heterogeneous Mendelian disorders. J Allergy Clin Immunol. 2017;139(1):232–45. PubMed PMID: 27577878. PMCID: PMC5222743. Epub 2016/09/01.
22. Heimall JR, Hagin D, Hajjar J, Henrickson SE, Hernandez-Trujillo HS, Tan Y, et al. Use of genetic testing for primary immunodeficiency patients. J Clin Immunol. 2018;38(3):320–9. PubMed PMID: 29675737. Epub 2018/04/21.
23. Uzzan M, Ko HM, Mehandru S, Cunningham-Rundles C. Gastrointestinal disorders associated with common variable immune deficiency (CVID) and chronic granulomatous disease (CGD). Curr Gastroenterol Rep. 2016;18(4):17. PubMed PMID: 26951230. PMCID: PMC4837890. Epub 2016/03/10.
24. Teachey DT, Lambert MP. Diagnosis and management of autoimmune cytopenias in childhood. Pediatr Clin N Am. 2013;60(6):1489–511. PubMed PMID: 24237984. PMCID: PMC5384653. Epub 2013/11/19.
25. Ghorbani M, Fekrvand S, Shahkarami S, Yazdani R, Sohani M, Shaghaghi M, et al. The evaluation of neutropenia in common variable immune deficiency patients. Expert Rev Clin Immunol. 2019;15:1–9. PubMed PMID: 31592698. Epub 2019/10/09.
26. Schimke LF, Rieber N, Rylaarsdam S, Cabral-Marques O, Hubbard N, Puel A, et al. A novel gain-of-function IKBA mutation underlies ectodermal dysplasia with immunodeficiency and polyendocrinopathy. J Clin Immunol. 2013;33(6):1088–99. PubMed PMID: 23708964. Epub 2013/05/28.
27. Torgerson TR, Ochs HD. Immune dysregulation, polyendocrinopathy, enteropathy, X-linked: forkhead box protein 3 mutations and lack of regulatory T cells. J Allergy Clin Immunol. 2007;120(4):744–50; quiz 51-2. PubMed PMID: 17931557. Epub 2007/10/13.

28. Conteduca G, Indiveri F, Filaci G, Negrini S. Beyond APECED: an update on the role of the autoimmune regulator gene (AIRE) in physiology and disease. Autoimmun Rev. 2018;17(4):325–30. PubMed PMID: 29427825. Epub 2018/02/11.
29. Soliani M, Cattalini M, Vitale A, Sota J, Cantarini L. Musculoskeletal manifestations in hereditary periodic fever syndromes. Clin Exp Rheumatol. 2018;36 Suppl 110(1):25–31. PubMed PMID: 29742055. Epub 2018/05/10.
30. Bates CA, Ellison MC, Lynch DA, Cool CD, Brown KK, Routes JM. Granulomatous-lymphocytic lung disease shortens survival in common variable immunodeficiency. J Allergy Clin Immunol. 2004;114(2):415–21. PubMed PMID: 15316526. Epub 2004/08/19.
31. Brodey PA, Wolff SM. Radiographic changes in the sacroiliac joints in familial Mediterranean fever. Radiology. 1975;114(2):331–3. PubMed PMID: 1110999. Epub 1975/02/01.
32. Salai M, Langevitz P, Blankstein A, Zemmer D, Chechick A, Pras M, et al. Total hip replacement in familial Mediterranean fever. Bull Hosp Jt Dis. 1993;53(1):25–8. PubMed PMID: 8374487. Epub 1993/01/01.
33. Sohar E, Pras M, Gafni J. Familial Mediterranean fever and its articular manifestations. Clin Rheum Dis. 1975;1(1):195–209.
34. Chase NM, Verbsky JW, Hintermeyer MK, Waukau JK, Tomita-Mitchell A, Casper JT, et al. Use of combination chemotherapy for treatment of granulomatous and lymphocytic interstitial lung disease (GLILD) in patients with common variable immunodeficiency (CVID). J Clin Immunol. 2013;33(1):30–9. PubMed PMID: 22930256. PMCID: PMC3557581. Epub 2012/08/30.
35. Choi HS, Ji MH, Kim SJ, Ahn HS. Platelet count recovery after intravenous immunoglobulin predicts a favorable outcome in children with immune thrombocytopenia. Blood Res. 2016;51(2):95–101. PubMed PMID: 27382553. PMCID: PMC4931943. Epub 2016/07/07.
36. Nugent DJ. IVIG in the treatment of children with acute and chronic idiopathic thrombocytopenic purpura and the autoimmune cytopenias. Clin Rev Allergy. 1992;10(1–2):59–71. PubMed PMID: 1606524. Epub 1992/01/01.
37. Gobert D, Bussel JB, Cunningham-Rundles C, Galicier L, Dechartres A, Berezne A, et al. Efficacy and safety of rituximab in common variable immunodeficiency-associated immune cytopenias: a retrospective multicentre study on 33 patients. Br J Haematol. 2011;155(4):498–508. PubMed PMID: 21981575. PMCID: PMC3428031. Epub 2011/10/11.
38. Fabre A, Marchal S, Barlogis V, Mari B, Barbry P, Rohrlich PS, et al. Clinical aspects of STAT3 gain-of-function germline mutations: a systematic review. J Allergy Clin Immunol Pract. 2019;7(6):1958–69. e9. PubMed PMID: 30825606. Epub 2019/03/03.
39. Bussone G, Mouthon L. Autoimmune manifestations in primary immune deficiencies. Autoimmun Rev. 2009;8(4):332–6. PubMed PMID: 1902860. Epub 2008/11/26.
40. Milner JD, Vogel TP, Forbes L, Ma CA, Stray-Pedersen A, Niemela JE, et al. Early-onset lymphoproliferation and autoimmunity caused by germline STAT3 gain-of-function mutations. Blood. 2015;125(4):591–9. PubMed PMID: 25359994. PMCID: PMC4304103. Epub 2014/11/02.
41. Neven B, Magerus-Chatinet A, Florkin B, Gobert D, Lambotte O, De Somer L, et al. A survey of 90 patients with autoimmune lymphoproliferative syndrome related to TNFRSF6 mutation. Blood. 2011;118(18):4798–807. PubMed PMID: 21885602. Epub 2011/09/03.
42. Cacoub P, Fremeaux-Bacchi V, De Lacroix I, Guillien F, Kahn MF, Kazatchkine MD, et al. A new type of acquired C1 inhibitor deficiency associated with systemic lupus erythematosus. Arthritis Rheum. 2001;44(8):1836–40. PubMed PMID: 11508436. Epub 2001/08/18.
43. Dupuis-Girod S, Medioni J, Haddad E, Quartier P, Cavazzana-Calvo M, Le Deist F, et al. Autoimmunity in Wiskott-Aldrich syndrome: risk factors, clinical features, and outcome in a single-center cohort of 55 patients. Pediatrics. 2003;111(5 Pt 1):e622–7. Epub 2003/05/03.
44. Coutinho A, Carneiro-Sampaio M. Primary immunodeficiencies unravel critical aspects of the pathophysiology of autoimmunity and of the genetics of autoimmune disease. J Clin Immunol. 2008;28(Suppl 1):S4–10. Epub 2008/02/23.

Chapter 14
Immune Dysregulation Leading to Autoimmunity

Melissa D. Gans and Rachel Eisenberg

Introduction

There are an increasing number of monogenic immune disorders that predominantly present with autoimmunity and immune dysregulation. In 2017, the International Union of Immunologic Societies (IUIS) recognized this expanding phenotype within its classification of primary immunodeficiency disorders [1]. The IUIS classifies immune dysregulatory diseases into two main groups: (1) hemophagocytic lymphohistiocytosis (HLH) and Epstein-Barr virus (EBV) susceptibility and (2) syndromes with autoimmunity and others. This chapter will focus on the latter, also known as primary immune regulatory disorders (PIRDs) (Table 14.1), in addition to other primary immunodeficiencies (Table 14.2) whose main defect is not immune dysregulation but who also have manifestations of immune dysregulation.

Pathophysiology

Immune dysregulation is caused by the failure of a self-tolerant immune system (Fig. 14.1). The development of a self-tolerant immune system is dependent on the ability of the immune system to differentiate a self-reactive lymphocyte from a non-self-reactive lymphocyte [2]. Failure in this process leads to the development of autoimmunity. This concept was first described in the mid-twentieth century by Paul Ehrlich who explained that antibodies directed against self, as opposed to pathogens, lead to host tissue damage and *horror autotoxicus* [3]. Today, there are

M. D. Gans · R. Eisenberg (✉)
Children's Hospital at Montefiore, Division of Allergy and Immunology,
Montefiore Medicinal Center, Bronx, NY, USA
e-mail: reisenbe@montefiore.org

Table 14.1 Examples of PIRDs

Disease	Inheritance	Typical clinical features	Immune dysregulation	Immunodeficiency
ALPS	Mostly AD, some somatic mutations	Young toddler with lymphoproliferation and autoimmune cytopenia [16, 17]	Mostly AIHA and ITP. Rarely, nephritis, hepatitis, primary biliary cirrhosis, colitis, arthritis, and vasculitis [90]	Rarely severe or recurrent infections secondary to impaired vaccine responses
APDS	AD	Toddlers with recurrent sinopulmonary infections, lymphadenopathy, neurodevelopmental delay, and viremia	Mostly enteropathy and cytopenia. Rarely, T1DM and arthritis [38]	Sinopulmonary infections secondary to hypogammaglobulinemia, poor vaccine responses, and low switch memory B cells. Herpesvirus infections (CMV/EBV)
CD25 deficiency	AR	Infants with autoimmune cytopenias, severe eczema, and severe invasive infections	Mostly cytopenias. Rarely, enteropathy and T1DM [49]	Severe viral, bacterial, and fungal infections
CTLA4 haplo-insufficiency	AD	Child with enteropathy, lymphadenopathy, cytopenia, interstitial lung disease, and lymphocytic infiltration of the brain	Enteropathy, cytopenia [26]	Sinopulmonary infections secondary to hypogammaglobulinemia
IL10/IL10R	AR	Child with enterocolitis with perianal disease, folliculitis, and sinopulmonary infections	Mostly enteropathy. Rarely, arthritis [55]	Sinopulmonary infections
IPEX	X-linked recessive	Male infants with severe diarrhea leading to failure to thrive, T1DM, dermatitis, and food allergies	Mostly enteropathy, endocrinopathy (T1DM, thyroid, adrenal insufficiency), and cytopenia. Rarely, nephropathy, hepatitis, alopecia, arthritis, and vasculitis [73]	Serious invasive infections, secondary hypogammaglobulinemia from protein losses

Table 14.1 (continued)

Disease	Inheritance	Typical clinical features	Immune dysregulation	Immunodeficiency
JAK1 GOF	AD	Young child with atopic dermatitis, hypereosinophilia with infiltration in liver and gastrointestinal tract, atopy, lymphoproliferation, and failure to thrive [91]	Thyroiditis [91]	Recurrent viral infections
LRBA deficiency	AR	Young toddler with enteropathy, lymphadenopathy, cytopenia, interstitial lung disease, and lymphocytic infiltration of the brain	Enteropathy, cytopenia [27]	Sinopulmonary infections secondary to hypogammaglobulinemia
STAT1 GOF	AD	Infant with chronic mucocutaneous candidiasis and recurrent sinopulmonary infections. Rarely, cerebral aneurysms	Rarely, thyroiditis, T1DM, cytopenia, and SLE [63]	Invasive *Candida* disease resistant to treatment, viral infections, and bacterial infections
STAT3 GOF	AD	Infant with endocrinopathy, enteropathy, short stature, atopic dermatitis, lymphoproliferation, and interstitial lung disease	Mostly cytopenia, T1DM, and enteropathy. Rarely, hypothyroidism, celiac disease, arthritis, alopecia, and hepatitis [32, 33]	Sinopulmonary infections secondary to hypogammaglobulinemia and low switch memory B cells
STAT5B LOF	AR	Toddler with dysmorphisms, enteropathy, atopic dermatitis, short stature resistant to growth hormone, and severe invasive infections [51, 52]	Mostly enteropathy. Rarely, ITP and arthritis [52]	Severe invasive infections

Table 14.2 Examples of primary immunodeficiencies associated with immune dysregulation

Disease	Typical clinical and immunological features	Autoimmune features	Mechanism for autoimmunity
22q11.2 deletion syndrome	Newborns with characteristic dysmorphic facies, congenital heart defects, velopharyngeal incompetence, hypocalcemia, sinopulmonary infections, and viral respiratory infections. Small to absent thymic tissue leads to variable T-cell deficiency and humoral deficiency	ITP, AIHA, arthritis, endocrinopathy, vitiligo, and enteropathy [92]	Decreased thymic tissue leads to decreased expression of AIRE [93]
Chronic granulomatous disease	Young toddlers with bacterial and fungal infections such as sepsis, pneumonia, superficial and deep abscesses, skin infections, septic arthritis, and osteomyelitis in addition to granulomas in multiple organs. Impaired phagocytosis leads to catalase-positive organism susceptibility	Enteropathy, SLE-like disease (particularly discoid lupus in female X-linked carriers), arthritis, vasculitis, and dermatomyositis [94, 95]	Unknown
CVID	Children or adults with recurrent sinopulmonary infections, lymphoproliferation, bronchiectasis, and granulomatous disease. Impaired B-cell differentiation leads to hypogammaglobulinemia, impaired vaccine responses, and low switch memory B cells	Cytopenia, endocrinopathy, vasculitis, SLE, arthritis, enteropathy, primary biliary cirrhosis, hepatitis, pernicious anemia, and gastritis. Seen in 25% of patients [41]	Impaired B-cell somatic hypermutation, reduced switched memory B cells, and reduced Tregs [96]
DOCK8 deficiency	Infants with severe atopic disease, skin abscesses, severe cutaneous viral infections, sinopulmonary infections, fungal disease, neurologic complications (e.g., central nervous system vasculitis), and malignancy. Elevated IgE, eosinophilia, T-cell lymphopenia, low IgM, and impaired vaccine responses	Cytopenia (AIHA, ITP), vasculitis, enteropathy, thyroid disease, uveitis/chorioretinitis [93]	Increased autoreactive B cells and poor Treg cell function [93]
Hyper IgM syndrome	Infants with sinopulmonary infections, invasive bacterial infections, viral infections, and lymphadenopathy. Impaired immunoglobulin class switching causes elevated IgM, low IgG, low IgA, and low IgE. Also presents with a defect in T lymphocyte function	Enteropathy, arthritis, cytopenia, hepatitis, and SLE [97]	Defective costimulatory signaling between B and T cells causes oligoclonal autoreactive TCR repertoire [97]

Table 14.2 (continued)

Disease	Typical clinical and immunological features	Autoimmune features	Mechanism for autoimmunity
Hypomorphic SCID	Infants with severe multiorgan autoimmunity and invasive bacterial, fungal, and viral infections. T-cell deficiency, hypogammaglobulinemia, and possibly NK cell deficiency (depending on etiology)	Cytopenia, alopecia, vitiligo, granulomas, myasthenia gravis, vasculitis, and psoriasis [98]	Low levels of enzyme activity needed for V(D)J recombination cause abnormal recombination and differentiation into an oligoclonal autoreactive BCR/TCR repertoire
Wiskott-Aldrich	Infants with thrombocytopenia, severe atopic dermatitis, viremia, and recurrent sinopulmonary infections later on developing lymphoma. T-cell deficiency, hypogammaglobulinemia, and small platelets	AIHA, AIN, vasculitis, arthritis, enteropathy, and IgA nephropathy [99]	Poor Treg function and impaired control of B-cell proliferation [99]

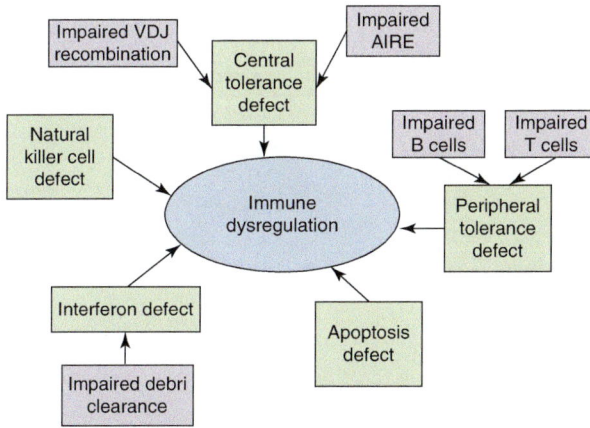

Fig. 14.1 Underlying defects causing immune dysregulation

over 100 monogenic defects (Table 14.3) leading to impaired self-tolerance and the development of autoimmunity, cytopenia, and enteropathy [4].

Development of a tolerant immune system depends on complex mechanisms occurring both centrally and peripherally. During early central development, lymphocytes that express the pre-B cell receptor (BCR) or pre-T-cell receptor (TCR) proliferate, maturate, and survive. Lymphocytes that do not express functional receptors die by apoptosis. Through VDJ recombination, lymphocytes form a complete TCR or BCR with a remarkably broad repertoire and then undergo positive and negative selection to ensure that only lymphocytes with antigen receptors that

Table 14.3 Monogenic diseases with evidence of immune dysregulation

Defect		Gene (protein)	Disease
Central tolerance	AIRE	AIRE	APECED
	VDJ recombination	DCLRE1C (Artemis) RAG1 RAG2	Classical SCID Leaky/hypomorphic SCID
		ZAP70	Leaky SCID ZAP70 GOF
	Thymic tissue	TBX1	22q11.2 deletion syndrome
Peripheral tolerance	T cells	BACH2	Mendelian BACH2-related immunodeficiency and autoimmunity
		BCL10	BCL10 deficiency
		CARD11	CARD11 haploinsufficiency
		CTLA4	CTLA4 haploinsufficiency
		DOCK8	Hyper IgE syndrome DOCK8 deficiency
		FOXP3	IPEX syndrome
		IKBKG	X-linked ectodermal dysplasia with immunodeficiency Incontinentia pigmenti
		IKKβ	IKKβ deficiency
		IL2RA (CD25)	CD25 deficiency
		IL10/IL10R	IL10/IL10R deficiency
		LRBA	LRBA deficiency
		MALT1	MALT1 deficiency
		OTULIN	OTULIN deficiency
		RMRP	Cartilage-hair hypoplasia
		RELA	RELA deficiency
		STAT1	STAT1 GOF
		STAT3	STAT3 GOF STAT3 LOF
		STAT5B	STAT5B LOF STAT5B GOF
		TTC7A	TTC7A deficiency
		WASP	Wiskott-Aldrich syndrome
		TRAC	TRAC deficiency
		JAK 1	JAK 1 GOF

14 Immune Dysregulation Leading to Autoimmunity

Table 14.3 (continued)

Defect		Gene (protein)	Disease
	B cells	ATP6AP1 BLK BLNK BTK CD19 CD21 CD79A/B CD81 CR2 (CD21) ICOS IGHM IGLL1 IKZF (IKAROS) IL21/IL21R IRF2BP2 NFKB1/2 MOGS (GCS1) MS4A1 (CD20) PIK3R1 PLCG2 PRKCD (PRKCδ) PTEN RAC2 TCF3 TNFRSF13B (TACI) TNFRSF13C (BAFF-R) TNFSF12 (TWEAK) TNFRSF7 (CD27) TRNT1 TTC37 VAV1	Agammaglobulinemia CVID
		AID CD40 CD40L UNG	Hyper-IgM syndrome
		CARD11	B-cell expansion with NF-κB and T-cell anergy syndrome
		INO80	INO80 deficiency
		ITCH	ITCH deficiency
		MSH6	MSH6 deficiency
		PIK3CD (PI3Kδ)	APDS
		TPP2	TPP2 deficiency

(continued)

Table 14.3 (continued)

Defect	Gene (protein)	Disease
Apoptosis	CASP8 CASP10 FADD FAS FASL NRAS	ALPS
	KRAS NRAS	RAS-associated autoimmune leukoproliferative disorder
	STK4 (MST1)	MST1 deficiency
Interferon	C1q C1r C1s C2 C4	Complement deficiency SLE
	CYBA (P22PHOX) CYBB (NOX2) NCF1 (P47PHOX) NCF2 (P67PHOX) NCF4 (P40PHOX)	Chronic granulomatous disease
	DNAse I	SLE
	IFIH1 (MDA5) SAMHD1 TREX1	Aicardi-Goutières syndrome
	NFAT5	NFAT5 haploinsufficiency
	PEPD	PEPD deficiency
	SCARF1	SCARF1 deficiency
	TMEM173 (STING)	Stimulator of interferon genes-associated vasculopathy with onset in infancy

Table 14.3 (continued)

Defect	Gene (protein)	Disease
NK cell dysfunction	AP3B1 AP3D1	Hermansky-Pudlak syndrome
	CD27 ITK	Lymphoproliferative syndrome
	CD70	CD70 deficiency
	CTPS1	CTPS1 deficiency
	GATA2	GATA2 deficiency
	FAAP24	FAAP24 deficiency
	LYST (CHS1)	Chediak-Higashi syndrome
	MAGT1	X-linked immunodeficiency with magnesium defect, EBV infection, and neoplasia disease
	MCM4	Immunodeficiency 54
	PRF1 STX11 STXBP2 (MUNC18-2) UNC13D (MUNC13-4)	Familial HLH
	RAB27A	Griscelli syndrome
	RASGRP1	RASGRP1 deficiency
	RLTPR (CARMIL2)	Immunodeficiency 58
	SH2D1A (SAP) XIAP (BIRC4)	X-linked lymphoproliferative disease
Unknown	POLE2	POLE2 deficiency
	PGM3	PGM3 deficiency

do not recognize self-survive. The binding strength of the BCR/TCR to antigen determines the fate of that lymphocyte. Lack of affinity leads to death by neglect. High affinity binding of both T and B lymphocytes will lead to negative selection. However, unique to B cells is their ability to change the specificity of their receptor with further editing to make a nonreactive receptor. Weak affinity to self-antigen permits T cells to develop into effector T cells (Teff) and B lymphocytes to mature further. Moderate affinity T cells will develop into T regulatory lymphocytes (Tregs), which are able to bind to self but produce an inhibitory response due to their unique set of receptors and cytokines. The bone marrow, where B cells mature, and the thymus, where T cells mature, contain mostly ubiquitous self-antigens. Therefore, B and T cells mostly encounter self-antigen during early maturation as opposed to foreign antigens, ensuring development of central tolerance. However, unique to the thymus is autoimmune regulator (AIRE) expression, which enables local expression of peripheral tissue-specific antigens. Therefore, central tolerance ensures that the naïve lymphocytes are incapable of responding to self-antigens that are expressed in central lymphoid organs. Defects at any point in this process can not only lead to primary immunodeficiency due to defective lymphocytes but also to the development of immune dysregulation and autoimmunity.

The process of central tolerance is imperfect and self-reactive lymphocytes may escape into the periphery. Mechanisms for peripheral tolerance include development of anergy, suppression via Treg cells, and death by apoptosis. Development of an anergic response occurs when there is lack of proper lymphocyte stimulation. Typically, two signals are required for the activation of T or B cells, the first being recognition of antigen and the second being a costimulatory signal. Common secondary signals include binding of CD28 on the TCR to CD80/86 on APCs or the binding of CD40 on the BCR to CD40L on the Teff cell. Prolonged signal one, as would be seen in continuously displayed self-antigen, in the absence of signal two leads to an anergic response. The secondary signal could also be inhibitory instead of activating, leading to an anergic response. An example would be expression of CTLA4 on the surface of the T cell, which binds to CD80/86 with a higher affinity and transmits an inhibitory signal.

Another mechanism of peripheral immune tolerance, and arguably the most important, is mediated by Tregs (Fig. 14.2). The constitutive expression of forkhead box P3 (FOXP3) transcription factor, a unique marker of the Treg cell, leads to expression of high affinity interleukin (IL) 2 receptor alpha (CD25) (see Fig. 14.1). CD25 consumes IL2, an important cytokine for the development of T cells, thereby depriving Teff of essential IL2 stimulation. Additionally, Tregs constitutively express inhibitory costimulatory molecules such as cytotoxic T-lymphocyte-associated protein 4 (CTLA4) and programmed cell death protein 1 (PD1). This is in contrast to Teff cells that place CTLA4 on its surface only upon activation to inhibit further signaling [5, 6]. Lipopolysaccharide-responsive beige-like anchor protein (LRBA) mediates the recycling of CTLA4 from the cell surface to an endosome and prevents the lysosomal degradation of CTLA4. Downstream effects of Treg activation are FOXP3 transcription of immunosuppressive cytokines IL10 and transforming growth factor beta (TGFβ). IL10's principal role is anti-inflammation, suppression of Teff cells, and limiting the immune response to pathogens [7]. TCRs on Treg cells bind to self-antigen and therefore it is imperative they display inhibitory receptors and anti-inflammatory cytokines in order to maintain tolerance. Defects in CTLA4 and LRBA both lead to significant autoimmunity. Defects in peripheral tolerance through Treg cells, specifically in FOXP3, CD25, and IL10, are notorious for causing immune dysregulation with significant enteropathy.

Programmed cell death through apoptosis is an additional mechanism by which immune tolerance is maintained. There are three mechanisms by which apoptosis can occur both centrally and peripherally in order to eliminate autoreactive lymphocytes [8]. One of the pathways, called the extrinsic or death receptor pathway, is mediated via Fas-FasL interaction, leading to recruitment of the adaptor Fas-associated protein with death domain (FADD) and cleavage of procaspase 8, which will activate caspase 3 [9]. Caspase 3 begins the execution phase of cell apoptosis whereby there is cell shrinkage, chromatin condensation, formation of apoptotic

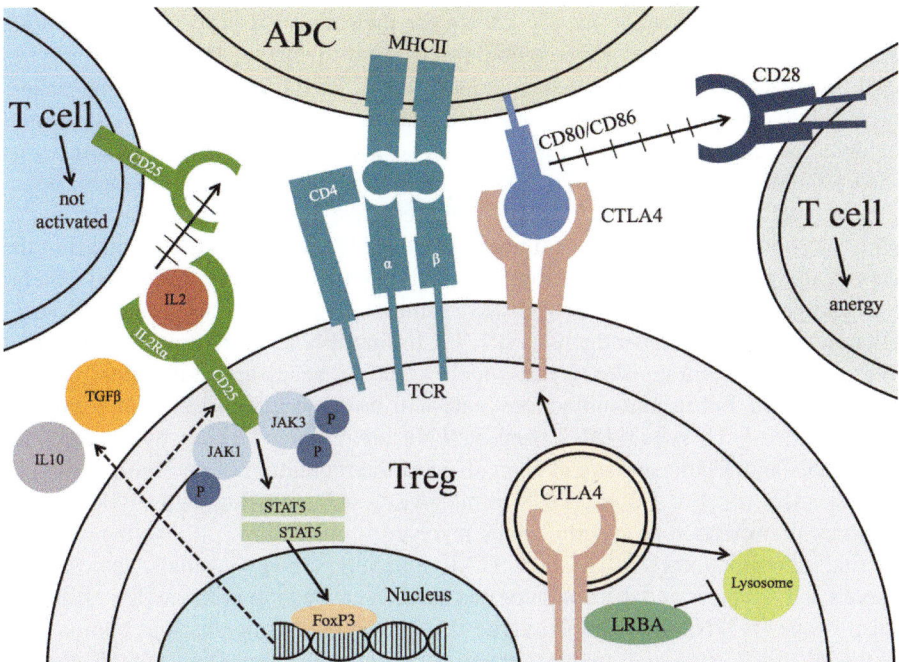

Fig. 14.2 The first signal for lymphocyte activation is MHC antigen presentation on an APC to the TCR on the T cell. The second signal is the binding of co-stimulatory molecules, such as CD80/CD86 on the APC to CD28 on the T cell. This figure represents how Tregs are able to inhibit the activation signaling process. Tregs constitutively express CTLA4, which has a higher affinity for CD80/CD86 than to CD28 on the T cell. The binding of CTLA4 to CD80/CD86 thereby inhibits the second signal required for activation. The T cell will become anergic if there is a continued first signal without a second signal. Additionally, Tregs consume IL2 in the microenvironment through their high affinity CD25 receptor, which is constitutively expressed. This deprives other T cells of IL2, which is required for T-cell activation. LRBA is essential for preventing lysosomal degradation of CTLA4 and allowing CTLA4 continued cycling to the cell surface. FOXP3 is a transcription factor in Tregs that upregulates anti-inflammatory cytokines, such as IL10 and TGFβ in addition to increased surface expression of CD25. Through these mechanisms, Tregs can inactivate neighboring T cells and other APCs from attacking self through the expression of surface markers and the microenvironment in which they create. PIRDs are due to defects in these mechanisms leading to IPEX syndrome (FOXP3 deficiency), CD25 deficiency, CTLA4 haploinsufficiency, LRBA deficiency, STAT5 deficiency, and IL10/IL10R deficiency

bodies, and lastly phagocytosis [8]. When mature T or B cells are overly activated, such as autoreactive T and B cells, they will express higher levels of Fas leading to apoptosis [10]. The other two apoptosis pathways include the granzyme/perforin pathway mediated by cytotoxic T cells and the intrinsic pathway signaled by hypoxia, toxins, or radiation [8]. All three pathways converge at caspase 3. Defects in the apoptosis pathway lead to the inability to clear cells that were marked as self-reactive and or were deemed to undergo apoptosis. This will lead to significant autoimmunity and lymphoproliferative findings given the inability of lymphocytes to undergo apoptosis and contract.

Interferons (IFN), while mostly known for their antiviral properties, also play a major role in maintaining immune homeostasis and tolerance. There are three types of IFNs, all necessary for immune regulation. Type I IFN, IFNα and IFNβ, are sensors of cytosolic nucleic acids, usually viral DNA. However, with increased cell death and/or defective nucleic acid metabolism, as is seen in systemic lupus erythematosus (SLE), there will be presence of excess self-cytosolic DNA. This leads to overproduction of type I IFNs, as the type I IFNs will recognize cytosolic nucleic acids, analogously to how they recognize viral nucleic acids [11]. The excess autoantigens in the debris, along with the presence of upregulated type I IFN, leads to continued generation and presentation of self-antigens to immune effector cells and eventual loss of tolerance to nuclear autoantigens [12, 13]. Chronic IFN also promotes expansion of Teff cells and downregulates Tregs, which would be necessary in the presence of a viral infection, but in a noninfectious state will promote inflammation and immune dysregulation [11]. Type II IFNs, namely, IFNγ, are produced mostly by natural killer (NK) cells and T cells and are also involved in the regulation of autoimmunity [14]. For instance, IFNγ activates STATs in the JAK-STAT signaling pathway leading to eventual transcription of specific genes involved in inhibiting cell division and promoting inflammation [15]. The JAK-STAT signaling pathway is a delicate system of checks and balances and disruption of this balance can lead to immune dysregulation. Lastly, type III IFNs (in addition to type II IFNs) signal through various components of the IL10R. IL10 is an immunosuppressive cytokine of Tregs. Defects in the regulation of IFNs can lead to autoimmunity and immune dysregulation.

Monogenic diseases leading to autoimmunity and immune dysregulation can be classified by the underlying defect in the process of developing a self-tolerant immune system (see Table 14.3). Many monogenic disorders have several underlying defects leading to immune dysregulation. Table 14.3 classifies diseases by the hypothesized predominant defect. Central tolerance defects include diseases in which there is production of a reactive T- or B-cell receptor. Peripheral tolerance defects can be due to impaired T-cell function, particularly Tregs, and encompass many disorders that predominantly present with enteropathy. Other peripheral tolerance defects include impaired B-cell function and can be associated with hypogammaglobulinemia. Defects in apoptosis can also affect tolerance, while interferonopathies and defects of debris clearance are known to be associated with immune dysregulation. Lastly, NK cell dysfunction leading to HLH is known to cause immune dysregulation (discussed in Chap. 19). Regardless of the underlying defect, the clinical presentations of various monogenic disorders of immune dysregulation have overlapping features. This is demonstrated by two example case presentations of patients with immune dysregulation and autoimmunity.

Case Presentation 1

A 3-year-old male presented with cow milk protein intolerance and persistent diarrhea from early infancy. He was diagnosed with autoimmune enteropathy with intraepithelial lymphocyte infiltration and eosinophilia on biopsy in addition to positive anti-goblet cell antibody in the serum. Multiple immunosuppressive therapies to control his bowel disease including tacrolimus, mycophenolic acid, and corticosteroids were ineffective. The patient had failure to thrive and required total parental nutrition. His infectious history was notable for chronic EBV viremia and cytomegalovirus (CMV) colitis without sinopulmonary infections and with normal pulmonary findings. The patient had diffuse lymphadenopathy and tonsillar hypertrophy as a toddler. The patient's parents are first cousins from Saudi Arabia and the patient's younger sister has a history of chronic idiopathic thrombocytopenic purpura (ITP), autoimmune neutropenia (AIN), EBV viremia, lymphadenopathy, and hepatosplenomegaly. There was a brother who died in early infancy of unknown causes. Extensive laboratory evaluation of the patient showed intact cellular and humoral immunity.

Diagnosis/Assessment

The differential diagnosis for a young child presenting with significant immune dysregulation is broad and includes many different PIRDs.

Autoimmune Lymphoproliferative Syndrome (ALPS)

ALPS is a PIRD caused by a variety of defects in the proteins involved in mediating apoptosis. ALPS patients present with lymphoproliferation, splenomegaly, and autoimmune cytopenia at a very young age, with a reported median age onset of 12 months [16, 17]. The autoimmune manifestations are mostly autoimmune hemolytic anemia (AIHA) and ITP, reported in up to 69% of ALPS patients. Other autoimmune disorders, such as the enteropathy found in the patient case, are rarer [18].

The revised diagnostic criteria for ALPS require that there is an increase in peripheral alpha beta double-negative T cells (CD3+, CD4-, CD8-) along with evidence of splenomegaly and/or chronic (>6 months) nonmalignant lymphadenopathy. There must also be evidence of one accessory criterion such as defective apoptosis or a genetic mutation. In the case of a somatic mutation leading to ALPS, sorted double-negative T cells must be sequenced. The term "probable ALPS" is reserved for patients with the required criteria but lacking an accessory criterion and instead has two secondary manifestations such as elevated soluble FAS ligand, elevated IL10, elevated vitamin B12, autoimmune cytopenia, and family history [19]. Although double-negative T cells are thought to be pathognomonic for ALPS, they can also be found in many other PIRDs [20]. While the exact consequence or cause of increased double-negative T cells is unknown, it is likely a nonspecific marker of immune dysregulation [21].

Immunosuppressive therapies such as mycophenolate mofetil, sirolimus, immunoglobulin, and rituximab are typically used to treat ALPS manifestations [22, 23]. Splenectomy may be very cautiously considered if the aforementioned therapies fail – given the increased risk for sepsis and death in splenectomized ALPS patients [23]. Bone marrow transplant is not generally recommended due to the low mortality in ALPS [24].

CTLA4 Haploinsufficiency

CTLA4 haploinsufficiency and LRBA deficiency can present very similarly to the patient's case. The common phenotype is autoimmunity, hypogammaglobulinemia, and lymphoproliferation of the lungs, gut, and brain [25, 26]. In a cohort of 21 CTLA4 haploinsufficiency patients described by Lo et al., the most common autoimmune findings were enteropathy (81%), ITP (43%), and AIHA (38%) – nearly identical to the LRBA cohort [26]. There are also significant infectious pulmonary complications in addition to noninfectious pulmonary manifestations in CTLA4 haploinsufficiency (e.g., chronic lung disease, digital clubbing). However, the pulmonary manifestations in LRBA deficiency are typically more severe compared to CTLA4 haploinsufficiency [26]. Pulmonary manifestations were not seen in this patient case, which is not unusual, because they are not necessarily seen in all CTLA4 haploinsufficiency or LRBA deficiency patients. LRBA deficiency also presents at a younger age on average than CTLA4 haploinsufficiency. LRBA deficiency presents in infancy and early childhood and CTLA4 haploinsufficiency commonly presents in children and young adults [26]. Other differences between the two diseases include a significantly increased risk for malignancy in CTLA4 haploinsufficiency compared to a lower risk in LRBA deficiency [4, 26, 27]. Lastly, LRBA deficiency displays complete penetrance whereas CTLA4 haploinsufficiency has incomplete penetrance with up to 40% of mutation positive family members being asymptomatic [25, 26]. Both diseases have variable expressivity [25, 26].

CTLA4 haploinsufficiency and LRBA deficiency are both rare diagnoses but are likely underreported and are also mimickers of common variable immunodeficiency (CVID). Among patients with a diagnosis of CVID who underwent whole exome sequencing (WES), about 4% were diagnosed with CTLA4 haploinsufficiency and 4% were found to have LRBA deficiency [28]. Both diseases can be treated with abatacept, a CTLA4 agonist, and bone marrow transplant [26, 29–31].

Genetic testing can confirm the diagnosis of CTLA4 haploinsufficiency. Haploinsufficiency of CTLA4 means that two functional allele copies of CTLA4 are necessary for CTLA4 function and loss of one allele copy (heterozygous) causes disease. This is distinct from dominant negative diseases where one defective allele copy (heterozygous) voids the other normal allele and causes disease. This is in contrast to LRBA deficiency, which will manifest as a homozygous mutation or compound heterozygous mutation, with two nonfunctional alleles.

STAT3 Gain of Function (GOF)

Germline STAT3 GOF patients typically present with very early onset of autoimmune endocrinopathy, followed by enteropathy, and then development of lymphoproliferation, autoimmune cytopenia, and interstitial lung disease [32–34]. The triad of early onset autoimmunity and lymphoproliferation in the context of severe growth failure should increase suspicion for STAT3 GOF. Type 1 diabetes (T1DM) or thyroid disease can occur within the first few months of life [34]. Autoimmune liver disease and gastrointestinal disease, including villous atrophy and lymphocytic infiltration, also present early in life with most being less than 2 years of age [34]. This is soon followed by lymphadenopathy, hepatosplenomegaly, and autoimmune cytopenias (AIHA, ITP, and AIN) [34]. Pulmonary manifestations including interstitial lung disease and sinopulmonary infections occur much later in the disease, typically in teenage years [34]. While the patient case had enteropathy and cytopenias, the characteristic endocrinopathies were not found. Of note, most STAT3 GOF patients will have more than one autoimmune manifestation, although the phenotype of STAT3 GOF is diverse and may only initially present with nonspecific inflammation or lymphoproliferation.

Laboratory findings in STAT3 GOF may reveal lymphopenia, hypogammaglobulinemia, decreased class-switched memory B cells, and expansion of double-negative T cells. Autoantibodies are typically not present, though celiac, anti-DNA, and anti-smooth muscle antibodies may be seen. Genetic sequencing will confirm diagnosis, though functional studies performed on a research basis can support the diagnosis or confirm a variant of unknown significance. Functional studies include in vitro STAT3 luciferase assay and suppressor of cytokine signaling 3 (SOCS3) expression levels [34].

Once STAT3 GOF immune dysregulation is recognized, this should prompt further assessment for related autoimmune conditions and when identified should be managed with specific therapies. STAT3 GOF immune dysregulation is theorized to be secondary to expansion of Th17 cells with contraction of Treg cells in the setting of excess STAT3 activity [35]. Inhibition of IL6, a cytokine that signals upstream STAT3 activation, has been successfully used in treating STAT3 GOF6 [36]. Jakinibs, which inhibit JAK/STAT signaling, have also been successfully used [36]. Bone marrow transplant is considered in difficult to control STAT3 GOF disease. Fabre et al. reviewed five cases of bone marrow transplant in STAT3 GOF disease where four patients died secondary to complications of transplant and one patient had complete remission of autoimmunity with improved growth [34].

Activated Phosphoinositide 3-Kinase δ (PI3Kδ) Syndrome (APDS)

Heterozygous gain of function mutations in the gene encoding the catalytic or regulatory subunits of PI3Kδ can cause a syndrome called APDS, which should also be considered in the differential diagnosis for the patient case presented [37]. PI3Kδ regulates B-cell proliferation and function. In APDS, there is uncontrolled B-cell proliferation leading to immune dysregulation and humoral deficiency. Patients with APDS typically present in early childhood with recurrent sinopulmonary infections (seen in almost all patients) along with findings of nonmalignant lymphadenopathy, herpesvirus infections, neurodevelopmental delay, and the propensity to develop lymphoma [38]. Autoimmune disease is seen in nearly half of APDS patients with the majority being autoimmune enteropathy and cytopenia [38]. While the patient case had characteristic autoimmunity as seen in APDS, there were no recurrent sinopulmonary infections. Lab findings that may be seen include hypogammaglobulinemia, poor vaccine responses, and decreased class-switched memory B cells [28]. Leniolisib, a targeted PI3Kδ inhibitor, has been shown effective for improving the immune dysregulation in a small number of APDS patients [39]. In a cohort of 11 APDS patients who underwent bone marrow transplant, there was 81% survival [40].

CVID

CVID is a heterogeneous diagnosis that encompasses many monogenic defects in B-cell immunity, many of which have yet to be discovered. The clinical features, lab findings, diagnosis and treatment are discussed in Chap. 2. Briefly, features of CVID include hypogammaglobulinemia, organomegaly, lymphoma, granulomatous disease, and lung findings such as bronchiectasis. Autoimmunity is found in about a quarter of CVID patients and the most common autoimmune findings in CVID, in order of prevalence, include: enteropathy, ITP, hepatitis, AIHA, pernicious anemia, AIN, thyroiditis, and vitiligo [41]. However, the presence of disease at a younger age, such as seen in the patient case, or signs of significant autoimmunity should prompt a search for an underlying monogenic PIRD.

Patient Diagnosis

In consideration of the multitude of monogenic defects that could present with the patient's clinical and laboratory history, the patient and his family underwent whole exome sequencing in search of a genetic diagnosis for his immune dysregulation. Testing revealed a homozygous deletion due to a frameshift mutation p.E81fs in the gene for LRBA. Both parents are heterozygous carriers of this variant and the sister was also homozygous for the variant (Fig. 14.3). The patient and patient's sister were diagnosed with LRBA deficiency. The patient was referred for bone marrow transplant at 4 years of age, which the parents refused, and the patient's family left the country and was lost to follow-up.

This patient case demonstrates that in patients with immune dysregulation, clinical history and immunological laboratory findings provide clues for a differential diagnosis. If available, flow cytometry and functional assessment may even provide further information. However, with the wide range of phenotypes in PIRDs, this

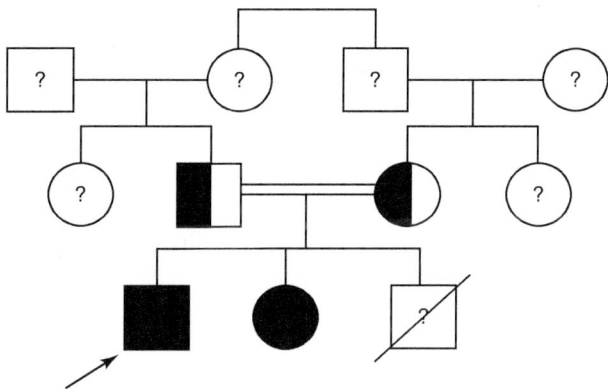

Fig. 14.3 Pedigree for patient case 1

may not be sufficient and genetic testing, particularly WES, may be more cost effective and timely. Genetic diagnosis can tremendously impact the management and outcome in patients with PIRDs.

Clinical History

Lopez Herrera et al. first discovered LRBA deficiency in 2012 as a syndrome of early onset hypogammaglobulinemia, autoimmunity, and inflammatory bowel disease [42]. However, since this initial discovery, the clinical spectrum of LRBA deficiency has been found to have a more varied presentation [27].

In a cohort of 93 LRBA-deficient patients described by Gamez-Diaz et al., the main clinical findings were immune dysregulation (95%), organomegaly (86%), and recurrent infections (71%) [27]. The most common manifestations of immune dysregulation were enteropathy (62%), AIHA (57%), and ITP (52%) [27]. Upper and lower respiratory infections were the major infectious complications (48% and 41%) with viral infections being the most frequent and often caused by CMV, adenovirus, and norovirus [27]. However, bacterial pathogens and fungal disease has also been described [27]. There was a significant incidence of severe parenchymal lung disease (52%) and lymphocytic interstitial pneumonia (38%); however, interestingly, hypogammaglobulinemia, initially described in all LRBA patients, was only seen in about half of the patients [27]. While malignancy was not described in the Gamez-Diaz et al. cohort, Cagdas et al. more recently described 14 patients with LRBA deficiency and Hodgkin's or non-Hodgkin's lymphoma in up to 27% of their patients [20]. The average time of onset of symptoms in LRBA-deficient patients is 4–7 years of age [20, 27].

The prognosis of LRBA deficiency can be poor and patients can die early in life from autoimmune, infectious, and therapeutic complications [20, 27]. Patients with LRBA deficiency need to be closely monitored for the known clinical sequelae of the disease and treated accordingly.

Laboratory Evaluation

LRBA deficiency is an autosomal recessive disease definitively diagnosed by genetic sequencing revealing pathogenic mutations in LRBA. However, there are immunological laboratory values that are characteristic for LRBA deficiency. Leukopenia is seen in about half of patients with LRBA deficiency [27]. There are typically normal or low total B-cell counts with a reduced memory compartment as evidenced by low switched memory B cells, suggesting defects in B-cell differentiation [27, 42]. Hypogammaglobulinemia is seen in about 57% of LRBA patients along with defects in specific antibody production [27, 42]. CD4 and CD8 T-cell subsets are typically normal; however, a significant number of patients in several of the cohorts displayed a double-negative alpha/beta T-cell repertoire and were initially diagnosed with an ALPS phenotype [20, 27]. Tregs may be decreased while circulating T follicular cells are increased [27]. Other defects include impaired T-cell activation and proliferation, decreased autophagy, and increased apoptosis in B cells with the latter two hypothesized to contribute to the significant autoimmunity seen in LRBA patients [20, 27, 42].

Rapid flow cytometry-based testing to diagnose LRBA deficiency is available on a research basis and has a reported sensitivity of 94% and a specificity of 80% [43]. However, LRBA-deficient patients with residual protein expression have been reported in several cohorts and, therefore, further analysis of CTLA4 shuttling and trans-endocytosis assays can be considered in these patients [44]. Lastly, with variants of unknown clinical significance in LRBA, rapid flow cytometry and functional assessment could be of clinical value [42].

Management/Outcome

Treatment

Given that LRBA deficiency leads to decreased CTLA4 cell surface expression, patients with LRBA deficiency are treated with abatacept, a CTLA4 immunoglobulin fusion drug. Abatacept acts as a replacement for the missing CTLA4 expression, thereby providing an inhibitory signal. Abatacept is able to restore immune tolerance leading to significant improvement in autoimmune symptoms and interstitial lung disease [44]. Abatacept can also completely control the lymphoproliferation and chronic diarrhea in LRBA-deficient patients [29].

Other therapies targeting immune dysregulation include corticosteroids and steroid-sparing agents such as sirolimus, cyclosporine, rituximab, and mycophenolate mofetil (Table 14.4) [27]. Sirolimus, a rapamycin inhibitor, has been studied in patients with both CTLA4 and LRBA deficiency given its ability to suppress Teff cells while allowing Treg expansion [26]. Some LRBA patients are able to obtain

Table 14.4 Common therapeutic modalities targeting autoimmunity in immune dysregulatory diseases

Method	Treatment	Mechanism of action
Removal of autoantibodies	Plasmapheresis	Removes pathogenic autoantibodies from patient's serum
	Splenectomy	Prevents clearance of autoantibody covered cells
	IVIG	1. Saturates neonatal fc receptors leading to increased clearance of autoantibody 2. Inhibits autoantibody binding to target antigen 3. Binds to activated complement components and precludes target surface deposition
Targeting of B cells	Rituximab	Anti-CD20 B-cell depletion, does not target plasma cells
	Belimumab	Anti-BAFF B-cell depletion, does not target plasma cells
	Bortezomib	Apoptosis of antibody producing plasma cells
Targeting of T cells	Sirolimus	mTOR inhibitor (mTOR is needed for translation of proteins that promote T-cell survival) preferentially targets T effector cells and double-negative T cells, allowing constriction of Teff cell and expansion of Treg cells
	Calcineurin inhibitors (cyclosporine and tacrolimus)	Inhibits IL2 synthesis by blocking gene transcription of cytokines such as IL2
	Basiliximab	Antibody against CD25 (alpha subunit of IL2R), inhibiting T-cell signaling
	Anti-thymocyte globulin	Anti-thymocyte globulin depleted circulated T cells
	Abatacept	CTLA4 agonist, binds to CD80/CD86 on an APC and prevents costimulatory binding of CD28 on naïve T cells
Targeting to B and T cell/nonspecific	Corticosteroids	Decrease lymphocyte recirculation, induce lymphocyte death, inhibit T-cell activation
	Azathioprine and MMF	Purine synthesis inhibitor leading to inhibition of T and B-cell DNA replication
	Leflunomide	Pyrimidine synthesis inhibitor leading to inhibition of T and B-cell DNA replication
	Methotrexate	Inhibits T and B-cell DNA replication
	Jakinibs	JAK inhibitor that suppresses JAK-STAT signaling cascade hyperactivation
	Leniolisib	PI3Kδ inhibitor, suppressing PI3Kδ hyperactivation
Other cytokine inhibition	Anti-cytokine for IL1, IL6, IL12, IL18, IL23, IL17A	Suppresses the activity of inflammatory cytokines that stimulate innate and adaptive immune cells

control of their immune dysregulation with the former discussed therapies, while others will require long-term therapy with associated therapeutic complications [27]. LRBA-deficient patients with hypogammaglobulinemia, poor specific antibodies, and clinical infections should be treated with replacement immunoglobulin [45].

While immunosuppressive therapy and immune modulating therapy may control some patients with LRBA deficiency, in those with severe resistant diarrhea, cytopenia, and/or viral infection, bone marrow transplant should be strongly considered. At least eight patients with CTLA4 haploinsufficiency and eight patients with LRBA deficiency have undergone bone marrow transplant. Eleven of 18 transplants were successful; however, one patient died two and a half years posttransplant and four had graft versus host disease [20, 27, 31].

Case Presentation 2

A 21-year-old male was referred for evaluation. The patient originally presented as an infant suffering from chronic diarrhea and recurrent episodes of otitis media. He was diagnosed with Coombs-positive AIHA at 16 months of age that was refractory to traditional treatments and required splenectomy. At 2 years of age, he was diagnosed with small bowel villous atrophy complicated by malabsorption, hemorrhagic colitis, cholecystitis, nephrolithiasis, and total parental nutrition dependence. He had many severe and invasive infections including viral encephalitis and repeat episodes of sepsis in addition to recurrent sinopulmonary infections. At 4 years of age, he was found to be panhypogammaglobulinemic after multiple rounds of rituximab and placed on replacement immunoglobulin. Throughout his childhood and teenage years, he also suffered from multiple organ autoimmunity: thyroiditis, pancreatitis, uveitis, chronic hepatitis, seizure disorder, and recurrent deep vein thromboses requiring anticoagulation. He was trialed on various other treatments for his uncontrolled autoimmunity including azathioprine, cyclophosphamide, corticosteroids, high-dose immunoglobulin, cyclosporine, tacrolimus, and plasmapheresis. The patient did not have dermatitis or any dermatological findings. Family history is notable for a healthy sister, several healthy maternal aunts, a male maternal distant cousin who died of unknown causes in early infancy, and many miscarriages in the family.

Diagnosis/Assessment

In a patient with many different autoimmune manifestations, severe enteropathy, and invasive infections, there are many disorders of immune dysregulation in the differential diagnosis.

Hypomorphic SCID

Classic severe combined immunodeficiency (SCID) is due to null mutations where there is no protein expression of the mutated genes, leading to complete absence of T cells (and often B and/or NK cells depending on the defect). This is in contrast to hypomorphic SCID (also known as leaky SCID) where there is residual protein expression of the mutated genes leading to the presence of T cells. However, the TCRs lack diversity and are autoreactive. Therefore, hypomorphic SCID patients will present with significant autoimmunity not seen in classical SCID [46]. Omenn syndrome is a subtype of hypomorphic SCID where there is enlarged lymphoid tissue, severe erythroderma, elevated IgE, and eosinophilia [47]. In Walter et al.'s cohort of 36 patients with RAG 1/2 mutations with hypomorphic activity who were not characterized as classic SCID, 89% displayed autoimmunity, most commonly AIHA, AIN, ITP, granulomas, enteropathy, and dermatitis [48]. Curative treatment is accomplished with bone marrow transplant, along with antimicrobial prophylaxis and immunoglobulin replacement prior to transplant [48]. As seen in hypomorphic SCID, the patient case displayed significant multiorgan autoimmunity, enteropathy, and recurrent bacterial and viral infections.

CD25 Deficiency

There are many features of the patient case that overlap with PIRDs, such as CD25 deficiency. CD25 deficiency is an extremely rare autosomal recessive disorder that can present with early onset enteropathy with villous atrophy, autoimmune cytopenia, severe eczema, and T1DM [49]. However, CD25-deficient patients are quite prone to viral, bacterial, and fungal infections with decreased T cells, abnormal mitogen-induced lymphocyte proliferation, and impaired IL10 expression [49, 50]. These profound infections are likely because the CD25 receptor is not only expressed on Tregs but also on Teff cells and allows the Teff cell to respond to IL2 in the presence of an immune response, such as an infection [49]. CD25 deficiency can be diagnosed by flow cytometry demonstrating decreased surface CD25 protein expression and confirmed by gene sequencing [49]. There have only been eight cases of CD25 deficiency diagnosis to date, and there are limited cases treated by bone marrow transplant [49].

STAT5B Loss of Function (LOF)/GOF

STAT5B LOF patients predominantly present with immune dysregulation (viz., enteropathy), eczema, and recurrent infections. These patients classically have other presenting features, such as short stature making the diagnosis more distinct and less alike to the patient case. In addition to STAT5B's role in the IL2R signaling cascade, which can explain the impairment of Tregs and autoimmunity, STAT5B is also important for growth hormone signal transduction. STAT5B LOF patients do not respond to supplemental growth hormone therapy causing dwarfism [51, 52]. STAT5B LOF patients are also dysmorphic with delayed puberty [51]. Infectious complications in STAT5B LOF are similar to CD25 deficiency and hypomorphic SCID, though STAT5B LOF patients often have hypergammaglobulinemia [51]. Bone marrow transplant has been shown in mice models to be effective in STAT5B LOF but has not been performed in humans to date [53].

STAT5B LOF is in contrast to STAT5B GOF disease, a recently described hypersensitivity syndrome of immune dysregulation [54]. STAT5B GOF presents with early onset non-clonal hypereosinophilia, eczema, food allergies, and failure to thrive [54]. In contrast to other STAT GOF diseases, STAT5B GOF has interestingly only been described as a somatic and not germline mutation, which would make this diagnosis less likely in the patient case where there is a suspect family history. Given that STAT5 GOF immune dysregulation is secondary to increased phosphorylation of STAT5, targeted therapy with jakinibs has been employed successfully (unpublished data).

IL10/IL10R Deficiency

While CD25 deficiency causes impaired IL10 expression, a primary defect in IL10 or IL10R also presents with a similar phenotype to the patient case [55]. IL10 and IL10R deficiency are autosomal recessive defects that predominantly present with enterocolitis with perianal disease, folliculitis, arthritis, and recurrent infections [56]. However, the patient family pedigree is more suspect for an X-linked disease. IL10 is very important for preventing inflammation in the gut, and IL10 or IL10R deficiency can cause very early onset inflammatory bowel disease. [55, 57] Bone marrow transplant is curative in these diseases, though data on efficacy is limited [58].

Autoimmune Polyendocrinopathy-Candidiasis-Ectodermal Dystrophy (APECED)

While CD25 deficiency, STAT5 deficiency, and IL10/IL10R deficiency share similar clinical features given the significant enteropathy, there are also several PIRDs that share overlapping autoimmune endocrinopathy features. For instance, APECED is an autosomal recessive defect in AIRE that classically presents with the triad of chronic mucocutaneous candidiasis, hypoparathyroidism, and Addison's disease [59]. AIRE enables thymic cells to express tissue antigens, and when autoreactive T cells bind to these tissue antigens they undergo apoptosis. Defects in AIRE cause the production of autoreactive TCRs and autoantibodies leading to the various autoimmune conditions associated with APECED such as vitiligo, keratosis, hepatitis, pancreatitis, T1DM, enteropathy, arthritis, neuropathy, and thyroiditis [59]. All patients with APECED will have chronic mucocutaneous candidiasis and about two-thirds will exhibit all three features of the classic triad, which is not consistent with the patient case's clinical presentation [59]. Candidiasis presents in early infancy while hypoparathyroidism and Addison's disease present later in childhood [59]. Additionally, patients with APECED can have respiratory infections and develop interstitial lung disease [59]. Lastly, APECED patients are at risk for septicemia as functional asplenia can occur in up to 20% of adult patients with APECED [59]. Various immunosuppressive treatments are used in APECED, particularly if there is development of autoimmune hepatitis. Hormone replacement therapies are employed if needed and antifungal therapy for candidiasis. Bone marrow transplant is generally not performed in APECED [60].

STAT1 GOF

Like APECED, STAT1 GOF disease characteristically also presents with chronic mucocutaneous candidiasis. Excess STAT1 shifts the balance away from STAT3 signaling which is required to drive T cells toward IL17 producing Th17 cells. IL17 is important for epithelial antifungal immunity and therefore these patients develop chronic mucocutaneous candidiasis [61, 62]. In a review of 274 patients with STAT1 GOF disease, Candida disease presented at an average age of onset of 1 year, and the fungal disease can become resistant to antifungal therapy [63]. Additionally, 74% of patients had bacterial and viral sinopulmonary infections with complications of lung damage [62]. A small subset of STAT1 GOF patients can have autoimmune manifestations such as hypothyroidism, T1DM, hematologic cytopenias, and SLE [63]. An unusual manifestation is the development of cerebral aneurysms in almost 6% of patients [62]. STAT1 GOF is an autosomal dominant condition and does not appear to affect FOXP3 levels or Treg expression [64]. However, in vitro data shows that swinging of the pendulum to excess STAT1 might lead to aberrant STAT5 phosphorylation in response to IL2 and this might explain the autoimmunity in STAT1 GOF disease [65]. There is also evidence that stronger IFN signaling can cause the immune dysregulation in STAT1 GOF [15]. While bone marrow transplant can be considered for STAT1 GOF patients, the success has been extremely poor in this PIRD particularly, with high rates of graft rejection [66]. There has been reported success in targeted therapy with jakinibs [36, 67].

Patient Diagnosis

With regard to the patient case, genetic analysis confirmed a pathogenic point mutation in forkhead box P3 (FOXP3) through targeted sanger sequencing, consistent with immunodysregulation polyendocrinopathy enteropathy X-linked (IPEX) syndrome (exon 11, g.1222G>A). Interestingly, the patient had normal percentage of FOXP3+ cells in the CD4 population by flow cytometry, though the number of FOXP3^{BRIGHT} cells was somewhat lower than normal controls. The patient was diagnosed with IPEX at 21 years of age, only a few years after FOXP3 was discovered

Fig. 14.4 Pedigree for patient case 2. Ectopic pregnancy (ECT), spontaneous abortion (SAB)

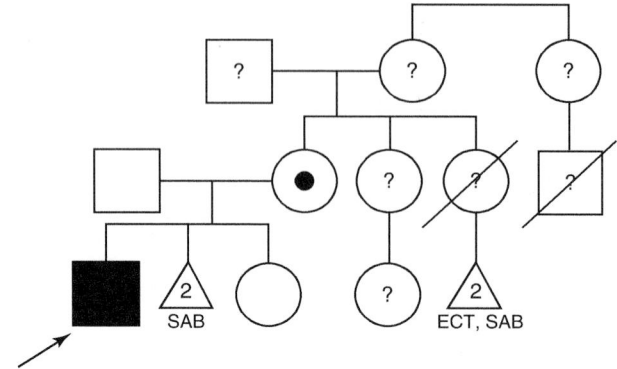

[68]. The patient's mother was found to be carrier of the same mutation (Fig. 14.4). He underwent evaluation for bone marrow transplant during which he died of urosepsis at 30 years of age.

This patient case demonstrates that when there is strong suspicion for a particular PIRD, targeted genetic testing can often provide the diagnosis. Additionally, bone marrow transplant is usually best performed at an early age as there is a high mortality in many PIRDs. Early diagnosis and referral to bone marrow transplant can be life-saving in some circumstances.

Clinical History

Patients with IPEX syndrome typically present with a triad of severe diarrhea, endocrinopathies, and dermatitis, often in the first year of life [69]. The mutation in FOXP3 causing IPEX syndrome is inherited in an X-linked recessive manner, and thus, affected patients are male. Female carriers with a pathogenic variant are unaffected. Pathogenic variants have been described across the entire FOXP3 gene and there is a wide range of manifestations within the same variant making a phenotype-genotype correlation difficult [70]. The phenotype will range from a fetal presentation with hydrops and echogenic bowel to a milder phenotype with autoimmunity presenting in adulthood [71, 72].

A multi-institutional review of 88 IPEX patients over more than 30 years provides valuable information regarding their presenting clinical history [73]. Diarrhea, usually enteropathy, is the most common presenting symptom of IPEX (97%) at an average presenting age of 8 months [73]. Small bowel biopsy findings typically show villous atrophy, and the enteropathy causes failure to thrive [73]. Food allergies are also common in IPEX patients [74].

Another hallmark symptom of the disease is endocrinopathy and occurs in 65% of IPEX patients [73]. The most common endocrinopathies include T1DM (49%), thyroid abnormalities (26%), and, more rarely, adrenal insufficiency [73]. For patients with T1DM, the average age of onset is 27 months, but T1DM can present as early as the first month of life [73, 75].

Skin findings are also common in IPEX patients – typically eczema (85%), alopecia (11%), or erythroderma (8%) [73]. Eczematous lesions usually present in the first month of life; however, fetal skin desquamation has also been reported [71]. Other rare skin manifestations described include pemphigoid nodularis and epidermolysis bullosa acquisita [76, 77].

Although IPEX patients do not have evidence of defective cellular or humoral immunity, they do experience infectious complications due to poor gut and skin barrier function [78]. Up to 47% of IPEX patients can have serious infections such as sepsis, meningitis, peritonitis, and pneumonia [73].

Autoimmune hematologic diseases occur in 42% of patients with IPEX [73]. Other less common abnormalities in IPEX include nephropathy, neurological manifestations, hepatitis, arthritis, vasculitis, and lymphadenopathy [73].

Prognosis of IPEX patients depends on the aggressiveness of treatment in early life. Without immunosuppressants for the immune dysregulation in early childhood, there is a high early mortality in IPEX patients from severe malabsorption or sepsis. In a long-term follow-up study of 88 patients with IPEX syndrome, survival to 30 years of age was 52% [73]. The type of mutation in FOXP3 is associated with increased or decreased survival with in-frame deletions having the best prognosis and polyadenylation site mutations the poorest prognosis [73].

Laboratory Evaluation

Common laboratory findings suggestive of IPEX in the context of an appropriate clinical picture include elevated IgE, eosinophilia, and autoimmune cytopenia [73]. Hypogammaglobulinemia secondary to protein loosing enteropathy or as a complication of treatment is also described in IPEX patients [73]. There are some reports of patients with IPEX presenting with hypogammaglobulinemia and a B-cell class-switching defect, though IPEX patients are not believed to have a primary humoral defect [79].

Autoantibodies are also pathognomonic for IPEX syndrome and typically correspond with the clinical presentation [80]. For instance, IPEX patients with T1DM can have antibodies against insulin, pancreatic islet cell, or anti-glutamate decarboxylase. IPEX patients with thyroiditis (even if normal thyroid function) can have anti-thyroglobulin and anti-microsome peroxidase antibodies. In cases of autoimmune cytopenia, the patients will have antibodies against that cell line. Anti-smooth muscle and anti-liver-kidney-muscle antibodies can be found in IPEX patients with hepatitis. Anti-enterocyte antibodies and anti-villin antibodies are associated with enteropathy [81, 82]. And lastly, anti-keratin antibodies could explain the skin findings in patients with IPEX [83]. IPEX patients can also have nonspecific antibodies such as antinuclear antibodies and anti-mitochondrial antibodies [84].

Flow cytometry can identify decreased numbers of FOXP3-expressing Tregs (CD4 + CD25 + FOXP3+) in IPEX patients. However, some pathogenic FOXP3 mutations can lead to normal expression of FOXP3 Tregs and therefore, flow cytometry cannot be relied upon for diagnosis of IPEX [75]. Additionally, other PIRDs display decreased CD4 + CD25 + FOXP3+ cells [73]. The diagnosis of IPEX syndrome is confirmed by genetic sequencing of FOXP3 revealing a hemizygous pathogenic variant. Given that some pathogenic mutations in IPEX are large deletions, confirmation requires deletion and duplication analysis [73]. Additionally, deletion of a noncoding exon has been described and sequencing of the FOXP3 region is necessary if clinical suspicion for IPEX is high [74].

Management/Outcome

Treatment

First-line treatment for IPEX patients targets the unregulated Teff cells that are implicated in the pathogenesis of IPEX. This is commonly accomplished by cyclosporine, tacrolimus, or sirolimus with or without glucocorticoids [85]. Other therapies that may be utilized include granulocyte colony stimulation factor (G-CSF) for AIN, rituximab for autoantibody mediated disease, and standard therapy for the associated endocrinopathies. Since the degree of enteropathy can cause severe malnourishment, particularly after immunosuppression, almost all patients with IPEX require nutritional support [69]. Control of dermatitis in IPEX patients is also important to prevent secondary superinfection. Lastly, prophylactic antibiotics for those with AIN or recurrent infections may be needed. However, despite the aforementioned therapeutic interventions, there is disease progression, complications from side effects, and high mortality in IPEX syndrome [69].

While there are promising results in mouse models using lentiviral gene therapy to suppress the autoimmunity in IPEX syndrome, there are no human clinical trials using gene therapy to date [86]. The only current available curative treatment for IPEX is bone marrow transplant [87, 88]. In a study of 40 IPEX patients who underwent bone marrow transplant, there was a 78% survival rate [73]. Another study of 58 transplanted IPEX patients showed a 73% survival rate at 15 years posttransplant [69]. Bone marrow transplant cannot only cure the severe enteropathy but can also lead to resolution of autoimmune cytopenia and autoimmune polyendocrinopathy. [69] The likelihood of resolution is greater in those that are transplanted before organ impairment has developed, with rare reversal of T1DM when present pretransplant [73, 89].

Clinical Pearls and Pitfalls

- Many patients with immunodeficiency also exhibit immune dysregulation.
- Patients presenting with early onset, refractory, or unusual presentations of autoimmune disease should be evaluated for primary immunodeficiencies and PIRDs (Table 14.5).
- Patients with a diagnosis of CVID or probable ALPS should be re-evaluated to assess for the possibility of a monogenic etiology of immune dysregulation.
- PIRDs may be identified through functional testing of the immune system and via flow cytometry looking for the presence of cell surface receptors.
- There are many monogenic etiologies for PIRDs and whole exome sequencing can help elucidate the diagnosis, screen for comorbidities, and aid in treatment.
- The penetrance and clinical expressivity varies vastly with many of the described diseases, even within the same families and with the same mutations.
- Targeted biologic therapies can treat the underlying monogenic defect in many PIRDs (see Table 14.4).
- Knowing the underlying PIRDs can aid in the decision of whether or not to pursue bone marrow transplantation as curative therapy.

Table 14.5 Differential diagnosis for case presentations

Patient case 1 Diagnosis: LRBA deficiency	Patient case 2 Diagnosis: IPEX syndrome
CTLA haploinsufficiency	IL10/IL10R deficiency
CVID	STAT5 LOF
IPEX syndrome	STAT3 GOF
STAT3 GOF	LRBA deficiency
ALPS	CD25 deficiency
APDS	CVID

References

1. Bousfiha A, Jeddane L, Picard C, Ailal F, Bobby Gaspar H, Al-Herz W, et al. The 2017 IUIS phenotypic classification for primary immunodeficiencies. J Clin Immunol. 2018;38(1):129–43. https://doi.org/10.1007/s10875-017-0465-8.
2. Nemazee D. Mechanisms of central tolerance for B cells. Nat Rev Immunol. 2017;17(5):281–94. https://doi.org/10.1038/nri.2017.19.
3. Fruton JS. The collected papers of Paul Ehrlich. Yale J Biol Med. 1957;29(6):1.
4. Grimbacher B, Warnatz K, Yong PFK, Korganow AS, Peter HH. The crossroads of autoimmunity and immunodeficiency: lessons from polygenic traits and monogenic defects. J Allergy Clin Immunol. 2016;137(1):3–17. https://doi.org/10.1016/j.jaci.2015.11.004.
5. Rowshanravan B, Halliday N, Sansom DM. CTLA-4: a moving target in immunotherapy. Blood. 2018;131(1):58–67. https://doi.org/10.1182/blood-2017-06-741033.
6. Egen JG, Allison JP. Cytotoxic T lymphocyte antigen-4 accumulation in the immunological synapse is regulated by TCR signal strength. Immunity. 2002;16(1):23–35.
7. Saraiva M, O'Garra A. The regulation of IL-10 production by immune cells. Nat Rev Immunol. 2010;10(3):170–81. https://doi.org/10.1038/nri2711.
8. Elmore S. Apoptosis: a review of programmed cell death. Toxicol Pathol. 2007;35(4):495–516. https://doi.org/10.1080/01926230701320337.
9. Dowdell KC, Niemela JE, Price S, Davis J, Hornung RL, Oliveira JB, et al. Somatic FAS mutations are common in patients with genetically undefined autoimmune lymphoproliferative syndrome. Blood. 2010;115(25):5164–9. https://doi.org/10.1182/blood-2010-01-263145.
10. Chervonsky AV. Apoptotic and effector pathways in autoimmunity. Curr Opin Immunol. 1999;11(6):684–8. https://doi.org/10.1016/s0952-7915(99)00037-0.
11. Srivastava S, Koch LK, Campbell DJ. IFNalphaR signaling in effector but not regulatory T cells is required for immune dysregulation during type I IFN-dependent inflammatory disease. J Immunol. 2014;193(6):2733–42. https://doi.org/10.4049/jimmunol.1401039.
12. Zharkova O, Celhar T, Cravens PD, Satterthwaite AB, Fairhurst AM, Davis LS. Pathways leading to an immunological disease: systemic lupus erythematosus. Rheumatology (Oxford). 2017;56(suppl_1):i55–66. https://doi.org/10.1093/rheumatology/kew427.
13. Son M, Diamond B, Santiago-Schwarz F. Fundamental role of C1q in autoimmunity and inflammation. Immunol Res. 2015;63(1–3):101–6. https://doi.org/10.1007/s12026-015-8705-6.
14. Eleftheriou D, Brogan PA. Genetic interferonopathies: an overview. Best Pract Res Clin Rheumatol. 2017;31(4):441–59. https://doi.org/10.1016/j.berh.2017.12.002.
15. Schindler C, Levy DE, Decker T. JAK-STAT signaling: from interferons to cytokines. J Biol Chem. 2007;282(28):20059–63. https://doi.org/10.1074/jbc.R700016200.
16. Teachey DT. New advances in the diagnosis and treatment of autoimmune lymphoproliferative syndrome. Curr Opin Pediatr. 2012;24(1):1–8. https://doi.org/10.1097/MOP.0b013e32834ea739.
17. Rieux-Laucat F, Le Deist F, Fischer A. Autoimmune lymphoproliferative syndromes: genetic defects of apoptosis pathways. Cell Death Differ. 2003;10(1):124–33. https://doi.org/10.1038/sj.cdd.4401190.
18. Price S, Shaw PA, Seitz A, Joshi G, Davis J, Niemela JE, et al. Natural history of autoimmune lymphoproliferative syndrome associated with FAS gene mutations. Blood. 2014;123(13):1989–99. https://doi.org/10.1182/blood-2013-10-535393.
19. Oliveira JB, Bleesing JJ, Dianzani U, Fleisher TA, Jaffe ES, Lenardo MJ, et al. Revised diagnostic criteria and classification for the autoimmune lymphoproliferative syndrome (ALPS): report from the 2009 NIH international workshop. Blood. 2010;116(14):e35–40. https://doi.org/10.1182/blood-2010-04-280347.
20. Cagdas D, Halacli SO, Tan C, Lo B, Cetinkaya PG, Esenboga S et al. A Spectrum of clinical findings from ALPS to CVID: several novel LRBA defects. J Clin Immunol. 2019. https://doi.org/10.1007/s10875-019-00677-6.

21. Russell TB, Kurre P. Double-negative T cells are non-ALPS-specific markers of immune dysregulation found in patients with aplastic anemia. Blood. 2010;116(23):5072–3. https://doi.org/10.1182/blood-2010-09-306910.
22. Rao VK, Oliveira JB. How I treat autoimmune lymphoproliferative syndrome. Blood. 2011;118(22):5741–51. https://doi.org/10.1182/blood-2011-07-325217.
23. Teachey DT, Seif AE, Grupp SA. Advances in the management and understanding of autoimmune lymphoproliferative syndrome (ALPS). Br J Haematol. 2010;148(2):205–16. https://doi.org/10.1111/j.1365-2141.2009.07991.x.
24. Rao VK, Oliveira JB. How I treat autoimmune lymphoproliferative syndrome. Blood. 2011;118(22):11.
25. Schubert D, Bode C, Kenefeck R, Hou TZ, Wing JB, Kennedy A, et al. Autosomal dominant immune dysregulation syndrome in humans with CTLA4 mutations. Nat Med. 2014;20(12):1410–6. https://doi.org/10.1038/nm.3746.
26. Lo B, Fritz JM, Su HC, Uzel G, Jordan MB, Lenardo MJ. CHAI and LATAIE: new genetic diseases of CTLA-4 checkpoint insufficiency. Blood. 2016;128(8):1037–42. https://doi.org/10.1182/blood-2016-04-712612.
27. Gamez-Diaz L, August D, Stepensky P, Revel-Vilk S, Seidel MG, Noriko M, et al. The extended phenotype of LPS-responsive beige-like anchor protein (LRBA) deficiency. J Allergy Clin Immunol. 2016;137(1):223–30. https://doi.org/10.1016/j.jaci.2015.09.025.
28. Maffucci P, Filion CA, Boisson B, Itan Y, Shang L, Casanova JL, et al. Genetic diagnosis using whole exome sequencing in common variable immunodeficiency. Front Immunol. 2016;7:220. https://doi.org/10.3389/fimmu.2016.00220.
29. Kiykim A, Ogulur I, Dursun E, Charbonnier LM, Nain E, Cekic S et al. Abatacept as a long-term targeted therapy for LRBA deficiency. J Allergy Clin Immunol Pract. 2019. https://doi.org/10.1016/j.jaip.2019.06.011.
30. Uzel G, Karanovic D, Su H, Rump A, Agharahimi A, Holland SM, et al. Management of cytopenias in CTLA4 haploinsufficiency using abatacept and sirolimus. Blood. 2018;132(Suppl 1):1.
31. Slatter MA, Engelhardt KR, Burroughs LM, Arkwright PD, Nademi Z, Skoda-Smith S, et al. Hematopoietic stem cell transplantation for CTLA4 deficiency. J Allergy Clin Immunol. 2016;138(2):615–9 e1. https://doi.org/10.1016/j.jaci.2016.01.045.
32. Flanagan SE, Haapaniemi E, Russell MA, Caswell R, Allen HL, De Franco E, et al. Activating germline mutations in STAT3 cause early-onset multi-organ autoimmune disease. Nat Genet. 2014;46(8):812–4. https://doi.org/10.1038/ng.3040.
33. Milner JD, Vogel TP, Forbes L, Ma CA, Stray-Pedersen A, Niemela JE, et al. Early-onset lymphoproliferation and autoimmunity caused by germline STAT3 gain-of-function mutations. Blood. 2015;125(4):591–9. https://doi.org/10.1182/blood-2014-09-602763.
34. Fabre A, Marchal S, Barlogis V, Mari B, Barbry P, Rohrlich PS, et al. Clinical aspects of STAT3 gain-of-function germline mutations: a systematic review. J Allergy Clin Immunol Pract. 2019;7(6):1958–69 e9. https://doi.org/10.1016/j.jaip.2019.02.018.
35. Hillmer EJ, Zhang H, Li HS, Watowich SS. STAT3 signaling in immunity. Cytokine Growth Factor Rev. 2016;31:1–15. https://doi.org/10.1016/j.cytogfr.2016.05.001.
36. Forbes LR, Vogel TP, Cooper MA, Castro-Wagner J, Schussler E, Weinacht KG, et al. Jakinibs for the treatment of immune dysregulation in patients with gain-of-function signal transducer and activator of transcription 1 (STAT1) or STAT3 mutations. J Allergy Clin Immunol. 2018;142(5):1665–9. https://doi.org/10.1016/j.jaci.2018.07.020.
37. Angulo I, Vadas O, Garcon F, Banham-Hall E, Plagnol V, Leahy TR, et al. Phosphoinositide 3-kinase delta gene mutation predisposes to respiratory infection and airway damage. Science. 2013;342(6160):866–71. https://doi.org/10.1126/science.1243292.
38. Coulter TI, Chandra A, Bacon CM, Babar J, Curtis J, Screaton N, et al. Clinical spectrum and features of activated phosphoinositide 3-kinase delta syndrome: a large patient cohort study. J Allergy Clin Immunol. 2017;139(2):597–606 e4. https://doi.org/10.1016/j.jaci.2016.06.021.

39. Rao VK, Webster S, Dalm V, Sediva A, van Hagen PM, Holland S, et al. Effective "activated PI3Kdelta syndrome"-targeted therapy with the PI3Kdelta inhibitor leniolisib. Blood. 2017;130(21):2307–16. https://doi.org/10.1182/blood-2017-08-801191.
40. Nademi Z, Slatter MA, Dvorak CC, Neven B, Fischer A, Suarez F, et al. Hematopoietic stem cell transplant in patients with activated PI3K delta syndrome. J Allergy Clin Immunol. 2017;139(3):1046–9. https://doi.org/10.1016/j.jaci.2016.09.040.
41. Agarwal S, Cunningham-Rundles C. Autoimmunity in common variable immunodeficiency. Ann Allergy Asthma Immunol. 2019. https://doi.org/10.1016/j.anai.2019.07.014.
42. Lopez-Herrera G, Tampella G, Pan-Hammarstrom Q, Herholz P, Trujillo-Vargas CM, Phadwal K, et al. Deleterious mutations in LRBA are associated with a syndrome of immune deficiency and autoimmunity. Am J Hum Genet. 2012;90(6):986–1001. https://doi.org/10.1016/j.ajhg.2012.04.015.
43. Gamez-Diaz L, Sigmund EC, Reiser V, Vach W, Jung S, Grimbacher B. Rapid flow cytometry-based test for the diagnosis of lipopolysaccharide responsive beige-like anchor (LRBA) deficiency. Front Immunol. 2018;9:720. https://doi.org/10.3389/fimmu.2018.00720.
44. Lo B, Zhang K, Lu W, Zheng L, Zhang Q, Kanellopoulou C, et al. AUTOIMMUNE DISEASE. Patients with LRBA deficiency show CTLA4 loss and immune dysregulation responsive to abatacept therapy. Science. 2015;349(6246):436–40. https://doi.org/10.1126/science.aaa1663.
45. Bonilla FA, Khan DA, Ballas ZK, Chinen J, Frank MM, Hsu JT, et al. Practice parameter for the diagnosis and management of primary immunodeficiency. J Allergy Clin Immunol. 2015;136(5):1186–205. e1–78. https://doi.org/10.1016/j.jaci.2015.04.049.
46. Villa A, Marrella V, Rucci F, Notarangelo LD. Genetically determined lymphopenia and autoimmune manifestations. Curr Opin Immunol. 2008;20(3):318–24. https://doi.org/10.1016/j.coi.2008.02.001.
47. Villa A, Notarangelo LD, Roifman CM. Omenn syndrome: inflammation in leaky severe combined immunodeficiency. J Allergy Clin Immunol. 2008;122(6):1082–6. https://doi.org/10.1016/j.jaci.2008.09.037.
48. Walter JE, Rosen LB, Csomos K, Rosenberg JM, Mathew D, Keszei M, et al. Broad-spectrum antibodies against self-antigens and cytokines in RAG deficiency. J Clin Invest. 2015;125(11):4135–48. https://doi.org/10.1172/JCI80477.
49. Vignoli M, Ciullini Mannurita S, Fioravanti A, Tumino M, Grassi A, Guariso G, et al. CD25 deficiency: a new conformational mutation prevents the receptor expression on cell surface. Clin Immunol. 2019;201:15–9. https://doi.org/10.1016/j.clim.2019.02.003.
50. Caudy AA, Reddy ST, Chatila T, Atkinson JP, Verbsky JW. CD25 deficiency causes an immune dysregulation, polyendocrinopathy, enteropathy, X-linked-like syndrome, and defective IL-10 expression from CD4 lymphocytes. J Allergy Clin Immunol. 2007;119(2):482–7. https://doi.org/10.1016/j.jaci.2006.10.007.
51. Bezrodnik L, Di Giovanni D, Caldirola MS, Azcoiti ME, Torgerson T, Gaillard MI. Long-term follow-up of STAT5B deficiency in three argentinian patients: clinical and immunological features. J Clin Immunol. 2015;35(3):264–72. https://doi.org/10.1007/s10875-015-0145-5.
52. Hwa V. STAT5B deficiency: impacts on human growth and immunity. Growth Hormon IGF Res. 2016;28:16–20. https://doi.org/10.1016/j.ghir.2015.12.006.
53. Snow JW, Abraham N, Ma MC, Goldsmith MA. Bone marrow transplant completely rescues hematolymphoid defects in STAT5A/5B-deficient mice. Exp Hematol. 2003;31(12):1247–52.
54. Ma CA, Xi L, Cauff B, DeZure A, Freeman AF, Hambleton S, et al. Somatic STAT5b gain-of-function mutations in early onset nonclonal eosinophilia, urticaria, dermatitis, and diarrhea. Blood. 2017;129(5):650–3. https://doi.org/10.1182/blood-2016-09-737817.
55. Zhu L, Shi T, Zhong C, Wang Y, Chang M, Liu X. IL-10 and IL-10 receptor mutations in very early onset inflammatory bowel disease. Gastroenterology Res. 2017;10(2):65–9. https://doi.org/10.14740/gr740w.

56. Kotlarz D, Beier R, Murugan D, Diestelhorst J, Jensen O, Boztug K, et al. Loss of interleukin-10 signaling and infantile inflammatory bowel disease: implications for diagnosis and therapy. Gastroenterology. 2012;143(2):347–55. https://doi.org/10.1053/j.gastro.2012.04.045.
57. Kole A, Maloy KJ. Control of intestinal inflammation by interleukin-10. Curr Top Microbiol Immunol. 2014;380:19–38. https://doi.org/10.1007/978-3-662-43492-5_2.
58. Engelhardt KR, Shah N, Faizura-Yeop I, Kocacik Uygun DF, Frede N, Muise AM, et al. Clinical outcome in IL-10- and IL-10 receptor-deficient patients with or without hematopoietic stem cell transplantation. J Allergy Clin Immunol. 2013;131(3):825–30. https://doi.org/10.1016/j.jaci.2012.09.025.
59. Kisand K, Peterson P. Autoimmune polyendocrinopathy candidiasis ectodermal dystrophy. J Clin Immunol. 2015;35(5):463–78. https://doi.org/10.1007/s10875-015-0176-y.
60. Shah M, Holland E, Chan CC. Resolution of autoimmune polyglandular syndrome-associated keratopathy with keratolimbal stem cell transplantation: case report and historical literature review. Cornea. 2007;26(5):632–5. https://doi.org/10.1097/ICO.0b013e3180415d1a.
61. Liu L, Okada S, Kong XF, Kreins AY, Cypowyj S, Abhyankar A, et al. Gain-of-function human STAT1 mutations impair IL-17 immunity and underlie chronic mucocutaneous candidiasis. J Exp Med. 2011;208(8):1635–48. https://doi.org/10.1084/jem.20110958.
62. Hambleton S. When the STATs are against you. Blood. 2016;127(25):3109–10. https://doi.org/10.1182/blood-2016-05-715029.
63. Toubiana J, Okada S, Hiller J, Oleastro M, Lagos Gomez M, Aldave Becerra JC, et al. Heterozygous STAT1 gain-of-function mutations underlie an unexpectedly broad clinical phenotype. Blood. 2016;127(25):3154–64. https://doi.org/10.1182/blood-2015-11-679902.
64. Uzel G, Sampaio EP, Lawrence MG, Hsu AP, Hackett M, Dorsey MJ, et al. Dominant gain-of-function STAT1 mutations in FOXP3 wild-type immune dysregulation-polyendocrinopathy-enteropathy-X-linked-like syndrome. J Allergy Clin Immunol. 2013;131(6):1611–23. https://doi.org/10.1016/j.jaci.2012.11.054.
65. Vargas-Hernandez A, Mace EM, Zimmerman O, Zerbe CS, Freeman AF, Rosenzweig S, et al. Ruxolitinib partially reverses functional natural killer cell deficiency in patients with signal transducer and activator of transcription 1 (STAT1) gain-of-function mutations. J Allergy Clin Immunol. 2018;141(6):2142–55 e5. https://doi.org/10.1016/j.jaci.2017.08.040.
66. Leiding JW, Okada S, Hagin D, Abinun M, Shcherbina A, Balashov DN, et al. Hematopoietic stem cell transplantation in patients with gain-of-function signal transducer and activator of transcription 1 mutations. J Allergy Clin Immunol. 2018;141(2):704–17 e5. https://doi.org/10.1016/j.jaci.2017.03.049.
67. Kiykim A, Charbonnier LM, Akcay A, Karakoc-Aydiner E, Ozen A, Ozturk G, et al. Hematopoietic stem cell transplantation in patients with heterozygous STAT1 gain-of-function mutation. J Clin Immunol. 2019;39(1):37–44. https://doi.org/10.1007/s10875-018-0575-y.
68. Bennett CL, Christie J, Ramsdell F, Brunkow ME, Ferguson PJ, Whitesell L, et al. The immune dysregulation, polyendocrinopathy, enteropathy, X-linked syndrome (IPEX) is caused by mutations of FOXP3. Nat Genet. 2001;27(1):20–1. https://doi.org/10.1038/83713.
69. Barzaghi F, Amaya Hernandez LC, Neven B, Ricci S, Kucuk ZY, Bleesing JJ, et al. Long-term follow-up of IPEX syndrome patients after different therapeutic strategies: an international multicenter retrospective study. J Allergy Clin Immunol. 2018;141(3):1036–49 e5. https://doi.org/10.1016/j.jaci.2017.10.041.
70. Seidel MG, Boztug K, Haas OA. Immune dysregulation syndromes (IPEX, CD27 deficiency, and others): always doomed from the start? J Clin Immunol. 2016;36(1):6–7. https://doi.org/10.1007/s10875-015-0218-5.
71. Khattri R, Cox T, Yasayko SA, Ramsdell F. An essential role for Scurfin in CD4+CD25+ T regulatory cells. Nat Immunol. 2003;4(4):337–42. https://doi.org/10.1038/ni909.

72. Hwang JL, Park SY, Ye H, Sanyoura M, Pastore AN, Carmody D, et al. FOXP3 mutations causing early-onset insulin-requiring diabetes but without other features of immune dysregulation, polyendocrinopathy, enteropathy, X-linked syndrome. Pediatr Diabetes. 2018;19(3):388–92. https://doi.org/10.1111/pedi.12612.
73. Gambineri E, Ciullini Mannurita S, Hagin D, Vignoli M, Anover-Sombke S, DeBoer S, et al. Clinical, immunological, and molecular heterogeneity of 173 patients with the phenotype of immune dysregulation, polyendocrinopathy, enteropathy, X-linked (IPEX) syndrome. Front Immunol. 2018;9:2411. https://doi.org/10.3389/fimmu.2018.02411.
74. Torgerson TR, Linane A, Moes N, Anover S, Mateo V, Rieux-Laucat F, et al. Severe food allergy as a variant of IPEX syndrome caused by a deletion in a noncoding region of the FOXP3 gene. Gastroenterology. 2007;132(5):1705–17. https://doi.org/10.1053/j.gastro.2007.02.044.
75. Gambineri E, Perroni L, Passerini L, Bianchi L, Doglioni C, Meschi F, et al. Clinical and molecular profile of a new series of patients with immune dysregulation, polyendocrinopathy, enteropathy, X-linked syndrome: inconsistent correlation between forkhead box protein 3 expression and disease severity. J Allergy Clin Immunol. 2008;122(6):1105–12 e1. https://doi.org/10.1016/j.jaci.2008.09.027.
76. McGinness JL, Bivens MM, Greer KE, Patterson JW, Saulsbury FT. Immune dysregulation, polyendocrinopathy, enteropathy, X-linked syndrome (IPEX) associated with pemphigoid nodularis: a case report and review of the literature. J Am Acad Dermatol. 2006;55(1):143–8. https://doi.org/10.1016/j.jaad.2005.08.047.
77. Bis S, Maguiness SM, Gellis SE, Schneider LC, Lee PY, Notarangelo LD, et al. Immune dysregulation, polyendocrinopathy, enteropathy, X-linked syndrome associated with neonatal epidermolysis bullosa acquisita. Pediatr Dermatol. 2015;32(3):e74–7. https://doi.org/10.1111/pde.12550.
78. Bacchetta R, Barzaghi F, Roncarolo MG. From IPEX syndrome to FOXP3 mutation: a lesson on immune dysregulation. Ann N Y Acad Sci. 2018;1417(1):5–22. https://doi.org/10.1111/nyas.13011.
79. Shamriz O, Patel K, Marsh RA, Bleesing J, Joshi AY, Lucas L, et al. Hypogammaglobulinemia with decreased class-switched B-cells and dysregulated T-follicular-helper cells in IPEX syndrome. Clin Immunol. 2018;197:219–23. https://doi.org/10.1016/j.clim.2018.10.005.
80. Barzaghi F, Passerini L, Bacchetta R. Immune dysregulation, polyendocrinopathy, enteropathy, x-linked syndrome: a paradigm of immunodeficiency with autoimmunity. Front Immunol. 2012;3:211. https://doi.org/10.3389/fimmu.2012.00211.
81. Kobayashi I, Kubota M, Yamada M, Tanaka H, Itoh S, Sasahara Y, et al. Autoantibodies to villin occur frequently in IPEX, a severe immune dysregulation, syndrome caused by mutation of FOXP3. Clin Immunol. 2011;141(1):83–9. https://doi.org/10.1016/j.clim.2011.05.010.
82. Moes N, Rieux-Laucat F, Begue B, Verdier J, Neven B, Patey N, et al. Reduced expression of FOXP3 and regulatory T-cell function in severe forms of early-onset autoimmune enteropathy. Gastroenterology. 2010;139(3):770–8. https://doi.org/10.1053/j.gastro.2010.06.006.
83. Huter EN, Natarajan K, Torgerson TR, Glass DD, Shevach EM. Autoantibodies in scurfy mice and IPEX patients recognize keratin 14. J Invest Dermatol. 2010;130(5):1391–9. https://doi.org/10.1038/jid.2010.16.
84. Tsuda M, Torgerson TR, Selmi C, Gambineri E, Carneiro-Sampaio M, Mannurita SC, et al. The spectrum of autoantibodies in IPEX syndrome is broad and includes anti-mitochondrial autoantibodies. J Autoimmun. 2010;35(3):265–8. https://doi.org/10.1016/j.jaut.2010.06.017.
85. Torgerson TR, Ochs HD. Regulatory T cells in primary immunodeficiency diseases. Curr Opin Allergy Clin Immunol. 2007;7(6):515–21. https://doi.org/10.1097/ACI.0b013e3282f1a27a.
86. Masiuk KE, Laborada J, Roncarolo MG, Hollis RP, Kohn DB. Lentiviral gene therapy in HSCs restores lineage-specific Foxp3 expression and suppresses autoimmunity in a mouse model of IPEX syndrome. Cell Stem Cell. 2019;24(2):309–17 e7. https://doi.org/10.1016/j.stem.2018.12.003.

87. Rao A, Kamani N, Filipovich A, Lee SM, Davies SM, Dalal J, et al. Successful bone marrow transplantation for IPEX syndrome after reduced-intensity conditioning. Blood. 2007;109(1):383–5. https://doi.org/10.1182/blood-2006-05-025072.
88. Zhan H, Sinclair J, Adams S, Cale CM, Murch S, Perroni L, et al. Immune reconstitution and recovery of FOXP3 (forkhead box P3)-expressing T cells after transplantation for IPEX (immune dysregulation, polyendocrinopathy, enteropathy, X-linked) syndrome. Pediatrics. 2008;121(4):e998–1002. https://doi.org/10.1542/peds.2007-1863.
89. Yamauchi T, Takasawa K, Kamiya T, Kirino S, Gau M, Inoue K et al. Hematopoietic stem cell transplantation recovers insulin deficiency in type 1 diabetes mellitus associated with IPEX syndrome. Pediatr Diabetes. 2019. https://doi.org/10.1111/pedi.12895.
90. Neven B, Magerus-Chatinet A, Florkin B, Gobert D, Lambotte O, De Somer L, et al. A survey of 90 patients with autoimmune lymphoproliferative syndrome related to TNFRSF6 mutation. Blood. 2011;118(18):4798–807. https://doi.org/10.1182/blood-2011-04-347641.
91. Del Bel KL, Ragotte RJ, Saferali A, Lee S, Vercauteren SM, Mostafavi SA, et al. JAK1 gain-of-function causes an autosomal dominant immune dysregulatory and hypereosinophilic syndrome. J Allergy Clin Immunol. 2017;139(6):2016–20 e5. https://doi.org/10.1016/j.jaci.2016.12.957.
92. McLean-Tooke A, Spickett GP, Gennery AR. Immunodeficiency and autoimmunity in 22q11.2 deletion syndrome. Scand J Immunol. 2007;66(1):1–7. https://doi.org/10.1111/j.1365-3083.2007.01949.x.
93. Biggs CM, Keles S, Chatila TA. DOCK8 deficiency: insights into pathophysiology, clinical features and management. Clin Immunol. 2017;181:75–82. https://doi.org/10.1016/j.clim.2017.06.003.
94. Battersby AC, Braggins H, Pearce MS, Cale CM, Burns SO, Hackett S, et al. Inflammatory and autoimmune manifestations in X-linked carriers of chronic granulomatous disease in the United Kingdom. J Allergy Clin Immunol. 2017;140(2):628–30 e6. https://doi.org/10.1016/j.jaci.2017.02.029.
95. Magnani A, Brosselin P, Beaute J, de Vergnes N, Mouy R, Debre M, et al. Inflammatory manifestations in a single-center cohort of patients with chronic granulomatous disease. J Allergy Clin Immunol. 2014;134(3):655–62 e8. https://doi.org/10.1016/j.jaci.2014.04.014.
96. Agarwal S, Cunningham-Rundles C. Autoimmunity in common variable immunodeficiency. Curr Allergy Asthma Rep. 2009;9(5):347–52.
97. Jesus AA, Duarte AJ, Oliveira JB. Autoimmunity in hyper-IgM syndrome. J Clin Immunol. 2008;28(Suppl 1):S62–6. https://doi.org/10.1007/s10875-008-9171-x.
98. Notarangelo LD, Kim MS, Walter JE, Lee YN. Human RAG mutations: biochemistry and clinical implications. Nat Rev Immunol. 2016;16(4):234–46. https://doi.org/10.1038/nri.2016.28.
99. Catucci M, Castiello MC, Pala F, Bosticardo M, Villa A. Autoimmunity in wiskott-Aldrich syndrome: an unsolved enigma. Front Immunol. 2012;3:209. https://doi.org/10.3389/fimmu.2012.00209.

Chapter 15
Dendritic Cells in Primary Immunodeficiency

Justin Greiwe

Introduction

Dendritic cells are a heterogenous group of highly specialized innate immune cells that initiate and regulate adaptive immune responses in the body. Providing a comprehensive overview of dendritic cell primary immunodeficiency disease (PID) is challenging since their role in immune dysfunction is not well described in the literature. Presenting relevant clinical cases is also problematic because there are so few documented cases of dendritic cell deficiency reported in the literature. Not surprising, although dendritic cells have been extensively researched in laboratory models, a clear role for dendritic cell deficiency in human disease is still poorly elucidated. This chapter will attempt to provide a brief overview of dendritic cells and further clarify their role in PID, specifically highlighting the recently described dendritic cell deficiency syndromes related to GATA binding protein 2 (GATA2) and interferon regulatory factor 8 (IRF8) mutations.

Case Presentation 1: Autosomal Recessive IRF8 Deficiency (K108E Individuals)

A 12-week-old male from Hong Kong presented to the pediatrician with impressive failure to thrive (significantly below 5th percentile), marked hepatosplenomegaly, and oral candidiasis. He is the youngest of three siblings who are all healthy. The child was well at birth with no evidence of congenital infection and received his

J. Greiwe (✉)
Bernstein Allergy Group, Inc., Cincinnati, OH, USA

Division of Immunology, Allergy, and Rheumatology, University of Cincinnati, Cincinnati, OH, USA standard Bacillus Calmette-Guérin (BCG) vaccination, which is mandatory for all newborns in Hong Kong. On exam the pediatrician noted a discharging Bacillus BCG scar and associated suppurative axillary lymphadenitis. The infant appeared healthy until the second month of life; family history is unremarkable for chronic illness or immunodeficiency. Subsequent laboratory evaluation revealed the following.

Parameter (units)	Value	Normal range (infant)
Hemoglobin (g/dL)	5.6	10.5–13.5
Platelets ($\times 10^9$/L)	65	150–450
White blood cells ($\times 10^9$/L)	120.5	6.0–17.5
Neutrophils ($\times 10^9$/L)	98	1.0–8.5
Lymphocytes ($\times 10^9$/L)	15.1	4–13.5
Monocytes ($\times 10^9$/L)	0.0	0.7–1.5
Eosinophils ($\times 10^9$/L)	1.8	0.3–0.8
Basophils ($\times 10^9$/L)	0.0	0.0–0.1
T lymphocytes (/μL)	8989	2300–6900
CD8+ T lymphocytes (/μL)	1649	400–2200
CD4+ T lymphocytes (/μL)	7235	1400–5300
NK lymphocytes (/μL)	2350	100–1400
B lymphocytes (/μL)	12,148	600–3000
IgG (g/L)	4.5	3.0–9.0
IgM (g/L)	2.1	0.4–1.6
IgA (g/L)	0.1	0.1–0.5
C-reactive protein (mg/L)	40	0–5
Erythrocyte sedimentation rate (mm/hr)	73	0–15
Renal function	Normal	
Liver function	Normal	

The patient was admitted to the hospital and excisional biopsy of the enlarged lymph node showed acid-fast bacilli on Ziehl-Neelsen stain and BCG was subsequently cultured. Broad-spectrum antibiotics and antimycobacterial therapy were instituted with a slow recovery over the subsequent weeks. Bone marrow biopsy showed granulocytic hyperplasia but no evidence of myelodysplasia or malignancy. After discharge the patient progressed well, meeting some developmental milestones. Progress was abruptly halted a few months later when he contracted a rhinovirus infection after being exposed to sick siblings at home. He was readmitted to the intensive care unit with high-spiking fevers, worsening hepatosplenomegaly, respiratory failure, and worsening cytopenias. A number of specialists were consulted due to concern for PID eventually resulting in the diagnosis of IRF8 deficiency. Due to the severity of his presentation, it was decided to proceed with a matched unrelated donor cord blood hematopoietic stem cell transplant at the age of 10 months. Although risk of myeloid malignancy in this clinical scenario is high, a good cure rate was demonstrated in previously published murine models with IRF8 deficiency post bone marrow transplantation. Close follow-up posttransplant has been encouraging. Fifteen months posttransplant the patient was doing well with no major infections, no hospital visits, and only mild developmental delay. Analysis of peripheral blood showed full donor reconstitution including monocytes, DC, and T lymphocytes.

Case Presentation 2: Autosomal Dominant IRF8 Deficiency (T80A Individuals)

An 18-month-old female born in South America was vaccinated with BCG vaccine at birth. She was full term and has been tracking nicely on the growth chart with no developmental abnormalities. She was an only child and the family recently moved to the USA. Since arriving, her parents noticed enlarged lymph nodes most prominently involving the left axilla. The pediatrician diagnosed her with suppurative lymphadenitis due to BCG vaccination. She was admitted to the hospital and treated with rifampin, isoniazid, and pyrazinamide for 6 months with improvement. No major issues occurred throughout childhood until 18 years of age when she was admitted to the hospital with fever and multiple lymphadenopathies (axillary and cervical). Given the patients history, isoniazid, rifampin, and pyrazinamide were empirically administered as the initial treatment. A tuberculin skin test with purified protein derivative was negative. She also had a normal nitroblue tetrazolium test, normal immunoglobulin counts, negative results for HIV testing, and normal CD4 and CD8 counts. An axillary lymph node was excised and histologic examination showed a tuberculoid granuloma, with visible acid-fast bacilli. Mycobacterium bovis BCG resistant to pyrazinamide was isolated from the lymph tissue. Pyrazinamide treatment was discontinued, and antibiotics were administered for approximately 1 year with clinical improvement. The patient, currently 26 years old, is well and has had no additional treatment or incidences of unusual infections.

Antigen-Presenting Cells

Dendritic cells are specialized antigen-presenting cells (APCs) that serve an essential role in linking innate and adaptive immunity. For antigens to trigger an adaptive immune response they must first be captured, processed, and presented in a recognizable form to T cells. The three professional APCs that the immune system uses to accomplish this purpose are macrophages, B lymphocytes, and dendritic cells. APCs perform four major functions outlined in Table 15.1.

Of all the APCs, dendritic cells have the broadest range of antigen presentation. Derived from hematopoietic stem cells in the bone marrow, dendritic cells develop discrete functions owing to their expression of specific pattern recognition receptors

Table 15.1 Major functions of antigen presenting cells [1]

1. *Monitoring the intracellular and extracellular environments*: APCs constantly sample the environment, both intracellular and extracellular, for potentially antigenic molecules
2. *Processing antigens through specific pathways*: APCs contain specialized intracellular machinery to break down these molecules and particles and present components of them on the cell surface in a form recognizable to T lymphocytes
3. *Transporting antigens from tissues to the peripheral lymphoid organs for interaction with T cells*: APCs shuttle antigens from tissues to the sites of lymphocyte priming, which are the peripheral lymphoid organs (i.e., lymph nodes, Peyer patches in the intestinal wall, tonsils and adenoids, appendix, and spleen)
4. *Providing activating signals to T cells*: APCs supply critical accessory signals without which T cells cannot become fully activated

(PRRs) and elaboration of specialized secretory products [2]. These PRRs are capable of distinguishing between microbes and self-tissues by recognizing highly conserved pathogen-associated molecular patterns (PAMPs), which are characteristic of a specific group of microbes (e.g., lipopolysaccharide, peptidoglycan, flagellin, microbial RNA and DNA, viral structures such as envelopes and capsids, as well as many other proteins, glycoproteins, and glycolipids). Upon recognition of endotoxin and other PAMPs, APCs like macrophages and dendritic cells promote the production of interleukin-12 (IL-12) and type 1 interferons (IFNs) alpha and beta to further enhance the adaptive immune response to antigens. These mediators are key regulators of dendritic cell development and the T helper type 1 (Th1) immune response leading to a robust host defense [3].

Dendritic Cell Overview

Dendritic cells are present in most tissues where they serve to detect pathogens and process extracellular and intracellular antigen for presentation to T cells in the context of major histocompatibility complex (MHC) molecules and the costimulatory molecules CD80 and CD86 [2]. Upon pathogen detection peripheral tissue dendritic cells activate and then migrate to T-cell areas of draining lymph nodes where they stimulate antigen-specific T-cell responses to induce adaptive immunity or tolerance to self-antigens [4]. In this context, dendritic cells are the primary cells that present antigen to naïve, unprogrammed T lymphocytes and induce their proliferation. Central to the antigen-specific adaptive immune response, these "migratory dendritic cells" are also able to interact with other immune cells including B and natural killer (NK) lymphocytes and innate lymphoid cells (ILCs) [4, 5]. Dendritic cells also act as effector cells, actively secreting IFN-gamma, which further primes dendritic cells to produce more IL-12 through a positive feedback loop as well as activating macrophages so that they are capable of killing intracellular mycobacteria [1].

Classification of Dendritic Cells

The mononuclear phagocyte system (MPS) has been defined as a family of cells comprising bone marrow progenitors, blood monocytes, and tissue macrophages. This system has historically been categorized into monocytes, dendritic cells, and macrophages based on functional and phenotypical characteristics. In the past, experts believed dendritic cells were derived from monocytes; however further research revealed these cells arise through a dedicated pathway of differentiation [6]. Guilliams et al. proposed an updated, unified nomenclature for the MPS classifying cells primarily by their ontogeny (monocyte or dendritic cell lineage) and secondarily by their location, function, and phenotype [7]. Dendritic cells can be divided into two main subsets: myeloid dendritic cells (mDC) and plasmacytoid dendritic cells (pDC). mDC, also known as conventional or classical dendritic cells, are the most numerous and function as professional APCs defined as either cDC1 (expressing CD141/BDCA3, Clec9A, XCR1) or cDC2 (expressing CD11c, CD1c/BDCA1). pDC (expressing CD123, CD303/BDCA2, CD304/BDCA4) mainly circulate and have a specialized role in generating type I interferon responses important for antiviral responses [8]. Both migratory and resident dendritic cells are found in lymph nodes while only cDC1 and cDC2 are found in nonlymphoid tissues (e.g., epithelia) [9]. Additional details of dendritic cell development and function are provided in Table 15.2 and Fig. 15.1 [2].

Table 15.2 Dendritic cell development and function [10–22]

Type	Dependent for differentiation	Functions
cDC1 (CD141/BDCA3, Clec9A, XCR1)	BATF3 and IRF8	Have superior cross-presenting ability via Clec9a and secrete TNFa, IFNg, and IFNl more abundantly than IL-12p40 on TLR3 ligation
cDC2 (CD11c, CD1c/BDCA1)	IRF4 and KLF4	Express TLR1, 2, 4, 5, and 8; produce IL-12 to prime CD4þ Th1 cells; proinflammatory cytokines IL-1b, TNFa, IL-23, and anti-inflammatory IL-10 can generate Th17 or Th2 responses to fungal antigens or allergens, respectively Tissue cDC2 can detect glycolipid antigens of mycobacteria through CD1a expression
pDC (CD123, CD303/BDCA2, CD304/BDCA4)	RUNX2, E2–2, BCL11A, IRF7, and IRF8	Major IFNa-producing cells in response to viral infection Can activate both Th1 and Th2 CD4þ responses and may induce Treg differentiation after viral infection and in the thymus

	Myeloid DCs				Inflammation
	cDC1	cDC2	pDC	LC	Monocyte-derived DC
Phenotype	CD141, Clec9A, XCR1,	CD1c, CD11b, CD11c, SIRPα	CD123, CD303, CD304, CD45RA	Langerin, CD1a, EpCam (Birbeck Granules–EM)	CD14 neg, CD1a, CD1c
TF	**IRF8**, BATF3, ID2	IRF4	**IRF8**, E22, RUNX2	RUNX3, ID2	KLF4
Location	Blood, lymph and non-lymph tissue	Blood, lymph and non-lymph tissue	Blood and lymph tissue	Epidermis, mucosae	Tissue inflammation
TLRs	TLR3 (TLR8)	TLR8 (TLR7, TLR9, TLR4)	TLR7, TLR9	TLR4, TLR9	TLR4, TLR9
Cytokines	IFN lambda (TLR3)	IL-12, IL-1b, TNFα (TLR8) IL-23 (TLR4 or TLR7/8) IL-10 (TLR4)	IFNα (TL7/9) IFN-III	IL-15	IL-12
T cell interactions	CD8+ responses cross present cellular Antigen and immune complexes	CD8+Th1 (IL-12) Th2 (allergens) Th17 (fungal) Location and environment dependent	CD4+/Th2 and CD8+/Th1 Granzyme B secretion	Amplify Th17 responses	CD8/Th1 (IL-12) TNFα, IL-1b, IL-6
Critical biological roles	Anti-tumour Anti-viral (ideal for vaccines)	Regulation of immune responses Tissue homeostasis Anti-mycobacterial	Anti-viral Anti-fungal Regulatory Treg induction after viral infection (HIV) via IDO production	Anti-viral Anti-fungal Lipid presentation via CD1a	Anti bacterial Anti mycobacterial

Fig. 15.1 Phenotype and function of human dendritic cell subsets. Characteristic phenotype, transcription factor requirements, Toll-like receptor (TLR) expression, cytokine production, T-cell interactions, and biological roles of human dendritic cell subsets. IDO, indoleamine 2,3-dioxygenase; RUNX2/3, runt-related transcription factor 2/3; SIRPα, signal regulatory protein alpha. Reproduced from Bigley et al. [2]. Open access article distributed under the Creative Commons Attribution License 4.0 (CCBY), which permits unrestricted use, distribution, and reproduction in any medium, provided the original work is properly cited

Table 15.3 Overview of dendritic cell (dc) deficiency [2]

Gene	Clinical phenotype	Cell phenotype	Effect on dendritic cells
Biallelic IRF8	Mycobacterial and viral infection; intracerebral calcification and developmental delay	Loss of all monocyte and DC subsets. Myeloproliferation	Complete absence of DC/monocyte but preservation of tissue macrophages and lymphoid cells
GATA2	Mycobacterial, viral (HPV) infection. Lymphedema, deafness, autoimmunity, malignancy, MDS/AML	Dendritic cell, monocyte, B and NK lymphoid (DCML) deficiency	Complete absence of DC/monocyte but preservation of tissue macrophages and lymphoid cells

Adapted from Bigley et al. [2]

Role in Immunodeficiency

Animal and human in vitro models suggest that dendritic cells play an important role in immunity; however their importance remains relatively unexplored in vivo. Given their central role as APCs and involvement in infection, autoimmunity, and maintenance of self-tolerance, deficiency or dysfunction of these cells would be expected to have significant clinical consequences. While many PIDs involving T and B lymphocytes are well known, dendritic cell deficiency or dysfunction has not been well described in the literature and is not a routine part of a primary immunodeficiency disease evaluation. Reasons for this lack of dendritic cell-specific PIDs are likely twofold: either dendritic cells are so essential for postnatal viability that a deficiency is not compatible with life or, conversely, dendritic cells only play a minor, partially redundant role in human immunity and therefore a deficiency is not clinically relevant [8]. This is a fairly simplistic explanation that doesn't take into account the practical challenges of studying dendritic cells. Reliably identifying and quantifying dendritic cells in vitro continues to be an issue due to various reasons including nonspecific cell surface markers, gaps in knowledge of hematopoietic precursors, and other technical limitations that preclude direct translation of results to the in vivo setting [8]. At least two forms of dendritic cell deficiency have been described, both leading to increased susceptibility to intracellular pathogens, most notably mycobacteria [23]. An overview of these conditions is provided in Table 15.3.

Mutation of Interferon Regulatory Factor 8

The first is the rarest dendritic cell deficiency and results in a mutation of interferon regulatory factor 8 (IRF8). Prior to the identification of IRF8 deficiency, there were no genetic disorders known to selectively impair dendritic cell development. As a predominately dendritic cell-mediated PID, IRF8 deficiency has provided valuable insight in the role dendritic cells play in human immunity [24]. IRF8 mutations have been reported in only a handful of patients; therefore our understanding is limited. Hambleton et al. described one case of biallelic IRF8 deficiency with an autosomal recessive K108E mutation in a newborn presenting at 10 weeks of age causing developmental defects in dendritic cells and monocytes leading to a complete absence of monocytes, circulating mDC and pDC, and a paucity of tissue-resident dermal dendritic cells [8, 24]. This patient suffered from a number of infections including disseminated infection with BCG following vaccination, severe respiratory viruses, oral candidiasis, and intracerebral calcification subsequently associated with developmental delay [2, 8]. BCG infection responded to transplantation with cord-blood stem cells along with complete donor cell repopulation and resolution of myeloproliferation. The complete lack of monocytes and dendritic cells with this deficiency suggests a common progenitor for these subsets in contrast to the autosomal dominant form defined by a heterozygous loss of function mutation in IRF8 (T8OA) leading to a more selective effect and less severe disease in adults. This single mutation appears to affect CD1c + mDC only resulting in increased susceptibility to BCG, emphasizing the theory that dendritic cells are critical for protection against mycobacteria [8]. Unlike biallelic IRF8 deficiency, the T80A mutation did not require stem cell transplantation and mycobacterial infection responded nicely to chemotherapy.

Mutation of GATA-Binding Factor 2

The second dendritic cell defect is a heterozygous mutation of GATA-binding factor 2 (GATA2) which comprises the largest group of cases [25–27]. This condition is extremely rare and has been described in about 30 patients worldwide [23]. GATA2 mutation leads to dendritic cell, monocyte, B and NK lymphoid deficiency, also known as DCML deficiency, characterized by the loss of all four cell lines in peripheral blood and tissue. Tissue macrophages and epidermal lymphoid cells on the other hand are well-maintained, but there is an almost complete absence of circulating and tissue dendritic cells [28]. GATA2 mutation in childhood is often linked to myelodysplastic syndrome (MDS)/chronic myelomonocytic leukemia (CMML), although immunodeficiency may also be present [29]. Despite the effect on multiple cell lines with this mutation, most patients survive undetected into adulthood (typically third decade of life) although this condition has a wide spectrum of age and phenotype at presentation. Unlike IRF8 deficiency, which most often presents with early developmental defects affecting patients in infancy, GATA2 mutation effects can remain dormant for decades suggesting an exhaustion of precursors over time; however, this phenotype, like IRF8 deficiency, remains poorly understood [8]. PID is the prominent feature of GATA2 defects when presenting in adults, putting patients at higher risk for infections to nontuberculous mycobacteria, opportunistic fungi, and some viruses, especially human papillomavirus (HPV) putting the patient at risk for HPV-driven malignancies. There is also an increased incidence of congenital deafness, primary lymphedema, and autoimmunity as well as a number of noninfectious life-threatening complications that do not relate directly to immunodeficiency including Emberger syndrome (primary lymphedema and MDS/acute myeloid leukemia [AML]), familial MDS/AML, and MonoMac syndrome (monocytopenia with *Mycobacterium avium* complex) [2]. For those patients who avoid developing early malignancies, survival into adulthood is oftentimes due to immune memory developed by a relatively intact immune system in childhood (normal class switched immunoglobulin, grossly intact T-cell compartment, and normal responses to childhood vaccines) [2]. Given the rarity of this condition, details about the influence of genetics, constitutive or acquired mutations, and environmental exposures on the pathogenesis and clinical phenotype are not fully understood [2].

PIDS That Impair Dendritic Cell Function

In addition to the mutations described above, there are several immunodeficiency disorders that have been associated with impaired dendritic cell quantity and function (Table 15.4). While dendritic cell dysfunction has been described in these disorders, the clinical significance of these defects remains unclear.

When to Test

Given the rarity of these conditions determining when to test for dendritic cell deficiency is very difficult. Cases of IRF8 and GATA2 mutations have provided a framework with which to guide clinical decision making as these defects are associated with increased susceptibility to tuberculosis and atypical mycobacteria, viral infections (particularly HPV and herpes simplex virus), pulmonary pathology (recurrent viral and bacterial infections), and autoimmunity. While these nonspecific features suggest global monocyte and dendritic cell loss, pretest risk cannot be accurately defined without a better model of the prevalence of these conditions. In order to advance our understanding of dendritic cell biology in humans, Bigley et al. recommend a more concerted effort to adopt universal survey level analysis (six-color flow cytometry) in all new patients with suspected immunodeficiency alongside typical T- and B-cell subset analysis [2]. A single-platform six-color method allows the analysis of multiple parameters on mDCs and pDCs simultaneously by using antibodies directed against a pool of lineage markers, specifically HLA-DR, CD11c, and CD123 [30]. Abnormal screening or a high index of suspicion would be followed by full immunophenotyping of myeloid mononuclear cells [2]. Using this approach could provide a wealth of new information, providing much needed insight into a part of the immune system that has not been well described.

Table 15.4 Immunodeficiency disorders that affect dendritic cell quantity and function [2]

PID	Mutation	Clinical phenotype	Effect on dendritic cells
Quantitative dendritic cell deficiency in other known disorders (pancytopenias)			
Reticular dysgenesis	Adenylate kinase 2 (AK2)	Neonatal fatal septicemia; hypoplasia of lymphoid organs	Global loss of monocytes, DCs and lymphoid cells
WHIM (warts, hypogammaglobulinemia, immunodeficiency, and myelokathexis)	CXCR4 mutation (CSC-chemokine receptor 4)	Warts (HPV), recurrent bacterial infections, carcinomas	Reduced numbers of monocytes and DCs
PIDs that impair dendritic cell function			
Bare lymphocyte syndrome	CIITA, RFXANK, RFX5, or RFXAP	Failure to thrive, diarrhea, respiratory tract infections, liver/biliary tract disease	Loss of MHC class II expression on leukocytes leads to deficient antigen presentation and failure to mount effective CD4+ T-cell responses
Wiskott-Aldrich syndrome (WAS)	WAS protein (WASp)	Thrombocytopenia, bacterial and viral infections, atopia, autoimmunity, IgA nephropathy, lymphoma	Cytoskeletal protein; affects DC migration and immune synapse with T cells. Impaired T-cell and antibody responses
CD40/CD40L deficiency	CD40 ligand (CD40L) gene (CD40LG)	Opportunistic infections; gastrointestinal and liver/biliary tract disease	Impaired DC signaling cytokine production and cross-presentation
Pitt-Hopkins syndrome	Transcription factor E2-2 (TCF4)	Recurrent infections in 35% of patients. Distinct facial features, epilepsy, intellectual disability	Impaired pDC IFNα responses in vitro
Hyper IgE-syndrome	STAT3 (signal transducer and activator of transcription 3)	Bacterial (*S. aureus*), Aspergillus, *Pneumocystis jirovecii*, mucocutaneous candidiasis, distinctive facial features	Impaired IL-10 responses in DCs

Adapted from Bigley et al. [2]

Conclusion

The few cases of IRF8 and GATA2 deficiencies reported to date have provided some understanding of basic dendritic cell biology and suggest that a loss of these cells has a selective effect on human immunity, specifically protection against mycobacteria. Additional cases of dendritic cell PID need to be identified and described so investigators can determine how these cells interact to induce T-cell memory and if these patients are at risk for additional infections or other autoimmune conditions. Further exploration of dendritic cell deficiency should clarify the genetic factors and cellular pathways of dendritic cell differentiation in human immunology that murine models have failed to elucidate. This combined with better screening practices could lead to improved identification of affected individuals as well as optimal treatment options.

Clinical Pearls and Pitfalls
- Dendritic cells are specialized antigen-presenting cells (APCs) that serve an essential role in linking innate and adaptive immunity.
- IRF8 deficiency causes complete absence of DC/monocyte but preservation of tissue macrophages and lymphoid cells.
- IRF8 deficiency leads to increased susceptibility to mycobacterial and viral infections as well as intracerebral calcification and developmental delay.
- GATA2 deficiency causes complete absence of DC/monocyte but preservation of tissue macrophages and lymphoid cells.
- GATA2 deficiency leads to increased susceptibility to mycobacterial and viral (HPV) infections as well as lymphedema, deafness, autoimmunity, malignancy, and MDS/AML.

References

1. Call ME. Antigen-presenting cells. In: Orange JS, editor. UpToDate. Waltham: UpToDate. Accessed 28 Jan 2020.
2. Bigley V, Barge D, Collina M. Dendritic cell analysis in primary immunodeficiency. Curr Opin Allergy Clin Immunol. 2016;16(6):530–40.
3. Kaplan JL, Shi HN, Walker WA. The role of microbes in developmental immunologic programming. Pediatr Res. 2011;69:465.
4. Segura E, Valladeau-Guilemond J, Donnadieu MH, Sastre-Garau X, Soumelis V, Amigorena S. Characterization of resident and migratory dendritic cells in human lymph nodes. J Exp Med. 2012;209:653–60.
5. Halim TY, Hwang YY, Scanlon ST, Zaghouani H, Garbi N, Fallon PG, et al. Group 2 innate lymphoid cells license dendritic cells to potentiate memory TH2 cell responses. Nat Immunol. 2016;17:57–64.
6. Schlitzer A, Sivakamasundari V, Chen J, Sumatoh HR, Schreuder J, Lum J, et al. Identification of cDC1- and cDC2-committed DC progenitors reveals early lineage priming at the common DC progenitor stage in the bone marrow. Nat Immunol. 2015;16:718–28.
7. Guilliams M, Ginhoux F, Jakubzick C, Naik SH, Onai N, Schraml BU, et al. Dendritic cells, monocytes and macrophages: a unified nomenclature based on ontogeny. Nat Rev Immunol. 2014;14:571–8.
8. Burns SO. Dendritic cell defects in primary immunodeficiency disorders. LymphoSign J. 2016;3(1):1–12.

9. Haniffa M, Ginhoux F, Wang XN, Bigley V, Abel M, Dimmick I, et al. Differential rates of replacement of human dermal dendritic cells and macrophages during hematopoietic stem cell transplantation. J Exp Med. 2009;206:371–85.
10. Grajales-Reyes GE, Iwata A, Albring J, Wu X, Tussiwand R, Kc W, et al. Batf3 maintains auto-activation of Irf8 for commitment of a CD8alpha(þ) conventional DC clonogenic progenitor. Nat Immunol. 2015;16:708–17.
11. Haniffa M, Shin A, Bigley V, McGovern N, Teo P, See P, et al. Human tissues contain CD141(hi) crosspresenting dendritic cells with functional homology to mouse CD103(þ) non-lymphoid dendritic cells. Immunity. 2012;37:60–73.
12. Lauterbach H, Bathke B, Gilles S, Traidl-Hoffmann C, Luber CA, Fejer G, et al. Mouse CD8alphaþ DCs and human BDCA3þ DCs are major producers of IFN-lambda in response to poly IC. J Exp Med. 2010;207:2703–17.
13. Hemont C, Neel A, Heslan M, Braudeau C, Josien R. Human blood mDC subsets exhibit distinct TLR repertoire and responsiveness. J Leukoc Biol. 2013;93:599–609.
14. Schlitzer A, McGovern N, Teo P, Zelante T, Atarashi K, Low D, et al. IRF4 transcription factor-dependent CD11bþ dendritic cells in human and mouse control mucosal IL-17 cytokine responses. Immunity. 2013;38:970–83.
15. Tussiwand R, Everts B, Grajales-Reyes GE, Kretzer NM, Iwata A, Bagaitkar J, et al. Klf4 expression in conventional dendritic cells is required for T helper 2 cell responses. Immunity. 2015;42:916–28.
16. Nizzoli G, Krietsch J, Weick A, Steinfelder S, Facciotti F, Gruarin P, et al. Human CD1cþ dendritic cells secrete high levels of IL-12 and potently prime cytotoxic T-cell responses. Blood. 2013;122:932–42.
17. Harman AN, Bye CR, Nasr N, Sandgren KJ, Kim M, Mercier SK, et al. Identification of lineage relationships and novel markers of blood and skin human dendritic cells. J Immunol. 2013;190:66–79.
18. Van Rhijn I, Ly D, Moody DB. CD1a, CD1b, and CD1c in immunity against mycobacteria. Adv Exp Med Biol. 2013;783:181–97.
19. Sawai CM, Sisirak V, Ghosh HS, Hou EZ, Ceribelli M, Staudt LM, et al. Transcription factor Runx2 controls the development and migration of plasmacytoid dendritic cells. J Exp Med. 2013;210:2151–9.
20. Cisse B, Caton ML, Lehner M, Maeda T, Scheu S, Locksley R, et al. Transcription factor E2-2 is an essential and specific regulator of plasmacytoid dendritic cell development. Cell. 2008;135:37–48.
21. Ippolito GC, Dekker JD, Wang YH, Lee BK, Shaffer AL 3rd, Lin J, et al. Dendritic cell fate is determined by BCL11A. Proc Natl Acad Sci U S A. 2014;111:E998–E1006.
22. Martin-Gayo E, Sierra-Filardi E, Corbi AL, Toribio ML. Plasmacytoid dendritic cells resident in human thymus drive natural Treg cell development. Blood. 2010;115:5366–75.
23. Collin M, Bigley V, Haniffa M, Hambleton S. Human dendritic cell deficiency: the missing ID? Nat Rev Immunol. 2011;11(9):575–83.
24. Hambleton S, Salem S, Bustamante J, Bigley V, Boisson-Dupuis S, Azevedo J, et al. IRF8 mutations and human dendritic-cell immunodeficiency. N Engl J Med. 2011;365(2):127–38.
25. Bigley V, Haniffa M, Doulatov S, Wang XN, Dickinson R, McGovern N, et al. The human syndrome of dendritic cell, monocyte, B and NK lymphoid deficiency. J Exp Med. 2011;208:227–34.
26. Dickinson RE, Griffin H, Bigley V, Reynard LN, Hussain R, Haniffa M, et al. Exome sequencing identifies GATA-2 mutation as the cause of dendritic cell, monocyte, B and NK lymphoid deficiency. Blood. 2011;118:2656–8.
27. Hahn CN, Chong CE, Carmichael CL, Wilkins EJ, Brautigan PJ, Li XC, et al. Heritable GATA2 mutations associated with familial myelodysplastic syndrome and acute myeloid leukemia. Nat Genet. 2011;43:1012–7.

28. Bigley V, Collin M. Dendritic cell, monocyte, B and NK lymphoid deficiency defines the lost lineages of a new GATA-2 dependent myelodysplastic syndrome. Haematologica. 2011;96:1081–3.
29. Wlodarski MW, Hirabayashi S, Pastor V, Starý J, Hasle H, Masetti R, et al. Prevalence, clinical characteristics, and prognosis of GATA2-related myelodysplastic syndromes in children and adolescents. Blood. 2016;127:1387–97.
30. Giannelli S, Taddeo A, Presicce P, Villa ML, Della BS. A six-color flow cytometric assay for the analysis of peripheral blood dendritic cells. Cytometry B Clin Cytom. 2008;74(6):349–55.

Part IV
Innate Immune Defects

Chapter 16
Congenital Neutropenia and Migration Defects

Thomas F. Michniacki, Saara Kaviany, and Kelly Walkovich

Abbreviations

AML	Acute myeloid leukemia
ANC	Absolute neutrophil count
CBCD	Complete blood count with differential
CGD	Chronic granulomatous disease
CHS	Chediak-Higashi syndrome
DADA2	Deficiency of adenosine deaminase 2
DEB	Diepoxybutane
DHR	Dihydrorhodamine
FISH	Fluorescence in situ hybridization
G-CSF	Granulocyte colony-stimulating factor
Hgb	Hemoglobin
HLH	Hemophagocytic lymphohistiocytosis
HSCT	Hematopoietic stem cell transplantation
MDS	Myelodysplastic syndrome
MMC	Mitomycin C (MMC)
MPO	Myeloperoxidase
SBDS	Shwachman-Bodian-Diamond syndrome
SCN	Severe congenital neutropenia
SDS	Shwachman-Diamond syndrome
WBC	White blood count

T. F. Michniacki (✉) · K. Walkovich
Division of Pediatric Hematology/Oncology, C.S. Mott Children's Hospital/University of Michigan, Ann Arbor, MI, USA
e-mail: tmich@med.umich.edu

S. Kaviany
Monroe Carell Jr. Children's Hospital at Vanderbilt, Nashville, TN, USA

Introduction

Congenital conditions caused by an absolute or functional deficiency of neutrophils are associated with considerable morbidity and mortality in children and adults. Quantitative neutrophil disorders include severe congenital neutropenia, cyclic neutropenia, and bone marrow failure syndromes, notably Shwachman-Diamond syndrome [1]. Phagocyte functional deficits result from myeloperoxidase deficiency, chronic granulomatous disease, the leukocyte adhesion disorders, Chediak-Higashi syndrome, and neutrophil-specific granule deficiency [2]. The focus of this chapter is to touch upon many of these disorders and provide clinicians with the knowledge necessary to effectively diagnose and manage these clinically important immunodeficiency conditions (Table 16.1).

Case Presentation 1

A 5-year-old boy was being evaluated by a pediatric hematologist for worsening of neutropenia since the age of 1 year. A routine complete blood cell count with platelets and differential (CBCPD) obtained at 12 months of age showed a white blood cell count (WBC) 3.6×10^3/uL (absolute neutrophil count (ANC) 0.8×10^3/uL), hemoglobin (Hgb) 12.1 g/dL, and platelets 389×10^3/uL. The initial moderate neutropenia was attributed to a recent viral illness and the patient was monitored with annual CBCPDs by his pediatrician. At well-child visits his mother noted that his stools were often loose and voluminous. His growth overall was poor with height falling below the 5th percentile for age. He had no history of bleeding symptoms, persistent adenopathy, or infections requiring hospitalizations. At a recent dental visit, he was found to have gingivitis and notable oral ulcers. Physical examination was without limb or nail abnormalities, significant bruising/petechiae, leukoplakia, or pulmonary crackles. A repeat CBCPD was obtained by the hematologist noting a WBC of 1.3×10^3/uL (ANC 0.3×10^3/uL), Hgb 9.8 g/dL, and platelets 178×10^3/uL. Given CBCD abnormalities a bone marrow examination was performed showing overall marrow hypocellularity (average of 40%) with granulocyte and erythroid hypoplasia but no evidence of dysplastic changes, malignancy, or ringed sideroblasts. Additional laboratory studies revealed a reduced pancreatic isoamylase level, no evidence of abnormal chromosomal breakage upon cellular exposure to mitomycin C (MMC) or diepoxybutane (DEB), and normal telomere lengths within lymphocytes and granulocytes by fluorescence in situ hybridization (FISH) testing.

Table 16.1 Congenital neutropenia and migration defect disorders

Condition	Mutation	Inheritance	Clinical manifestations	Diagnostic testing	Management
Chediak-Higashi syndrome	LYST	AR	Ocular and cutaneous albinism, neurologic decline, large granules within granulocytes, recurrent infections, bleeding, risk of hemophagocytic lymphohistiocytosis (HLH)	Platelet aggregation studies, neurologic imaging, EMG/EEG, peripheral smear review, HLH evaluation studies, light microscopy of hair shafts, genetic testing	Antimicrobial prophylaxis, G-CSF, +/− interferon gamma, therapies targeting HLH, HSCT improves hematologic/immune dysfunction but fails to slow progression of neurologic abnormalities
Chronic granulomatous disease	CYBB CYBA NCF1 NCF2 NCF4 CYBC1	XL AR AR AR AR AR	Catalase-positive organism infections, autoimmunity including granuloma formation/oral ulcers/urologic difficulties/colitis, hepatic dysfunction, risk of fungal disease and mulch pneumonitis	Neutrophil functional testing (DHR preferred), ESR/CRP trending, imaging to evaluate for infections with inflammatory marker elevations, genetic testing	Prophylaxis with TMP-SMX and itraconazole, +/− interferon-gamma, aggressive infection management with broad-spectrum antimicrobials, glucocorticoids for liver granulomas and mulch/nocardia pneumonitis, immunosuppression for significant auto-inflammation, HSCT
Cyclic neutropenia	ELANE	AD	Neutropenia every 14–35 days with associated monocytosis, severe bacterial and fungal infections (including *Clostridium*), osteopenia, oral ulcers and gingivitis, less risk of malignant conversion than severe congenital neutropenia	Bone marrow biopsy, frequent CBCDs to evaluate neutrophil count pattern, genetic testing	G-CSF, HSCT in severe refractory cases

(continued)

Table 16.1 (continued)

Condition	Mutation	Inheritance	Clinical manifestations	Diagnostic testing	Management
Leukocyte adhesion deficiency	ITGB2	AR	Neutrophilia, umbilical cord separation delay, recurrent bacterial infections, inadequate wound healing, severe periodontitis/gingivitis, skin ulcerations, colitis, HPV infections	Absence of functional CD18 and CD11 on leukocytes via flow cytometry, genetic testing	Ustekinumab (IL-23/IL-12 antibody), quality oral hygiene, antimicrobial prophylaxis, GM-CSF not useful, HSCT in those with severe phenotypes
	SLC35C1	AR	Neutrophilia, recurrent infections, developmental delay, short stature with depressed nasal bridge, Bombay (hh) blood phenotype, no delay in umbilical cord separation, periodontal disease	Analysis of blood phenotype, absence of sialyl Lewis X (CD15a) on leukocytes via flow cytometry, genetic testing	Antimicrobial prophylaxis, quality oral hygiene, fucose supplementation (limited evidence)
	FERMT3	AR	Neutrophilia, recurrent bacterial infections, bleeding due to dysfunctional platelet aggregation, osteoporosis-like bone irregularities, delayed umbilical cord separation	Evaluation of integrin activation and expression on leukocytes, functional neutrophil and platelet assays, genetic testing	Antimicrobial prophylaxis, platelet transfusions in those with bleeding, HSCT
Myeloperoxidase deficiency	MPO	AR	Frequently asymptomatic, Candida or other fungal infections in the setting of diabetes or additional immunodeficiency	Histochemical staining for MPO, DHR	Antimicrobial prophylaxis in those with recurrent infections, excellent control of blood glucose levels in diabetics
Severe congenital neutropenia	ELANE HAX1 WAS G6PC3 JAGN1	AD AR XL AR AR	Severe neutropenia (often <200/uL), bone marrow biopsy with absence of myeloid precursors, recurrent bacterial/fungal infections, lack of dysmorphic features, risk of MDS/AML progression	Bone marrow biopsy, CBCDs, genetic testing	G-CSF daily, HSCT with severe disease

Disease	Gene	Inheritance	Clinical features	Diagnostic evaluation	Management
Shwachman-Diamond syndrome	SDBS, EFL1, DNAJC21, SRP54	AR, AR, AR, AD	Bone marrow hypocellularity with pancytopenia, pancreatic exocrine insufficiency, steatorrhea, skeletal abnormalities, hepatic disease, short stature, failure to thrive, elevated risk for MDS/AML	Bone marrow evaluation, ultrasound of pancreas, serum trypsinogen (<3yo) or isoamylase (>3yo), genetic screening	G-CSF, annual bone marrow evaluations, pancreatic enzyme and fat-soluble vitamin replacement, HSCT in those with severe disease
Specific granule defects	CEBPE, SMARCD2	AR, AR	Recurrent bacterial/fungal infections, absence of specific granules within leukocytes, bleeding, frequent bi-lobed neutrophils (pseudo Pelger-Huet anomaly), risk of progression to MDS/AML	Light/electron microscopy evaluation of neutrophils, biochemical measurements of granule proteins, abnormal neutrophil chemotaxis, prolonged bleeding time, genetic testing	Aggressive management of infections, antimicrobial prophylaxis, GM-CSF with severe infections, HSCT in those with significant disease
Wiskott-Aldrich syndrome	WAS	XL	Immunodeficiency with recurrent infections, neutropenia, eczema, malignancy risk, bleeding, lymphadenopathy, hepatosplenomegaly, autoimmunity including immune-mediated thrombocytopenia	WAS protein analysis via flow cytometry on lymphocytes, reduced T lymphocytes and immunoglobulins, decreased mean platelet value, genetic testing	Platelet transfusions (irradiated), prophylactic antimicrobials, IVIG for hypogammaglobulinemia, low-dose IL-2 therapy, rituximab in those with autoimmune cytopenias, HSCT, gene therapy

AD autosomal dominant, *AML* acute myeloid leukemia, *AR* autosomal recessive, *CBCD* complete blood count with differential, *CRP* C-reactive protein, *DHR* dihydrorhodamine, *EEG* electroencephalogram, *EMG* electromyography, *ESR* erythrocyte sedimentation rate, *FISH* fluorescence in situ hybridization, *G-CSF* granulocyte colony-stimulating factor, *GM-CSF* granulocyte-macrophage colony-stimulating factor, *HLH* hemophagocytic lymphohistiocytosis, *HSCT* hematopoietic stem cell transplantation, *IL-2* interleukin-2, *IVIG* intravenous immunoglobulin, *MDS* myelodysplastic syndrome, *MPO* myeloperoxidase, *NBT* nitroblue tetrazolium, *TMP-SMX* trimethoprim-sulfamethoxazole, *XL* X-linked

Diagnosis/Assessment

Signs and Symptoms

Congenital bone marrow failure conditions can present at any age with cytopenias. The diagnosis of Shwachman-Diamond syndrome (SDS) most frequently manifests with intermittent and waxing/waning neutropenia during childhood [3, 4]. Anemia and thrombocytopenia may be present in patients with SDS but may be intermittent and asymptomatic. Bone marrow biopsy often reveals hypocellularity and hematopoietic cell line maturation delay/hypoplasia. Progression to aplastic anemia can occur with additional transformation to myelodysplastic syndrome and acute myeloid leukemia possible. Overall the risk in SDS for having malignant transformation is significant (18–36% at 30 years) but less so than patients with Fanconi anemia (40% by age 50) [3, 5]. SDS-associated neutropenia increases the risk of infections, including severe sepsis, in individuals diagnosed with the condition with additional neutropenic findings of oral ulcerations and gingivitis possible on physical examination. Quantitative and qualitative B- and T-cell defects may also be seen on laboratory analysis, further increasing infectious risk [5, 6].

Classically SDS is associated with exocrine pancreatic dysfunction causing poor growth, insufficient nutrient absorption, steatorrhea, and voluminous stool output, although these findings might not always be present [3, 6]. Asymptomatic patients may still have fatty infiltration within the pancreas on ultrasound imaging and show abnormal pancreatic enzyme testing (reduced fecal elastase, serum trypsinogen, or serum pancreatic isoamylase levels) [3]. The absence of ringed sideroblasts on marrow assessment assists in differing the condition from Pearson syndrome, which additionally has pancreatic dysfunction [7]. Interestingly, pancreatic abnormalities may spontaneously improve as patients age. Hepatic manifestations have also been reported, including hepatomegaly with transaminitis and hyperbilirubinemia findings consistent with cholestasis [3, 5].

Physical examination or imaging may reveal skeletal abnormalities, including metaphyseal dysplasia and thoracic/pelvic dystrophies [3, 6]. Malformed upper extremities and thumbs may be seen but less frequently than in other congenital bone marrow failure syndromes, such as Fanconi anemia, Diamond-Blackfan anemia, or congenital amegakaryocytic thrombocytopenia [8, 9]. Finally, behavioral and neurocognitive manifestations can be present in those with SDS, with some individuals having developmental delay or neuropsychological disorders [5, 6].

Diagnostic Testing

Bone marrow biopsy assists in verifying suspected marrow hypocellularity and evaluating for promyelocytic arrest (a phenomenon associated with severe congenital neutropenia) as well as ruling out additional causes of cytopenias, including malignancy and autoimmune processes. Marrow analysis should include diagnostic pathology, flow cytometry, karyotyping, and FISH screening for dysplastic genetic rearrangements. Telomere length testing is usually normal, unlike in dyskeratosis congenita, and chromosomal breakage upon exposure to DEB and MMC is unremarkable, which differs from Fanconi anemia [8, 10]. Idiopathic or acquired causes of aplastic anemia may manifest similarly with bone marrow hypocellularity but typically present with more pronounced acute anemia and thrombocytopenia and a lack of significant gastrointestinal concerns [11, 12]. Testing for deficiency of adenosine deaminase 2 (DADA2) through quantitative enzyme analysis should be considered as such patients may present with bone marrow failure but typically manifest with early-onset stroke and rheumatologic complaints [13]. In children with pancreatic dysfunction and pulmonary symptoms, cystic fibrosis, often through sweat chloride testing, should be ruled out [14]. Serum trypsinogen testing is most accurate in those <3 years of age, while pancreatic isoamylase analysis is superior if 3 years of age or greater [3, 6].

Genetic testing may verify a suspected diagnosis of SDS. The condition is autosomal recessive in nature with most patients (around 90%) having mutations involving the Shwachman-Bodian-Diamond syndrome (SBDS) gene on chromosome 7q.11. However, up to 10% of patients may fail to have abnormal genetic testing [3, 5]. The SBDS protein appears to have important functions in ribosomal biogenesis, mitotic spindle function. and maintenance of the bone marrow stromal environment. It is still fully unclear how deficits in the abovementioned functions of SBDS lead to the varied clinical manifestations of SDS [5]. Recent studies have shown that additional genes involved in ribosomal biogenesis, DNAJC21, ELF1, and SRP54, may also be associated with a SDS phenotype [6, 15–17].

Management/Outcome

Given the significant clinical variability between patients and the rarity of the disorder, the natural history of SDS is overall poorly defined [3, 6]. CBCPDs should be monitored frequently (at least every 3 months) given risk of progression to significant bone marrow failure and possibility of transformation to dysplasia or myeloid neoplasm. Annual bone marrow evaluations should be strongly considered. Patients with clinically significant neutropenia and a history of recurrent infections may benefit from daily or intermittent dosing of granulocyte colony-stimulating factor (G-CSF) [3, 5]. The need for blood product transfusions is rare with SDS unless considerable marrow hypocellularity is present. Pancreatic enzyme replacement and supplementation of fat-soluble vitamins is necessary in those with significant pancreatic dysfunction but may be discontinued in patients who have resolution of their pancreatic phenotype as they age [3, 5].

Hematopoietic stem cell transplantation should be considered in those with SDS-associated severe aplastic anemia and is often necessary in patients who have progressed to myelodysplastic syndrome (MDS) or acute myeloid leukemia (AML) [5]. Outcomes posttransplantation were previously poor in this population but have improved recently with optimization of supportive care, usage of reduced intensity conditioning regimens, and enhanced prevention of graft-versus-host disease measures, although those with AML continue to have a poor prognosis [6, 18, 19].

Case Presentation 2

An 18-year-old female is hospitalized for her second bout of *Candida* sepsis. She additionally had a history of frequent mucocutaneous fungal infections and polyarthritis and was recently diagnosed with type 1 diabetes mellitus. CBCPDs obtained during admission showed neutrophilia and normal absolute lymphocyte counts. Quantitative T- and B-cell subsets showed normal absolute values with proliferation of T cells to antigens and mitogens additionally unremarkable. Immunoglobulin levels, including IgE, were normal. Dihydrorhodamine oxidation (DHR) testing was abnormal but genetic testing for mutated genes associated with chronic granulomatous disease was negative.

Diagnosis/Assessment

Signs and Symptoms

Myeloperoxidase (MPO) is abundantly found within neutrophils and enzymatically reacts with hydrogen peroxide and chloride to produce hypochlorous acid as part of the respiratory burst pathway that facilitates destruction of phagocytosed microbes [20]. MPO deficiency is one of the most common primary phagocytic disorders but very frequently manifests without any clinical symptoms [21]. Those with complete MPO deficiency may present with an elevated risk of disseminated or invasive candidiasis infections. A concurrent diabetes mellitus diagnosis further increases this risk. Human MPO-deficient neutrophils appear to have a reduced ability to kill *Aspergillus fumigatus*, but patients with MPO deficiency seem to have a less significant risk of *Aspergillus* infection than those with chronic granulomatous disease (CGD) [22, 23]. MPO deficiency is further associated with autoimmune clinical symptoms, revealing the enzyme's importance in regulation of inflammation [24, 25].

Diagnostic Testing

Given that oxidation of DHR to rhodamine 123 requires the presence of hydrogen peroxide, a diagnosis of MPO deficiency can yield abnormal DHR results. Such a finding could lead the clinician to assume a diagnosis of chronic granulomatous disease in this patient. However, abnormal DHR testing may also be present with significant glucose-6-phosphate dehydrogenase deficiency [26]. Histochemical staining for MPO within neutrophils and a normal nitroblue tetrazolium assay result may aid in making the correct diagnosis [22, 26]. Additional disorders of neutrophil function, such as the leukocyte adhesion defect disorders, Chediak-Higashi syndrome, and neutrophil-specific granule deficiency, should also be considered within the differential diagnosis [2].

Human immunodeficiency virus (HIV) should be ruled out in those with severe disseminated fungal infections and a history of chronic mucocutaneous *Candida* infection [27]. Further causes of such infections, including CARD9 and STAT3 deficiencies, should be considered [28, 29]. Even in those found to have a deficiency of MPO, additional causes of the patient's symptomology should be ruled out given the overwhelming majority of MPO-deficient patients are asymptomatic, as incorrectly attributing a patient's clinical manifestations to MPO deficiency may result in overlooking the true cause of their immunodeficiency.

Management/Outcome

Most individuals with MPO deficiency do well and are asymptomatic. Therefore, treatment interventions are often unnecessary. Aggressive management of acute infections in those with a history of invasive organisms should be undertaken. In such individuals, prophylactic antifungal therapy may be helpful. Specific treatments targeting the pathologic cause of the disorder, MPO deficiency, are lacking. Supportive care options include optimal control of serum glucose values in diabetic patients and avoidance when possible, of therapies such as corticosteroids that further exacerbate the risk of fungal infections [22].

Case Presentation 3

An 8-month-old female was hospitalized for her second episode of suppurative lymphadenitis. She also had a history of numerous bouts of pneumonia, as well as persistent stomatitis. During these episodes CBCPDs obtained demonstrated significant neutropenia (absolute neutrophil counts ranging from 0.1×10^9/L to 0.3×10^9/L). Both episodes of lymphadenitis were confirmed to be caused by *Staphylococcus aureus*. She had a normal evaluation of circulating B, T, and NK cells. Her immunoglobulin (IgA, IgM, and IgG) serum concentrations were normal.

Diagnosis/Assessment

Signs and Symptoms

Severe congenital neutropenia (SCN) is characterized by severe neutropenia, with absolute neutrophil counts (ANC) less than 0.2×10^9/L on at least three separate occasions in a one-month time period [1, 30]. Clinically, these patients present with severe bacterial infections early in life. Genetic evaluations have detected both inherited (autosomal dominant, X-linked, or recessive in situations frequently with consanguinity) and spontaneous mutations. Dominant forms are caused by neutrophil elastase (*ELANE*) mutations, while patients with X-linked inheritance will manifest mutations in the Wiskott-Aldrich syndrome (*WAS*) gene. Kostmann syndrome is the autosomal recessive form of the disorder due to pathogenic variants in *HAX1*, characterized by early stage maturation arrest of myeloid differentiation [31]. The incidence of SCN is approximately one in one million [1]. Phenotypically, these patients may present with mouth sores, gingivitis, otitis media, respiratory infections, cellulitis, and skin abscesses. They also may have mild hepatosplenomegaly on exam [1, 30].

Diagnostic Testing

Frequent CBCPD testing over a month period is required for the diagnosis of SCN and to rule out cyclic patterns to the neutropenia. Cyclic neutropenia is an autosomal dominant congenital granulopoietic disorder caused by mutations in the *ELANE* gene as well [1, 32, 33]. This disorder is characterized by periods of normal neutrophil counts oscillating with severe neutropenia classically within a 21-day cycle with 5–7 days of profound neutropenia. Cyclic neutropenia is estimated to effect approximately 0.6 per 1 million people. At times of the neutropenic nadir, reciprocal monocytosis is observed. Clinically, these patients may experience oral ulcers, stomatitis, or cutaneous infections during periods of neutropenia. Diagnosis is made by obtaining CBCPD approximately two to three times a week, for 2 months [1, 33]. Genetic testing confirming pathogenic variants in *ELANE* can also support the diagnosis. Treatment is focused on utilizing G-CSF to minimize the length of neutropenia per cycle such that cycles are typically reduced to 9–11 day cycles with 1–2 days of profound neutropenia [1].

Severe congenital neutropenia patients may demonstrate peripheral blood eosinophilia and monocytosis on the CBCPDs obtained at the time of diagnosis and also during times of profound neutropenia. They may also demonstrate mild thrombocytosis and anemia of chronic disease [1, 30]. Their bone marrow evaluation will demonstrate arrest of myeloid cell maturation at the promyelocytic stage. This maturation arrest in the bone marrow is not seen in immune or idiopathic neutropenia making this assessment a key component of evaluation. Antineutrophil antibody testing may additionally be positive on testing in those suspected of an immune-mediated neutropenia, although a negative result does not rule out a diagnosis of the condition and a positive result does not rule out a diagnosis of congenital conditions, such as SCN [34].

Management/Outcome

The incidence of fatal disease in SCN has decreased tremendously due to the use of G-CSF. The vast majority (95%) of patients respond well to G-CSF, although dosing can be quite variable between patients [1, 30]. In SCN patients requiring extremely high G-CSF dosing (greater than 8–10 mcg/kg/day) or those with severe infections despite apparently adequate G-CSF dosing, hematopoietic stem cell transplant should be considered [35, 36].

Approximately 10–20% of patients with the initial diagnosis of SCN will go on to develop MDS/AML [1, 37]. The development of MDS or AML does not appear to be related to the use of G-CSF. The development of MDS may present with subtle changes in platelet count or hemoglobin or pathologically flawed bone marrow failing to respond appropriately to increases in the dosing of G-CSF. Due to the risk of MDS/AML, annual bone marrow evaluations and every three-month CBCPD are recommended in patients with SCN [37]. In patients who demonstrate cytogenetic abnormalities or MDS on bone marrow evaluation, stem cell transplantation should be pursued, as traditional chemotherapy agents are not effective in these patients [1, 35, 36].

Case Presentation 4

A 2-year-old boy was admitted to the local hospital for evaluation of fever and abdominal pain. His previous history included frequent respiratory infections, recurrent ear infections, and occasional episodes of high fevers. He was noted to have significant lymphadenopathy and hepatosplenomegaly on exam, in addition to pallor and areas of skin hypopigmentation. His laboratory evaluation demonstrated pancytopenia, coagulopathy, and elevated transaminases. In particular, his lymphocytes were noted to have rod-shaped cytoplasmic organelles with a central linear density. His bone marrow evaluation also demonstrated giant intracytoplasmic inclusions in the myeloid cells, as well as evidence of hemophagocytosis.

Diagnosis/Assessment

Signs and Symptoms

Chediak-Higashi syndrome (CHS) is an autosomal recessive disorder caused by mutations in the lysosomal trafficking regulator (*LYST*), leading to formation of giant lysosomes or lysosome-related organelles [38]. Phenotypically, CHS is defined by immunodeficiency, oculocutaneous albinism, and hemophagocytic lymphohistiocytosis (HLH). Patients with CHS also have bleeding phenomena as a result of deficient platelet dense bodies [39, 40]. The immunodeficiency is characterized by incomplete degranulation and chemotaxis defects of neutrophils [41].

To aid in clinical diagnosis, these patients typically have partial albinism with hair colors ranging from gray to white, as well as eye pigmentation changes that can result in photosensitivity. The infections associated with CHS are typically pyogenic, especially involving the respiratory tract and skin. Due to the abovementioned platelet defects, they may have easy bruising and mucosal bleeding. Their neurologic manifestations can include weakness, ataxia, sensory defects, and neurodegeneration [40].

Diagnostic Testing

The hallmark of a CHS diagnosis is the presence of large cytoplasmic granules in granulocytes. Platelet aggregation studies reflect on the deficient platelet granules. Evaluation of hair shafts demonstrates large, speckled pigment clumps [39]. The classic bone marrow evaluation demonstrates abnormal granules in all stages of myeloid cell maturation, as well as evidence of hemophagocytic lymphohistiocytosis. Ultimately genetic testing of the *CHS1/LYST* gene can confirm diagnosis [40].

Other similar disorders include Griscelli syndrome, which also results in partial albinism, respiratory tract infections, hypogammaglobulinemia, and variable cellular immunodeficiency [42]. Griscelli syndrome type 2 patients also demonstrate immunodeficiency phenotypes and hemophagocytic lymphohistiocytosis but these patients do not have the giant granules as seen in CHS [43]. Hermansky-Pudlak also results in oculocutaneous albinism and bleeding phenotypes despite a normal platelet count due to the absent platelet dense bodies. This syndrome, however, does not involve neutrophils or natural killer cell dysfunction or result in the accelerated phase seen in CHS [44].

Other conditions with chemotactic defects of neutrophils include hyperimmunoglobulin (hyper-Ig) E syndrome. Patients present with elevated IgE levels (typically >200 IU-mL), as well as recurrent *Staphylococcal* infection of the respiratory tract and lung [45]. Skeletal and dental abnormalities, in addition to dermatitis, are also seen in patients with hyper-IgE [46].

Management/Outcome

Diagnostic workup is important to identify CHS patients prior to development of the "accelerated phase" if possible. Approximately 85% of patients with CHS will enter this phase, which can occur anytime between birth and early childhood. In the accelerated phase, patients demonstrate fever, pancytopenia, hepatosplenomegaly, lymphadenopathy, coagulopathy, and jaundice. This accelerated phase is a nonmalignant infiltrate of lymphohistiocytes across multiple organs [39, 40]. It is typically precipitated by infection, in particular Epstein-Barr virus infections [40, 47]. Unfortunately, development of the accelerated phase can be fatal as result of severe anemia, bleeding complications, or infectious complications. In patients who do survive past the first decade of life (<20%), progressive neurological dysfunction typically leads to further complications [39, 40].

Supportive care including prophylactic antibiotics given immune dysfunction is key in patients with CHS. Treatment of the hematologic and immune defects of CHS is bone marrow transplant; however the neurological outcomes are not improved after transplantation. Higher mortality is associated with patients who enter transplant at the time of the accelerated phase [48, 49].

Case Presentation 5

A 3-year-old girl was referred to pediatric hematology for evaluation of a persistent mild-moderate leukocytosis in the setting of recurrent *Staphylococcal aureus* skin infections. In review of her history, she was hospitalized for the first 2 weeks of life due to omphalitis and a presumed leukemoid reaction. With intravenous antibiotics, her omphalitis resolved, and her leukocytosis improved, although her parents note she had persistent neutrophilia even at discharge. In addition, she has received antibiotics three additional times for extensive skin abscesses. Incision and drainage of each abscess was attempted and yielded positive growth of *Staphylococcal aureus* but no pus. The complete blood count obtained at her 1-year well-child visit showed her white blood cell count (WBC) was 21.8×10^3/uL (absolute neutrophil count (ANC) 17.2×10^3/uL), hemoglobin (Hgb) 12.1 g/dL, and platelets 482×10^3/uL. A dihydrorhodamine flow assay previously demonstrated a normal oxidative burst. Physical exam was notable for poor dentition with diffuse gingival hyperemia and two ulcerative skin lesions on her left leg. Flow cytometric analysis for CD18 expression on neutrophils was decreased and CD11b expression was nearly absent.

Diagnosis/Assessment

Signs and Symptoms

Patients with leukocyte adhesion deficiency 1 (LAD1), particularly those with severe disease, routinely present in the newborn period often with omphalitis, delayed umbilical cord separation and recurrent infections, especially with *Staphylococcus aureus* and gram-negative bacilli. Of note, delayed umbilical cord separation is not reported in other forms of LAD but is frequently found in patients with urachal anomalies [50]. Moreover, delayed umbilical cord separation is not uniformly seen in patients with LAD1. Laboratory evaluation of LAD1 patients demonstrates a neutrophil predominant leukocytosis that may be subtle during periods of wellness but exuberant with infections. The physical exam is notable for the lack of pus formation and poor wound healing. Older patients have near universal periodontal disease secondary to dysregulation of the IL17/23 axis [51] with many patients suffering complete loss of their teeth by late adolescence. Additionally, LAD1 patients are prone to inflammatory skin lesions that are pyoderma gangrenosum-like in appearance although notably on biopsy do not have a neutrophilic infiltrate [52], inflammatory bowel disease [53], and HPV-related warts [54].

The differential diagnosis for patients with suspected LAD1 includes LADII (impaired fucosylation of macromolecules, especially selections) and LADIII (defective beta integrin activation) as well as other related defects that share a common link of a defect in adhesion protein or flawed regulation of adhesion proteins that do not allow phagocytes to migrate from the peripheral blood across the endothelium and into tissue. Importantly, LADII patients can be clinically distinguished by the high frequency of neurologic manifestations, craniofacial anomalies, and the presence of the rare Bombay erythrocyte phenotype, while LADIII is accompanied by bleeding diatheses.

Diagnostic Testing

Criteria for the diagnosis of LAD1 was published in 1999 and relies heavily on the decreased expression of CD18 on leukocytes (<5% expression) in the appropriate clinical setting of recurrent or deep-seated infections, delayed umbilical cord separation, poor wound healing, and leukocytosis [55]. Updated flow cytometric analysis for LAD1 suggests that both the assessment of CD18 and CD11 (through either CD11a, CD11b, or CD11c) expression on leukocytes be routinely performed as some patients with LAD1 may have expression or residual function of CD18; however, all LAD1 patients have near absent expression of CD11 subunits. Utilizing both CD18 and CD11a measurements increases the sensitivity of the assay and minimizes the risk of delayed or missed diagnoses [56]. Beyond functional testing, genetic sequencing is being increasingly utilized to identify biallelic pathogenic variants in the common beta chain of the beta-2 integrin family (*ITGB2*). Identification of familial pathogenic variants is being increasingly used in prenatal counseling.

LADII patients can be diagnosed through flow cytometric analysis of peripheral blood leukocytes to assess for the absence of properly fucosylated macromolecules, particularly of sialyl Lewis X expression, i.e., CD15a. Confirmation of LADII is obtained through sequencing the gene encoding the GDP-fucose transporter. LADIII patients primarily rely on identification of pathogenic variants in the kindlin-3 gene, although functional assessment of integrin function is also useful.

Management/Outcomes

Optimal management of LAD1 is dependent on the severity of disease. Historically, severity of clinical features and the magnitude of functional defects have been directly related to the degree of CD18 expression [57], although the correlation is imperfect as several cases of LAD1 are now recognized to have normal expression of CD18, albeit nonfunctional.

Patients are generally classified into severe and moderate subgroups with a relative assignment of less than 2% CD18 expression of the β2 integrins considered severe disease. Patients with severe disease have historically been assigned a very poor prognosis with most patients dying in the first decade of life without hematopoietic stem cell transplant (HSCT) [58]. HSCT is the only current curative option for LAD1, although gene therapy has been explored [59]. Patients with mild/moderate disease respond to conservative measures including optimizing oral hygiene, aggressive antimicrobial therapy for infections, and prevention of infection through prophylactic antibiotics as needed and vaccination, particularly immunization against HPV.

For the management of periodontal and/or skin disease related to LAD1, ustekinumab, a monoclonal antibody of the p40 subunit common to IL-12 and IL-23, has been used with favorable results [51]. LADII management relies on the use of antibiotics and fucose supplementation, while LADIII management is focused on management of bleeding complications and consideration of HSCT [60].

Conclusion

Congenital neutropenia and migration defect disorders may manifest with various phenotypes, but all can cause an elevated risk of serious bacterial, fungal, and even viral infections. Early diagnosis is essential to decreasing the morbidity and mortality of these conditions with crucial diagnostic laboratory analyses including functional neutrophil studies, flow cytometry, and direct pathologic evaluation of the bone marrow and peripheral blood. Supportive care often entails usage of antimicrobial prophylaxis, aggressive management of infectious complications, and regular administration of G-CSF. Frequently hematopoietic stem cell transplantation can be curative but is not without risks.

Clinical Pearls/Pitfalls
- Congenital bone marrow failure syndromes may present with a reduction in only one cell line and may not diagnostically become apparent until adulthood.
- Abnormal physical exam findings may be crucial to assisting in the diagnosis of congenital neutropenia and migration defect disorders.
- Significant enzymatic deficiencies in MPO and glucose-6-phosphate dehydrogenase may lead to abnormal DHR testing results, leading to an incorrect presumed diagnosis of chronic granulomatous disease.
- Clinically asymptomatic and well-appearing African-Americans may present with ANC values less than 500/microL which is likely consistent with a diagnosis of Duffy null benign ethnic neutropenia, rather than severe congenital neutropenia.
- Griscelli syndrome may present similarly to Chediak-Higashi syndrome with albinism, immunodeficiency, and hemophagocytosis but Chediak-Higashi syndrome may be differentiated by microscopic examination of patient hair shaft and peripheral blood granulocytes.
- Delayed umbilical cord detachment should raise suspicion for LAD1, but evaluation for urachal anomalies should also be considered.
- HSCT remains the only curative therapy for leukocyte adhesion defects, but IL-23 directed therapy with ustekinumab has shown promise in improving oral and skin manifestations of LAD1.
- Patients with LADII can be easily differentiated from LAD1 patients by the presence of the rare Bombay blood group in patients with LADII.

References

1. Walkovich K, Boxer LA. How to approach neutropenia in childhood. Pediatr Rev. 2013;34:173–84.
2. Amulic B, Cazalet C, Hayes GL, Metzler KD, Zychlinsky A. Neutrophil function: from mechanisms to disease. Annu Rev Immunol. 2012;30:459–89.
3. Myers KC, Bolyard AA, Otto B, Wong TE, Jones AT, Harris RE, et al. Variable clinical presentation of Shwachman-Diamond syndrome: update from the North American Shwachman-Diamond Syndrome Registry. J Pediatr. 2014;164:866–70.
4. Lachowiez C, Meyers G. Identifying unexpected inherited marrow failure syndromes in adults presenting with Aplastic Anemia, MDS or solid tumors. Blood. 2016;128:5071–1.
5. Myers KC, Davies SM, Shimamura A. Clinical and molecular pathophysiology of Shwachman-Diamond syndrome: an update. Hematol Oncol Clin North Am. 2013;27:117–128, ix.
6. Nelson AS, Myers KC. Diagnosis, treatment, and molecular pathology of Shwachman-Diamond Syndrome. Hematol Oncol Clin North Am. 2018;32:687–700.
7. Farruggia P, Di Marco F, Dufour C. Pearson syndrome. Expert Rev Hematol. 2018;11:239–46.
8. Triemstra J, Pham A, Rhodes L, Waggoner DJ, Onel K. A review of Fanconi anemia for the practicing pediatrician. Pediatr Ann. 2015;44:444–5, 448, 450 passim.
9. Dokal I, Vulliamy T. Inherited aplastic anaemias/bone marrow failure syndromes. Blood Rev. 2008;22:141–53.
10. Savage SA. Human telomeres and telomere biology disorders. Prog Mol Biol Transl Sci. 2014;125:41–66.
11. Young NS. Aplastic Anemia. N Engl J Med. 2018;379:1643–56.
12. Kallen ME, Dulau-Florea A, Wang W, Calvo KR. Acquired and germline predisposition to bone marrow failure: diagnostic features and clinical implications. Semin Hematol. 2019;56:69–82.
13. Michniacki TF, Hannibal M, Ross CW, Frame DG, DuVall AS, Khoriaty R, et al. Hematologic manifestations of deficiency of adenosine deaminase 2 (DADA2) and response to tumor necrosis factor inhibition in DADA2-associated bone marrow failure. J Clin Immunol. 2018;38:166–73.
14. VanDevanter DR, Kahle JS, O'Sullivan AK, Sikirica S, Hodgkins PS. Cystic fibrosis in young children: a review of disease manifestation, progression, and response to early treatment. J Cyst Fibros. 2016;15:147–57.
15. Dhanraj S, Matveev A, Li H, Lauhasurayotin S, Jardine L, Cada M, et al. Biallelic mutations in DNAJC21 cause Shwachman-Diamond syndrome. Blood. 2017;129:1557–62.
16. Carapito R, Konantz M, Paillard C, Miao Z, Pichot A, Leduc MS, et al. Mutations in signal recognition particle SRP54 cause syndromic neutropenia with Shwachman-Diamond-like features. J Clin Invest. 2017;127:4090–103.
17. Bezzerri V, Cipolli M. Shwachman-diamond syndrome: molecular mechanisms and current perspectives. Mol Diagn Ther. Epub ahead of print 9 November 2018. https://doi.org/10.1007/s40291-018-0368-2.
18. Cesaro S, Oneto R, Messina C, Gibson BE, Buzyn A, Steward C, et al. Haematopoietic stem cell transplantation for Shwachman-Diamond disease: a study from the European group for blood and marrow transplantation. Br J Haematol. 2005;131:231–6.
19. Dalle J-H, Peffault de Latour R. Allogeneic hematopoietic stem cell transplantation for inherited bone marrow failure syndromes. Int J Hematol. 2016;103:373–9.
20. Aratani Y. Myeloperoxidase: its role for host defense, inflammation, and neutrophil function. Arch Biochem Biophys. 2018;640:47–52.
21. Parry MF, Root RK, Metcalf JA, Delaney KK, Kaplow LS, Richar WJ. Myeloperoxidase deficiency: prevalence and clinical significance. Ann Intern Med. 1981;95:293–301.
22. Ren R, Fedoriw Y. The molecular pathophysiology, differential diagnosis, and treatment of MPO deficiency. J Clin Exp Pathol;2. Epub ahead of print 2012. https://doi.org/10.4172/2161-0681.1000109.

23. Falcone EL, Holland SM. Invasive fungal infection in chronic granulomatous disease: insights into pathogenesis and management. Curr Opin Infect Dis. 2012;25:658–69.
24. Neutrophil-mediated regulation of innate and adaptive immunity: the role of myeloperoxidase. https://www.hindawi.com/journals/jir/2016/2349817/. Accessed 15 Oct 2019.
25. Kutter D, Devaquet P, Vanderstocken G, Paulus JM, Marchal V, Gothot A. Consequences of total and subtotal myeloperoxidase deficiency: risk or benefit ? Acta Haematol. 2000;104:10–5.
26. Milligan KL, Mann D, Rump A, Anderson VL, Hsu AP, Kuhns DB, et al. Complete myeloperoxidase deficiency: beware the 'false-positive' dihydrorhodamine oxidation. J Pediatr. 2016;176:204–6.
27. Blood GA. Human immunodeficiency virus (HIV). Transfus Med Hemother. 2016;43:203–22.
28. Corvilain E, Casanova J-L, Puel A. Inherited CARD9 deficiency: invasive disease caused by Ascomycete Fungi in previously healthy children and adults. J Clin Immunol. 2018;38:656–93.
29. Farmand S, Kremer B, Häffner M, et al. Eosinophilia and reduced STAT3 signalling affect neutrophil cell death in autosomal-dominant Hyper-IgE syndrome. Eur J Immunol. Epub ahead of print 13 October 2018. https://doi.org/10.1002/eji.201847650.
30. Welte K, Zeidler C, Dale DC. Severe congenital neutropenia. Semin Hematol. 2006;43:189–95.
31. Boztug K, Klein C. Genetics and pathophysiology of severe congenital neutropenia syndromes unrelated to neutrophil elastase. Hematol Oncol Clin North Am. 2013;27:43–60, vii.
32. Horwitz MS, Corey SJ, Grimes HL, Tidwell T. ELANE mutations in cyclic and severe congenital neutropenia: genetics and pathophysiology. Hematol Oncol Clin North Am. 2013;27:19–41, vii.
33. Lange RD, Jones JB. Cyclic neutropenia. Review of clinical manifestations and management. Am J Pediatr Hematol Oncol. 1981;3:363–7.
34. Newburger PE, Dale DC. Evaluation and management of patients with isolated neutropenia. Semin Hematol. 2013;50:198–206.
35. Carlsson G, Winiarski J, Ljungman P, Ringdén O, Mattsson J, Nordenskjöld M, et al. Hematopoietic stem cell transplantation in severe congenital neutropenia. Pediatr Blood Cancer. 2011;56:444–51.
36. Fioredda F, Iacobelli S, van Biezen A, Gaspar B, Ancliff P, Donadieu J, et al. Stem cell transplantation in severe congenital neutropenia: an analysis from the European Society for Blood and Marrow Transplantation. Blood. 2015;126:1885–92; quiz 1970.
37. Skokowa J, Dale DC, Touw IP, Zeidler C, Welte K. Severe congenital neutropenias. Nat Rev Dis Primers. 2017;3:17032.
38. Gil-Krzewska A, Saeed MB, Oszmiana A, Fischer ER, Lagrue K, Gahl WA, et al. An actin cytoskeletal barrier inhibits lytic granule release from natural killer cells in patients with Chediak-Higashi syndrome. J Allergy Clin Immunol. 2018;142:914–927.e6.
39. Introne W, Boissy RE, Gahl WA. Clinical, molecular, and cell biological aspects of Chediak-Higashi syndrome. Mol Genet Metab. 1999;68:283–303.
40. Kaplan J, De Domenico I, Ward DM. Chediak-Higashi syndrome. Curr Opin Hematol. 2008;15:22–9.
41. Clark RA, Kimball HR. Defective granulocyte chemotaxis in the Chediak-Higashi syndrome. J Clin Invest. 1971;50:2645–52.
42. Mancini AJ, Chan LS, Paller AS. Partial albinism with immunodeficiency: Griscelli syndrome: report of a case and review of the literature. J Am Acad Dermatol. 1998;38:295–300.
43. Minocha P, Choudhary R, Agrawal A, Sitaraman S. Griscelli syndrome subtype 2 with hemophagocytic lympho-histiocytosis: a case report and review of literature. Intractable Rare Dis Res. 2017;6:76–9.
44. El-Chemaly S, Young LR. Hermansky-Pudlak Syndrome. Clin Chest Med. 2016;37:505–11.
45. Dinauer MC. Disorders of neutrophil function: an overview. Methods Mol Biol. 2007;412:489–504.
46. Al-Shaikhly T, Ochs HD. Hyper IgE syndromes: clinical and molecular characteristics. Immunol Cell Biol. 2019;97:368–79.

47. Merino F, Henle W, Ramírez-Duque P. Chronic active Epstein-Barr virus infection in patients with Chediak-Higashi syndrome. J Clin Immunol. 1986;6:299–305.
48. Thakor A, Geng B, Liebhaber M, Moore T, Wang K, Roberts RL. Successful stem cell transplantation in Chediak-Higashi syndrome. J Allergy Clin Immunol Pract. 2015;3:271–2.
49. Eapen M, DeLaat CA, Baker KS, Cairo MS, Cowan MJ, Kurtzberg J, et al. Hematopoietic cell transplantation for Chediak-Higashi syndrome. Bone Marrow Transplant. 2007;39:411–5.
50. Razvi S, Murphy R, Shlasko E, Cunningham-Rundles C. Delayed separation of the umbilical cord attributable to urachal anomalies. Pediatrics. 2001;108:493–4.
51. Moutsopoulos NM, Zerbe CS, Wild T, Dutzan N, Brenchley L, DiPasquale G, et al. Interleukin-12 and interleukin-23 blockade in leukocyte adhesion deficiency type 1. N Engl J Med. 2017;376:1141–6.
52. Simpson AM, Chen K, Bohnsack JF, Lamont MN, Siddiqi FA, Gociman B. Pyoderma gangrenosum-like wounds in leukocyte adhesion deficiency: case report and review of literature. Plast Reconstr Surg Glob Open. 2018;6:e1886.
53. Uzel G, Kleiner DE, Kuhns DB, Holland SM. Dysfunctional LAD-1 neutrophils and colitis. Gastroenterology. 2001;121:958–64.
54. Leiding JW, Holland SM. Warts and all: human papillomavirus in primary immunodeficiencies. J Allergy Clin Immunol. 2012;130:1030–48.
55. Conley ME, Notarangelo LD, Etzioni A. Diagnostic criteria for primary immunodeficiencies. Representing PAGID (Pan-American Group for Immunodeficiency) and ESID (European Society for Immunodeficiencies). Clin Immunol. 1999;93:190–7.
56. Levy-Mendelovich S, Rechavi E, Abuzaitoun O, Vernitsky H, Simon AJ, Lev A, et al. Highlighting the problematic reliance on CD18 for diagnosing leukocyte adhesion deficiency type 1. Immunol Res. 2016;64:476–82.
57. Anderson DC, Schmalsteig FC, Finegold MJ, Hughes BJ, Rothlein R, Miller LJ, et al. The severe and moderate phenotypes of heritable Mac-1, LFA-1 deficiency: their quantitative definition and relation to leukocyte dysfunction and clinical features. J Infect Dis. 1985;152:668–89.
58. Etzioni A. Genetic etiologies of leukocyte adhesion defects. Curr Opin Immunol. 2009;21:481–6.
59. Qasim W, Cavazzana-Calvo M, Davies EG, Davis J, Duval M, Eames G, et al. Allogeneic hematopoietic stem-cell transplantation for leukocyte adhesion deficiency. Pediatrics. 2009;123:836–40.
60. Stepensky PY, Wolach B, Gavrieli R, Rousso S, Ben Ami T, Goldman V, et al. Leukocyte adhesion deficiency type III: clinical features and treatment with stem cell transplantation. J Pediatr Hematol Oncol. 2015;37:264–8.

Chapter 17
Chronic Granulomatous Disease

Danielle E. Arnold and Jennifer R. Heimall

Introduction

Chronic granulomatous disease (CGD) is a rare inherited primary immunodeficiency due to mutations in any of the critical subunits of the phagocyte NADPH oxidase complex, resulting in impaired oxidase activity of neutrophils, monocytes, and tissue macrophages. It is characterized by increased susceptibility to recurrent and severe infections with a subset of microorganisms, granuloma formation, and inflammatory disease. CGD was first described by Janeway et al. in 1954 [1] and was dubbed "fatal granulomatous disease of childhood" in 1959 [2], with most patients historically succumbing to infection or other complications of disease by 10 years of age. However, with increasing awareness of disease, widespread use of prophylactic antimicrobials, and advancements in hematopoietic stem cell transplantation (HSCT), outcomes have improved dramatically and many patients now live well into adulthood.

Mechanism of Neutrophil Dysfunction

Neutrophils play a key role in the defense against invading pathogens primarily by engulfing and rapidly killing microbes within phagocytic vacuoles via activation of the NADPH oxidase complex and the resultant "respiratory burst" during which

---

D. E. Arnold (✉) · J. R. Heimall
Immune Deficiency – Cellular Therapy Program, National Cancer Institute, National Institutes of Health, Bethesda, MD, USA
e-mail: danielle.arnold@nih.gov

reactive oxygen species (ROS) are generated and microbicidal proteases are activated. The NADPH oxidase complex is assembled from both membrane-bound proteins embedded in the walls of secondary granules and distinct cytosolic proteins (Fig. 17.1). The membrane-bound heterodimer cytochrome b558 is composed of the catalytic glycoprotein gp91phox and the non-glycosylated protein p22phox. Upon phagocyte activation, the cytosolic proteins p47phox, p67phox, and p40phox translocate to cytochrome b558 and recruit Rac1/2 to form the activated NADPH oxidase complex. Upon formation of the activated NADPH oxidase complex, gp91phox undergoes a conformational change to expose the protein's catalytic component, which then shuttles electrons from cytosolic NADPH to molecular oxygen in the phagolysosome, leading to the formation of superoxide ions. Superoxide ions are used to generate reactive oxygen species (ROS) such as hydrogen peroxide, hypochlorous acid, hydroxyl radicals, and secondary amines that participate in the direct killing of phagocytosed microorganisms. The creation of the hydroxyl radical also results in an overall negative charge within the phagolysosome, triggering the rapid influx of potassium,

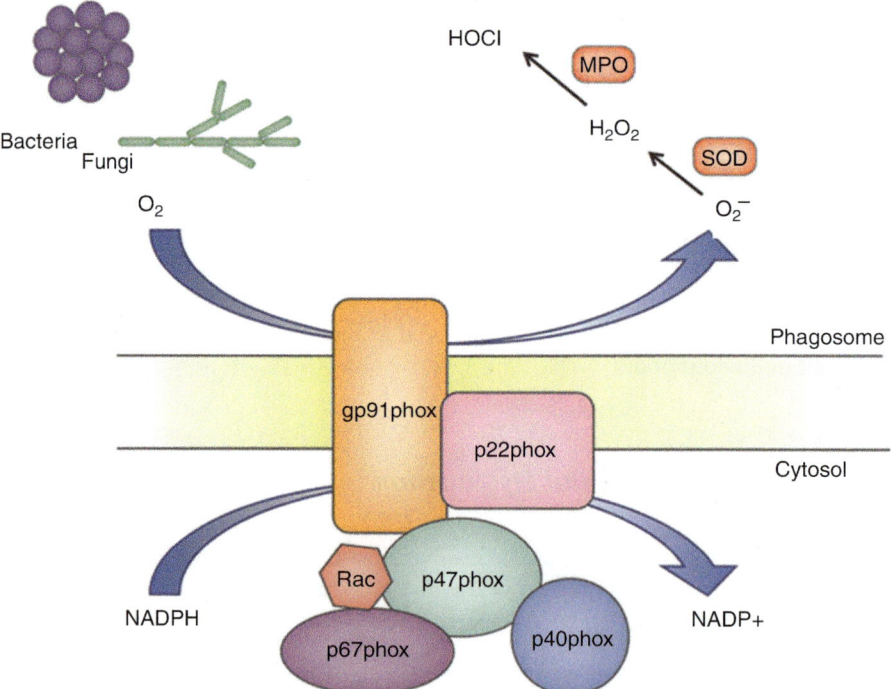

Fig. 17.1 The activated NADPH oxidase complex. Upon phagocyte activation, the various components of NADPH oxidase come together to form the activated NADPH oxidase complex. Gp91phox shuttles electrons from cytosolic NADPH to molecular oxygen in the phagolysosome, resulting in the formation of superoxide ion (O_2^-). Superoxide ion is converted to hydrogen peroxide (H_2O_2) either spontaneously or by superoxide dismutase (SOD), and hydrogen peroxide is converted to hypochlorous acid (HOCl, bleach) by myeloperoxidase. Bleach is then able to directly kill engulfed pathogens

which in turns leads to activation of intraphagosomal proteases that further contribute to microbial clearance [3]. Additionally, the NADPH oxidase complex is required for the activation of neutrophil extracellular traps (NETs) [4], which are webs of chromatin filaments and antimicrobial peptides that are released from apoptotic neutrophils and entrap extracellular pathogens to facilitate clearance by the immune system.

Of note, neutrophils are essential for the elimination of a wide spectrum of microorganisms; however, patients with CGD are at increased risk of infection almost exclusively with catalase-positive pathogens. This is thought to be because the distal mechanisms of the bactericidal pathway, including myeloperoxidase, remain intact in patients with CGD. Catalase-positive organisms, however, can degrade host-produced hydrogen peroxide before it is converted to hypochlorous acid by myeloperoxidase, thus escaping this mechanism of killing. That being said, only a subset of catalase-positive microorganisms is responsible for the majority of infections seen in CGD, the reasons for which remain unclear.

Epidemiology

The incidence of CGD varies significantly worldwide. A large retrospective review of a national registry reported an incidence of about 1:200,000–250,000 live births in the United States [5]. Interestingly, the incidence of CGD is quite variable across Europe, ranging from 1:133,000 in the United Kingdom to 1:100,000 in Italy [6, 7]. Published rates of CGD by country are shown in Table 17.1 [5–11].

Genetics

Mutations in any of the five structural subunits of the NADPH oxidase complex result in defective ROS production and the clinical presentation of CGD (Table 17.2). Mutations in the *CYBB* gene, which encodes the transmembrane glycoprotein gp91phox and is the located on the X chromosome, is the most common cause of

Table 17.1 Reported rates of CGD worldwide

Country	Rate of CGD
United States [5]	1:200,000–250,000
United Kingdom [6]	1:133,000
Italy [7]	1:1,000,000
Sweden [8]	1:450,000
Greece [9]	1:45,450
Japan [10]	1:300,000
Israel [11]	
Jews	1:100,000
Arabs	1:67,000

Table 17.2 Genetic etiology of CGD in the United States and Western Europe

Gene	Protein	Mode of inheritance	Proportion of CGD
CYBB	gp91phox	X-linked	67%
CYBA	p22phox	AR	5%
NCF1	p47phox	AR	20–25%
NCF2	p67phox	AR	5%
NCF4	p40phox	AR	26 cases
CYBC1	CYBC1/Eros	AR	9 cases

AR autosomal recessive

CGD worldwide and accounts for approximately two-thirds of cases of CGD in North America and Europe [5–7, 12–14]. Biallelic pathogenic mutation in *NCF1* (p47phox) is the most common cause of autosomal recessive CGD and accounts for between 20% and 25% of CGD, and mutations in *CYBA* (p22phox) and *NCF2* (p67phox) each account for about 5% of cases. There have been 26 reported cases of CGD due to *NCF4* (p40phox) mutations [15, 16]. Interestingly, these patients suffered from significant autoinflammatory disease but none of the patients had the recurrent infections characteristic of the other genetic forms of CGD. Of note, in countries with high rates of consanguinity, the incidence of autosomal recessive CGD often exceeds that of X-linked CGD.

Recently, biallelic loss-of-function mutations in *CYBC1* were identified as the genetic cause of CGD in a cohort of eight patients from Iceland and in one patient from Saudi Arabia [17, 18]. Most of the patients suffered from recurrent infections and several had autoinflammatory disease, including colitis and histopathological evidence of granuloma formation. *CYBC1* is not directly involved in the respiratory burst but was found to be essential for the expression of the gp91phox/p22phox heterodimer and formation of the NADPH oxidase complex. All patients had an impaired neutrophil oxidative burst on whom testing was performed.

Finally, *CYBB* is located at Xp21.1, and patients with large deletions in the X chromosome may have other monogenic disorders in addition to CGD. The *XK* gene, which encodes the Kx blood group, is immediately telomeric to *CYBB*, and the loss of *XK* results in McLeod syndrome, the most common syndrome seen with CGD. Patients with McLeod syndrome are severely restricted for receiving transfusions, which may have implications for those patients under consideration for HSCT. Larger deletions may also result in loss of *RPGR* (retinitis pigmentosa), *DMD* (Duchenne muscular dystrophy), and *OTC* (ornithine transcarbamylase deficiency).

Case Presentation 1

A 6-year-old boy with a history of recurrent cutaneous abscesses and one prior episode of *Aspergillus fumigatus* pneumonia at 4 years of age presents to the ED with 3 days of low-grade fever and vague abdominal pain. The boy appeared tired, and physical exam was notable for slight guarding on palpation of the right upper quadrant and a liver edge palpable 2 cm below the right costal margin. Labs were remarkable for an elevated white blood cell count at $12.6 \times 10^3/\mu L$ and an elevated C-reactive protein level at 9.8 mg/dL (normal < 1.0). Transaminases, bilirubin, and albumin levels were all normal. A right upper quadrant ultrasound demonstrated a loculated collection of fluid 6.2 cm in diameter in the right hepatic lobe, and the patient was empirically started on piperacillin-tazobactam plus metronidazole. He underwent percutaneous drainage of the abscess, and cultures returned positive for methicillin-sensitive *Staphylococcus aureus* at 9 h. Antibiotics were transitioned to oxacillin monotherapy at that time. Immunology was consulted given the patient's infectious history, and the new unusual diagnosis of a *Staphylococcal* liver abscess. Immune workup demonstrated normal quantitative immunoglobulin levels and lymphocyte subset counts with protective vaccine titers. Dihydrorhodamine assay demonstrated a broad-based histogram peak with a modest shift of the fluorescence signal in stimulated neutrophils characteristic of autosomal recessive CGD. After 9 days on antibiotic therapy, the patient continued to spike intermittent fevers, and his CRP remained elevated despite broadening antibiotics to vancomycin and meropenem. Repeat ultrasound demonstrated that the abscess had increased in size to 8.4 cm in diameter, and so methylprednisolone 1 mg/kg/day was initiated given the patient's new diagnosis of CGD. The patient defervesced, and repeat ultrasound 3 days later demonstrated shrinking of the abscess. The liver abscess resolved over the next 6 weeks, and glucocorticoids were weaned off over a period of 5 months. Genetic testing ultimately demonstrated a deleterious mutation in the *NCF1* gene, and the patient was started on trimethoprim-sulfamethoxazole and itraconazole prophylaxis.

Diagnosis/Assessment

This patient's clinical presentation is characteristic for CGD with onset of symptoms at an early age and a history of recurrent often unusual infections. In general, patients with X-linked CGD have a more severe disease course with earlier age of onset (9–14 months) and diagnosis (2.1–4.9 years) compared to patients with autosomal recessive disease (mean age of onset 30–41 months and diagnosis 5.8–8.8 years) [5–7, 11, 12]. Most patients present with infection, as this patient did, and infection remains the leading cause of death in patients with CGD despite the use of appropriate antimicrobial prophylaxis [5, 19].

Infections in CGD

Infections are primarily with a subset of catalase-positive microorganisms, and the most common sites of infection are the lungs, skin, lymph nodes, and liver (Table 17.3). Osteomyelitis and bacteremia/fungemia are also common. In North America, the majority of infections are due to *Aspergillus* spp., *Staphylococcus*

Table 17.3 Most common infections in CGD

Infection	Percent of patients affected
Pneumonia	79–87%
Aspergillus species	
Staphylococcus aureus	
Burkholderia cepacia	
Nocardia species	
Subcutaneous abscess	42%
Staphylococcus aureus	
Serratia marcescens	
Liver abscess	27–32%
Staphylococcus aureus	
Lymphadenitis	25–53%
Staphylococcus aureus	
Serratia marcescens	
Osteomyelitis	25%
Serratia marcescens	
Aspergillus	
Bacteremia/fungemia	18%
Burkholderia cepacia	
Lung abscess	16%
Aspergillus species	
Staphylococcus aureus	
Nocardia species	
Brain abscess	3%
Aspergillus species	

aureus, *Burkholderia* spp., *Serratia marcescens*, and *Nocardia* spp. About 80% of patients have at least one episode of pneumonia, and *Aspergillus*, *Staphylococcus*, *Burkholderia*, and *Nocardia* are the pathogens most commonly identified in cases of pneumonia [5, 19]. *Staphylococcus* and *Serratia* are the most common causes of lymphadenitis and skin abscesses, and *Staphylococcus* is the most common cause of liver abscesses [5, 19]. Liver abscesses ultimately affect about one-third of patients with CGD and are often recurrent and difficult to treat [5, 19]. *Burkholderia* is the most common cause of sepsis and is associated with a high fatality rate [19, 20]. Europe and Israel also have high rates of infection with *Salmonella* spp. and *Salmonella* spp., which are frequent causes of septicemia in these regions [11, 12, 21]. In addition to the aforementioned pathogens, local or disseminated infections due to bacille Calmette-Guerin (BCG) have been reported at rates of 16.6–59.2% in CGD patients in countries where the BCG vaccine is routinely administered [22–25]. *Mycobacterium tuberculosis* infections are also reported at higher rates than what is considered usual for people living in areas endemic for tuberculosis [26, 27].

There are a number of unusual and virtually pathognomonic bacterial infections that have been identified in CGD patients in recent years. *Chromobacterium violaceum* and *Francisella philomiragia* are both gram-negative bacteria found in brackish water (i.e., water resulting from the mixing of seawater with freshwater, as in estuaries) and have been reported to cause skin and deep tissue abscesses as well as sepsis in CGD [28–30]. *Granulibacter bethesdensis* is a ubiquitous gram-negative rod found in soil and organic decay that has been isolated from patients with chronic necrotizing lymphadenitis, sepsis, and meningitis [31].

Patients with CGD have one of the highest rates of invasive fungal infection among all primary immunodeficiencies, with *Aspergillus* spp. being isolated at some point in about 40% of patients [5, 19]. The lungs and chest wall are the most common sites of *Aspergillus* infection. *Aspergillus* is also a major cause of osteomyelitis and brain abscesses [5, 32]. *A. fumigatus* followed by *A. nidulans* are the most frequently identified Aspergillus species [19, 33–35]. Of note, *A. fumigatus* was previously the leading cause of mortality in CGD, but with the advent of azole antifungal treatment, death from *A. fumigatus* is now uncommon [35]. However, the incidence of infection with *A. nidulans* and other *Aspergillus* species (e.g., *A. viridinutans*, *A. tanneri*, *A. niger*, and *A. terreus*) has increased with widespread use of azole antifungal prophylaxis. Unfortunately, these *Aspergillus* species generally cause more severe, refractory, and invasive disease that are difficult to treat and associated with high mortality rates [32–39]. Other fungi frequently seen in CGD include *Rhizopus* spp., *Trichosporon* spp., *Paecilomyces* spp., *Phellinus tropicalis*, *Geosmithia argillacea*, and *Neosartorya udagawae*, among others [40–46]. *Candida* infections are also common [5, 19]. Of note, dimorphic mold infections such as histoplasmosis and blastomycosis as well as the yeast infection cryptococcosis are not seen at increased rates in CGD, and mucormycosis is typically seen only in the setting of significant iatrogenic immunosuppression [47].

Diagnostic Testing

CGD should be in the differential diagnosis for all patients with severe or recurrent cutaneous abscesses, lymphadenitis, and pneumonia and any instance of deep tissue abscess, especially in the lungs or liver. Infections with organisms such as *Aspergillus* spp., *B. cepacia*, *Nocardia* spp., and *Serratia marcescens* should also prompt evaluation for CGD, and infection with any of the other rare or pathognomonic pathogens referenced above should be considered CGD until proven otherwise.

Dihydrorhodamine Assay

There are a number of diagnostic tests available to assess NADPH oxidase function in stimulated neutrophils. The nitroblue tetrazolium (NBT) reduction test was used historically, and the ferricytochrome c oxidase assay has been used on a research basis; however, the dihydrorhodamine (DHR) assay is currently considered the gold standard for diagnosis given the ease, wide availability, and high sensitivity of the assay. In the DHR assay, neutrophils are incubated with DHR-123 and stimulated with phorbol 12-myristate 13-acetate (PMA). Functional neutrophils produce superoxide radicals that oxidize DHR-123 to rhodamine, which fluoresces green and can be detected by flow cytometry. This allows for the enumeration of the proportion of rhodamine-positive (i.e., oxidase-positive) neutrophils (Fig. 17.2). In addition to diagnosing CGD, the DHR assay can also distinguish between those with absent and those with residual NADPH oxidase activity. Mechanistically, the survival of patients with CGD is strongly associated with residual superoxide production independent of the specific gene affected [14]. In general, patients with X-linked CGD have absent and those with AR CGD have residual NADPH oxidase activity. Carriers of X-linked CGD typically have two distinct populations of neutrophils on the DHR assay: a rhodamine-positive and a rhodamine-negative subset. The relative proportions of these populations can be used to evaluate degree of lyonization (i.e., X chromosome inactivation). Of note, there are a number of medical conditions that can result in a false-positive DHR assay, including severe G6PD deficiency, myeloperoxidase deficiency, and the syndrome of synovitis, acne, pustulosis, hyperostosis, and osteitis (SAPHO). Granulocytic ehrlichiosis, an infection

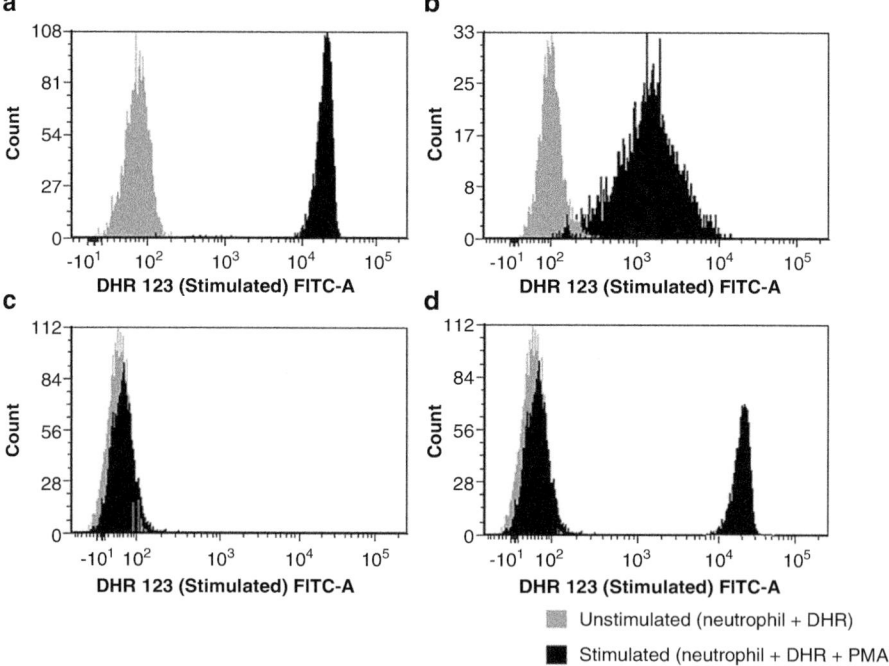

Fig. 17.2 The DHR-123 assay. Typical DHR histograms from a (**a**) healthy donor, patients with (**b**) autosomal recessive and (**c**) X-linked CGD, and a (**d**) carrier of X-linked CGD. Patients with autosomal recessive CGD classically have residual oxidase activity while patients with X-linked CGD are typically oxidase null. Carriers of X-linked CGD have two distinct populations of neutrophils – a rhodamine-negative and a rhodamine-positive population

caused the *Ehrlichia* bacterium primarily transported by the lone star tick, has also been reported to decrease neutrophil oxidase activity and may be associated an abnormal DHR assay [48–51].

Genetic Testing

Patients with an abnormal neutrophil function test should undergo confirmatory genetic testing. In general, patients with nonsense, frameshift, and splice site variants or deletions are more likely to be associated with absent or severely decreased residual NADPH oxidase activity and worse clinical outcomes than patients with missense mutations. Of note, the *NCF1* gene is flanked by highly homologous (>98%) pseudogenes, which may complicate genetic testing in patients with suspected p47phox deficiency. Western blot assays and flow cytometry have both been used on a research basis to evaluate for p47phox protein expression in patients with inconclusive genetic testing as a confirmatory diagnostic measure [52, 53].

Management/Outcome

Prophylaxis

All patients diagnosed with CGD should be promptly started on trimethoprim-sulfamethoxazole (5 mg/kg/d div BID up to 320 mg trimethoprim a day) and itraconazole (5 mg/kg/d up to 200 mg daily) prophylaxis, and prophylaxis should be continued lifelong or until the patient has successfully undergone definitive curative therapy. Trimethoprim-sulfamethoxazole has been shown to markedly reduce the incidence of bacterial infections in patients with CGD [54–58]; in one large retrospective study, trimethoprim-sulfamethoxazole prophylaxis decreased the rate of bacterial infection from 15.8 to 6.9 per 100 patient-months in patients with X-linked disease and from 7.1 to 2.4 per 100 patient-months in those with autosomal recessive disease [58]. Trimethoprim alone, dicloxacillin, ciprofloxacin, and quinolones are alternative options for patients with sulfamethoxazole allergy or G6PD deficiency.

The advent of azole antifungals and the widespread adoption of itraconazole prophylaxis have led to improved overall survival rates for patients with CGD around the world. In a seminal trial of 39 patients with CGD randomized to receive either placebo or itraconazole, only one patient receiving itraconazole had a serious fungal infection compared to seven in the placebo group over a follow-up period of approximately 113 patient-years [59]. For those unable to tolerate itraconazole, posaconazole has been shown to be safe and effective [60]. Of note, azole antifungal therapy may be complicated by transaminitis, and as such, liver function tests should be periodically monitored. Azole absorption is also quite variable, so many clinicians choose to monitor drug levels, especially in patients with gastrointestinal disease.

IFN-gamma has been shown to stimulate superoxide production and bactericidal activity of neutrophils in vitro, and in one large randomized, double-blind, placebo-controlled trial of 128 patients with CGD from the National Institutes of Health (NIH), IFN-gamma prophylaxis was associated with a decrease in both the number and severity of infections compared to controls [61]. Furthermore, long-term follow-up of 9 years demonstrated sustained benefit [62]. However, a large prospective Italian study found that long-term IFN-gamma prophylaxis did not significantly decrease the rate of infection [7], and there was no significant difference in the number of fungal infections between patients receiving IFN-gamma and those not receiving it in the itraconazole study discussed above [59]. Additionally, side effects are common, including fever, malaise, chills, fatigue, and injection site swelling and/or tenderness, and as such, many patients do not tolerate IFN-gamma injections. For these reasons, the use of IFN-gamma prophylaxis remains variable. However, when used, IFN-gamma is started at a dose of 50 µg/m^2 (or 1.5 µg/kg if BSA is <0.5 m^2) administered subcutaneously three times weekly.

In addition to antimicrobial prophylaxis, patients with CGD should receive all routine childhood immunizations except for the BCG vaccine. They should also be counseled to avoid decaying organic matter (e.g., mulch, hay, dead leaves), where fungal spores are often found, and brackish water as described above. CGD patients may otherwise participate in all normal activities without restriction.

Management of Acute Infections

Patients with CGD have reported rates of significant infection of around 0.3 per year despite appropriate antimicrobial prophylaxis [7, 19]. As such, all CGD patients with fever or any other signs or symptoms concerning for infection should be promptly evaluated with a thorough physical and laboratory evaluation. It should be noted that some patients with CGD, particularly young children, may not present with classic signs and symptoms of infection, and laboratory values may be falsely reassuring. Therefore, there should be a low threshold for imaging, particularly of the chest and/or abdomen, and when in doubt, one should err on the side of treating empirically with antimicrobials. Initial antibiotic therapy should provide good coverage for both *S. aureus* and gram-negative bacteria, including *B. cepacia* (e.g., combination of vancomycin/clindamycin/oxacillin and ceftazidime/carbapenem depending on local resistance patterns). The addition of treatment strength dosing of trimethoprim-sulfamethoxazole to cover ceftazidime-resistant *B. cepacia* and *Nocardia* spp. and voriconazole to cover *Aspergillus* spp. may also be considered as part of initial empiric therapy. If patients do not improve within 24–48 h, and an infectious agent has not been identified, voriconazole should be started if not already done so, and more aggressive diagnostic procedures should be considered. Of note, *Aspergillus* serological tests (e.g., *Aspergillus* galactomannan), the (1-3)-beta-D-glucan assay, and bronchoalveolar lavage all have low sensitivity in patients with CGD, and therefore, invasive sampling of involved tissues is often needed [35]. However, even with invasive sampling, a causative pathogen is only identified about

50% of the time [19, 20]. Surgical intervention is often necessary, and patients frequently require prolonged treatment courses extending for several months.

Granulocyte transfusions have also been used successfully for patients with severe and/or refractory infections unresponsive to antimicrobials [63]. The number of infused granulocytes is typically about 10^9–10^{10} per transfusion with variable dosing schedules, ranging from daily to a few times per week which are sometimes limited by granulocyte availability. Adverse events are common, most frequently manifested as chills and fever but hypotension, respiratory distress, and transfusion-related acute lung injury have also been reported. Many patients develop alloimmunization [64–66], and as such, granulocyte transfusions should be used cautiously for those patients being considered for HSCT. Some centers have used sirolimus with granulocyte transfusions to decrease the risk of alloimmunization, and rituximab has been used to treat alloimmunization, although the effectiveness of these measures has not been well described.

In general, glucocorticoids are typically avoided in patients with active infection; however, one of the hallmarks of CGD is an exuberant and aberrant inflammatory response to infection. As such, glucocorticoids are sometimes used for CGD patients with severe and/or refractory infections [67, 68]. In particular, glucocorticoids in addition to appropriate antimicrobial agents are recommended for the treatment of liver abscesses [69, 70], as was done for the patient described in the case above. Liver abscesses are dense, caseous, and often difficult to drain, and traditionally, CGD patients often required surgical resection. However, in a case series from the NIH, nine patients who received glucocorticoids for the treatment of *Staphylococcal* liver abscesses refractory to conventional therapy all experienced resolution of the liver abscesses without the need for surgical intervention [69]. Glucocorticoids are typically dosed at 1 mg/kg/day for 2–3 weeks, followed by a taper over several months (on average 5 months).

Case Presentation 2

An otherwise healthy boy developed abdominal pain; bloody, mucousy stools; and failure to thrive at 18 months of age and was diagnosed at age 24 months with very early-onset inflammatory bowel disease based on results from an endoscopy and flexible sigmoidoscopy. Inflammatory bowel disease was complicated by recurrent perirectal abscesses and multiple enterocutaneous fistulae requiring surgical intervention. Colitis was poorly responsive to multiple therapies, including azathioprine, methotrexate, infliximab (anti-TNF-alpha), anakinra (anti-IL-1), and vedolizumab (anti-alpha 4 beta 7 integrin), and the patient ultimately underwent partial colectomy with diverting ileostomy at 8 years of age. The patient was referred to immunology for evaluation at 12 years of age given the early onset and severe nature of his inflammatory bowel disease. At time of evaluation, he was on methotrexate, ustekinumab (anti-IL-12/IL-23), and prednisone 10 mg daily with moderate control of disease. His height and weight were both at the third percentile. Infectious history was not significant. The patient's mother had systemic lupus erythematous, but family history was otherwise unremarkable. A DHR assay demonstrated absent neutrophil oxidative burst consistent with X-linked CGD, and genetic testing identified a pathogenic mutation in *CYBB*. The decision was made at that time to pursue curative HSCT. Fortunately, the patient's younger brother was found to be a full 10/10 HLA-identical match, and the patient underwent HSCT at 13 years of age with reduced-toxicity myeloablative conditioning. His posttransplant course was overall unremarkable, and the patient had full resolution of CGD colitis by 3 months posttransplant. Growth also improved, and the patient is now at the tenth percentile for height and weight 2 years posttransplant.

Diagnosis/Assessment

Inflammatory Complications of CGD

In addition to recurrent and severe infections, CGD is characterized by immune dysregulation with high rates of autoinflammation, particularly of the GI tract, lungs, and liver. Importantly, patients may present with inflammatory disease as their only disease manifestation in the absence of a significant infectious history, as was the case for the patient described above. Autoinflammation is seen with all genotypes, but in general, severe inflammatory disease occurs more commonly in patients with X-linked CGD than in those with autosomal recessive disease [71]. Furthermore, up to 18% of CGD patients reaching adulthood develop autoimmune disease, including lupus-like symptoms, sarcoidosis, IgA nephropathy, and rheumatoid arthritis, among others [5, 12, 72].

Inflammatory bowel disease or colitis is the most common inflammatory disease seen in patients with CGD. In a series of 140 pediatric patients with CGD at the NIH, 32.8% had colitis [73], and rates as high as 60% have been reported in other series [71]. The median age of onset of GI disease was 5 years in the NIH cohort, although symptoms may develop at any point. Furthermore, the GI symptoms may be nonspecific, including abdominal pain, noninfectious diarrhea, nausea and vomiting, and failure to thrive. Any portion of the GI tract may be involved, but the colon is the most common site affected, and colitis is often fistulizing [73, 74]. Perirectal disease, frequently with recurrent and/or severe perirectal abscesses, is also particularly common. Many patients develop failure to thrive due to poorly controlled disease; in the aforementioned NIH study, 32% of patients had delayed growth [73]. In addition to colitis, about 50% of patients also develop gastrointestinal granulomas, which may be obstructive [71, 73, 75].

Other common sites of inflammatory disease include the lungs, liver, genitourinary tract, eyes and skin. About 20–30% of patients surviving into adulthood develop inflammatory lung disease [71, 76], and granulomatous disease, with or without lymphocyte infiltration, interstitial lung disease, pulmonary nodules, pleural thickening and/or effusions, and chronic obstructive pulmonary disease have all been reported [71, 76, 77]. Of note, inflammatory lung disease may occur independently from or simultaneously with infection, and infection may be the trigger for onset of inflammatory disease. Inflammatory liver disease is also common in CGD patients. In one review from the NIH, granulomas, venopathy of the portal vein, and nodular regenerative hyperplasia were all reported [78]. Poorly controlled liver disease may progress to non-cirrhotic pulmonary hypertension; the development of thrombocytopenia in this setting is associated with especially poor outcomes [79]. Inflammatory genitourinary symptoms are not uncommon, and granuloma formation in the genitourinary tract may result in ureteral or bladder outlet obstruction [71, 80]. Eosinophilic cystitis is also a rare complication that has also been reported [81, 82]. Ocular manifestations of CGD include chorioretinitis, uveitis, and ocular granulomas [71]. Common dermatologic manifestations include severe and/or granulomatous acne, inflammatory nodular lesions, and cutaneous lymphocytic infiltration [71, 72]. Poor wound healing with increased risk of wound dehiscence has also been described [83, 84]. Furthermore, macrophage activation syndrome or hemophagocytic lymphohistiocytosis has been reported in CGD patients and may be life-threatening [85–88].

Finally, patients with CGD may develop an entity known as mulch pneumonitis, which is due to an exuberant inflammatory response to inhalation of fungal elements in decaying organic matter (e.g., mulch, hay, and dead leaves) [89–91]. Symptoms typically occur 1–10 days after exposure to fungal elements, and symptoms tend to progress rapidly. Chest x-ray characteristically demonstrates diffuse interstitial infiltrates. Mulch pneumonitis is associated with a high mortality rate if not identified early and should be considered for all CGD patients who present with acute onset of fever, dyspnea, and hypoxia.

X-Linked Carriers

The patient's mother in the case above reported a history of systemic lupus erythematosus, which may be related to her presumed status as a carrier of X-linked CGD. Female carriers of X-linked CGD have a dual phagocyte population due to lyonization, and in some cases, severe skewing of X chromosome inactivation may lead to the clinical syndrome of CGD. Furthermore, female carriers may have progressive skewing with age and may develop manifestations of CGD later in life. However, recent studies from the United Kingdom and the NIH also indicate that female carriers are at increased risk of medical complications, particularly autoimmune disease, regardless of degree of lyonization.

In a UK survey of 94 female carriers of X-linked CGD [92], cutaneous symptoms, most frequently photosensitivity but also malar-like lupus rash and eczema, were reported by 63 (79%) women. Skin abscesses were reported by 14 (17%), and gastrointestinal symptoms were reported by 40 (42%) women. Twenty-four (26%) women also met criteria for systemic lupus erythematosus. The NIH study [93], which included 162 female carriers of X-linked CGD, also found high rates of cutaneous symptoms and autoimmune disease, at 25% and 19%, respectively. Fifteen percent of women also had a history of severe CGD-related infections. There was a clear correlation between history of infection and neutrophil oxidative capacity in the NIH study; women with less than 10–20% oxidase-positive neutrophils were at increased risk of infection. Interestingly, in both studies, there was no relationship between autoimmune disease and neutrophil respiratory oxidative burst.

In addition to an increased rate of the medical complications described above, a recent publication, also from the United Kingdom, reported impaired emotional health with high rates of anxiety and significantly reduced quality of life scores in female carriers of X-liked CGD [94]. Taken together, these studies suggest that female carriers should be monitored long term, and in general, experts recommend antimicrobial prophylaxis for those with less than 10% oxidase-positive neutrophils. Furthermore, based on the increased risk of autoimmune disease and potential skewing of X inactivation with time, many centers prefer not to use female carriers as donors for HSCT in their affected family members, although HSCT outcomes using female carrier donors have not been published.

Diagnostic Testing

Patients with granulomatous inflammation, early-onset inflammatory bowel disease, or any of the unusual inflammatory complications described above should be screened for CGD regardless of infectious history. In particular, all patients with early-onset inflammatory bowel disease should receive a DHR assay at presentation, as a diagnosis of CGD may influence treatment decisions.

Management/Outcome

Treatment of Autoinflammation

Glucocorticoids are the mainstay of treatment of inflammatory disease in patients with CGD, and they are often effective for the treatment of granulomatous lesions. However, CGD colitis, interstitial lung disease, and other inflammatory manifestations of CGD are often difficult to treat, and additional immunomodulators are often necessary. This raises a dilemma for CGD patients, as iatrogenic immunosuppression increases their already high risk of infection and may be associated with significant morbidity and mortality.

Patients with CGD colitis typically respond to glucocorticoids, but relapse is common, and many patients become glucocorticoid dependent [71, 73]. Infliximab may be effective at treating colitis, but has been associated with increased risk of infection and death in patients with CGD, and as such, infliximab and other TNF-alpha inhibitors are generally strictly avoided [94]. Patients have variable response to the typical glucocorticoid-sparing agents used for the treatment of inflammatory bowel disease, including salicylic acid derivatives, antimetabolites such as azathioprine, and 6-mercaptopurine. Anakinra, ustekinumab, and vedolizumab have all been used in small numbers of patients with CGD colitis with varying degrees of success [95–98]. Ultimately, many patients remain refractory to treatment and fail multiple therapies as described in the case above, and their only curative option is hematopoietic stem cell transplantation and possibly gene therapy.

Hematopoietic Cell Transplantation

Allogeneic HSCT is the only widely available definitive treatment for CGD with the potential for resolution of both infectious and inflammatory complications. Initial studies showed that HSCT for CGD was possible, but rates of graft failure were high and overall survival outcomes were poor [100–102]. However, with optimization of clinical status pre-HSCT, fine-tuning of conditioning regimens, and improved supportive care peri- and post-HSCT, outcomes have improved significantly over the last two decades (Table 17.4). Overall survival rates are now consistently near or >90% for pediatric patients less than 14 years regardless of donor source [103–109], and pediatric patients who undergo HSCT have fewer infections, improved growth parameters and performance scores, and higher quality of life measures compared to those treated conventionally [110–112]. Adolescents and adults have traditionally been difficult to transplant; however, there have been several studies in recent years reporting high disease-free survival rates in adolescents and adult patients, including those with severe infection and/or uncontrolled inflammatory disease at time of transplantation [66, 113–117].

There remains debate as to the optimal conditioning regimen for CGD, and practice varies significantly from center to center. Many centers throughout the world have adopted a highly successful reduced-toxicity myeloablative conditioning regimen reported by Güngör and others in 2014 [113] that includes customized busulfan dosing with pharmacokinetic analysis, fludarabine, and antithymocyte globulin. However, some centers have subsequently reported an increased incidence of graft rejection, late graft failure, and mixed myeloid chimerism [119]. This is notable, as data on female carriers of X-linked CGD suggests the level of neutrophil oxidase activity that protects a CGD patient from infection may be different than that which protects against autoinflammation [92, 93], and the degree of myeloid chimerism needed to protect against new-onset inflammatory and autoimmune disease posttransplant is unknown.

Furthermore, the role of autoinflammation on HSCT outcomes also remains incompletely understood. Encouragingly, one recent study report from the Primary Immunodeficiency Treatment Consortium that included 49 CGD patients with IBD and 96 patients without IBD who underwent allogeneic HSCT reported a 5-year overall survival was equivalent for patients with and without colitis at 80% and 83%, respectively [120]. Furthermore, colitis was not associated with an increased risk of graft-versus-host disease and all surviving patients with a history of colitis had resolution of disease posttransplant. However, further studies are needed to fully elucidate how the presence of autoinflammation and accompanying organ

Table 17.4 Published HSCT outcomes in patients with CGD

Reference	N	Age in years, median (range)	Donor source	Conditioning regimen	Overall survival (%)	Disease-free survival (%)	Median follow-up (years)
Horowitz et al. [99]	10	15 (5–36)	MRD	RIC	70	60	1.4
Seger et al. [101]	27	8.5 (0.8–38.7)	MRD (25) URD (2)	MAC (23) RIC (4)	85	81	2
Soncini et al. [103]	20	6.25 (1.25–21)	MRD (9) URD (9) UCB (2)	MAC (16) RIC (4)	90	90	5
Schuetz et al. [102]	12	9.5 (4–20)	MRD (3) URD (9)	MAC (9) RIC (3)	75	58	4.4
Martinez et al. [105]	11	3.8 (1–13)	MRD (4) URD (7)	MAC	100	100	4
Tewari et al. [106]	12	4.95 (0.67–11.6)	MRD (5) UCB (7)	MAC	100	83.3	5.8
Gungor et al. [113]	56	12.7 (0.8–40)	MRD (21) URD (35)	RTC	93	89	1.75
Khandelwal et al. [114]	18	3.18 (0.45–19.39)	MRD (3) URD (15)	MAC (14) RIC (4)	83	83	1.65
Morillo-Gutierrez et al. [107]	70	8.9 (3.8–19.3)	MRD (13) URD (55) UCB (1) Haplo (1)	RTC	91.4	84	2.8
Fox et al. [115]	11	19 (17–28)	MRD (3) URD (8)	RIC	81.8	81.8	2.69
Parta et al. [116]	40	16 (4–32)	MRD (4) URD (36)	RIC	82.5	80	3.4
Genenry et al. [118]	55	5.3 (0.6–18)	MRD (20) URD (31) Haplo (4)	MAC (25) RTC (30)	89	77	6.5

MRD matched related donor, *URD* unrelated donor, *UCB* umbilical cord blood, *Haplo* haploidentical donor, *MAC* myeloablative conditioning, *RIC* reduced-intensity conditioning, *RTC* reduced-toxicity myeloablative conditioning

dysfunction at time of HSCT impacts overall survival, engraftment, immune reconstitution, and risk of post-HSCT complications.

Gene Therapy

As with all monogenic diseases, gene therapy is an appealing alternative to HSCT, providing an option for patients without an HLA-identical donor and eliminating the risk of graft-versus-host disease. The first gene therapy trials for CGD took place at the NIH in the 1990s [121], and several small trials have subsequently been conducted to treat gp91phox deficiency using gamma-retroviral vectors and reduced-intensity conditioning [122–126]. Notably, many of the patients had active and refractory severe infection at time of gene therapy. All trials demonstrated initial engraftment of transduced neutrophils at 10–30% of circulating neutrophils, and most patients experienced full or partial resolution of infection. However, cell engraftment progressively decreased with time, and several patients developed myelodysplastic syndrome (MDS) due to insertional activation of proto-oncogenes [123, 125].

In response to the high incidence of MDS seen with γ-retroviral vectors, gene therapy trials are currently underway using self-inactivating (SIN) lentiviral vectors. Encouragingly, a recent report from a multicenter trial using a SIN lentiviral vector and near-myeloablative conditioning demonstrated sustained persistence of 12–46% oxidase positive neutrophils and no new infections in six of seven patients (aged at 7–27 years) at 1–2.5-year follow-up [127]. Furthermore, one of these patients had a history of colitis that resolved completely following gene therapy.

Ultimately, long-term outcomes with gene therapy are unknown, and as with HSCT, it is unclear what level of oxidase-positive neutrophils is necessary for resolution of preexisting autoinflammation and to prevent new-onset inflammatory and autoimmune disease.

Conclusion

Overall, CGD outcomes have improved markedly over the past few decades. In 2000, Winkelstein et al. reported a mortality rate for 5% per year for X-linked CGD and 2% per year for autosomal recessive CGD[5]. However, several large registries have subsequently reported survival rates approaching 90% by age 10 years, largely attributed to the widespread adoption of itraconazole prophylaxis [6, 7, 14]. Current long-term survival rates are unknown, however, as recognition and management of disease and transplant outcomes continue to improve with time. Furthermore, there remain no standard long-term treatment guidelines for patients with CGD. Indications for HSCT remain controversial, particularly for patients with residual oxidase activity, and transplant procedures for CGD patients vary markedly from center to center. Thus, additional large, multicenter studies are needed to further optimize HSCT procedures, and long-term follow-up is needed to clarify the role of gene therapy for CGD.

Clinical Pearls and Pitfalls

- All patients with severe or recurrent cutaneous abscesses, lymphadenitis, and/or pneumonia, any instance of deep tissue abscess, and infection with *Aspergillus* spp., *B. cepacia*, *Nocardia* spp., and *Serratia marcescens* should be evaluated for CGD.

- All patients with early-onset inflammatory bowel disease (<10 years of age), particularly those with perirectal and/or difficult to control disease, should be screened for CGD, particularly before starting infliximab or other anti-TNF-alpha agents.
- CGD patients should be counseled to avoid decaying organic matter (e.g., hay, mulch, dead leaves) and brackish water (i.e., water resulting from the mixing of seawater with freshwater, as in estuaries).
- CGD patients with fever or any signs or symptoms of infection should be evaluated promptly with a thorough physical and laboratory evaluation even if symptoms are mild and guardians/patients report that they are overall well appearing.
- *Aspergillus galactomannan*, (1-3)-beta-D-glucan, and bronchoalveolar lavage all have poor sensitivity in CGD, and negative results do not exclude fungal infection.
- CGD patients often require prolonged antimicrobial courses with courses 4–6 months or longer in duration common.
- Glucocorticoids may be necessary in addition to antimicrobial therapy for the treatment of the hyperactive inflammatory response frequently seen in CGD patients with infection.
- Female relatives of patients with X-linked CGD should be screened for carrier status and, if positive, followed long term. Those with <10% oxidase-positive neutrophils on DHR assay should be started on antimicrobial prophylaxis.
- Definitive therapy with allogeneic hematopoietic cell transplantation should be considered for all patients with CGD. Transplant should not be delayed, as outcomes are better for younger patients before they develop severe infection or autoinflammation with resultant organ dysfunction.

References

1. Janeway CA, Craig J, Davison M, et al. Hypergammaglobulinemia associated with severe, recurrent, and chronic non-specific infection. Am J Dis Child. 1954;88:388–92.
2. Bridges RA, Berendes H, Good RA. A fatal granulomatous disease of childhood; the clinical, pathological, and laboratory features of a new syndrome. AMA J Dis Child. 1959;97(4):387–408.
3. Reeves EP, Lu H, Jacobs HL, et al. Killing activity of neutrophils is mediated through activation of proteases by K+ flux. Nature. 2002;416(6878):291–7.
4. Fuchs TA, Abed U, Goosmann C, et al. Novel cell death program leads to neutrophil extracellular traps. J Cell Biol. 2007;176(2):231–41.
5. Winkelstein JA, Marino MC, Johnston RB, et al. Chronic granulomatous disease: report on a national registry of 368 patients. Medicine. 2000;79(3):155–69.
6. Jones LB, McGrogan P, Flood TJ, et al. Special article: chronic granulomatous disease in the United Kingdom and Ireland: a comprehensive national patient-based registry. Clin Exp Immunol. 2008;152(2):211–8.

7. Martire B, Rondelli R, Soresina A, et al. Clinical features, long-term follow-up and outcome of a large cohort of patients with chronic granulomatous disease: an Italian multicenter study. Clin Immunol. 2008;126(2):155–64.
8. Åhlin A, de Boer M, Roos D, et al. Prevalence, genetics and clinical presentation of chronic granulomatous disease in Sweden. Acta Paediatr. 1995;84(2):1386–94.
9. Raptaki M, Varela I, Spanou K, et al. Chronic granulomatous disease: a 25-year patient registry based on a multistep diagnostic procedure, from the referral center for primary immunodeficiencies in Greece. J Clin Immunol. 2013;33(8):1302–9.
10. Hasui M, Hayakawa H, Kanegasaki S, et al. Chronic granulomatous disease in Japan: incidence and natural history. Pediatr Int. 1999;41(5):589–93.
11. Wolach B, Gavrieli R, de Boer M, et al. Chronic granulomatous disease: clinical, functional, molecular, and genetic studies. The Israeli experience with 84 patients. Am J Hematol. 2017;92(1):28–36.
12. van den Berg J, van Koppen E, Ahlin A, et al. Chronic granulomatous disease: the European experience. PLoS ONE. 2009;4(4):e5234.
13. Roos D, Kuhns DB, Maddalena A, et al. Hematologically important mutations: the autosomal recessive forms of chronic granulomatous disease (second update). Blood Cell Mol Dis. 2010;44(4):291–9.
14. Kuhns DB, Alvord WG, Heller T, et al. Residual NADPH oxidase and survival in chronic granulomatous disease. N Engl J Med. 2010;363(27):2600–10.
15. Matute JD, Arias AA, Wright NAM, et al. A new genetic subgroup of chronic granulomatous disease with autosomal recessive mutations in p40 phox and selective defects in neutrophil NADPH oxidase activity. Blood. 2009;114(5):3309–15.
16. van de Geer A, Nieto-Patlán A, Kuhns DB, et al. Inherited p40 phox deficiency differs from classic chronic granulomatous disease. J Clin Invest. 2018;128(9):3957–75.
17. Thomas DC, Charbonnier LM, Schejtman A, et al. EROS/CYBC1 mutations: decreased NADPH oxidase function and chronic granulomatous disease. J Allergy Clin Immunol. 2019;143(2):782–5.
18. Arnadottir GA, Norddahl GL, Gudmundsdottir S, et al. A homozygous loss-of-function mutation leading to CYBC1 deficiency causes chronic granulomatous disease. Nat Commun. 2018;9(1):4447.
19. Marciano BE, Spalding C, Fitzgerald A, et al. Common severe infections in chronic granulomatous disease. Clin Infect Dis. 2015;60(8):1176–83.
20. Bortoletto P, Lyman K, Camacho A, et al. Chronic granulomatous disease: a large, single-center US experience. Pediatr Infect Dis J. 2015;34(10):1110–4.
21. Wolach B, Gavrieli R, de Boer M, et al. Chronic granulomatous disease in Israel: clinical, functional and molecular studies of 38 patients. Clin Immunol. 2008;129(1):103–14.
22. Baba LA, Ailal F, el Hafidi N, et al. Chronic granulomatous disease in Morocco: genetic, immunological, and clinical features of 12 patients from 10 kindreds. J Clin Immunol. 2014;34(4):452–8.
23. de Oliveira-Junior EB, Zurro NB, Prando C, et al. Clinical and genotypic spectrum of chronic granulomatous disease in 71 Latin American patients: first report from the LASID registry. Pediatr Blood Cancer. 2015;62(12):2102–7.
24. Fattahi F, Badalzadeh M, Sedighipour L, et al. Inheritance pattern and clinical aspects of 93 Iranian patients with chronic granulomatous disease. J Clin Immunol. 2011;31(5):792–801.
25. Zhou Q, Hui X, Ying W, et al. A cohort of 169 chronic granulomatous disease patients exposed to BCG vaccination: a retrospective study from a single center in Shanghai, China (2004–2017). J Clin Immunol. 2018;38(3):260–72.
26. Lee PPW, Chan KW, Jiang L, et al. Susceptibility to mycobacterial infections in children with x-linked chronic granulomatous disease: a review of 17 patients living in a region endemic for tuberculosis. Pediatr Infect Dis J. 2008;27(3):224–30.
27. Conti F, Lugo-Reyes SO, Blancas Galicia L, et al. Mycobacterial disease in patients with chronic granulomatous disease: a retrospective analysis of 71 cases. J Allergy Clin Immunol. 2016;138(1):241–8.

28. Sirinavin S, Techasaensiri C, Benjaponpitak S, Pornkul R, Vorachit M. Invasive Chromobacterium violaceum infection in children: case report and review. Pediatr Infect Dis J. 2005;24(6):559–61.
29. Meher-Homji Z, Mangalore RP, D R Johnson P, Y L Chua K. Chromobacterium violaceum infection in chronic granulomatous disease: a case report and review of the literature. JMM Case Rep. 2017;4(1):e005084.
30. Mailman TL, Schmidt MH. Francisella philomiragia adenitis and pulmonary nodules in a child with chronic granulomatous disease. Can J Infect Dis Med Microbiol. 2005;16(4):245–8.
31. Greenberg DE, Shoffner AR, Zelazny AM, et al. Recurrent granulibacter bethesdensis infections and chronic granulomatous disease. Emerg Infect Dis. 2010;16(9):1341–8.
32. Dotis J, Roilides E. Osteomyelitis due to Aspergillus species in chronic granulomatous disease: an update of the literature. Mycoses. 2011;54(6):e686–96.
33. Falcone EL, Holland SM. Invasive fungal infection in chronic granulomatous disease: insights into pathogenesis and management. Curr Opin Infect Dis. 2012;25(6):658–69.
34. Beauté J, Obenga G, le Mignot L, et al. Epidemiology and outcome of invasive fungal diseases in patients with chronic granulomatous disease: a multicenter study in France. Pediatr Infect Dis J. 2011;30(1):57–62.
35. Blumental S, Mouy R, Mahlaoui N, et al. Invasive mold infections in chronic granulomatous disease: a 25-year retrospective survey. Clin Infect Dis. 2011;53(12):e159–69.
36. Vinh DC, Shea YR, Jones PA, et al. Chronic invasive aspergillosis caused by Aspergillus viridinutans. Emerg Infect Dis. 2009;15(8):1292–4.
37. Sugui JA, Peterson SW, Clark LP, et al. Aspergillus tanneri sp. nov., a new pathogen that causes invasive disease refractory to antifungal therapy. J Clin Microbiol. 2012;50(10):3309–17.
38. Kaltenis P, Mudäniene V, Maknavičius S, Šeinin D. Renal amyloidosis in a child with chronic granulomatous disease and invasive aspergillosis. Pediatr Nephrol. 2008;23(5):831–4.
39. Mortaz E, Sarhifynia S, Marjani M, et al. An adult autosomal recessive chronic granulomatous disease patient with pulmonary Aspergillus terreus infection. BMC Infect Dis. 2018;18(1):552.
40. Dotis J, Pana ZD, Roilides E. Non-Aspergillus fungal infections in chronic granulomatous disease. Mycoses. 2013;56(4):449–62.
41. Silliman CC, Lawellin DW, Lohr JA, Rodgers BM, Donowitz LG. Paecilomyces lilacinus infection in a child with chronic granulomatous disease. J Infect. 1992;24(2):191–5.
42. Wang SM, Shieh CC, Liu CC. Successful treatment of Paecilomyces variotii splenic abscesses: a rare complication in a previously unrecognized chronic granulomatous disease child. Diagn Microbiol Infect Dis. 2005;53(2):149–52.
43. Ramesh M, Resnick E, Hui Y, et al. Phellinus tropicalis abscesses in a patient with chronic granulomatous disease. J Clin Immunol. 2014;34(2):130–3.
44. Haidar G, Zerbe CS, Cheng M, et al. Phellinus species: an emerging cause of refractory fungal infections in patients with X-linked chronic granulomatous disease. Mycoses. 2017;60(3):155–60.
45. de Ravin SS, Challipalli M, Anderson V, et al. Geosmithia argillacea: an emerging cause of invasive mycosis in human chronic granulomatous disease. Clin Infect Dis. 2011;52(6):e136–43.
46. Vinh DC, Shea YR, Sugui JA, et al. Invasive Aspergillosis due to Neosartorya udagawae. Clin Infect Dis. 2009;49(1):102–11.
47. Vinh DC, Freeman AF, Shea YR, et al. Mucormycosis in chronic granulomatous disease: association with iatrogenic immunosuppression. J Allergy Clin Immunol. 2009;123(6):1411–3.
48. Siler U, Romao S, Tejera E, et al. Severe glucose-6-phosphate dehydrogenase deficiency leads to susceptibility to infection and absent NETosis. J Allergy Clin Immunol. 2017;139(1):212–9.
49. Mauch L, Lun A, O'Gorman MRG, et al. Chronic granulomatous disease (CGD) and complete myeloperoxidase deficiency both yield strongly reduced dihydrorhodamine 123 test signals but can be easily discerned in routine testing for CGD. Clin Chem. 2007;53(5):890–6.

50. Ferguson PJ, Lokuta MA, El-Shanti HI, et al. Neutrophil dysfunction in a family with a SAPHO syndrome-like phenotype. Arthritis Rheum. 2008;58(10):3264–9.
51. Banerjee R, Anguita J, Roos D, Fikrig E. Cutting edge: infection by the agent of human granulocytic ehrlichiosis prevents the respiratory burst by down-regulating gp91phox. J Immunol. 2000;164(8):3946–9.
52. Kuhns DB, Wu X, Hsu AP, et al. Characterization of patients and carriers of p47phox chronic granulomatous disease by flow cytometric analysis of p47phox expression and droplet digital PCR analysis of NCF1. J Clin Immunol. 2018;38(3):349.
53. Kuhns DB, Hsu AP, Sun D, et al. NCF1 (p47 phox)-deficient chronic granulomatous disease: comprehensive genetic and flow cytometric analysis. Blood Adv. 2019;3(2):136–47.
54. Gallin JI, Buescher ES, Seligmann BE, et al. NIH conference. Recent advances in chronic granulomatous disease. Ann Intern Med. 1983;99(5):657–74.
55. Forrest CB, Forehand JR, Axtell RA, Roberts RL, Johnston RB. Clinical features and current management of chronic granulomatous disease. Hematol Oncol Clin N Am. 1988;2(2):253–66.
56. Weening RS, Kabel P, Pijman P, Roos D. Continuous therapy with sulfamethoxazole-trimethoprim in patients with chronic granulomatous disease. J Pediatr. 1983;103(1):127–30.
57. Mouy R. Chronic septic granulomatosis. Clinical and therapeutic aspects. Ann Pediatr. 1989;36(6):374–8.
58. Margolis DM, Melnick DA, Alling DW, Gallin JI. Trimethoprim-sulfamethoxazole prophylaxis in the management of chronic granulomatous disease. J Infect Dis. 1990;162(3):723–6.
59. Gallin JI, Alling DW, Malech HL, et al. Itraconazole to prevent fungal infections in chronic granulomatous disease. N Engl J Med. 2003;348(24):2416–22.
60. Segal BH, Barnhart LA, Anderson VL, et al. Posaconazole as salvage therapy in patients with chronic granulomatous disease and invasive filamentous fungal infection. Clin Infect Dis. 2005;40(11):1684–8.
61. Gallin JI, Malech HL, Weening RS, et al. A controlled trial of interferon gamma to prevent infection in chronic granulomatous disease: the international chronic granulomatous disease cooperative study group. N Engl J Med. 1991;324(8):509–16.
62. Marciano BE, Wesley R, de Carlo ES, et al. Long-term interferon-therapy for patients with chronic granulomatous disease. Clin Infect Dis. 2004;39(5):692–9.
63. Marciano BE, Allen ES, Conry-Cantilena C, et al. Granulocyte transfusions in patients with chronic granulomatous disease and refractory infections: the NIH experience. J Allergy Clin Immunol. 2017;140(2):622–5.
64. Stroncek DF, Leonard K, Eiber G, et al. Alloimmunization after granulocyte transfusions. Transfusion. 1996;75(3):744–55.
65. Heim KF, Fleisher TA, Stroncek DF, et al. The relationship between alloimmunization and posttransfusion granulocyte survival: experience in a chronic granulomatous disease cohort. Transfusion. 2011;51(6):1154–62.
66. Parta M, Kelly C, Kwatemaa N, et al. Allogeneic reduced-intensity hematopoietic stem cell transplantation for chronic granulomatous disease: a single-center prospective trial. J Clin Immunol. 2017;37(6):548–58.
67. Yamazaki-Nakashimada MA, Stiehm ER, Pietropaolo-Cienfuegos D, Hernandez-Bautista V, Espinosa-Rosales F. Corticosteroid therapy for refractory infections in chronic granulomatous disease: case reports and review of the literature. Ann Allergy Asthma Immunol. 2006;97(2):257–61.
68. Freeman AF, Marciano BE, Anderson VL, et al. Corticosteroids in the treatment of severe nocardia pneumonia in chronic granulomatous disease. Pediatr Infect Dis J. 2011;30(9):806–8.
69. Leiding JW, Freeman AF, Marciano BE, et al. Corticosteroid therapy for liver abscess in chronic granulomatous disease. Clin Infect Dis. 2012;54(5):694–700.
70. Straughan DM, McLoughlin KC, Mullinax JE, et al. The changing paradigm of management of liver abscesses in chronic granulomatous disease. Clin Infect Dis. 2018;66(9):1427–34.

71. Magnani A, Brosselin P, Beauté J, et al. Inflammatory manifestations in a single-center cohort of patients with chronic granulomatous disease. J Allergy Clin Immunol. 2014;134(3):655–62.
72. Dunogué B, Pilmis B, Mahlaoui N, et al. Chronic granulomatous disease in patients reaching adulthood: a nationwide study in France. Clin Infect Dis. 2017;64(6):767–75.
73. Marciano BE, Rosenzweig SD, Kleiner DE, et al. Gastrointestinal involvement in chronic granulomatous disease. Pediatrics. 2004;114(2):462–8.
74. Alimchandani M, Lai JP, Aung PP, et al. Gastrointestinal histopathology in chronic granulomatous disease a study of 87 patients. Am J Surg Pathol. 2013;37(9):1365–72.
75. Johnson FE, Humbert JR, Kuzela DC, Todd JK, Lilly JR. Gastric outlet obstruction due to X-linked chronic granulomatous disease. Surgery. 1975;78(2):217–23.
76. Salvator H, Mahlaoui N, Catherinot E, et al. Pulmonary manifestations in adult patients with chronic granulomatous disease. Eur Respir J. 2015;45(6):1613–23.
77. Mahdaviani SA, Mohajerani SA, Rezaei N, et al. Pulmonary manifestations of chronic granulomatous disease. Expert Rev Clin Immunol. 2013;9(2):153–60.
78. Hussain N, Feld JJ, Kleiner DE, et al. Hepatic abnormalities in patients with chronic granulomatous disease. Hepatology. 2007;45(3):675–83.
79. Feld JJ, Hussain N, Wright EC, et al. Hepatic involvement and portal hypertension predict mortality in chronic granulomatous disease. Gastroenterology. 2008;134(7):1917–26.
80. Walther MM, Malech H, Berman A, et al. The urological manifestations of chronic granulomatous disease. J Urol. 1992;147(5):1314–8.
81. Barese CN, Podestá M, Litvak E, Villa M, Rivas EM. Recurrent eosinophilic cystitis in a child with chronic granulomatous disease. J Pediatr Hematol Oncol. 2004;26(3):209–12.
82. Claps A, della Corte M, Gerocarni Nappo S, et al. How should eosinophilic cystitis be treated in patients with chronic granulomatous disease? Pediatr Nephrol. 2014;29(11):2229–33.
83. Eckert JW, Abramson SL, Starke J, Brandt ML. The surgical implications of chronic granulomatous disease. Am J Surg. 1995;169(3):320–3.
84. Feingold PL, Quadri HS, Steinberg SM, et al. Thoracic surgery in chronic granulomatous disease: a 25-year single-institution experience. J Clin Immunol. 2016;36(7):677–83.
85. Akagi K, Kawai T, Watanabe N, et al. A case of macrophage activation syndrome developing in a patient with chronic granulomatous disease-associated colitis. J Pediatr Hematol Oncol. 2014;36(3):e169–72.
86. Valentine G, Thomas TA, Nguyen T, Lai YC. Chronic granulomatous disease presenting as hemophagocytic lymphohistiocytosis: a case report. Pediatrics. 2014;134(6):e1727–30.
87. Parekh C, Hofstra T, Church JA, Coates TD. Hemophagocytic lymphohistiocytosis in children with chronic granulomatous disease. Pediatr Blood Cancer. 2011;56(3):460–2.
88. Bode SFN, Ammann S, Al-Herz W, et al. The syndrome of hemophagocytic lymphohistiocytosis in primary immunodeficiencies: implications for differential diagnosis and pathogenesis. Haematologica. 2015;100(7):978–88.
89. Siddiqui S, Anderson VL, Hilligoss DM, et al. Fulminant mulch pneumonitis: an emergency presentation of chronic granulomatous disease. Clin Infect Dis. 2007;45(6):673–81.
90. Ameratunga R, Woon ST, Vyas J, Roberts S. Fulminant mulch pneumonitis in undiagnosed chronic granulomatous disease: a medical emergency. Clin Pediatr. 2010;49(12):1143–6.
91. Maaloul I, Ben Ameur S, Chabchoub I, et al. Fulminant mulch pneumonitis in a previously healthy child. Arch Pediatr. 2018;25(8):495–6.
92. Battersby AC, Braggins H, Pearce MS, et al. Inflammatory and autoimmune manifestations in X-linked carriers of chronic granulomatous disease in the United Kingdom. J Allergy Clin Immunol. 2017;140(2):628–30.
93. Marciano BE, Zerbe CS, Falcone EL, et al. X-linked carriers of chronic granulomatous disease: illness, lyonization, and stability. J Allergy Clin Immunol. 2018;141(1):365–71.
94. Battersby A, Braggins H, Pearce M, et al. Health-related quality of life and emotional health in X-linked carriers of chronic granulomatous disease in the United Kingdom. J Clin Immunol. 2019;39(2):195–9.
95. de Luca A, Smeekens SP, Casagrande A, et al. IL-1 receptor blockade restores autophagy and reduces inflammation in chronic granulomatous disease in mice and in humans. Proc Natl Acad Sci U S A. 2014;111(9):3526–31.

96. Hahn KJ, Ho N, Yockey L, et al. Treatment with Anakinra, a recombinant IL-1 receptor antagonist, unlikely to induce lasting remission in patients with CGD colitis. Am J Gastroenterol. 2015;110(6):938–9.
97. Butte MJ, Park KT, Lewis DB. Treatment of CGD-associated colitis with the IL-23 blocker ustekinumab. J Clin Immunol. 2016;36(7):619–20.
98. Campbell N, Chapdelaine H. Treatment of chronic granulomatous disease–associated fistulising colitis with vedolizumab. J Allergy Clin Immunol Pract. 2017;5(6):1748–9.
99. Horwitz ME. Stem-cell transplantation for inherited immunodeficiency disorders. Pediatr Clin North Am. 2000;47(6):1371–87. https://doi.org/10.1016/s0031-3955(05)70276-5. Pediatr Clin North Am. 2000. PMID: 11131001.
100. Horwitz ME, Barrett AJ, Brown MR, et al. Treatment of chronic granulomatous disease with nonmyeloablative conditioning and a T-cell-depleted hematopoietic allograft. N Engl J Med. 2001;344(12):881–8.
101. Seger RA, Gungor T, Belohradsky BH, et al. Treatment of chronic granulomatous disease with myeloablative conditioning and an unmodified hemopoietic allograft: a survey of the European experience, 1985–2000. Blood. 2002;100(13):4344–50.
102. Schuetz C, Hoenig M, Gatz S, et al. Hematopoietic stem cell transplantation from matched unrelated donors in chronic granulomatous disease. Immunol Res. 2009;44(1–3):35–41.
103. Soncini E, Slatter MA, Jones LBKR, et al. Unrelated donor and HLA-identical sibling haematopoietic stem cell transplantation cure chronic granulomatous disease with good long-term outcome and growth. Br J Haematol. 2009;145(1):73–83.
104. Goździk J, Pituch-Noworolska A, Skoczeń S, et al. Allogeneic haematopoietic stem cell transplantation as therapy for chronic granulomatous disease-single centre experience. J Clin Immunol. 2011;31(3):322–7.
105. Martinez CA, Shah S, Shearer WT, et al. Excellent survival after sibling or unrelated donor stem cell transplantation for chronic granulomatous disease. J Allergy Clin Immunol. 2012;129(1):176–83.
106. Tewari P, Martin PL, Mendizabal A, et al. Myeloablative transplantation using either cord blood or bone marrow leads to immune recovery, high long-term donor chimerism and excellent survival in chronic granulomatous disease. Biol Blood Marrow Transplant. 2012;18(9):1368–77.
107. Morillo-Gutierrez B, Beier R, Rao K, et al. Treosulfan-based conditioning for allogeneic HSCT in children with chronic granulomatous disease: a multicenter experience. Blood. 2016;128(21):2585.
108. Mehta B, Mahadeo K, Kapoor N, Abdel-Azim H. Low-dose total-body irradiation and alemtuzumab-based reduced-intensity conditioning regimen results in durable engraftment and correction of clinical disease among children with chronic granulomatous disease. Pediatr Transplant. 2015;19(4):408–12.
109. Lum SH, Flood T, Hambleton S, et al. Two decades of excellent transplant survival for chronic granulomatous disease: a supraregional immunology transplant center report. Blood. 2019;133(23):2547–9.
110. Cole T, Pearce MS, Cant AJ, et al. Clinical outcome in children with chronic granulomatous disease managed conservatively or with hematopoietic stem cell transplantation. J Allergy Clin Immunol. 2013;132(5):1150–5.
111. Cole T, McKendrick F, Titman P, et al. Health related quality of life and emotional health in children with chronic granulomatous disease: a comparison of those managed conservatively with those that have undergone haematopoietic stem cell transplant. J Clin Immunol. 2013;33(1):8–13.
112. Yonkof JR, Gupta A, Fu P, Garabedian E, Dalal J. Role of allogeneic hematopoietic stem cell transplant for chronic granulomatous disease (CGD): a report of the United States Immunodeficiency Network. J Clin Immunol. 2019;39:448–58.
113. Güngör T, Teira P, Slatter M, et al. Reduced-intensity conditioning and HLA-matched haemopoietic stem-cell transplantation in patients with chronic granulomatous disease: a prospective multicentre study. Lancet. 2014;383(9915):436–48.

114. Khandelwal P, Bleesing JJ, Davies SM, et al. A Single-Center Experience Comparing Alemtuzumab, Fludarabine, and Melphalan Reduced-Intensity Conditioning with Myeloablative Busulfan, Cyclophosphamide, and Antithymocyte Globulin for Chronic Granulomatous Disease. Biol Blood Marrow Transplant. 2016;22(11):2011–8. https://doi.org/10.1016/j.bbmt.2016.08.013. Epub 2016. Biol Blood Marrow Transplant. 2016. PMID: 27543157.
115. Fox TA, Chakraverty R, Burns S, et al. Successful outcome following allogeneic hematopoietic stem cell transplantation in adults with primary immunodeficiency. Blood. 2018;131(8):917–31.
116. Parta M, Kelly C, Kwatemaa N, et al. Allogeneic Reduced-Intensity Hematopoietic Stem Cell Transplantation for Chronic Granulomatous Disease: a Single-Center Prospective Trial. J Clin Immunol. 2017;37(6):548–58. https://doi.org/10.1007/s10875-017-0422-6. Epub 2017 Jul 28. J Clin Immunol. 2017. PMID: 28752258.
117. Arnold DE, Sullivan KE, Jyonouchi S, et al. Immune reconstitution in six adolescents with chronic granulomatous disease following hematopoietic stem cell transplant. J Allergy Clin Immunol Pract. 2017;7(3):1052–4.
118. Lum SH, Flood T, Hambleton S, et al. Two decades of excellent transplant survival for chronic granulomatous disease: a supraregional immunology transplant center report. Blood. 2019;133(23):2546–9. https://doi.org/10.1182/blood.2019000021. Epub 2019 Apr 5. Blood. 2019. PMID: 30952673.
119. Oshrine B, Morsheimer M, Heimall J, Bunin N. Reduced-intensity conditioning for hematopoietic cell transplantation of chronic granulomatous disease. Pediatr Blood Cancer. 2015;62(2):359–61.
120. Marsh RA, Leiding JW, Logan BR, et al. Chronic granulomatous disease-associated IBD resolves and does not adversely impact survival following allogeneic HCT. J Clin Immunol. 2019;39(7):653–67.
121. Malech HL, Maples PB, Whiting-Theobald N, et al. Prolonged production of NADPH oxidase-corrected granulocytes after gene therapy of chronic granulomatous disease. Proc Natl Acad Sci U S A. 1997;94(22):12133–8.
122. Ott MG, Schmidt M, Schwarzwaelder K, et al. Correction of X-linked chronic granulomatous disease by gene therapy, augmented by insertional activation of MDS1-EVI1, PRDM16 or SETBP1. Nat Med. 2006;12(4):401–9.
123. Stein S, Ott MG, Schultze-Strasser S, et al. Genomic instability and myelodysplasia with monosomy 7 consequent to EVI1 activation after gene therapy for chronic granulomatous disease. Nat Med. 2010;16(2):198–204.
124. Bianchi M, Hakkim A, Brinkmann V, et al. Restoration of NET formation by gene therapy in CGD controls aspergillosis. Blood. 2009;114(13):2619–22.
125. Siler U, Paruzynski A, Holtgreve-Grez H, et al. Successful combination of sequential gene therapy and rescue allo-HSCT in two children with X-CGD – importance of timing. Curr Gene Ther. 2015;15(4):416–27.
126. Kang HJ, Bartholomae CC, Paruzynski A, et al. Retroviral gene therapy for X-linked chronic granulomatous disease: results from phase I/II trial. Mol Ther. 2011;19(11):2092–101.
127. Malech HL, Booth C, Kang EM, et al. Lentiviral vector gene therapy for X-linked chronic granulomatous disease corrects neutrophil function. J Clin Immunol. 2019;39(Suppl 1):S45.

Chapter 18
Primary Immunodeficiencies of Complement

Peter D. Arkwright

Case Presentation 1

Two brothers aged 13 and 14 years old, both with a history of group Y *Neisseria meningitidis* septicemia during the previous 12 months, were referred for investigation of a possible underlying immunodeficiency. The boys presented to hospital on separate occasions with a fever and a non-blanching petechial rash. They had no circulatory compromise and no clinical features suggestive of meningitis. They were treated with intravenous ceftriaxone and required no respiratory or circulatory support. The family were white European, and there was no history of consanguinity. Two other siblings were well with no significant infections.

Both boys had a history of tonsillitis and recurrent suppurative otitis media. There was no history of skin or chest infections. Previous chickenpox had been mild with only a few spots. On examination, both boys looked well with clear lungs and skin. One still had signs of a perforated left tympanic membrane but no discharge. Blood count and serum immunoglobulins were normal and tetanus antibody titers protective. However, both CH50 and AH50 hemolysis were undetectable. Complement C7 protein was absent when measured by immunoprecipitation. Gene sequencing revealed a homozygous c.1561C>A (R499S) mutation in the *C7* gene of the complement membrane attack complex in both patients. Parents were heterozygous for the gene mutation.

The family were provided with advice and written information about primary complement deficiency, as well as contact details for the national patient support group. They were also given genetic counseling and open access to the children's ward in case of further infections. The two other siblings were tested and had normal CH50 and AH50. The boys were commenced on prophylactic amoxicillin and

---

P. D. Arkwright (✉)
Lydia Becker Institute of Immunology and Inflammation, University of Manchester, Manchester, UK
e-mail: peter.arkwright@nhs.net

given the conjugate quadrivalent A, C, W, and Y meningococcal vaccine, as well as booster doses of *Haemophilus influenzae* type b (Hib) and Prevnar vaccines. Meningococcal B (MenB) vaccine was not yet available.

Four months after the first clinic appointment, the older brother presented to hospital with PCR positive MenB disease associated with fever and rash, but again no circulatory compromise. He was treated with a 7-day course of intravenous ceftriaxone in accordance with local antibiotic guidelines. When seen in clinic 1 month later, the patient admitted he had not taken his antibiotic prophylaxis. He and his brother were followed up in the pediatric clinic until they were both over 17 years old. At that point, they failed to attend their hospital appointments and were referred to colleagues in the adult service. They did attend their first appointment in the adult clinic, where again both admitted not taking their prophylactic antibiotics. A booster dose of the quadrivalent meningococcal vaccine was given. They have failed to attend further follow-up in the past decade.

Discussion of Case Presentation 1

There are several important learning points to be gleaned from this case of terminal complement pathway deficiency which classically presents with invasive meningococcal disease. Disorders of terminal complement components C5–C9, involved in the formation of the membrane attack complex create pores in the bacterial membrane leading to their lysis, are typically associated with invasive *Neisseria meningitidis* infections. Patients often present with recurrent meningococcal sepsis due to unusual serotypes. They may also have a clinical history of bacterial sinopulmonary or skin infections. Immunity to viruses is normal. Less than half of patients present in the first decade of life. Three quarters will present by the end of the second decade [1]. Recommended screening is CH50 and AH50, which are often absent. C3 and C4 is typically normal. As these diseases are inherited in an autosomal recession pattern and the risk of other siblings being affected is one in four, all siblings should be screened. Vaccination against meningococcal serotypes using conjugate quadrivalent A, C, W, Y, and the B vaccines will help to protect patients from severe invasive disease, although protection is not absolute and therefore patients will still need access to acute medical services to treat septic episodes. Life-long prophylactic antibiotics are recommended, but patient compliance is variable, particularly in the higher-risk teenage and young adult age group. Intermittent antibiotic use may increase the risk of antibiotic resistance. Long-term follow-up is important to ensure that antibody protection against meningococcal serotypes is maintained but may be challenging in patients who are well.

Case Presentation 2

A 10-year-old Asian boy from a highly consanguineous family was referred for an immunological opinion while in hospital with an acute CNS vasculopathy. He had presented with global dysphagia, quadra- and bulbar paresis, generalized

Fig. 18.1 Early-onset SLE in boy with C1q deficiency demonstrating classical malar rash of lupus erythematosus

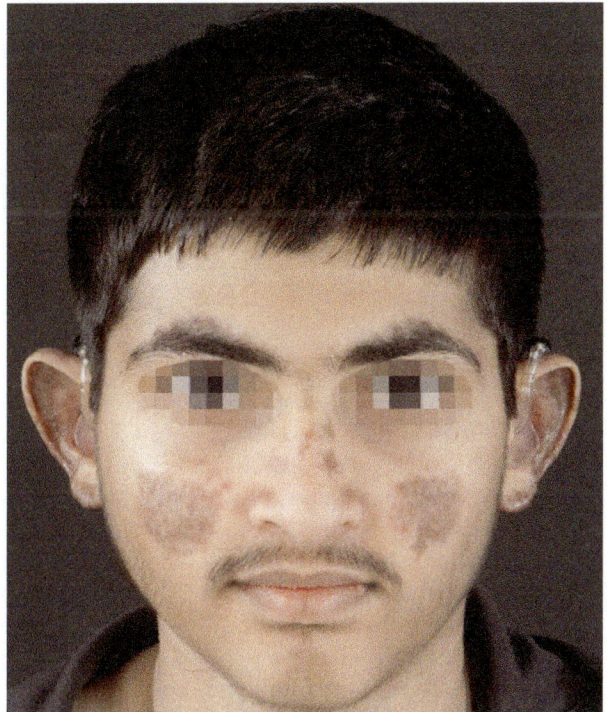

hypertonia, and a resting tremor. Prior to admission, he had a 5-week history of fevers, vomiting, and diarrhea. No pathogens had been isolated from his stools, blood, or CSF. At 3 years old, he has suffered from *Streptococcus pneumoniae* meningitis requiring intensive care, which had left him with sensorineural deafness and learning difficulties. On examination, he had a malar rash typical of lupus (Fig. 18.1). An MRI scan of his brain showed bilateral infarcts in his basal ganglia consistent with a small vessel vasculitis. Anti-Sm, SS-A60 (Ro), and cardiolipin IgG antibodies were positive, but dsDNA autoantibodies were consistently negative. CSF protein and interferon-α were raised [2].

The patient responded to high-dose intravenous corticosteroids, but his clinical condition deteriorated when the drug dose was weaned. Pulse intravenous cyclophosphamide was added, in accordance with recommended treatment for neuropsychiatric SLE and he made a steady improvement. Immunosuppressive therapy was continued using oral prednisolone, hydroxychloroquine, and azathioprine.

The patient had five brothers, one of whom had died at 17 months of age of *Streptococcus pneumoniae* meningitis, another had signs of discoid lupus [3]. His father had died at 38 years old of congestive cardiac failure after suffering from renal failure secondary to chronic glomerulonephritis at 18 years old, requiring renal transplantation.

CH50 hemolysis was absent in the proband, his father, and three of his brothers. The brother who died at 17 months had not been tested. Further testing confirmed a defect in the C1q component of the classical complement cascade. Because of the severity of the proband's disease he underwent successful hematopoietic stem cell transplantation (HSCT) from an HLA-matched but unaffected brother [4] and at the age of 24, 7 years posttransplant, remains well with normal C1q levels and no evidence of clinical or laboratory evidence of autoimmunity.

Unfortunately, one of his affected brothers subsequently developed acute CNS vasculitis, which left him in a vegetative state despite aggressive immunosuppressive therapy and he died at 17 years old. His other affected brothers remain asymptomatic in their thirties and currently require no treatment.

Discussion of Case Presentation 2

This case describes a deficiency of the classical component pathway component, C1q, and illustrates how classical pathway component deficiencies are associated with a complex interplay between infection and autoimmunity. Disorders of the classical complement pathway are more likely to be associated with invasive pneumococcal than meningococcal disease. This is because C1q, C2, and C4 promote opsonization and phagocytosis, which are more important than pore formation in pneumococcal immunity. CH50 is the screening test of choice for patients suspected of having a deficiency of the classical complement pathway. C1q deficiency prevents normal clearance of immune complexes by monocytes [2]. Immune complexes are thus taken up by dendritic cells, which induce proinflammatory responses, endothelial damage, and vasculitis resembling SLE. Renal and CNS vasculitis cause serious morbidity and mortality, even with prompt instigation of systemic immunosuppressants. Twenty percent of patients with C1q deficiency die by the age of 20 years, although 50% remain healthy and well into middle age. Vasculitis is usually anti-dsDNA autoantibody negative, while anti-Sm, anti-SSA (Ro), and anti-cardiolipin autoantibodies are often positive. As these diseases are inherited in an autosomal recessive pattern and the risk of other siblings being affected is one in four, all siblings should be screened. Unlike other complement factors, C1q is produced by bone marrow-derived monocytes and is potentially curable by hematopoietic stem cell transplant (HSCT). Deciding on the best course of management is challenging, as the clinical course is variable, even among affected members of the same family. Patients need to be managed on a case-by-case basis.

A Complement Pathway Primer

An understanding of disease pathogenesis and therapy depends on knowledge of the underlying biology and this is true also for complement disorders. A summary of important concepts is provided in the following section (Fig. 18.2). The complement pathway in humans has evolved through the integration of previously functionally diverse ancestral proteins into a unifying cascade [5–7].

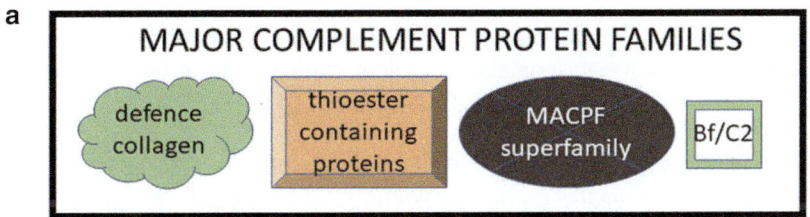

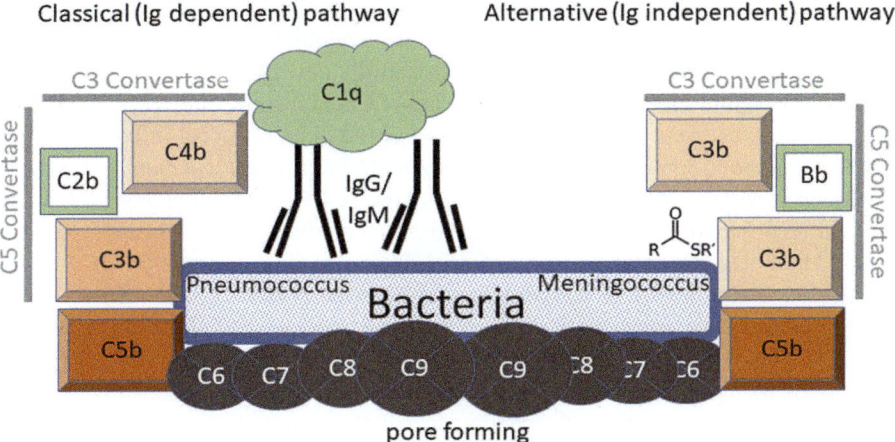

Fig. 18.2 Complement system components. (**a**) Major complement protein families. (**b**) Major complement activation pathways

Complement factor C1 inhibitor deficiency (hereditary angioedema) occurs in 1/10,000 individuals. It is not associated with an infection or autoimmunity risk, but rather skin and soft tissue, bowel, and laryngeal edema, the latter which is associated with upper airway obstruction and death in a third of unrecognized/untreated cases. C1 inhibitor deficiency can be confused with allergy but does not respond to antihistamines or intramuscular epinephrine. It requires specific treatment with C1 inhibitor replacement or bradykinin receptor blockade. This complement deficiency is not discussed further in this chapter.

1. *Pore-forming terminal complement components mediate bacterial lysis.* Complement factors C6–C9 of the terminal complement cascade induce bacterial lysis. They are all members of the membrane attack complex/perforin (MACPF) protein superfamily, pore-forming toxins that punch holes in the membranes of gram-negative bacteria and are particularly important for immunity against meningococcus. Phylogenetically, they are related to cholesterol-dependent cytolysins (streptolysin O, pneumolysin) secreted by gram-positive bacteria that punch holes in mammalian cell membranes containing cholesterol [8]. Deficiencies of these terminal complement pathway components are mainly associated with recurrent invasive meningococcal infections.

2. *C3 thioester-containing proteins orchestrate terminal pathway activation, opsonization, and phagocyte recruitment.* At the functional heart of the complement cascade is C3, a thioester-containing protein, with structural homology to C4 and C5. Cleavage and activation of C3 results in C3b with its characteristic short-acting, highly reactive thioester chemical group. The relevance of the thioester group is that it mediates covalent binding of C3b to bacteria and other membrane surfaces in the immediate vicinity, initiating a local inflammatory response with minimal bystander damage. C3b is a key component of C5 convertase, which activates C5 and subsequently C6–C9-induced lysis [9]. Protein fragments C3a and C5a released during the activation of C3 and C5 by binding to their respective receptors on the vascular endothelium function as chemoattractants, increasing local vascular permeability and allowing ingress of phagocytic cells into local tissues. Deficiencies of C3, C5, and C4 are associated with primarily recurrent invasive meningococcal and pneumococcal infections.
3. *Activation of C3 by defense collagen proteins of the classical and mannose-binding lectin complement pathways.* C1q binds to the Fc CH2 domain of aggregated IgG and IgM within immune complexes [10]. This binding alters its tertiary structure and thus activates serine proteases C1r and C1s, the C3 convertase (C4bC2b), and subsequently the rest of the complement pathway [11]. C1q thus forms a direct link between the innate and acquired immune systems. C1q also binds apoptotic cells, nucleic acids, and bacteria, including *Streptococcus pneumoniae* [12], promoting their clearance by macrophages. C1q deficiency is more likely to be associated with recurrent invasive pneumococcal than meningococcal infections. In addition, the inability to clear immune complexes, nucleic acids, and apoptotic cells leads to an immune complex, SLE-like vasculitis in 80% of patients. Mannose-binding lectin (MBL) is also a defense collagen protein. Unlike C1q, it does not require immunoglobulin, but binds direct to bacteria via mannose-containing glycoproteins to activate the C4bC2b C3 convertase. MBL seems to be largely redundant in humans, as 25% of healthy Eurasians and 50–60% of people from sub-Sahara have reduced or absent MBL expression [13]. However, some studies suggest that patients with MBL deficiency may experience more severe septic episodes, necessitating a more vigilant approach to monitoring and treating these patients with appropriate antibiotics at the first sign of infection [14].
4. *Auto-activation of C3.* Small amounts of C3b are continually being produced by the spontaneous breakdown of C3. This process is augmented by binding of C3b to Factor B (a C2 homolog) leading to the formation of C3bBb (a C3 convertase). Cleavage of Factor B to active Bb occurs by Factor D [15]. Subsequent binding of a second C3b molecule to the C3bBb complex leads to the formation of a C5 convertase (C3bBbC3b) and the activation of the C6–C9 complex of the terminal pathway. Properdin stabilizes the C3bBb complex, increasing the half-life of C3b from 2 to 18 min. This "alterative pathway" of complement activation functions independently of prior antibody production to specific microbes and can be thought of a pure and thus rapid innate immune response to infection. Deficiencies of Factor B, Factor D, or properdin are associated with recurrent invasive infections with meningococcus and pneumococcus [15–17].

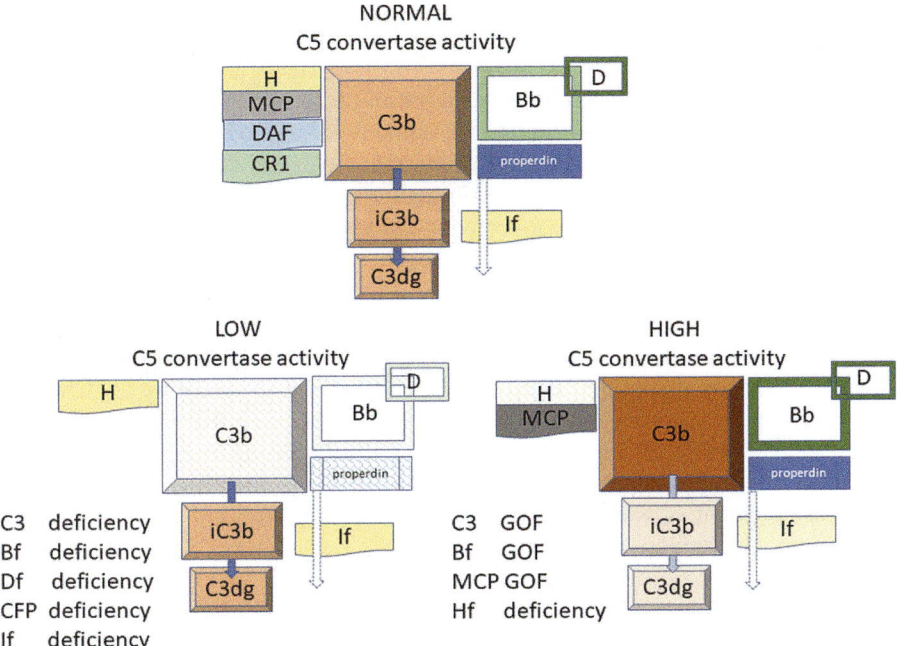

Fig. 18.3 Regulation of C3 in health and diseases associated with reduced or overactivity

5. *Regulation of C3 activity.* C3b is essential for immunity to encapsulated bacteria, but its activity needs to be tightly regulated to prevent excessive autoactivation, which causes damaging autoinflammation, particularly in the vasculature. C3b activity is modulated by a number of regulatory proteins, which either neutralize C3b activity (Factor H, decay acceleration factor (DAF, CD55), CR1, and membrane cofactor protein (MCP, CD46)) or promote its degradation to iC3b and C3dg (Factor I) (Fig. 18.3). Deficiency of Factor H or MCP results in C3b overactivity and chronic inflammation particularly involving the renal vasculature leading to atypical hemolytic uremic syndrome (aHUS) or membranoproliferative glomerulonephritis (MPGN). Interestingly, despite Factor I promoting degradation of C3b, complete Factor I deficiency is associated with recurrent invasive bacterial infections, while partial deficiency leads to recurrent sterile neuroinflammation [18].

Diagnosis/Assessment

Key to the diagnosis of complement deficiencies is, firstly, to consider the possibility within the clinical differential and, secondly, to request the correct screening test. As primary complement diseases are very uncommon, most clinicians are likely to see only a few patients with these diseases over their career.

Role and Responsibility of Primary Care Physicians

Symptomatic patients will almost always present to hospital and therefore physicians solely working in the community are unlikely to have to diagnose complement disorders. The major caveat is that as primary complement deficiencies are inherited, it is important that birth of a new sibling into a family where there is already a history of complement deficiency prompts the primary care physician to refer the baby to a specialist for testing soon after birth. In published series, two thirds of children with complement deficiencies have a family history, and important questions to ask parents are "Is there a family history of immune problems?" and "Does anyone else in the immediate family (particularly brothers or sisters) suffer from an immune problem?" [19]. The consequences of not doing so can be tragic. Children can die of meningococcal septicemia in the first year of life despite prompt commencement of intravenous antibiotics, if the family, the obstetrician, or primary care physician does not notify appropriate infectious disease specialists knowledgeable about complement deficiencies after the birth of a high-risk child so that prompt therapeutic interventions can be implemented.

Role and Responsibilities of Secondary Care/ Hospital-Based Physicians

Table 18.1 highlights important clinical features which should prompt hospital-based clinicians to consider a complement deficiency. Classical complement pathway defects should be considered in patients presenting with *Streptococcus pneumoniae* pneumonia or blood-borne infections, particularly if recurrent where serum immunoglobulin concentrations are normal.

Table 18.1 Clinical features of complement pathway defects: similarities and differences

	Classical pathway defects	Alternative pathway defects	C3b dysregulation
Examples	Deficiencies of C1q, C2, C4	Deficiencies of C3, Factor B, properdin, C5–C9	C3 or Factor B gain of function, deficiencies of Factor H, Factor I, membrane cofactor protein
Infections	Invasive/recurrent pneumococcal rather than meningococcal infections predominate	Invasive/recurrent meningococcal rather than meningococcal infections predominate	No inherent predisposition to infection. Risk of meningococcal disease with eculizumab
Autoimmunity	Immune complex SLE-like disease with raised anti-Sm autoantibodies (esp. with C1q)	None	aHUS, membrano-proliferative/dense deposit glomerulopathy
Family history	Often present	Often present	Often present

Both children and adults may alternatively present with immune complex disease affecting the skin (discoid lupus), kidneys, brain, and other organs. Particularly in prepubertal children presenting with florid signs of SLE, an underlying immunodeficiency or immune dysregulatory disorder should be considered, including defects in C1q, C2, C4 of the classical complement cascade, as well as defects in other pathways such as nucleic acid sensing and degradation, proteasome function, and type I interferon signaling [20]. Of the complement deficiencies, C1q is most likely to be associated with early-onset SLE. A review of 45 patients from 31 families with C1q deficiency found that 80% suffered from clinical features suggestive of SLE. Nine (20%) of the patients died, all but one before 20 years old. A detailed family history should be taken. CH50 is the primary screening test and if normal rules out a classical complement pathway defect.

Alternative pathway defects often present with *Neisseria meningitidis* infections involving uncommon or unencapsulated strains, particularly if recurrent or associated with an additional history of sinopulmonary or skin infections [1]. Again, a detailed family history should be taken. Autoimmunity is unusual in patients with terminal complement component defects (C5–C9). CH50 and AH50 are the primary screening tests and if normal rule out an alternative pathway defect.

Clinicians managing patients with aHUS, as well as membranoproliferative/dense deposit glomerulopathy or recurrent IgA vasculitis (Henoch-Schönlein purpura), should consider underlying complement deficiencies. Infection-induced HUS is the more common form of HUS and is triggered by Shiga toxin-producing *Escherichia coli* (STEC). Risk factors are eating contaminated meat or swimming in fecal-contaminated water. In contrast, non-infection-induced aHUS is found to be associated with either an acquired (autoantibody) or a constitutional dysregulation of the complement alternative pathway in more than 60% of patients. Primary complement deficiencies causing aHUS, membranoproliferative/dense deposit glomerulopathy, and recurrent IgA vasculitis (Henoch-Schönlein purpura) include Factor H (25%), Factor I (5–10%), or membrane cofactor protein (CD46) with gain of function C3 (10%) [21–23]. In these patients either gain of function mutations in C3 or deficiencies in complement regulatory factors result in C3b overactivity driving endothelial inflammation and injury. Atypical HUS is associated with 3% mortality in children and 10% mortality in adults over a 5-year follow-up. The risk of renal failure requiring dialysis is one-third of pediatric patients and half of adults [24].

Laboratory Testing for Patients with Possible Complement Deficiencies

Screening Tests

Most clinicians requesting complement tests select C3 and C4 measurements. These tests are inappropriate for the vast majority of patients with primary complement deficiencies. The correct screening tests are CH50 and AH50. As with screening for the coagulation defects, CH50 and AH50 assess the function of the whole complement cascade, rather than a specific component. CH50 assesses the activity of the classical, immunoglobulin-dependent pathway, while AH50 assesses the activity of the alternative, immunoglobulin-independent pathway. Classical pathway (CH50) activation is reported as the reciprocal of the serum dilution at which 50% of sheep erythrocytes pre-coated with rabbit anti-sheep red blood cell antibody lyse. The degree of hemolysis is quantified by measuring the absorbance of the hemoglobin released into the supernatant at 540 nm. Activity of the alternative pathway (AH50) is measured using unsensitized rabbit (or guinea pig) erythrocytes, which, unlike sheep erythrocytes, are lysed by human complement without the need for pre-coating with immunoglobulin [25].

Some laboratories measure CH100 and AP100 (100% lysis of erythrocytes by the patient's serum) rather than CH50 and AH50 (50% lysis). CH100 and AP100 utilize a plate rather than tube screening method.

If CH50 and/or AH50 are low (typically undetectable), then after confirming that the abnormality is not due to a technical error by repeating the test, relevant specific complement components should be tested, followed by targeted gene mutation screening of the specific complement protein. When repeating the assay, it may be prudent to send the sample to a different reference lab as assay reliability may differ between laboratories.

Reasons for Falsely Low CH50 and AH50 Activity

Abnormally low CH50 and AH50 activity may occur if blood samples are not taken and processed correctly. It is important that blood is sampled from a free-flowing venipuncture. Poor sampling, including finger or heal prick samples from infants and children, is likely to induce activation of the complement cascade resulting in falsely low, sometimes undetectable levels. Additionally, complement factors are a group of enzymes which degrade spontaneously, even at room temperature. Blood samples should ideally be transferred on ice and be received by the laboratory within 4 h. Delay in receipt of blood samples by the laboratory, particularly if overnight or after a weekend, is likely to result in falsely low levels, making interpretation difficult and thus requiring a repeat blood test. Where there is no local laboratory that can measure CH50 and AH50, separation and freezing of the serum, before sending the frozen serum on dry ice, may be required.

Patients with Complement System Dysregulation Rather than Deficiency

For patients with aHUS or membranoproliferative glomerulopathy due to complement pathway dysregulation rather than deficiency, CH50 and AH50 may be normal. For patients with these clinical presentations, candidate gene testing (mutation analysis for *C3*, Factor B (*CFB*), Factor H (*CFH*), Factor I (*CFI*), and membrane cofactor protein (*CD46*)) is the investigation of choice.

Autoantibody Testing in Cases of SLE-Like Disease

When investigating the possibility of SLE-like disease in patients with C1q deficiency, anti-double-stranded (ds)DNA antibodies may be normal. It is more common to find raised ANA with a speckled appearance, positive anti-Sm, anti-SSA (Ro), and anti-cardiolipin IgG antibodies [3, 4].

Supplementary Immune Tests

The word "complement" derives from the fact that this system of blood proteins *complements* the antibody system, promoting opsonization and phagocytosis of encapsulated bacteria. Thus, in patients where there is a deficiency of complement, the risk of life-threatening invasive infections due to encapsulated organisms, particularly *Neisseria meningitidis* and *Streptococcus pneumoniae*, can be partly mitigated by immunization against these organisms. An important part of monitoring patients to prevent infectious complications is regular 1–2 yearly measurement of vaccine responses to these bacteria and booster immunization with conjugate, rather than polysaccharide, vaccines when antibody levels start to wane below protective levels. Ideally serotype-specific responses to pneumococci and meningococci should be measured, as they more directly reflect the effectiveness of the specific vaccine.

Management/Outcome

Diseases of the Classical Pathway

Classical pathway defects carry a significant morbidity and mortality from *Streptococcus pneumoniae* infections and, particularly in C1q deficiency, the potential for serious immune complex-mediated vasculitis affecting the brain and kidneys, as the second clinical case illustrates. Immunization with conjugate pneumococcal vaccines helps protect against infection. Autoimmune complications in C1q deficiency are unpredictable, sometimes fulminant, and may be poorly responsive to high-dose corticosteroids, cyclophosphamide, and rituximab routinely used to treat SLE, particularly if there is a delay in recognition and commencement of therapy [26].

Most complement components are produced by liver hepatocytes. The exception is C1q, which is produced by bone marrow-derived monocytes. Thus, in families where the patient or their close relatives have died or have suffered from serious complications, HSCT may be considered as a potentially curative therapeutic option in C1q deficiency. HSCT should only be carried out in a center with sufficient throughput and experience in managing patients with a range of nonmalignant diseases. The risk of exacerbating vascular inflammation and graft versus host disease can be reduced by using reduced intensity conditioning and up-front serotherapy to remove autoreactive T-lymphocytes [4]. The dilemma for clinicians is to determine which patients would benefit from HSCT and which patients may go through life without any major medical complications. Current statistics suggest that 20% of patients with C1q deficiency die by the age of 20 years old, while 50% may survive into middle age [26]. Benefits and risks need to be weighed up and discussed for individual patients based on their previous clinical course and current clinical status, family history, and availability of a well-matched HLA donor.

Diseases of the Terminal Complement Pathway (Membrane Attack Complex)

The main risk for patients with terminal complement components (C5–C9) deficiencies is recurrent meningococcal rather than pneumococcal infections. Autoimmune complications are not a significant problem. With the advent of conjugate quadrivalent MenA, C, W, Y, and MenB vaccines, the infection risk can be reduced but not completely mitigated by immunization and booster vaccines when meningococcal serotype titers drop below the protective range. A study of 45 Russian patients with terminal component deficiencies showed that meningococcal vaccination reduced the risk of infection and also its severity [27].

Because protective levels of antibodies to pneumococcus and meningococcus do not guarantee protection against potentially life-threatening sepsis, prophylactic antibiotics such as amoxicillin are recommended in all patients. The challenge, as illustrated in the first clinical case, is the problem of noncompliance, not only with antibiotic prophylaxis but general follow-up. It should be assumed that many patients will not take their prophylactic antibiotics regularly and emphasizing the importance of seeking urgent medical attention in case of a high fever or other signs of sepsis is an important part of the management plan.

Complement C3 Deficiencies and Dysregulatory Disorders

C3 is at the heart of the complement pathway activity. Complete lack of C3 is associated with a high risk of recurrent sinopulmonary infections and meningitis caused by encapsulated bacteria, particularly pneumococcus and meningococcus, as documented in 80% of 40 C3-deficient patients [28] of whom 15% also had SLE-like disease. Symptom onset was in the first few years of life and 29% of children died before their second birthday.

For patients with defects in C3b regulation due to a deficiency in one of the regulatory factors (e.g., Factor H, Factor I, MCP), the main risk is renal vascular disease leading to renal failure requiring dialysis, rather than an inherent risk of infection directly caused by the complement deficiency. These patients are typically managed by renal physicians. Unlike patients with other causes of end-stage renal disease, where renal transplantation is preferred to long-term dialysis, the risk of recurrent disease after transplant is 30–60%, as the defect in C3b activity remains. Anti-C5 monoclonal antibody (Eculizumab) therapy was introduced in 2011 as first-line treatment for aHUS to reverse the underlying overactivity of the complement pathway. Eculizumab is effective but expensive. Furthermore, because it neutralizes the activity of C5, there is an increased risk of meningococcal disease [29, 30]. For that reason, knowledge of this group of diseases is also within the realm of immunology and infectious disease specialists. As with primary C5–C9 deficiency, this infection risk can be partly offset by vaccination, which increases titers of protective antibodies to the meningococcus and therefore offsets the complement deficiency. Even with protective antibody levels against meningococcus it is recommended that patients take prophylactic antibiotics.

Checklist During Clinical Review

After Initial Diagnosis

Once the diagnosis of a complement deficiency is made, the patient and the family should be provided with advice regarding the natural history, potential complications, and measures required to reduce this risk. Table 18.2 provides a checklist, which should be completed after diagnosis.

- The patient and their caregivers need to understand the risk of invasive pneumococcal and meningococcal disease. They should be given written advice that they can show to attending physicians if they have a septic episode and provided with open access to acute medical services.
- Vaccine responses (pneumococcal and meningococcal serotypes) to encapsulated bacteria should be checked and additional booster vaccines given where these responses are inadequate or when the patient has not been previously vaccinated against these bacterial strains. Despite protective antibody levels, long-term antibiotic prophylaxis is recommended for all patients with complement deficiency as additional protection against potentially life-threatening sepsis.
- For patients with C1q deficiency, clinical examination and investigations should be performed looking for evidence of an SLE-like disorder.

Table 18.2 Checklist for management of newly diagnosed patients

	Classical pathway defects	Alternative pathway defects
Education	Explain implications of diagnosis (infection, autoimmune, risk to other siblings) Provide written information if available and links to patient support group	Explain implications of diagnosis (infection, autoimmune, risk to other siblings) Provide written information if available and links to patient support group
Address infection risk	Pneumococcal conjugate (not polysaccharide) primary vaccines or booster Provide letter to patient (upload as image on cellphone) indicating that symptoms of sepsis should prompt physician review and prompt commencement of IV antibiotics while waiting blood culture and PCR results Consider providing open access to local hospital ward in case of sepsis	Meningococcal quadrivalent conjugate (not polysaccharide) and MenB primary vaccine or boosters. Life-long prophylactic antibiotics. Provide letter to patient (upload as image on cellphone) indicating that symptoms of sepsis should prompt physician review and prompt commencement of IV antibiotics while waiting blood culture and PCR results Consider providing open access to local hospital ward in case of sepsis
Screen for autoimmune disease	C1q deficiency: blood pressure, skin examination, joint examination, urinalysis, renal function, autoimmune screen for evidence of SLE (ESR, CBC, anti-dsDNA, anti-Sm, Ro, cardiolipin IgG)	In patients with C3b dysregulation: blood pressure, urinalysis, renal function, CBC and differential, coagulation profile, C3
Address possibility that other siblings or relatives may be affected	Genetic counseling Screen other siblings, even if asymptomatic Highlight to parents and primary care physician that any newborn siblings need to be screened and given prophylactic antibiotics until clear/ vaccinated	Genetic counseling Screen other siblings, even if asymptomatic (in properdin deficiency consider screening male relatives on maternal side of the family) Highlight to parents and primary care physician that any newborn siblings need to be screened and given prophylactic antibiotics until clear/ vaccinated

- A detailed family history should be taken and genetic counseling arranged so that the patient understands the potential implications of the diagnosis for siblings and other family members.
- Written literature on the disease can usually be provided by national patient support groups, if it is not available locally.
- All siblings, whether healthy or with a history of previous infections, should be screened for the complement deficiency, initially with CH50 and AH50 as their risk of having the disease is typically one in four.

Table 18.3 Checklist of management of patients being followed up

	Classical pathway defects	Alternative pathway defects
Education	Review understanding of implications of diagnosis (infection, autoimmune, risk to other siblings) Remind patient about links to patient support group	Review understanding of implications of diagnosis (infection, autoimmune, risk to other siblings) Remind patient about links to patient support group
Address infection risk	Consider checking pneumococcal serotype responses and providing pneumococcal conjugate (not polysaccharide) booster if low Check that patient has letter (upload as image on cellphone) indicating that symptoms of sepsis should prompt physician review and prompt commencement of IV antibiotics while waiting blood culture and PCR results Check access to local hospital ward in case of sepsis Consider and discuss pros/cons of antibiotic prophylaxis, particularly if serotype titers inadequate	Consider checking meningococcal serotype responses and providing meningococcal conjugate (not polysaccharide) booster if low Check that patient has letter to patient (upload as image on cellphone) indicating that symptoms of sepsis should prompt physician review and prompt commencement of IV antibiotics while waiting blood culture and PCR results Check access to local hospital ward in case of sepsis Discuss importance of antibiotic prophylaxis
Screen for autoimmune disease	C1q deficiency: blood pressure, skin examination, joint examination, urinalysis, renal function, autoimmune screen for evidence of SLE (ESR, CBC, anti-dsDNA, anti-Sm, Ro, cardiolipin IgG)	In patients with C3b dysregulation: blood pressure, urinalysis, renal function, CBC and differential, coagulation profile, C3, stools for *E. coli* O157:H7
Address possibility that other siblings and relatives may be affected	Check understanding of inheritance Check if mother is pregnant or if other siblings have been born since patient last seen Highlight to parents and primary care physician that any newborn siblings need to be screened and given prophylactic antibiotics until clear/vaccinated	Check understanding of inheritance Check if mother is pregnant or if other siblings have been born since patient last seen Highlight to parents and primary care physician that any newborn siblings need to be screened and given prophylactic antibiotics until clear/vaccinated
Transition	Ensure smooth transition to adult/other service if appropriate	Ensure smooth transition to adult/other service if appropriate

Additional Follow-Up Visits

It is recommended that patients are followed up regularly. For patients with terminal complement deficiencies this may only be at yearly intervals, but particularly for patients with C1q deficiency and disorders of complement dysregulation, depending on comorbidities, this is likely to be more frequently (Table 18.3).

- The patient and their family's understanding of the disease should be reviewed, as should vaccine responses, compliance with antibiotic prophylaxis, and access to medical services for acute septic episodes.
- Direct questioning, particularly in patients with young parents as to whether there are any new additions to the family or any planned pregnancies, in which case, newborns should be screened and covered with prophylactic amoxicillin, at least until screening and the infant vaccine schedule has been completed at the end of the first year of life.
- For patients reaching adulthood, or families who are planning to move out of the area, arrangements for smooth transition to alternative specialist services are important.

Clinical Pearls and Pitfalls

- Although rare, primary complement deficiencies often affect more than one family member and therefore a detailed family history and testing of siblings is important.
- Complement deficiencies are largely inherited as autosomal recessive diseases and the risk of siblings also being affected is one in four.
- Invasive meningococcal infections are a common presentation in patients with terminal complement defects (C5–C9), while invasive pneumococcal infections predominate in patients with classical pathway defects (C1, C2, C4).
- Eighty percent of patients with C1q deficiency have SLE-like immune complex disease of the skin, kidneys, and brain. Anti-dsDNA antibodies are classically negative in these patients.
- The appropriate screening test for the majority of patients with complement deficiencies is CH50 and AH50, not C3 and C4 unless associated with aHUS or membranoproliferative glomerulonephritis.
- Although most complement proteins are synthesized by the liver, the exception is C1q which is produced by bone marrow monocytes, making this complement deficiency amenable to cure with HSCT.

References

1. Hoare S, El-Shazali O, Clark JE, Fay A, Cant AJ. Investigation for complement deficiency following meningococcal disease. Arch Dis Child. 2002;86:215–7.
2. Santer DM, Hall BE, George TC, Tangsombatvisit S, Liu CL, Arkwright PD, et al. C1q deficiency leads to the defective suppression of IFN-alpha in response to nucleoprotein containing immune complexes. J Immunol. 2010;185:4738–49.
3. Vassallo G, Newton RW, Chieng SE, Haeney MR, Shabani A, Arkwright PD. Clinical variability and characteristic autoantibody profile in primary C1q complement deficiency. Rheumatology (Oxford). 2007;46:1612–4.

4. Arkwright PD, Riley P, Hughes SM, Alachkar H, Wynn RF. Successful cure of C1q deficiency in human subjects treated with hematopoietic stem cell transplantation. J Allergy Clin Immunol. 2014;133:265–7.
5. Nonaka M. Evolution of the complement system. Subcell Biochem. 2014;80:31–43.
6. Elvington M, Liszewski MK, Atkinson JP. Evolution of the complement system: from defense of the single cell to guardian of the intravascular space. Immunol Rev. 2016;274:9–15.
7. Morgan PB, Boyd C, Bubeck D. Molecular cell biology of complement membrane attack. Semin Cell Dev Biol. 2017;72:124–32.
8. Moreno-Hagelsieb G, Vitug B, Medrano-Soto A, Saier MH. The membrane attack complex/perforin superfamily. J Mol Microbiol Biotechnol. 2017;27:252–67.
9. Ricklin D, Reis ES, Mastellos DC, Gros P, Lambris JD. Complement component C3 – the "Swiss Army Knife" of innate immunity and host defense. Immunol Rev. 2016;274:33–58.
10. Casals C, García-Fojeda B, Minutti CM. Soluble defense collagens: sweeping up immune threats. Mol Immunol. 2019;112:291–304.
11. Sontheimer RD, Racila E, Racila DM. C1q: its functions within the innate and adaptive immune responses and its role in lupus autoimmunity. J Invest Dermatol. 2005;125:14–23.
12. Agarwal V, Ahl J, Riesbeck K, Blom AM. An alternative role of C1q in bacterial infections: facilitating Streptococcus pneumoniae adherence and invasion of host cells. J Immunol. 2013;191:4235–45.
13. Dahl M, Tybjaerg-Hansen A, Schnohr P, Nordestgaard BG. A population-based study of morbidity and mortality in mannose-binding lectin deficiency. J Exp Med. 2004;199:1391–9.
14. De Pascale G, Cutuli SL, Pennisi MA, Antonelli M. The role of mannose-binding lectin in severe sepsis and septic shock. Mediat Inflamm. 2013;2013:625803.
15. Fijen CA, van den Bogaard R, Schipper M, Mannens M, Schlesinger M, Nordin FG, et al. Properdin deficiency: molecular basis and disease association. Mol Immunol. 1999;36:863–7.
16. Slade C, Bosco J, Unglik G, Bleasel K, Nagel M, Winship I. Deficiency in complement factor B. N Engl J Med. 2013;369:1667–9.
17. Biesma DH, Hannema AJ, van Velzen-Blad H, Mulder L, van Zwieten R, Kluijt I, et al. A family with complement factor D deficiency. J Clin Invest. 2001;108:233–40.
18. Shields AM, Pagnamenta AT, Pollard AJ, OxClin WGS, Taylor JC, Allroggen H, et al. Classical and non-classical presentations of complement factor I deficiency: two contrasting cases diagnosed via genetic and genomic methods. Front Immunol. 2019;10:1150.
19. Subbarayan A, Colarusso G, Hughes SM, Gennery AR, Slatter M, Cant AJ, et al. Clinical features that identify children with primary immunodeficiency diseases. Pediatrics. 2011;127:810–6.
20. Alperin JM, Ortiz-Fernández L, Sawalha AH. Monogenic lupus: a developing paradigm of disease. Front Immunol. 2018;9:2496.
21. Turley AJ, Gathmann B, Bangs C, Bradbury M, Seneviratne S, Gonzalez-Granado LI, et al. Spectrum and management of complement immunodeficiencies (excluding hereditary angioedema) across Europe. J Clin Immunol. 2015;35:199–205.
22. Kavanagh D, Goodship TH, Richards A. Atypical hemolytic uremic syndrome. Semin Nephrol. 2013;33:508–30.
23. Sethi S, Fervenza FC. Membranoproliferative glomerulonephritis – a new look at an old entity. N Engl J Med. 2012;366:1119–31.
24. Wijnsma KL, Duineveld C, Wetzels JFM, van de Kar NCAJ. Eculizumab in atypical hemolytic uremic syndrome: strategies toward restrictive use. Pediatr Nephrol. 2018;34:2261–77.
25. Platts-Mills TA, Ishizaka K. Activation of the alternate pathway of human complements by rabbit cells. J Immunol. 1974;113:348–58.
26. van Schaarenburg RA, Schejbel L, Truedsson L, Topaloglu R, Al-Mayouf SM, Riordan A, et al. Marked variability in clinical presentation and outcome of patients with C1q immunodeficiency. J Autoimmun. 2015;62:39–44.
27. Platonov AE, Vershinina IV, Kuijper EJ, Borrow R, Käyhty H. Long term effects of vaccination of patients deficient in a late complement component with a tetravalent meningococcal polysaccharide vaccine. Vaccine. 2003;21:4437–47.

28. Okura Y, Kobayashi I, Yamada M, Sasaki S, Yamada Y, Kamioka I, et al. Clinical characteristics and genotype-phenotype correlations in C3 deficiency. J Allergy Clin Immunol. 2016;137:640–644.e1.
29. Kirschfink M, Mollnes TE. Modern complement analysis. Clin Diagn Lab Immunol. 2003;10:982–9.
30. Ladhani SN, Campbell H, Lucidarme J, Gray S, Parikh S, Willerton L, et al. Invasive meningococcal disease in patients with complement deficiencies: a case series (2008–2017). BMC Infect Dis. 2019;19:522.

Chapter 19
Natural Killer Cell Defects

Natalia S. Chaimowitz and Lisa R. Forbes

Natural killer (NK) cells are innate lymphocytes that play a critical role in defense against viral infection and in tumor surveillance [1, 2]. NK cells originate in the bone marrow and make up approximately 3–15% of all lymphocytes in peripheral blood [3, 4]. Although characterized as lymphocytes, NK cells are also considered part of the innate immune system because typically they do not require previous exposure to foreign, pathogenic, or dangerous material to function [5].

NK cells distinguish themselves from other lymphocytes by expressing CD56, a neural cell adhesion molecule, and they do not display other lymphocyte surface markers such as CD3, CD4, or CD19. In the peripheral blood, there are two major circulating NK cell populations characterized by their CD56 expression. The minor population express very high levels of CD56 and is referred to as "CD56^{bright}", whereas the majority population is referred to as "CD56^{dim}." CD56^{bright} cells are responsible for cytokine production but can mediate weak cytotoxicity. In addition, CD56^{bright} NK cells are considered developmentally immature and have been shown to be a precursor to the mature CD56^{dim} NK cells [6]. CD56^{dim} NK cells express CD16, the Fc-gamma-RIIIa receptor for immunoglobulin (Ig) G, and are considered mature effectors of NK cell spontaneous cytotoxicity and antibody-dependent cellular cytotoxicity (ADCC).

An important function of NK cells is cellular killing or cytotoxicity. NK cells survey surrounding cells for abnormalities and kill those that fail to display various signatures of healthy cells, particularly virally infected and malignant cells. The two primary mechanisms utilized by NK cells are NK cell spontaneous cytotoxicity and ADCC. Both mechanisms involve the release of lytic granule contents which

---

N. S. Chaimowitz
Section of Immunology, Allergy and Retrovirology, Department of Pediatrics, Texas Children's Hospital, Houston, TX, USA

L. R. Forbes (✉)
Texas Children's Hospital, Section of Immunology, Allergy and Retrovirology, Department of Pediatrics, Baylor College of Medicine, Houston, TX, USA
e-mail: lisa.forbes@bcm.edu

contain the pore-forming molecule perforin, as well as cell death-inducing enzymes, such as granzyme [3, 7]. The importance of NK cells in human host defense is highlighted by a small number of human diseases in which NK cells are absent or do not function properly. These conditions are primarily characterized by severe, recurrent, or atypical infections with herpes viruses.

Primary immunodeficiency disorders (PIDDs) occur when genetic abnormalities impacting immunity lead to immune dysregulation, immune impairment, or both. There are currently more than 350 described monogenic disorders of immunity that can cause PIDDs [8]. These diseases may affect single cell subsets or may affect multiple immune cell lineages. There are currently seven primary immunodeficiencies that affect NK cells primarily. In addition, there are approximately 50 described diseases in which the impairment of NK cells is one of the features of the disease [9]. In this chapter we will discuss both primary NK cell disorders and disorders in which NK cell defects contribute to the patient's clinical disease.

Primary NK Cell Disorders

Case Presentation 1

A 13-year-old girl with a past medical history significant for recurrent otitis media which resulted in perforated tympanic membranes presented to the emergency room with disseminated and life-threatening varicella virus infection. The patient was treated with acyclovir and was discharged home. Three years later, she developed life-threatening systemic cytomegalovirus (CMV) infection followed by disseminated herpes simplex virus (HSV) infection. Due to the nature of her infections, immunology was consulted. The patient had normal antibody responses and normal lymphocyte proliferation. Her lymphocyte subsets showed normal CD4 and CD8 T cell normal and a complete absence of CD3$^-$CD56^{bright} and a marked decrease in the CD3$^-$CD56^{dim}CD16$^+$ lymphocytes resulting in absent NK cell cytotoxicity. The decision was made to perform a hematopoietic cell transplantation due to the invasive and refractory nature of her herpes viral disease as well as the severity of the impairment revealed in her immune evaluation [10]. She died during bone marrow transplantation and genetic testing postmortem revealed a mutation [c.1026insGCCG; pA342GfsX41] in the GATA2 gene [11].

Diagnosis and Assessment

Clinical features of NK cell disorders include severe, recurrent, or atypical infections with herpes viruses (cytomegalovirus (CMV), varicella-zoster virus (VZV) highlighted in the case above, herpes simplex viruses (HSV) I and II, and Epstein-Barr virus (EBV)) and cutaneous wart-causing papilloma viruses [12].

NK cell deficiencies can be divided into classical NK cell or functional NK cell deficiency. Classical NK cell deficiency results from an absence or profound decrease in CD3⁻CD56⁺ NK cell numbers, specifically defined as NK cells making up less than 1% of peripheral blood lymphocytes. In these disorders, NK cell development and/or homeostasis is impaired. In functional NK cell deficiency, the NK cells are present, but their functional activities are impaired [13]. When a classical and/or functional NK cell deficiency is suspected, it is important to assess both NK cell numbers and NK cell function (Fig. 19.1).

The number of NK cell, B cell, and T cell can be determined by flow cytometry panels on peripheral blood. Some hospitals can also provide information regarding NK cell subsets (CD56^{bright} and CD56^{dim}). The normal ratio of bright to dim NK cells is 1:10. A ratio higher than 1:5 should be considered abnormal. Evaluating NK cell subsets is particularly important because all classical NK cell deficiencies have abnormal NK cell subset distribution (Table 19.1).

NK function is assessed by cytotoxicity testing of peripheral blood lymphocytes. A chromium release assay using ^{51}Cr is the preferred method. If cytotoxicity testing is abnormal, the testing should be repeated on three separate occasions, at least 1 month apart because the results can be compromised by many external variables, such as active illness, medications, and physiologic stress.

The results of the above testing can help narrow the diagnosis. If NK cells were found to be less than 1% of lymphocytes and NK cell cytotoxicity is severely depressed or absent, the patient can be diagnosed as having a classical NK cell deficiency. To date, six causes of classical NK cell deficiency have been described: *GATA2*, *MCM4*, *MCM10*, *RTEL1*, *IRF8*, and *GINS1*.

GATA2 is a diversely expressed hematopoietic transcription factor. It is required for the maintenance and survival of the hematopoietic stem cell pool and the formation of early blood and lymphatic vessels [14, 15]. GATA2 deficiency is also known as GATA2 haploinsufficiency, meaning one copy of the gene is inactivated or deleted and the remaining functional copy of the gene is not adequate to preserve normal function of the gene product, GATA2 protein in this case. This impairment of GATA2 function leads to a complex autosomal dominant disorder with heterogenous disease manifestations that affect multiple organ systems. The mechanism by which GATA2 regulates the progression through the developmental stages of NK cell development is poorly understood. The presentation of GATA2 haploinsufficiency can typically be associated with primary lymphedema, aplastic anemia, myelodysplasia, myelodysplastic syndrome, and/or acute myeloid leukemia. While the overall prevalence of GATA2 haploinsufficiency is unknown, the prevalence of GATA2 haploinsufficiency in a cohort of children with myelodysplastic syndrome and refractory cytopenias is 14% and 17%, respectively [16]. Patients are susceptible to atypical mycobacterial infections, fungal infections, and severe and recalcitrant viral infections. Classically, the immune phenotype reveals severe monocytopenia, thrombocytopenia, B cell, and CD4+ cell lymphopenia in addition to the primary NK cell defect. With regard to NK cells, patients with GATA2 haploinsufficiency have reduced numbers of NK cells and are completely deficient in the CD56^{bright} NK cell subset [11, 17, 18]. The finding of CD56^{bright} NK cell deficiency is pathognomonic for GATA2 deficiency.

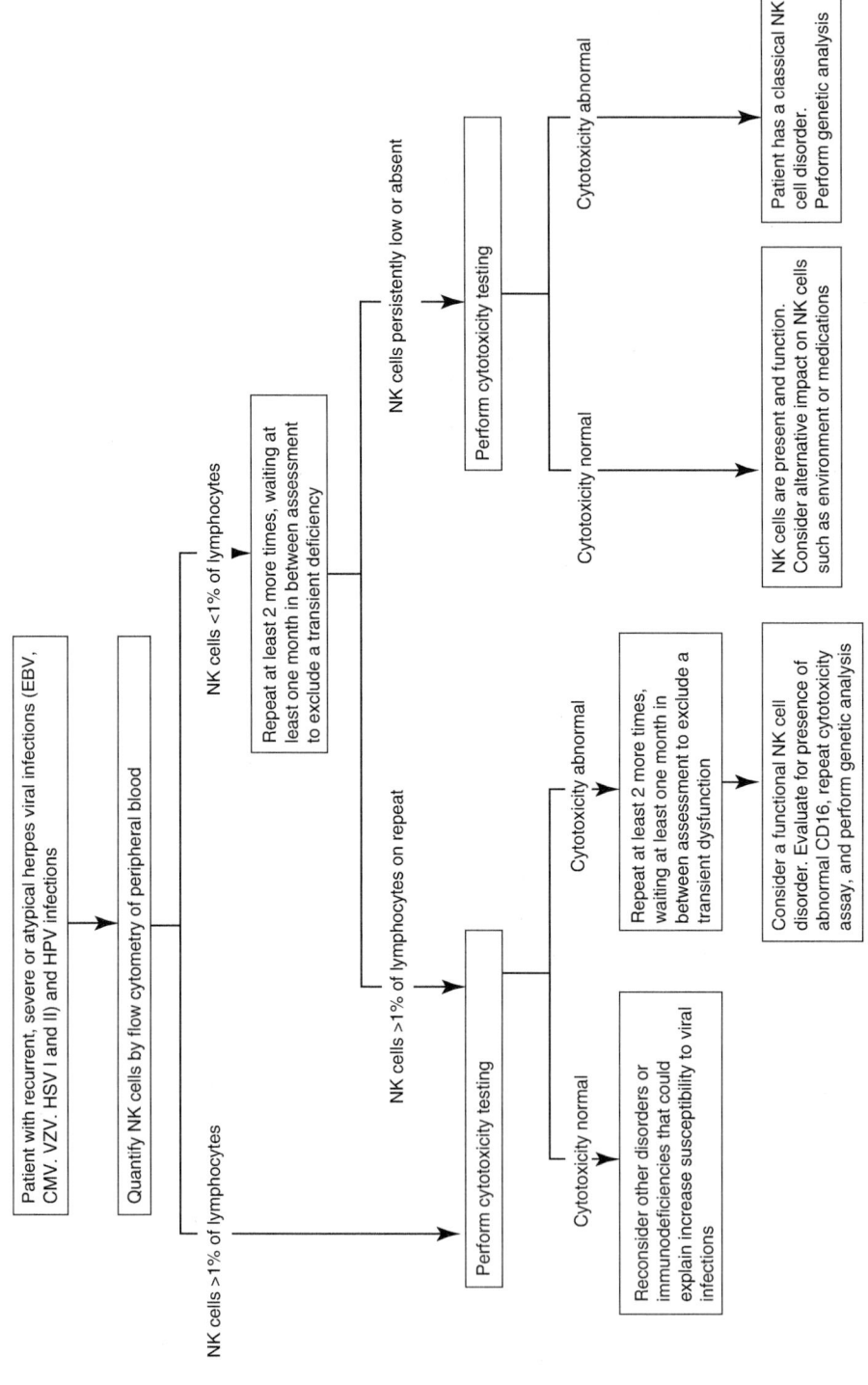

Fig. 19.1 Evaluation of NK cell quantity and function in a patient suspected of having an NK cell deficiency syndrome

Table 19.1 Human NK cell deficiencies and their effects on NK cell subsets and function

Gene	Inheritance	NK cell number	CD56^{dim} number	CD56^{bright} number	NK cell lytic function	Other features	Reference
Classical NK cell deficiency							
GATA2	AD	Normal or ↓	Normal or ↓	↓↓↓	↓	Primary lymphedema, aplastic anemia, myelodysplasia, myelodysplastic syndrome, and/or acute myeloid leukemia	[16]
IRF8	AR	↓	↓	Normal or ↑	↓	Lack of monocytes and dendritic cells	[78, 79]
MCM4	AR	↓	↓	Normal or ↑	↓	Adrenal insufficiency, developmental delay and short stature	[18]
MCM10	AR	↓	↓	Normal or ↑	↓	Reduced effector and memory T cells. Hemaphagocytic lymphohistiocytosis (HLH)	[20]
GINS1	AR	↓	↓	↓	↓	Intrauterine and post-natal growth retardation, chronic neutropenia	[26]
RTEL1	AR	↓	Not done	Not done	↓	Dyskeratosis congenita, bone marrow failure, and immunodeficiency	[28]
Functional NK cell deficiency							
FCGR3A	AR	Normal or ↓	Normal or ↓	Normal	↓ (ADCC is preserved)		[29]

AR autosomal recessive, *AD* autosomal dominant

Unlike GATA2 haploinsufficiency, MCM4 deficiency and IRF8 deficiency are characterized by a decreased in the CD56^{dim} NK cell population. Minichromosome maintenance complex component 4 (MCM4) is a DNA helicase that is required for DNA duplication and is important for chromosomal maintenance. MCM4 deficiency is characterized as a classical NK cell deficiency with associated adrenal insufficiency, developmental delay, and short stature [19, 20]. MCM10 on the other hand, was found in a child with severe and fatal CMV infection. The NK cell phenotype is similar to that of MCM4 [20]. Interferon regulatory factor 8 (IRF8) is a member of the IRF family of transcription factors that help shape the inflammatory response, particularly to viral infections. IRF8 plays a critical role in lineage determination of hemopoietic cells and governs the development of granulocytes, dendritic cells, monocytes, B cells, and NK cells [21, 22]. Recent studies in mice have demonstrated that IRF8 is upregulated early in the course of viral infections and that it is required for NK cell-mediated host protection against viral infections [23]. Patients with biallelic mutations in IRF8 are susceptible to severe viral infections. The CD56^{dim} subset of IRF8-deficient patients demonstrate decreased frequency causing an overall decrease in total NK cell number. These data along with human in vitro functional data add to the evidence that IRF8 is a critical regulator of NK cell terminal maturation [24, 25].

Go-Ichi-Ni-San (GINS) complex subunit 1 (*GINS1*) is a component of the GINS complex, a group of proteins that are essential for DNA replication, and like MCM4 and MCM10, it is important for chromosomal maintenance. Recently, autosomal recessive, partial GINS1 deficiency has been described. These patients were noted to have intrauterine and postnatal growth retardation, chronic neutropenia, and NK cell deficiency. Unlike other classical NK cell deficiencies, the number and percentage of both CD56^{dim} and CD56^{bright} is decreased [26]. The fifth classical NK cell deficiency is the regulator of telomere elongation helicase I deficiency (RTEL1). RTEL1 deficiency has been reported to cause Hoyeraal-Hreidarsson syndrome, which presents with dyskeratosis congenita, bone marrow failure, and immunodeficiency. RTEL1 is an essential DNA helicase that disassembles DNA secondary structures and maintains telomere integrity [27]. RTEL1 deficiency was described in a patient who presented with severe disseminated VZV infection and found to have markedly reduced NK cell cytotoxicity. The patient had normal proportions of B cells and T cells, normal B cell and T-cell mitogen-induced proliferation, and normal immunoglobulin levels. Given that the NK cell phenotype was the main immunologic parameter impaired, the authors concluded that RTEL1 deficiency was responsible for the patient's susceptibility to severe viral infections [28]. NK cell phenotyping was not carried out, so it is unknown which NK cell subsets are most affected by RTEL1 deficiency. The effect of deficiencies in proteins involved in DNA stability, such as MCM4, MCM10, GINS1, and RTEL1, suggests a specific sensitivity of human NK cells to DNA damage.

While a normal NK cell number and subset distribution rules out a classical NK cell deficiency, a functional NK cell deficiency remains on the differential. There is only one cause of functional NK deficiency reported to date. This deficiency results from mutation in *FCGR3A*, the gene encoding for the low-affinity IgG Fc receptor found on NK cells and macrophages (Fc gamma RIIIA, CD16). The Fc receptor essential for antibody-dependent cellular cytotoxicity (ADCC) is CD16. In ADCC, NK cells via CD16 recognize and bind to the Fc portion of an IgG antibody that is bound to the surface of a pathogen-infected target cell. This binding leads to NK cell activation and the release of lytic granules resulting on the death of the target cells [29]. *FCGR3A* defects have been described in two patients. One patient presented with recurrent HSV infections while the other patient presented with recurrent EBV-associated Castleman's disease and HPV infections. Despite low normal to normal NK cell numbers these patients had impaired cytotoxicity. Interestingly, ADCC was not impaired. Elegant experiments showed that the portion of the CD16 receptor abrogated is important for facilitating natural spontaneous cytotoxicity and not where the CD16 molecule recognizes the Fc portion of the bound antibody.

Therefore, these patients had normal antibody-mediated cell cytotoxicity, but impaired natural cytotoxicity [30, 31]. While this is the only functional NK cell deficiency described, there are many patients with functional NK cell defects in which the pathogenesis remains unknown.

Management and Outcomes

As previously mentioned, NK cell disorders are characterized by susceptibility to severe and/or recurrent viral infections, including VZV, HSV I and II, EBV, and CMV. Prophylactic antiviral medications should be considered in all patients with known or suspected primary NK cell deficiencies, either classical or functional. Serologic testing should be performed in order to assess if the NK-deficient patient has experienced infections with known herpesviruses. Patients should also be screened for active infections with nucleic acid polymerase chain reaction (PCR) in peripheral blood. Evidence of past viral exposure by serology without viremia demonstrates that the patient is able to control that infection; therefore, viral prophylaxis against that organism is not needed. However, NK cell-deficient patients that are naïve to HSV or CMV should receive viral prophylaxis, to be continued indefinitely.

Patients with NK cell deficiencies are also at increased risk of severe human papillomavirus (HPV) infections. The administration of recombinant HPV to both male and female patients is recommended. Live attenuated viral vaccines, such as MMR and varicella vaccine, are not recommended since they may place the NK cell-deficient patient at risk for disseminated infection.

The only curative treatment is hematopoietic stem cell transplantation. This option is considered for patients with history of life-threatening infection. The severity of the patient's illness must be balanced against the risk of transplantation. Successful transplants have been reported in patients with GATA2 haploinsufficiency and RTEL1 deficiency [32, 33]. Hematopoietic stem cell transplant for the treatment of MCM4 deficiency, MCM10 deficiency, IRF8 deficiency, and GINS1 deficiency has not been reported.

Primary Immunodeficiency Diseases with an NK Cell Abnormality

Case Presentation 2

A 2-week-old male born full term to non-consanguineous parents was referred to immunology with very low T-cell receptor excision circles (TRECs) on the newborn screen for severe combined immunodeficiency (SCID). At time of evaluation, the patient was well appearing and in no acute distress. He did not have any dysmorphic features and physical exam was normal. His mother reported that he had been formula feeding without complication and had already returned to birth weight. Upon evaluation, lymphocyte phenotyping demonstrated lymphopenia with undetectable T cells and NK cells. Genetic testing demonstrated a known pathogenic variant in IL-2 receptor gamma chain gene, confirming the diagnosis of X-linked SCID.

Diagnosis and Assessment

Disorders affecting NK cells can be categorized as those affecting NK cell development, proliferation and survival, as well as diseases impairing the mechanics and signaling required for cytotoxicity. Patients with disorders affecting NK cells can present with susceptibility to herpesvirus infection, but, in addition, might be susceptible to fungal and bacterial infections, as well as be susceptible to autoimmunity and immune dysregulation, depending on the specific genetic defect.

Severe combined immunodeficiency (SCID) is characterized by impaired T-cell development. In some forms of SCID, B cell and/or NK cell development is also impacted by the molecular defect. The gene *IL2RG* encodes for the common gamma chain of the IL-2 receptor (IL-2Rγ). The common gamma chain is shared by several cytokine receptors critical for T-cell development and in some cases NK cell development. For example, IL-2Rγ is part of the subunit of the IL-15 receptor and IL-15 is essential for NK development, proliferation, and survival. Therefore, a mutation in *IL2RG* (X-linked SCID) disrupts IL-15 signaling through JAK3, a signaling molecule downstream of IL-15 receptor, required for development and survival of NK cells. Patients affected by this form of SCID are susceptible to bacterial, fungal, and viral infections. NK cells are affected in other forms of SCID, for example, adenosine deaminase (ADA) deficiency, Janus kinase 3 (JAK3) deficiency, and adenylate kinase-2 (AK2) deficiency, also known as reticular dysgenesis [34, 35]. In these diseases, NK cell deficiency results from an impairment in NK cell differential and development; however, defect is not isolated to NK cells. These patients previously presented as young infants with life-threatening infections. However, in the United States all 50 states have TREC newborn screening. Therefore, they are now being detected while they are healthy and without morbidity [36].

If SCID is suspected, initial testing includes a complete blood count (CBC) with differential to evaluate absolute lymphocyte count. Typically, patients with SCID have a lymphocyte count less than 2500 cells/μL. Lymphocyte phenotyping by flow cytometry is important to assess T-cell, B cell, and NK cell counts. The diagnostic criteria for SCID is an absolute T-cell count of less than 300 cells/μL. Genetic testing via targeted gene panels or whole exome sequencing is now the final step in the evaluation of a patient with SCID to determine the molecular diagnosis. However, the diagnosis does not require a molecular defect as long as the patient meets diagnostic criteria.

SCID is just one example of diseases in which multiple lymphocyte subsets can be affected. There is a large number of combined immunodeficiencies in which NK cell function is also impaired. Cellular killing by NK cells is mediated through the release of lytic granules toward a bound target cell at the immunologic synapse [29]. Lytic granules are a type of secretory lysosome that undergo a regulated secretion process. In the case of NK cells and cytotoxic T cells (effector cells), the secretory lysosome contains perforin and granzymes, the ammunition needed for cell death. The release of lytic granules requires the effector cell to form a synapse with the target cell so when the lytic granules traffic to the cell surface they can release the toxic mediators to induce cell death [37]. This process is in part mediated by actin organization. When the actin cytoskeletal organization and/or the trafficking of secretory granules is impaired, the cytotoxic capacity of the cell is diminished [29]. Primary immunodeficiency diseases with absent or diminished NK cell cytotoxicity can be caused by defects in the contents of lytic granules, formation and maturation of lytic granules, defective lytic granule docking and priming at the immunologic synapse, and actin reorganization [29].

NK cell degranulation requires rearrangement of the cytoskeleton and is particularly dependent on actin. Impaired cytotoxicity is usually a feature in disorders in which actin function is affected. Wiskott-Aldrich syndrome (WAS) is an X-linked disorder caused by mutation in the gene that encodes the Wiskott-Aldrich syndrome protein (WASp). WASp is expressed in the cytoplasm of hematopoietic cells and is critical for actin cytoskeleton remodeling [38]. Absolute NK cell numbers are normal, but cytotoxicity in WASp-deficient NK cells is impaired [39]. The classical triad of WAS includes microthrombocytopenia, eczema, and susceptibility to infections [40]. Screening for WASp expression in lymphocytes can be done via flow cytometry [41]. It should be noted, however, that a subset of patients has normal WASp expression but impaired function. Therefore, even if WASp expression is normal, and WAS is suspected, *WAS* gene sequencing should be carried out for diagnosis.

In order for NK cells to secrete their secretory granules and kill target cells, NK cells need to be activated. Disorders that impair NK cell activation lead to impaired cytotoxicity. Calcium release-activated channel (CRAC) deficiency, secondary to mutations in *ORAI1* gene, leads to compromised activation-induced calcium flux, thus resulting in impaired NK cell degranulation. The patients with CRAC deficiency not only have abnormal NK cell cytotoxicity but also impaired T-cell responses [42]. Laboratory findings typically include normal to slightly reduced lymphocyte counts, and immunoglobulin levels are normal to elevated. However, T-cell proliferative responses to mitogens and antigens, NK cell cytotoxicity, and specific antibody responses to vaccination are impaired. Patients usually present with invasive bacterial, fungal, mycobacterial, and opportunistic infections [43]. Nuclear factor-kB (NFkB) is a master regulatory transcription factor important for both innate and adaptive immune responses. The NFkB essential modulator (NEMO) is a key regulator of NFkB signaling. In NK cells, NFkB is important for NK maturation, cytotoxicity, and IFN-gamma production [44, 45]. NFkB essential modulator (NEMO), also known as inhibitor of nuclear facto kappa-B gamma, is the regulatory subunit of the IkB kinase complex, which results in NFkB activation. Laboratory findings in NEMO deficiency typically include hypogammaglobulinemia with poor specific antibody production, either elevated IgM or IgA and low NK cell function [46]. Patients with NEMO deficiency are at risk for mycobacteria, and bacterial and viral infection, particularly CMV [47]. Analysis of toll-like receptor function, a component of the innate immune system, may reveal defects due to impaired NFkB signaling. In both of these disorders, and many others, definitive diagnosis is carried out by genetic sequencing.

In addition to viral susceptibility, another consequence of a defect in the cascade necessary for the function and release of lytic granules is hemophagocytic lymphohistiocytosis (HLH). The diagnosis of HLH is based on having five out of the following eight laboratory and clinical findings: fever >38.5C; splenomegaly; peripheral blood cytopenia of at least two cell lines; hypertriglyceridemia and/or hypofibrinogenemia; hemophagocytosis in bone marrow, spleen, lymph node, or liver; low or absent NK cell activity; elevated ferritin >500 ng/mL; and elevated soluble CD25 (soluble IL-2 receptor alpha) [48]. Familial HLH is a genetically heterogenous disorder caused by mutations in genes specifically related to the various steps in the process of docking and priming of lytic granules as well as the release of toxic mediators from lytic granules [49]. The two most common causes of familial HLH are perforin deficiency and Munc13-4 deficiency. Perforin is a pore-forming molecule contained in lytic granules and when released essentially pokes a hole in the target cell's membrane so the toxic mediators can pass through the immunologic synapse and induce cell death. Although NK cell numbers are normal, NK cell function is grossly impaired due to perforin deficiency [50]. *UNC13D* gene encodes for Munc13-4, a protein involved in the priming of secretory granules, and facilitates their fusion with the plasma membrane. Munc13-4 deficiency impairs the release of perforin and granzyme into the synaptic cleft, thus leading to impaired NK cell cytotoxicity [51]. Other gene defects that cause familial HLH are *STX11* and *STXBP2* [52]. Both of these genes encode for proteins important for the release of lytic granules and their deficiency results in reduced NK cell degranulation. As a result of the abrogated cytotoxic cell function, macrophages and histiocytes become overstimulated and begin to phagocytose white and red blood cells leading to a clinical phenotype characterized by long-lasting fevers, hepatosplenomegaly, cytopenia, elevated ferritin, elevated triglycerides, elevated alpha-chain of the soluble interleukin-2 receptor (sCD25), and low fibrinogen [53].

It is important to mention that other cell types outside of the immune system utilize secondary granule mechanisms similar to lytic granules used by NK cells. Melanocytes are a specialized skin cell that produce the skin-darkening melanin. Melanin is contained within granules and these granules are transferred to other cells within the skin and hair [54]. While the contents of the granules are different between NK cells and melanocytes, these cells are both dependent on secretory granules for their function. There are three syndromes with defective secretory/lytic granules where both the cytotoxic mechanism and the delivery of pigment is affected leading to HLH and partial albinism. Chediak-Higashi syndrome (CHS) is caused by mutations in the *LYST* gene which encodes for a protein important for lysosomal trafficking. Clinically, CHS is characterized by albinism, bleeding tendency, recurrent bacterial infections, neurologic dysfunction, impaired NK cell function, and HLH. The presence of giant inclusion bodies of lysosomal origin in granule-containing cells such as hematopoietic cells and melanocytes is a hallmark of the disease [55]. Griscelli syndrome is a rare autosomal-recessive disorder characterized by partial oculocutaneous albinism and HLH caused by mutations in *RAB27A* gene encoding for a protein that is involved in vesicle trafficking within the cell. Cytotoxic defects in both NK cells and CD8 T cells result from the inability of cytotoxic granules to dock to the plasma membrane and hypopigmentation is due to defective release of melanosomes from melanocyte dendrites [56]. Hermansky-Pudlak syndrome (HPS) is an autosomal recessive genetic disorder that results from mutations in the gene encoding for adaptor protein-3 (AP-3) complex. This heterotetrameric protein complex recognizes sorting signals for trafficking of membrane proteins to lysosomes. Patients with HPS have oculocutaneous albinism, bleeding disorder, and recurrent infections secondary to both congenital neutropenia and impaired cytotoxic activity [57].

Management and Outcomes

The management of disorders affecting NK cells among other cells of the immune system is very dependent on the underlying molecular diagnosis. For SCID, such as X-linked SCID or AK2 deficiency, prophylactic antibiotics, such as trimethoprim sulfamethoxazole to prevent *P. jirovecii* pneumonia, prophylactic acyclovir to prevent herpes simplex infection, and prophylactic azithromycin to prevent mycobacterial infections are sometimes used. The only available definite treatment, however, is a hemopoietic stem cell transplant [34, 58]. For patients with other T-cell lymphopenia syndromes including the profound defect observed in patients with CRAC deficiency, prophylactic antibiotics, immunoglobulin replacement therapy, and hematopoietic stem cell transplantation are also the best therapy for these patients [59]. Survival is excellent in patients that undergo bone marrow transplantation prior to the onset of infections [60]. Gene therapy for X-linked SCID is under study and recent clinical trials have demonstrated promising results [61].

The management of combined immunodeficiencies often is tailored to the patient's presentation and underlying molecular diagnosis. In WAS, for example, prophylactic antibiotics are often used as described above. Moreover, patients sometimes require platelet transfusions to treat major bleeding episodes. Those patients with significant antibody deficiency are treated with intravenous immune globulin. Similarly, to SCID disorders, hematopoietic cell transplantation is the only available curative treatment and excellent patient outcomes have been reported [62–64]. Gene therapy for WAS is also under investigation as an alternative to hematopoietic cell transplantation [65]. In the case of NEMO, treatment typically includes immunoglobulin replacement therapy and antimycobacterial prophylaxis. If a patient's presentation is severe, hematopoietic stem cell transplant should be considered [46].

The treatment of HLH generally consists of immunosuppressive and chemotherapeutic agents. Typically, a regimen of dexamethasone and etoposide is the mainstay treatment in North America based on the HLH-1994 and HLH-2004 study protocols [66]. Recently, emapalumab, a monoclonal antibody directed against interferon-gamma, a cytokine highly upregulated in HLH, has been approved for the management of HLH in patients with refractory, recurrent, or progressive disease or intolerance to standard HLH therapy [67]. Most patients with primary HLH are candidates for hematopoietic cell transplantation. The outcomes of hematopoietic cell transplantation are generally better if HLH is in remission at time of transplantation [68].

Environmental Effects on NK Cell Function

While inborn errors in the immune system are rare, most commonly NK cell number and function are affected by medications and environmental exposures. Studies have demonstrated that NK cell cytotoxicity in vitro is increased at fever-range temperatures and in cold temperatures, suggesting that NK cells are capable of responding to temperature [69, 70]. The role of travel in NK cell function has been studied; while spending time in the forest environment enhances NK cell function, long-duration spaceflight is associated with a decline in NK cell cytotoxicity [71, 72]. A recent study compared NK cell cytotoxicity in overweight individuals with or without comorbidities such as hypertension, hyperlipidemia, and impaired glucose tolerance where they found that patients who were overweight with comorbidities had decreased NK cytotoxicity [73]. These results suggest that NK cell function can be affected by metabolic disorders. A small study assessed in vitro cytotoxicity from NK cells isolated from peripheral blood mononuclear cells in smokers, former smokers, and nonsmokers. The study demonstrated that the percentage of NK cells in total lymphocytes was significantly lower in smokers than nonsmokers. Moreover, NK cell cytotoxicity was lower in smokers than nonsmokers. Interestingly, former smokers had comparable NK cell cytotoxicity than nonsmoker [74]. In addition to toxins like cigarettes, medications can also affect NK cell number and function. Several immunosuppressive medications have been studied for the effect on NK cell function in vitro. Treatment of NK cells with mycophenolic acid, prednisone, azathioprine, 6-mercaptopurine, or cyclosporine leads to decreased NK cells [75–77].

In summary, NK cells play a critical role in host defense against viral infections and are primed and ready to react to infectious, malignant, and environmental triggers. While primary NK cell deficiencies are rare, NK cells are affected in >50 primary immunodeficiency diseases. NK cell defects, whether primary or as part of a broader immunodeficiency, are an essential piece of our immune system defense and should be suspected in any patient with severe, recurrent, and/or refractory viral infections as well as HLH.

Clinical Pearls and Pitfalls
- Natural killer (NK) cells are innate lymphocytes that play a critical role in defense against viral infection and in tumor surveillance.
- Patients with disorders affecting NK cells are susceptible to viral infections, particularly those in the herpes virus family. In addition, for disorders in which NK cells are affected, patients are at risk for autoimmunity and immune dysregulation, depending on the specific genetic defect.
- Classical NK cell deficiency results from an absence or profound decrease in $CD3^-CD56^+$ NK cell numbers while functional NK cell deficiency results from impaired NK cell function.
- Evaluation of NK cell disorders requires both quantification of NK cell numbers and NK cell cytotoxicity.
- NK cell number and function can be affected by medications and environmental factors; therefore, repeated assessment of NK cell number and function is needed prior to diagnosing NK cell deficiency.

References

1. Vivier E, Tomasello E, Baratin M, Walzer T, Ugolini S. Functions of natural killer cells. Nat Immunol. 2008;9(5):503–10.
2. Gregoire C, Chasson L, Luci C, Tomasello E, Geissmann F, Vivier E, et al. The trafficking of natural killer cells. Immunol Rev. 2007;220:169–82.
3. Benson DM Jr, Yu J, Becknell B, Wei M, Freud AG, Ferketich AK, et al. Stem cell factor and interleukin-2/15 combine to enhance MAPK-mediated proliferation of human natural killer cells. Blood. 2009;113(12):2706–14.
4. Angelo LS, Banerjee PP, Monaco-Shawver L, Rosen JB, Makedonas G, Forbes LR, et al. Practical NK cell phenotyping and variability in healthy adults. Immunol Res. 2015;62(3):341–56.
5. Bryceson YT, Long EO. Line of attack: NK cell specificity and integration of signals. Curr Opin Immunol. 2008;20(3):344–52.
6. Marcenaro E, Notarangelo LD, Orange JS, Vivier E. Editorial: NK cell subsets in health and disease: new developments. Front Immunol. 2017;8:1363.
7. Watzl C, Long EO. Signal transduction during activation and inhibition of natural killer cells. Curr Protoc Immunol. 2010;Chapter 11:Unit 11 9B.
8. Bousfiha A, Jeddane L, Picard C, Ailal F, Bobby Gaspar H, Al-Herz W, et al. The 2017 IUIS phenotypic classification for primary immunodeficiencies. J Clin Immunol. 2018;38(1):129–43.
9. Mace EM, Orange JS. Emerging insights into human health and NK cell biology from the study of NK cell deficiencies. Immunol Rev. 2019;287(1):202–25.
10. Biron CA, Byron KS, Sullivan JL. Severe herpesvirus infections in an adolescent without natural killer cells. N Engl J Med. 1989;320(26):1731–5.
11. Mace EM, Hsu AP, Monaco-Shawver L, Makedonas G, Rosen JB, Dropulic L, et al. Mutations in GATA2 cause human NK cell deficiency with specific loss of the CD56(bright) subset. Blood. 2013;121(14):2669–77.
12. Abel AM, Yang C, Thakar MS, Malarkannan S. Natural killer cells: development, maturation, and clinical utilization. Front Immunol. 2018;9:1869.

13. Mace EM, Orange JS. Genetic causes of human NK cell deficiency and their effect on NK cell subsets. Front Immunol. 2016;7:545.
14. Dickinson RE, Griffin H, Bigley V, Reynard LN, Hussain R, Haniffa M, et al. Exome sequencing identifies GATA-2 mutation as the cause of dendritic cell, monocyte, B and NK lymphoid deficiency. Blood. 2011;118(10):2656–8.
15. Lopez-Soto A, Lorenzo-Herrero S, Gonzalez S. Biallelic IRF8 mutations causing NK cell deficiency. Trends Mol Med. 2017;23(3):195–7.
16. Hambleton S, Salem S, Bustamante J, Bigley V, Boisson-Dupuis S, Azevedo J, et al. IRF8 mutations and human dendritic-cell immunodeficiency. N Engl J Med. 2011;365(2):127–38.
17. Gineau L, Cognet C, Kara N, Lach FP, Dunne J, Veturi U, et al. Partial MCM4 deficiency in patients with growth retardation, adrenal insufficiency, and natural killer cell deficiency. J Clin Invest. 2012;122(3):821–32.
18. Cottineau J, Kottemann MC, Lach FP, Kang YH, Vely F, Deenick EK, et al. Inherited GINS1 deficiency underlies growth retardation along with neutropenia and NK cell deficiency. J Clin Invest. 2017;127(5):1991–2006.
19. Hanna S, Beziat V, Jouanguy E, Casanova JL, Etzioni A. A homozygous mutation of RTEL1 in a child presenting with an apparently isolated natural killer cell deficiency. J Allergy Clin Immunol. 2015;136(4):1113–4.
20. Mace EM, Dongre P, Hsu HT, Sinha P, James AM, Mann SS, et al. Cell biological steps and checkpoints in accessing NK cell cytotoxicity. Immunol Cell Biol. 2014;92(3):245–55.
21. Tsai FY, Keller G, Kuo FC, Weiss M, Chen J, Rosenblatt M, et al. An early haematopoietic defect in mice lacking the transcription factor GATA-2. Nature. 1994;371(6494):221–6.
22. Kazenwadel J, Secker GA, Liu YJ, Rosenfeld JA, Wildin RS, Cuellar-Rodriguez J, et al. Loss-of-function germline GATA2 mutations in patients with MDS/AML or MonoMAC syndrome and primary lymphedema reveal a key role for GATA2 in the lymphatic vasculature. Blood. 2012;119(5):1283–91.
23. Novakova M, Zaliova M, Sukova M, Wlodarski M, Janda A, Fronkova E, et al. Loss of B cells and their precursors is the most constant feature of GATA-2 deficiency in childhood myelodysplastic syndrome. Haematologica. 2016;101(6):707–16.
24. Hsu AP, Sampaio EP, Khan J, Calvo KR, Lemieux JE, Patel SY, et al. Mutations in GATA2 are associated with the autosomal dominant and sporadic monocytopenia and mycobacterial infection (MonoMAC) syndrome. Blood. 2011;118(10):2653–5.
25. Hughes CR, Guasti L, Meimaridou E, Chuang CH, Schimenti JC, King PJ, et al. MCM4 mutation causes adrenal failure, short stature, and natural killer cell deficiency in humans. J Clin Invest. 2012;122(3):814–20.
26. Tamura T, Kurotaki D, Koizumi S. Regulation of myelopoiesis by the transcription factor IRF8. Int J Hematol. 2015;101(4):342–51.
27. Shukla V, Lu R. IRF4 and IRF8: governing the virtues of B lymphocytes. Front Biol (Beijing). 2014;9(4):269–82.
28. Adams NM, Lau CM, Fan X, Rapp M, Geary CD, Weizman OE, et al. Transcription factor IRF8 orchestrates the adaptive natural killer cell response. Immunity. 2018;48(6):1172–82 e6.
29. Fleisher G, Starr S, Koven N, Kamiya H, Douglas SD, Henle W. A non-x-linked syndrome with susceptibility to severe Epstein-Barr virus infections. J Pediatr. 1982;100(5):727–30.
30. Mace EM, Bigley V, Gunesch JT, Chinn IK, Angelo LS, Care MA, et al. Biallelic mutations in IRF8 impair human NK cell maturation and function. J Clin Invest. 2017;127(1):306–20.
31. Vannier JB, Sarek G, Boulton SJ. RTEL1: functions of a disease-associated helicase. Trends Cell Biol. 2014;24(7):416–25.
32. de Vries E, Koene HR, Vossen JM, Gratama JW, von dem Borne AE, Waaijer JL, et al. Identification of an unusual Fc gamma receptor IIIa (CD16) on natural killer cells in a patient with recurrent infections. Blood. 1996;88(8):3022–7.
33. Grier JT, Forbes LR, Monaco-Shawver L, Oshinsky J, Atkinson TP, Moody C, et al. Human immunodeficiency-causing mutation defines CD16 in spontaneous NK cell cytotoxicity. J Clin Invest. 2012;122(10):3769–80.

34. Tholouli E, Sturgess K, Dickinson RE, Gennery A, Cant AJ, Jackson G, et al. In vivo T-depleted reduced-intensity transplantation for GATA2-related immune dysfunction. Blood. 2018;131(12):1383–7.
35. Bhattacharyya R, Tan AM, Chan MY, Jamuar SS, Foo R, Iyer P. TCR alphabeta and CD19-depleted haploidentical stem cell transplant with reduced intensity conditioning for Hoyeraal-Hreidarsson syndrome with RTEL1 mutation. Bone Marrow Transplant. 2016;51(5):753–4.
36. Buckley RH, Schiff RI, Schiff SE, Markert ML, Williams LW, Harville TO, et al. Human severe combined immunodeficiency: genetic, phenotypic, and functional diversity in one hundred eight infants. J Pediatr. 1997;130(3):378–87.
37. Pannicke U, Honig M, Hess I, Friesen C, Holzmann K, Rump EM, et al. Reticular dysgenesis (aleukocytosis) is caused by mutations in the gene encoding mitochondrial adenylate kinase 2. Nat Genet. 2009;41(1):101–5.
38. Puck JM. Neonatal screening for severe combined immunodeficiency. Curr Opin Pediatr. 2011;23(6):667–73.
39. Blott EJ, Griffiths GM. Secretory lysosomes. Nat Rev Mol Cell Biol. 2002;3(2):122–31.
40. Blundell MP, Worth A, Bouma G, Thrasher AJ. The Wiskott-Aldrich syndrome: the actin cytoskeleton and immune cell function. Dis Markers. 2010;29(3–4):157–75.
41. Orange JS, Ramesh N, Remold-O'Donnell E, Sasahara Y, Koopman L, Byrne M, et al. Wiskott-Aldrich syndrome protein is required for NK cell cytotoxicity and colocalizes with actin to NK cell-activating immunologic synapses. Proc Natl Acad Sci U S A. 2002;99(17):11351–6.
42. Aldrich RA, Steinberg AG, Campbell DC. Pedigree demonstrating a sex-linked recessive condition characterized by draining ears, eczematoid dermatitis and bloody diarrhea. Pediatrics. 1954;13(2):133–9.
43. Chiang SCC, Vergamini SM, Husami A, Neumeier L, Quinn K, Ellerhorst T, et al. Screening for Wiskott-Aldrich syndrome by flow cytometry. J Allergy Clin Immunol. 2018;142(1):333–5 e8.
44. Maul-Pavicic A, Chiang SC, Rensing-Ehl A, Jessen B, Fauriat C, Wood SM, et al. ORAI1-mediated calcium influx is required for human cytotoxic lymphocyte degranulation and target cell lysis. Proc Natl Acad Sci U S A. 2011;108(8):3324–9.
45. Feske S, Gwack Y, Prakriya M, Srikanth S, Puppel SH, Tanasa B, et al. A mutation in Orai1 causes immune deficiency by abrogating CRAC channel function. Nature. 2006;441(7090):179–85.
46. Lougaris V, Patrizi O, Baronio M, Tabellini G, Tampella G, Damiati E, et al. NFKB1 regulates human NK cell maturation and effector functions. Clin Immunol. 2017;175:99–108.
47. Lougaris V, Tabellini G, Vitali M, Baronio M, Patrizi O, Tampella G, et al. Defective natural killer-cell cytotoxic activity in NFKB2-mutated CVID-like disease. J Allergy Clin Immunol. 2015;135(6):1641–3.
48. Orange JS, Jain A, Ballas ZK, Schneider LC, Geha RS, Bonilla FA. The presentation and natural history of immunodeficiency caused by nuclear factor kappaB essential modulator mutation. J Allergy Clin Immunol. 2004;113(4):725–33.
49. Orange JS, Brodeur SR, Jain A, Bonilla FA, Schneider LC, Kretschmer R, et al. Deficient natural killer cell cytotoxicity in patients with IKK-gamma/NEMO mutations. J Clin Invest. 2002;109(11):1501–9.
50. Jordan MB, Allen CE, Weitzman S, Filipovich AH, McClain KL. How I treat hemophagocytic lymphohistiocytosis. Blood. 2011;118(15):4041–52.
51. Chinn IK, Eckstein OS, Peckham-Gregory EC, Goldberg BR, Forbes LR, Nicholas SK, et al. Genetic and mechanistic diversity in pediatric hemophagocytic lymphohistiocytosis. Blood. 2018;132(1):89–100.
52. Stepp SE, Dufourcq-Lagelouse R, Kumar V. Pillars article: perforin gene defects in familial hemophagocytic lymphohistiocytosis. Science. 1999;286:1957–9. J Immunol. 2015;194(11):5044–6.
53. Rudd E, Bryceson YT, Zheng C, Edner J, Wood SM, Ramme K, et al. Spectrum, and clinical and functional implications of UNC13D mutations in familial haemophagocytic lymphohistiocytosis. J Med Genet. 2008;45(3):134–41.

54. Zur Stadt U, Beutel K, Kolberg S, Schneppenheim R, Kabisch H, Janka G, et al. Mutation spectrum in children with primary hemophagocytic lymphohistiocytosis: molecular and functional analyses of PRF1, UNC13D, STX11, and RAB27A. Hum Mutat. 2006;27(1):62–8.
55. Marsh RA, Haddad E. How I treat primary haemophagocytic lymphohistiocytosis. Br J Haematol. 2018;182(2):185–99.
56. Cichorek M, Wachulska M, Stasiewicz A, Tyminska A. Skin melanocytes: biology and development. Postepy Dermatol Alergol. 2013;30(1):30–41.
57. Karim MA, Suzuki K, Fukai K, Oh J, Nagle DL, Moore KJ, et al. Apparent genotype-phenotype correlation in childhood, adolescent, and adult Chediak-Higashi syndrome. Am J Med Genet. 2002;108(1):16–22.
58. Meeths M, Bryceson YT, Rudd E, Zheng C, Wood SM, Ramme K, et al. Clinical presentation of Griscelli syndrome type 2 and spectrum of RAB27A mutations. Pediatr Blood Cancer. 2010;54(4):563–72.
59. Dell'Acqua F, Saettini F, Castelli I, Badolato R, Notarangelo LD, Rizzari C. Hermansky-Pudlak syndrome type II and lethal hemophagocytic lymphohistiocytosis: case description and review of the literature. J Allergy Clin Immunol Pract. 2019;7(7):2476–8 e5.
60. Roberts JL, Lengi A, Brown SM, Chen M, Zhou YJ, O'Shea JJ, et al. Janus kinase 3 (JAK3) deficiency: clinical, immunologic, and molecular analyses of 10 patients and outcomes of stem cell transplantation. Blood. 2004;103(6):2009–18.
61. Feske S, Picard C, Fischer A. Immunodeficiency due to mutations in ORAI1 and STIM1. Clin Immunol. 2010;135(2):169–82.
62. Pai SY, Logan BR, Griffith LM, Buckley RH, Parrott RE, Dvorak CC, et al. Transplantation outcomes for severe combined immunodeficiency, 2000–2009. N Engl J Med. 2014;371(5):434–46.
63. Mamcarz E, Zhou S, Lockey T, Abdelsamed H, Cross SJ, Kang G, et al. Lentiviral gene therapy combined with low-dose busulfan in infants with SCID-X1. N Engl J Med. 2019;380(16):1525–34.
64. Pai SY, DeMartiis D, Forino C, Cavagnini S, Lanfranchi A, Giliani S, et al. Stem cell transplantation for the Wiskott-Aldrich syndrome: a single-center experience confirms efficacy of matched unrelated donor transplantation. Bone Marrow Transplant. 2006;38(10):671–9.
65. Filipovich AH, Stone JV, Tomany SC, Ireland M, Kollman C, Pelz CJ, et al. Impact of donor type on outcome of bone marrow transplantation for Wiskott-Aldrich syndrome: collaborative study of the International Bone Marrow Transplant Registry and the National Marrow Donor Program. Blood. 2001;97(6):1598–603.
66. Ozsahin H, Cavazzana-Calvo M, Notarangelo LD, Schulz A, Thrasher AJ, Mazzolari E, et al. Long-term outcome following hematopoietic stem-cell transplantation in Wiskott-Aldrich syndrome: collaborative study of the European Society for Immunodeficiencies and European Group for Blood and Marrow Transplantation. Blood. 2008;111(1):439–45.
67. Hacein-Bey Abina S, Gaspar HB, Blondeau J, Caccavelli L, Charrier S, Buckland K, et al. Outcomes following gene therapy in patients with severe Wiskott-Aldrich syndrome. JAMA. 2015;313(15):1550–63.
68. Bergsten E, Horne A, Arico M, Astigarraga I, Egeler RM, Filipovich AH, et al. Confirmed efficacy of etoposide and dexamethasone in HLH treatment: long-term results of the cooperative HLH-2004 study. Blood. 2017;130(25):2728–38.
69. Vallurupalli M, Berliner N. Emapalumab for the treatment of relapsed/refractory hemophagocytic lymphohistiocytosis. Blood. 2019;134(21):1783–6.
70. Messina C, Zecca M, Fagioli F, Rovelli A, Giardino S, Merli P, et al. Outcomes of children with hemophagocytic lymphohistiocytosis given allogeneic hematopoietic stem cell transplantation in Italy. Biol Blood Marrow Transplant. 2018;24(6):1223–31.
71. Ostberg JR, Dayanc BE, Yuan M, Oflazoglu E, Repasky EA. Enhancement of natural killer (NK) cell cytotoxicity by fever-range thermal stress is dependent on NKG2D function and is associated with plasma membrane NKG2D clustering and increased expression of MICA on target cells. J Leukoc Biol. 2007;82(5):1322–31.

72. Lackovic V, Borecky L, Vigas M, Rovensky J. Activation of NK cells in subjects exposed to mild hyper- or hypothermic load. J Interf Res. 1988;8(3):393–402.
73. Tsao TM, Tsai MJ, Hwang JS, Cheng WF, Wu CF, Chou CK, et al. Health effects of a forest environment on natural killer cells in humans: an observational pilot study. Oncotarget. 2018;9(23):16501–11.
74. Bigley AB, Agha NH, Baker FL, Spielmann G, Kunz HE, Mylabathula PL, et al. NK cell function is impaired during long-duration spaceflight. J Appl Physiol (1985). 2019;126(4):842–53.
75. Kim M, Kim M, Yoo HJ, Lee JH. Corrigendum: natural killer cell activity and interleukin-12 in metabolically healthy versus metabolically unhealthy overweight individuals. Front Immunol. 2018;9:2179.
76. Inoue C, Takeshita T, Kondo H, Morimoto K. Cigarette smoking is associated with the reduction of lymphokine-activated killer cell and natural killer cell activities. Environ Health Prev Med. 1996;1(1):14–9.
77. Meehan AC, Mifsud NA, Nguyen TH, Levvey BJ, Snell GI, Kotsimbos TC, et al. Impact of commonly used transplant immunosuppressive drugs on human NK cell function is dependent upon stimulation condition. PLoS ONE. 2013;8(3):e60144.
78. Orandi AB, Vogel TP, Keppel MP, Utterson EC, Cooper MA. Azathioprine-associated complete NK cell deficiency. J Clin Immunol. 2017;37(6):514–6.
79. Yusung S, McGovern D, Lin L, Hommes D, Lagishetty V, Braun J. NK cells are biologic and biochemical targets of 6-mercaptopurine in Crohn's disease patients. Clin Immunol. 2017;175:82–90.

Chapter 20
Mucocutaneous Candidiasis

William K. Dolen, Laura S. Green, and Betty B. Wray

Case Presentation 1

A 43-year-old African-American male was first seen at age 8 years for evaluation of persistent oral white plaques that at times were painful. He was otherwise well. His mother had a history of chronic onychomycosis on four fingers of each hand. She intermittently had oral plaques of candidiasis for which she used nystatin swish and swallow with little benefit. Otherwise she was healthy and working every day. He was followed intermittently thereafter, and as he developed thickening and scaling of several nails on his hands and feet, he was treated with oral ketoconazole. He was lost to follow-up until age 33, when he presented with extensive onychomycosis of two nails on his right hand, all toes of both feet, and recurrent oral candidiasis (Fig. 20.1). He denied having had pneumonia or any chronic infections. He was prescribed oral antifungals and topical agents for his feet with little improvement. He wanted his nails removed because they interfered with his ability to get a job. At age 42 he presented with persistent cough. A chest x-ray showed bibasilar infiltrates that improved dramatically after antibiotic therapy. His cough also cleared. A CBC was normal except for mild anemia (hemoglobin 12 g/dL) and slight eosinophilia (6%). An IL-17 level was less than 5 pg/mL (normal greater than or equal to 13 pg/mL). He convinced a surgeon to remove his infected nails. Subsequently, he was seen in the ED for paronychia but no other infections. He has not kept regular appointments but returns when he feels it necessary. He has twin daughters, and at

---

W. K. Dolen (✉) · B. B. Wray
Medical College of Georgia at Augusta University, Augusta, GA, USA
e-mail: bdolen@augusta.edu

L. S. Green
The Allergy, Asthma and Sinus Center, Knoxville, TN, USA

Fig. 20.1 The CMC patient's hands and feet

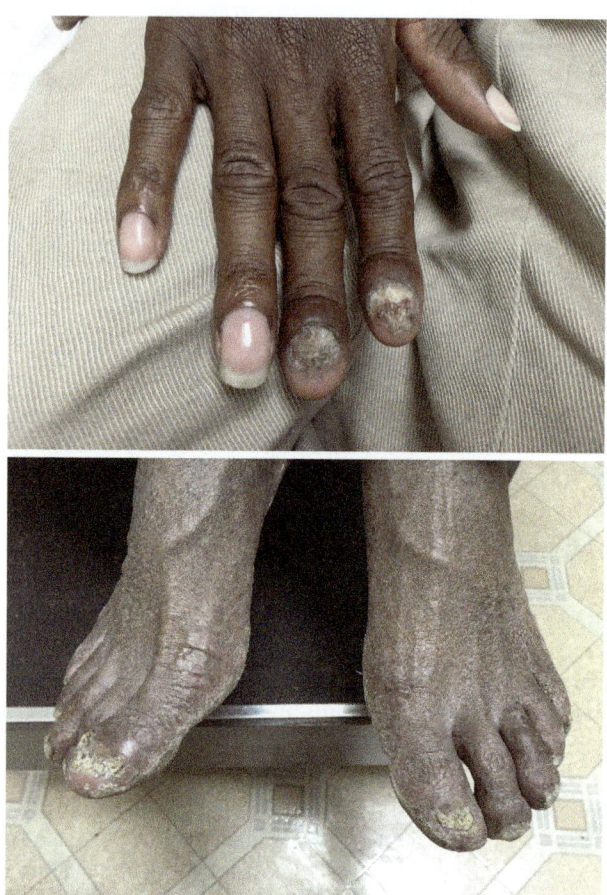

age 2 neither shows any signs of fungal infection. This patient, although the clinical information is incomplete, has features of an autosomal dominant form of familial chronic mucocutaneous candidiasis.

Case Presentation 2 [1]

A 5-year-old female fell at school and had hypertonicity of the upper extremities lasting for about 20 s. She was taken to an emergency department, where a positive Chvostek sign was noted on physical examination. Laboratory evaluation revealed calcium 4.8 mg/mL (8.8–10.8 mg/mL), phosphorus 12.3 mg/dL (4.1–5.4 mg/dL), and magnesium 1.6 mg/mL (1.8–2.3 mg/mL). In the intensive care unit, she had refractory hypocalcemia despite intravenous calcium gluconate and magnesium sulfate. Her parathyroid hormone level was <4.0 pg/mL (8.5–72.5 pg/mL), and her calcium level normalized after she was given parathyroid hormone. In the previous 3 weeks, she had several episodes of possible seizure activity, which was being evaluated on an outpatient basis. Past history indicated that pregnancy, labor, and delivery were normal. As an infant, she developed recurrent candida diaper rashes that responded to topical antifungal medications. At age 4 years, she developed onychomycosis of the nails of the right foot and right thumb. This did not respond well to topical or oral antifungal therapy. Gene sequencing revealed *AIRE* gene mutations in the patient and both parents.

Chronic Mucocutaneous Candidiasis

The dimorphic yeast *Candida albicans* is a normal component of the human microbiome. The innate and adaptive immune systems collaborate to prevent or limit candidal infection. Particularly in infancy, or following antibiotic or corticosteroid therapy, candidiasis can occur in immunologically normal individuals, but severe candidiasis in children and adults warrants evaluation for primary or secondary immunodeficiency and other comorbidities (Table 20.1).

The term "chronic mucocutaneous candidiasis" (CMC) loosely describes a number of very rare primary immunodeficiency disorders. Depending on the defect, prevalence ranges from a few individuals in case reports (e.g., CANDF6) to several hundred reported cases. Patients typically present with chronic or recurrent candidal infections of the nails, skin, oral, and genital mucosae. Some patients have associated autoimmune endocrinopathies and other types of infections. The clinical presentation helps distinguish the diagnosis and primary cause of CMC.

Once thought to be a specific T lymphocyte defect, CMC can be caused by a number of different defects in the dectin and Th17 pathways of innate immunity. There are many known underlying genetic causes (Table 20.2), and basic laboratory testing and genetic testing are needed to establish and confirm the diagnosis. Genetic testing focuses on the pathways of the innate immune system (see Fig. 20.1) that

Table 20.1 Underlying causes of chronic candidiasis[a]

Infancy
Long-term antibiotic use
Long-term inhaled steroid use
Immunosuppressive therapy
Diabetes mellitus
Neoplasia, including lymphoreticular malignancy
HIV1 infection; AIDS
SCIDs, other combined immunodeficiency
If the above are excluded or unlikely, consider chronic mucocutaneous candidiasis, with or without endocrinopathy

[a]Adapted from Green and Dolen [2]

Table 20.2 Known causes of chronic mucocutaneous candidiasis[a]

Disorder	Gene	Inheritance	MIM entry (gene)	MIM entry (disease)
CANDF4 (dectin-1 deficiency)	CLEC7A	AR	*606264	#613108
CANDF2	CARD9	AR	*607212	#212050
AD hyper IgE syndrome (HIGE1)	STAT3	AD	*102582	#147060
AR hyper IgE syndrome (DOCK8)	DOCK8	AR	*611432	#243700
CANDF7 (immunodeficiency 31C)	STAT1 (gain of function)	AD	*600555	#614162
Immunodeficiency 42 (RORγ and RORγt)	RORC	AR	*602943	#616622
CANDF6	IL17F	?	*606496	#613956
CANDF5 (immunodeficiency 51)	IL17RA	AR	*605461	#613953
CANDF9	IL17RC	AR	*610925	#616445
CANDF8	TRAF3IP2	AR	*607043	#615527
CANDF3 (with ICAM1 deficiency)	Unknown (11p13–q12)	AD	n/a	%607644
CANDF1	Unknown (2p22.3–p21)	AD	n/a	%114580
APS1/APECED	AIRE	AR (AD reported)	*607358	#240300

[a]Adapted from Green and Dolen [2]
MIM numbers are from Online Mendelian Inheritance in Man (OMIM) [3]

involve the dectin-1 pattern recognition receptor (PRR), Th17 cells, the Th17 cytokines, IL-17 and IL-22, and their receptors. Individual genetic tests and testing panels are available from reference laboratories.

The Dectin Pathway

Defects in the dectin and Th17 pathways (Figs. 20.2 and 20.3) cause the familial forms of CMC. The PRR dectin-1 is a C-type lectin receptor found on phagocytic cells that binds the β-glucan component of the candidal cell wall. A dectin-1 defect [4] causes the form of CMC termed CANDF4. In a signaling cascade, dectin-1 activates the signaling molecule CARD9 (caspase recruitment domain-containing protein 9), which if defective causes the CANDF2 form of CMC [5] (see Fig. 20.2). CARD9-deficient patients are also at risk for subcutaneous phaeohyphomycosis, deep dermatophytosis, meningoencephalitis, and colitis. Patients may also develop other chronic invasive fungal infections, including *Aspergillus* spp., *Pneumocystis jirovecii*, and *Cryptococcus neoformans*. When activated, CARD9 couples with

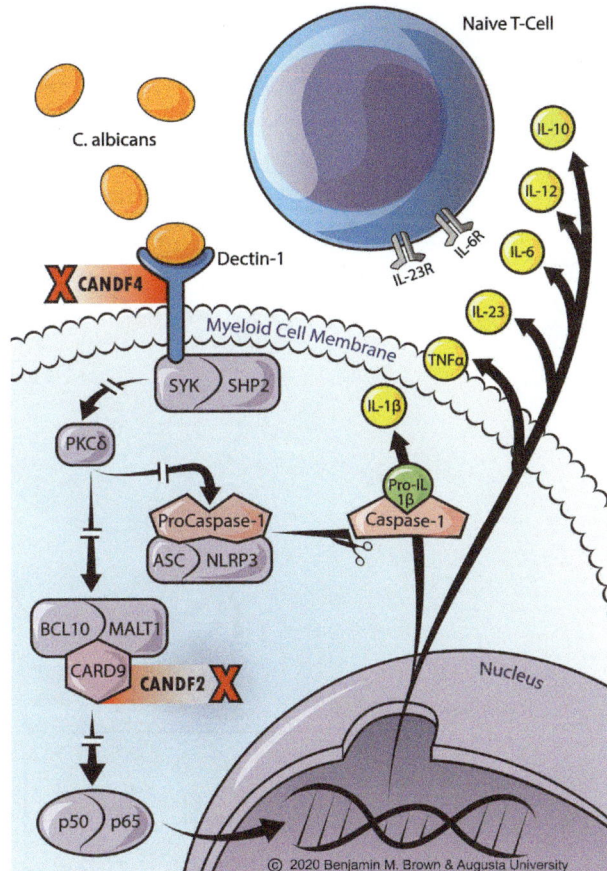

Fig. 20.2 The dectin pathway. (Printed with permission from © 2020 Augusta University and Benjamin M. Brown)

BCL10 and MALT-1 (see Fig. 20.2), inducing activation of nuclear factor-κB (NF-κB) and eventually (see Fig. 20.2) initiating production of pro-inflammatory cytokines (IL-6, IL-23, TNF-alpha, IL-1β). As depicted in Fig. 20.3, IL-6 induces the transcription factor STAT3 (signal transducer and activator of transcription 3) which induces T lymphocytes to differentiate into Th17 cells that produce IL-17 and other cytokines. STAT3 deficiency produces the classic form of autosomal dominant hyper IgE syndrome that is associated with CMC.

The Hyper IgE Syndromes

The major cause of autosomal dominant hyper IgE syndrome is a mutation in STAT3 [6], an important component of the Th17 pathway (see Fig. 20.3). Patients have low levels of IL-17A and IL-22-producing T cells. CMC is seen in up to 83% of patients with the STAT3 form of AD HIES, commonly presenting with oral,

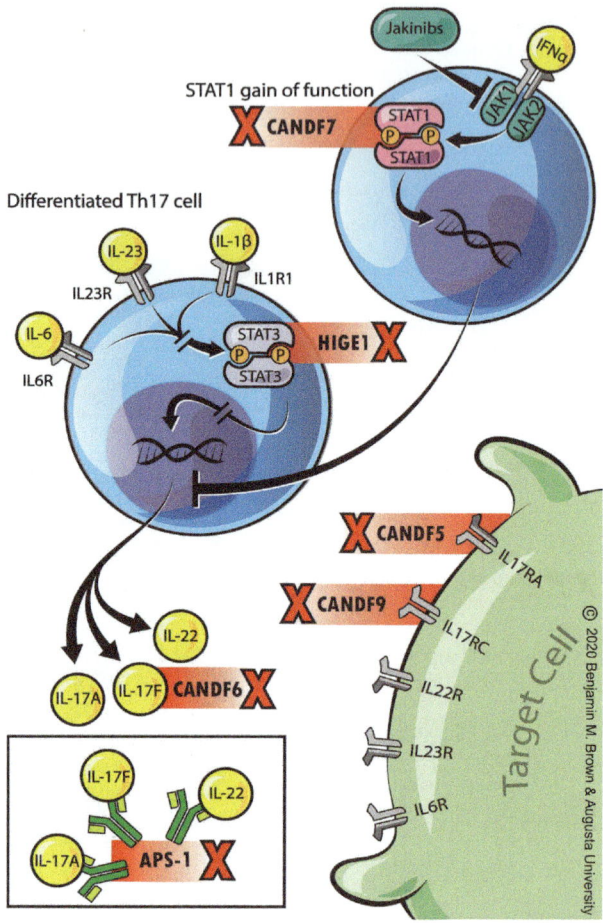

Fig. 20.3 The IL-17 pathway. (Printed with permission from © 2020 Augusta University and Benjamin M. Brown)

genital, or cutaneous candidiasis or onychomycosis. Systemic candida infections are rare. DOCK8 (dedicator of cytokinesis 8) is a regulator of the actin skeleton of cells. A defect produces an autosomal recessive form of hyper IgE syndrome, often with chronic candidiasis [7]. Patients can also have associated asthma, food allergy, and viral skin infections.

STAT1 Gain of Function

Gain of function mutations in STAT1 (signal transducer and activator of transcription 1) cause the majority of cases of familial candidiasis, termed CANDF7 [8, 9] (see Fig. 20.3). Inheritance is autosomal dominant. These mutations cause STAT1 to be hyperphosphorylated upon activation by Janus kinases (JAKs), increasing STAT1-dependent responses to cytokines, especially IL-6 and IL-21, and resulting in inhibition of STAT3 and the IL-17 pathway (IL-17A, IL-17F, and IL-22) which is important in the skin and mucosal response (see Fig. 20.3). Nearly all patients with a STAT1 gain of function mutation will present with CMC, with onset usually in infancy or early childhood. Patients initially develop mild candidiasis affecting the nails and oral mucosa, but the disease progresses to more severe and persistent oropharyngeal, esophageal, and genital involvement in adulthood. Patients also have increased susceptibility to dermatophytic infections of the scalp, skin, or nails and can develop features of combined immunodeficiency, including invasive candidiasis, disseminated coccidioidomycosis, histoplasmosis, or disseminated mucormycosis [10]. Patients are also at risk for recurrent bacterial pneumonias, chronic sinusitis, and otitis media and for recurrent viral infections. Some patients manifest autoimmune disease, including thyroid disease, type I diabetes mellitus, vitiligo, psoriasis, autoimmune hepatitis, and autoimmune cytopenias. They are also at risk for developing aneurysms and malignancy.

IL12B and IL12RB1

Interleukin 12 (IL-12) is a heterodimer encoded by IL12A (the p35 subunit) and IL12B (the p40 subunit). The p40 subunit is also part of the IL-23 heterodimer. Defects in the p40 subunit are associated with Mendelian susceptibility to mycobacterial disease (MSMD); some patients have associated chronic candidiasis. The IL-12 receptor is also a heterodimer, formed by IL-12Rβ1 and IL-12Rβ2 subunits. A defect in the IL12RB1 gene is the most common cause of MSMD, with chronic candidiasis found in about 25% of patients [11].

The Th17 Pathway

The *RORC* gene encodes retinoid-related orphan receptor gamma (RORγ) and RORγt. RORγt interacts with STAT3 and is a key transcription factor for Th17 cytokine production. Patients have impaired production of IL-17A, IL-17F, and IL-22, as well as impaired T lymphocyte function [12]. In addition to chronic candidiasis, patients have severe mycobacteriosis.

IL-17 Cytokine and Receptor Defects

Defects in Th17 cytokine receptors and related molecules also cause CMC [2] (see Fig. 20.3). IL17F gene mutations cause CANDF6. An IL17RA gene defect causes CANDF5, and an IL17RC defect causes CANDF9. The TRAF3IP2 gene encodes for TRAF3 interacting protein 2, an adaptor molecule that interacts with members of the IL17R family to activate various pathways that result in gene induction.

Other Defects

The molecular basis of CANDF3 and CANDF1, listed in Online Mendelian Inheritance in Man [3], is not known. CANDF3 is associated with ICAM1 deficiency. Patients typically have only mild candidiasis of the nails of the fingers and toes.

Autoimmune Polyendocrinopathy Syndrome Type 1

Defects in the AIRE (autoimmune regulator) gene cause a rare condition termed "autoimmune polyendocrinopathy syndrome type 1" (APS1) or "autoimmune-polyendocrinopathy-candidiasis-ectodermal dystrophy" (APECED) [13–15], also termed Whitaker syndrome. Several hundred patients have been reported worldwide [1]. Most patients present with a classic triad of adrenal insufficiency (Addison disease), hypoparathyroidism, and CMC. The presence of two of these is required for a working diagnosis. Other endocrinopathies, including hypergonadotropic hypogonadism, type 1 diabetes mellitus, autoimmune thyroiditis, chronic hepatitis, pernicious anemia, and pituitary failure, have been reported [1]. Associated ectodermal disturbances include vitiligo, alopecia, keratoconjunctivitis, dental enamel hypoplasia, pitted nail dystrophy, and tympanic membrane calcification. Patients are also at risk of developing oral squamous cell carcinoma. CMC, which is the most common presenting feature, usually appears in infancy or early childhood, sequentially followed by hypoparathyroidism and adrenal insufficiency [16]. Because the *AIRE* gene is directly involved in development of T-cell tolerance to self-antigens, and indirectly involved in B-cell tolerance to self-antigens, patients with AIRE defects produce high-affinity autoantibodies to various cytokines, including type I interferons, IL-17A, IL-17F, and IL-22 (see Fig. 20.3), to other interleukins, and to various enzymes involved in endocrine function [17].

Diagnosis

Diagnosis of CMC requires a thorough history, physical examination, and selected basic laboratory tests. For a patient presenting with chronic candidiasis, the clinician would first evaluate to rule out conditions listed in Table 20.1, for these are more common than CMC. In the diagnosis of CMC, a good family history and a detailed review of systems with endocrinologic focus are important. Basic laboratory tests would include a CBC with differential, a complete metabolic panel, fungal culture, and levels of IgG, IgA, IgM, and IgE. Other tests, such as screening for endocrinopathies, should be ordered as indicated.

A working diagnosis can be confirmed by genetic testing. Consultation with a geneticist or a pathologist will determine whether individual gene testing or ordering a CMC genetic testing panel would be more cost-effective. Since a STAT1 gain of function mutation is the most common cause of familial CMC, and specific therapy (albeit off-label) is available for refractory cases, evaluation might start with this single test. If STAT1 is normal, one might consider a CMC panel. If this is normal, the diagnosis should be reevaluated before ordering whole exome or other types of sequencing. When a defect is identified, family members should be offered genetic counselling and screening.

Management

Patients with familial chronic mucocutaneous candidiasis require long-term management with antifungal agents, with monitoring for and treatment of comorbidities. When topical antifungal therapy is unsuccessful (as is often the case), systemic therapy will be required. Unfortunately, antifungal resistance can, and does, occur and relapse can be expected on cessation of antifungal therapy. As part of general care, excellent oral hygiene is important [14]; abstinence from tobacco use, limited alcohol consumption, and avoidance of irritant toothpastes are recommended. Hematopoietic stem cell transplantation has been successful in some cases [18]. Management of APS-1 is a collaborative effort between endocrinology, focusing on treating the endocrinopathies, and infectious disease, with focus on the chronic candidiasis.

Multiple case reports suggest that some patients with chronic mucocutaneous candidiasis caused by STAT1 gain of function mutation may respond to jakinibs (Janus kinase inhibitors), a new class of drugs that inhibit JAK1/2, signaling molecules in the cytokine receptor JAK-STAT pathway. JAK1/2 inhibition reduces abnormal phosphorylation of STAT1. Ruxolitinib is an orally given jakinib that reduces abnormal phosphorylation of STAT1 [19–23]. It is approved for treatment of myelofibrosis and polycythemia vera in adults, for corticosteroid-refractory acute graft-versus-host disease in persons age 12 years and older. In one case report, oral candidiasis and alopecia responded promptly to ruxolitinib, and the candidiasis returned 2 weeks after the medication was stopped [22]. Baricitinib, another orally given jakinib, has also been reported as beneficial [24]. It is approved for treatment of rheumatoid arthritis in adults. The use of a jakinib to treat CMC with the STAT1 GOF mutation is off-label, but it is a reasonable alternative to consider when conventional therapies have failed.

Conclusion

Candidiasis can occur in immunologically normal infants, children, and adults. Predisposing factors are listed in Table 20.1. Patients with unusually severe chronic candidiasis unresponsive to conventional antifungal therapy warrant evaluation for CMC. Evaluation begins with a careful history, examination, and selected laboratory tests to exclude the more common causes of chronic candidiasis. Confirmation of CMC requires genetic testing to identify the underlying cause (Table 20.2). Management can be frustrating for both the patient and clinician. Standard therapy involves the use of chronic antifungal medications. For more severe cases, hematopoietic stem cell transplantation has been successful, and emerging case reports indicate that oral jakinib therapy may help individuals with the STAT1 GOF mutation.

References

1. Sanford E, Watkins K, Nahas S, Gottschalk M, Coufal NG, Farnaes L, et al. Rapid whole-genome sequencing identifies a novel AIRE variant associated with autoimmune polyendocrine syndrome type 1. Cold Spring Harb Mol Case Stud. 2018;4(5):1–8.
2. Green L, Dolen WK. Chronic candidiasis in children. Curr Allergy Asthma Rep. 2017;17:1–6. https://doi.org/10.1007/s11882-017-0699-9.
3. Online Mendelian Inheritance in Man, OMIM® [database on the Internet]. McKusick-Nathans Institute of Genetic Medicine. Available from: https://omim.org.
4. Taylor PR, Tsoni SV, Willment JA, Dennehy KM, Rosas M, Findon H, et al. Dectin-1 is required for beta-glucan recognition and control of fungal infection. Nat Immunol. 2007;8(1):31–8. https://doi.org/10.1038/ni1408.
5. Whibley N, Jaycox JR, Reid D, Garg AV, Taylor JA, Clancy CJ, et al. Delinking CARD9 and IL-17: CARD9 protects against Candida tropicalis infection through a TNF-alpha-dependent, IL-17-independent mechanism. J Immunol. 2015;195(8):3781–92. https://doi.org/10.4049/jimmunol.1500870.
6. Freeman AF, Holland SM. The hyper-IgE syndromes. Immunol Allergy Clin N Am. 2008;28(2):277–91, viii. https://doi.org/10.1016/j.iac.2008.01.005.
7. Engelhardt KR, Gertz ME, Keles S, Schaffer AA, Sigmund EC, Glocker C, et al. The extended clinical phenotype of 64 patients with dedicator of cytokinesis 8 deficiency. J Allergy Clin Immunol. 2015;136(2):402–12. https://doi.org/10.1016/j.jaci.2014.12.1945.
8. Akarcan SE, Severcan EU, Karaca NE, Isik A, Aksu G, Migaud M, et al. Gain-of-function mutations in STAT1: a recently defined cause for chronic mucocutaneous candidiasis disease mimicking combined immunodeficiencies. Case Rep Immunol. 2017; https://doi.org/10.1155/2017/2846928.
9. Toubiana J, Okada S, Hiller J, Oleastro M, Lagos Gomez M, Aldave Becerra JC, et al. Heterozygous STAT1 gain-of-function mutations underlie an unexpectedly broad clinical phenotype. Blood. 2016;127(25):3154–64. https://doi.org/10.1182/blood-2015-11-679902.
10. Baris S, Alroqi F, Kiykim A, Karakoc-Aydiner E, Ogulur I, Ozen A, et al. Severe early-onset combined immunodeficiency due to heterozygous gain-of-function mutations in STAT1. J Clin Immunol. 2016;36(7):641–8.
11. de Beaucoudrey L, Samarina A, Bustamante J, Cobat A, Boisson-Dupuis S, Feinberg J, et al. Revisiting human IL-12Rbeta1 deficiency: a survey of 141 patients from 30 countries. Medicine (Baltimore). 2010;89(6):381–402. https://doi.org/10.1097/MD.0b013e3181fdd832.
12. Okada S, Markle JG, Deenick EK, Mele F, Averbuch D, Lagos M, et al. IMMUNODEFICIENCIES. Impairment of immunity to Candida and Mycobacterium in humans with bi-allelic RORC mutations. Science (New York, NY). 2015;349(6248):606–13. https://doi.org/10.1126/science.aaa4282.
13. Kisand K, Peterson P. Autoimmune polyendocrinopathy candidiasis ectodermal dystrophy. J Clin Immunol. 2015;35(5):463–78. https://doi.org/10.1007/s10875-015-0176-y.

14. Humbert L, Cornu M, Proust-Lemoine E, Bayry J, Wemeau JL, Vantyghem MC, et al. Chronic Mucocutaneous candidiasis in autoimmune polyendocrine syndrome type 1. Front Immunol. 2018;9:2570.
15. Constantine GM, Lionakis MS. Lessons from primary immunodeficiencies: autoimmune regulator and autoimmune polyendocrinopathy-candidiasis-ectodermal dystrophy. Immunol Rev. 2019;287(1):103–20. https://doi.org/10.1111/imr.12714.
16. Weiler FG, Dias-da-Silva MR, Lazaretti-Castro M. Autoimmune polyendocrine syndrome type 1: case report and review of literature. Arq Bras Endocrinol Metab. 2012;56:54–66.
17. Meyer S, Woodward M, Hertel C, Vlaicu P, Haque Y, Kämer J, et al. AIRE-deficient patients harbor unique high-affinity disease-ameliorating autoantibodies. Cell. 2016;166:582–95.
18. Leiding JW, Okada S, Hagin D, Abinun M, Shcherbina A, Balashov DN, et al. Hematopoietic stem cell transplantation in patients with gain-of-function signal transducer and activator of transcription 1 mutations. J Allergy Clin Immunol. 2018;141(2):704–17. https://doi.org/10.1016/j.jaci.2017.03.049.
19. Higgins E, Al Shehri T, McAleer MA, Conlon N, Feighery C, Lilic D, et al. Use of ruxolitinib to successfully treat chronic mucocutaneous candidiasis caused by gain-of-function signal transducer and activator of transcription 1 (STAT1) mutation. J Allergy Clin Immunol. 2015;135(2):551–3.
20. Mossner R, Diering N, Bader O, Forkel S, Overbeck T, Gross U, et al. Ruxolitinib induces interleukin 17 and ameliorates chronic mucocutaneous candidiasis caused by STAT1 gain-of-function mutation. Clin Infect Dis. 2016;62(7):951–3.
21. Weinacht KG, Charbonnier LM, Alroqi F, Plant A, Qiao Q, Wu H, et al. Ruxolitinib reverses dysregulated T helper cell responses and controls autoimmunity caused by a novel signal transducer and activator of transcription 1 (STAT1) gain-of-function mutation. J Allergy Clin Immunol. 2017;139(5):1629–40.e2.
22. Bloomfield M, Kanderova V, Parackova Z, Vrabcova P, Svaton M, Fronkova E, et al. Utility of Ruxolitinib in a child with chronic mucocutaneous candidiasis caused by a novel STAT1 gain-of-function mutation. J Clin Immunol. 2018;38(5):589–601.
23. Vargas-Hernandez A, Mace EM, Zimmerman O, Zerbe CS, Freeman AF, Rosenzweig S, et al. Ruxolitinib partially reverses functional natural killer cell deficiency in patients with signal transducer and activator of transcription 1 (STAT1) gain-of-function mutations. J Allergy Clin Immunol. 2018;141(6):2142–55.
24. Meesilpavikkai K, Dik WA, Schrijver B, Nagtzaam NMA, Posthumus-van Sluijs SJ, van Hagen PM, et al. Baricitinib treatment in a patient with a gain-of-function mutation in signal transducer and activator of transcription 1 (STAT1). J Allergy Clin Immunol. 2018;142(1):328–30.e2.

Part V
Secondary Immunodeficiency

Chapter 21
Immunodeficiency Secondary to Malignancies and Biologics

S. Shahzad Mustafa

The vast majority of individuals have normally functioning immune systems, but there is a subset of individuals at increased risk of infection due to a heterogeneous group of immunodeficiencies. Whereas primary immunodeficiency (PIDD) arises from inherited or sporadic genetic mutations, secondary immunodeficiency (SID) is more common and caused by a myriad of factors (Table 21.1). Malnutrition is the most common worldwide cause of SID [1]. HIV leading to AIDS is the most common infectious cause of SID. Other causes of SID include extremes of age, pregnancy, metabolic conditions (diabetes, cirrhosis, and renal dysfunction), conditions leading to protein loss (nephrotic syndrome, protein-losing enteropathy), physiologic stressors (surgery, trauma), and environmental exposures (radiation, exposure to toxic chemicals). Medications can also lead to SID, with systemic glucocorticoids being a common culprit [2]. With the increasing arsenal of chemotherapeutics and B-cell depleting therapies, biologic agents are becoming increasingly recognized for their risk of SID. Lastly, malignancies can lead to SID, particularly B-cell disorders such as non-Hodgkin's lymphoma, multiple myeloma, and chronic lymphocytic leukemia. This chapter will focus on SID caused by malignancies and biologics.

Case Presentation 1

A 64-year-old gentleman with past medical history of hypothyroidism, hypertension, and non-Hodgkin's lymphoma presents for evaluation of recurrent sinusitis and possible allergies. The patient reports one to two sinus infections annually for

S. S. Mustafa (✉)
Division of Allergy, Immunology, Rheumatology, Rochester Regional Health,
University of Rochester School of Medicine and Dentistry, Rochester, NY, USA
e-mail: shahzad.mustafa@rochesterregional.org

© Springer Nature Switzerland AG 2021
J. A. Bernstein (ed.), *Primary and Secondary Immunodeficiency*,
https://doi.org/10.1007/978-3-030-57157-3_21

Table 21.1 Common causes of secondary immunodeficiency

Malignancy	Medications	Other
Chronic lymphocytic leukemia	B cell depleting therapies[a]	Organ transplantation
Lymphoma	Systemic corticosteroids	Nephrotic syndrome
Multiple myeloma	Anti-epileptic agents	Protein-losing enteropathy
	Phenytoin	Celiac disease
	Carbamazepine	Crohn's disease
	Valproic acid	Ulcerative colitis
	Lamotrigine	
Leukemia	Purine analogs	Physiologic stressors
	Fludarabine	Surgery
	Azathioprine	Trauma
Myelodysplastic syndrome	Tyrosine kinase inhibitors	Metabolic disorders
	Imatinib	Diabetes mellitus
	Ibrutinib	Cirrhosis
	Dasatinib	
Waldenstrom's macroglobinemia		Infections
		HIV/AIDS
Solid tumors	[a]Please see Table 21.2	Burns
		Malnutrition
		Radiation
		Pregnancy
		Extremes of age
		Toxic chemicals

Table 21.2 Biologics associated with secondary immunodeficiency

Anti-CD20	Anti-CD19	Anti-CD22	Anti-CD52	Anti-CD38	Anti-BAFF
Rituximab	Binatumumab	Epratuzumab	Alemtuzumab	Daratumumab	Belimumab
Ofatumumab	Targeted chimeric antigen receptor T cells (CAR-T)			Isatuximab	
Veltuzumab					
Ocrelizumab					
Obinutuzumab					
Ublituximab					

the past 4 years. He describes the episodes as presenting with marked sinus pressure and discomfort, often associated with tooth pain and discolored nasal discharge. He is febrile during the episodes, and the symptoms significantly affect his daily activity for 3–5 days. Each episode is successfully treated with oral antibiotics.

He cannot recall being treated with systemic glucocorticoids. In between the episodes of sinusitis, the patient reports minimal nasal congestion, rhinorrhea, or postnasal drip. He denies anosmia, lingering respiratory symptoms, or reactions to NSAIDs. He also reports one hospitalization 2 years ago for community-acquired pneumonia complicated by a para-pneumonic effusion requiring drainage with a chest tube, with isolation of *Streptococcus pneumoniae* on microbial culture. He denies a history of additional infections and denies chronic diarrhea. He feels generally well otherwise.

The patient reports that his lymphoma was diagnosed in 2002 when he presented with night sweats and a pathologic left femur fracture. At that time, he underwent eight cycles of therapy with R-CHOP (rituximab, cyclophosphamide, doxorubicin hydrochloride, vincristine, prednisolone) followed by 2 years of maintenance therapy with rituximab. The patient did well until 2016 when he experienced recurrence of lymphoma, at which time he was treated with bendamustine and rituximab for six cycles followed by maintenance therapy with rituximab for 2 years. His last dose of rituximab was 18 months ago. The patient currently takes levothyroxine for his hypothyroidism and diltiazem for hypertension. He does not use any supplements or over-the-counter medications. He does not smoke cigarettes. With the exception of his sinus complaints, he feels like he is in good health. Physical exam is largely unremarkable, with normal nasal turbinates and no evidence of polyps, no oropharyngeal erythema, no lymphadenopathy, no adventitious breath sounds, and no hepatosplenomegaly. Skin prick testing to aeroallergens completed by a previous allergist was negative, and a CT sinus was also unremarkable.

Diagnosis/Assessment

This case highlights the importance of a detailed history when evaluating individuals for immunodeficiency. Individuals with immunodeficiency commonly present with recurrent sinopulmonary infections, and this patient's history of recurrent bacterial sinusitis along with a community-acquired pneumonia complicated by a parapneumonic effusion requiring drainage and extended inpatient hospitalization raises the possibility of underlying immunodeficiency. Recognizing and addressing immunodeficiency in a timely manner has been associated with improved morbidity and mortality, particularly in the setting of bronchiectasis [3–5]. There are important distinguishing factors between primary and secondary immunodeficiency. Although SID is up to 30 times more common than PIDD [6], this group of heterogeneous disorders is generally poorly defined in the medical literature, making true prevalence difficult to ascertain. Although PIDDs are relatively uncommon, they are generally better defined than SIDs, and international registries are improving knowledge of these conditions, most notably with common variable immunodeficiency (CVID) [7]. PIDD generally presents at a much younger age as compared to SID, with CVID having a bimodal presentation in childhood and young adulthood, whereas SID due to malignancy and chemotherapeutics often presents later in life, often beyond the fifth decade. In a cohort of patients with SID, Duraisingham et al. showed the most frequent cause to be previous chemotherapy for B-cell lymphoma, most commonly therapy with rituximab [8]. Additionally, patients with SID had similar IgG levels as patients with PIDD, but significantly higher IgA and IgM levels, making these immunologic measurements an important distinguishing factor between SID and PIDD [8]. Despite these differences, both PIDD and SID typically present with an increased risk of non-neutropenic bacterial infections, and both are responsive to therapy with prophylactic antibiotics and/or immunoglobulin replacement (IgR) therapy.

The patient in Case 1 has multiple risk factors for developing SID, including a history of lymphoma, along with multiple cycles of rituximab in conjunction with additional chemotherapeutic agents. Although multiple biologic agents have been associated with SID (Table 21.2), rituximab is a commonly used B-cell depleting therapy associated with SID. Rituximab is a chimeric IgG1 anti-CD20 monoclonal antibody used to treat B-cell neoplasms and autoimmune conditions, including rheumatologic conditions such as rheumatoid arthritis, systemic lupus erythematosus, systemic vasculitides, autoimmune cytopenias such as idiopathic thrombocytopenic purpura, and autoimmune skin diseases such as pemphigus vulgaris and bullous pemphigoid [9]. Rituximab depletes peripheral B cells, with normalization being poorly understood and highly variable, ranging from months to years [10, 11]. Although it does not affect Ig-producing circulating plasma cells due to their lack of CD20 expression, rituximab has been associated with causing clinically significant hypogammaglobulinemia [12]. The degree of immune suppression caused by rituximab depends on multiple factors, including the type of underlying illness for which it is being used. Patients treated with rituximab for malignancy appear to be more susceptible to hypogammaglobulinemia as compared to patients treated with rituximab for rheumatologic disease [13]. Casulo et al. reported that 38% of patients treated with rituximab for lymphoma developed hypogammaglobulinemia, with a much smaller percentage needing Ig replacement therapy [14]. As compared to patients with malignancy, rates of hypogammaglobulinemia and clinically significant non-neutropenic bacterial infections were much lower in patients with rheumatoid arthritis who were treated with rituximab [15]. In addition to the underlying condition, additional risk factors for hypogammaglobulinemia due to rituximab include lower pre-treatment IgG levels, increasing number of doses and duration of therapy with rituximab, and use of concomitant chemotherapies, particularly fludarabine [16, 17].

Previous literature illustrates that hypogammaglobulinemia in patients treated with B-cell depleting therapies has an increased risk of infection. Van Vollenhoven et al. reviewed over 2500 patients with rheumatoid arthritis and showed sinopulmonary infections, including community-acquired pneumonia, to be the most commonly reported infectious complication [15]. There are a host of additional reported infections, including urinary tract infections [18], skin infections, reactivation of hepatitis B [12], and otomastoiditis [19]. Nonbacterial infections such as cytomegalovirus CMV) have also been reported [12]. Similarly, ibrutinib has also been associated with increased risk of infection in the setting of B-cell malignancies [20].

Given that rituximab and other B-cell depleting therapies are associated with hypogammaglobulinemia and increased risk of infection, immunologists strongly encourage clinicians to check baseline immunoglobulin levels (IgG, IgM, IgA) and peripheral B cell prior to initiating therapy with these medications. This baseline information can be particularly helpful in uncovering underlying PIDD, as this may present with malignancy and/or autoimmunity. Unfortunately, consensus guidelines are lacking, and this information is still routinely missing from the medical record in patients treated with rituximab and similar B-cell depleting agents [21]. The degree of secondary hypogammaglobulinemia from rituximab also varies with the underlying disease state. In a retrospective review of a small cohort of patients treated with rituximab who were referred for further immune evaluation, 19 were referred for hypogammaglobulinemia, with a mean IgG = 342 ± 40 mg/dL. IgM and IgA were also reduced, and all patients had decreased or absent B cells while having no evidence of neutropenia. Patients most commonly presented with recurrent sinopulmonary infections, and there was one patient with bacterial meningitis leading to death. All but one of the 19 patients required IgR therapy [22]. Casulo et al. demonstrated similar frequency of hypogammaglobulinemia in patients with non-Hodgkin's lymphoma, along with similar severity of Ig suppression, and resulting infectious complication and therapeutic outcomes [14]. Similar literature is lacking for other B-cell depleting therapies.

Although checking baseline immunoglobulin levels initiates an immune evaluation, assessing for functional status of humoral immunity requires evaluating vaccine responses. Whereas evaluating vaccine responses is a routine part of the evaluation of PIDD, this practice is variably used in the setting of SID, including SID due to B-cell depleting therapies [23]. Previous studies have shown that rituximab can impair vaccine responses even in the setting of normal to modestly decreased Ig levels [24–26]. Vaccine responses should be checked for peptide and polysaccharide antigens, namely, *Streptococcus pneumoniae* (Table 21.3). Commonly used peptide

Table 21.3 Use of vaccine responses in evaluating immunodeficiency

Vaccine	T-cell independent or dependent	Protective response
Haemophilus influenza	Dependent	2-fold increase to >1.0 µg/ml
Diphtheria	Dependent	2-fold increase to >0.1 IU/ml
Tetanus	Dependent	2-fold increase to >0.15 IU/ml
Rabies	Dependent	2-fold increase to 0.5 IU/ml
Meningococcal conjugate	Dependent	2-fold increase to 2.0 µg/ml
Meningococcal polysaccharide	Independent	2-fold increase to 2.0 µg/ml (2 of 4 serotypes)
Pneumococcal polysaccharide (PPV23)	Independent	If baseline < 1.3 µg/ml, increase 2-fold to >1.3 µg/ml OR increase 4-fold
		If baseline > 1.3 µg/ml, increase 2-fold
		Responses need to be demonstrated by 70% of serotypes
Pneumococcal conjugate (PCV13)	Dependent	If baseline < 1.3 µg/ml, increase 2-fold to >1.3 µg/ml OR increase 4-fold
		If baseline > 1.3 µg/ml, increase 2-fold
		Responses need to be demonstrated by 70% of serotypes

vaccines include those for *Corynebacterium diphtheriae* (diphtheria), *Haemophilus influenza*, *Neisseria meningitides*, and *Clostridium tetani* (tetanus). Patients treated with rituximab may preserve their response to peptide antigens while having a decreased response to polysaccharide antigens [26] or can demonstrate a suboptimal response to both peptides and polysaccharides [27]. These studies demonstrate the importance of evaluating vaccine responses to increase the sensitivity of diagnosing SID due to rituximab and other B-cell depleting therapies, since many patients preserve their immunoglobulin levels while lacking vaccine responses, hypothetically making them more susceptible to non-neutropenic bacterial infections.

Case Presentation 1 Revisited

The patient in case 1 has multiple risk factors for developing SID, including a history of malignancy, along with multiple doses and prolonged duration of therapy with rituximab in conjunction with addition chemotherapeutic agents, resulting in recurrent sinopulmonary infections along with a life-threatening community-acquired pneumonia complicated with a para-pneumonic effusion. He therefore warrants evaluation for SID. The patient's laboratory evaluation is as follows:

- CBC normal
- Comprehensive metabolic panel normal
- IgG = 487 mg/dL (650–1600 mg/dL)
- IgM = 18 mg/dL (50–300 mg/dL)
- IgA = 235 mg/dL (40–350 mg/dL)
- CD19 = 0 absolute cells (110–660), 0% of cells (6–29%)
- Pre-vaccination diphtheria IgG = 0.57 IU/mL, post-vaccination diphtheria IgG = 0.67 IU/mL
- Pre-vaccination tetanus IgG = 0.91 IU/mL, post-vaccination tetanus IgG = 0.99 IU/mL
- Pre-vaccination *Streptococcus pneumoniae* IgG > 1.3 μg/ml for 1/23 serotypes
- Post-vaccination *Streptococcus pneumoniae* IgG > 1.3 μg/ml for 1/23 serotypes

Normal vaccine responses are defined as follows [28]:

- Diphtheria: twofold increase and must be into protective range
- Tetanus: twofold increase and must be in protective range
- *Streptococcus pneumoniae* (based on response to PPV23):
  - If < 1.3 μg/ml, twofold increase to > 1.3 μg/ml OR fourfold increase.
  - If > 1.3 μg/ml, twofold increase.
  - For adults, responses must be demonstrated by 70% of serotypes.

Although there remains debate and a lack of consensus of what constitutes an adequate response to vaccination with *Streptococcus pneumoniae*, an impaired vaccine response is generally defined as an abnormal response to any of the above antigens. The patient's laboratory evaluation reveals absent B cells and moderate hypogammaglobulinemia affecting IgG and IgM with preserved levels of IgA. Importantly, the patient demonstrates poor vaccine responses to both peptide (diphtheria and tetanus) and polysaccharide (*Streptococcus pneumoniae*) antigens, consistent with humoral immunodeficiency that is consistent with his increased burden of non-neutropenic bacterial infections.

Management/Outcome

It is important to note that this patient continues to have evidence of SID despite having received his last dose of rituximab 18 months ago. The lack of recovery after this period of time puts him at risk for long-lasting humoral dysfunction and thus at increased risk for ongoing non-neutropenic bacterial infections. Management options for his SID include prophylactic vaccination, prophylactic antibiotics, or immunoglobulin replacement (IgR) therapy.

Given the well-documented impairment on vaccine responses due to rituximab, all medically indicated vaccines should ideally be administered prior to initiation of therapy with rituximab and likely all B-cell depleting therapies. Live vaccines are contraindicated in cases of significant immunodeficiency, but there is minimal data on the safety of live vaccines in SID due to B-cell depleting therapies. Consideration regarding live vaccination should therefore likely be made on a case by case basis depending on the risk of infectious complications. As has been previously shown, rituximab affects humoral immunity and subsequent vaccine responses. In general, conjugated vaccines such as influenza and PCV13 are therefore more likely to elicit an immune response, due to the role of T-cell immunity, which presumably remains intact despite therapy with rituximab. Svensson et al. demonstrated PCV13 to be superior to PPV23 in patients with lymphoma treated with rituximab [29]. If patients treated with rituximab receive routine vaccinations, evaluating post-vaccination titers is particularly helpful to assess efficacy, given the variability in response to vaccination.

Although there is a paucity of literature to support the use of prophylactic antibiotics in the management of SID, this is a commonly used treatment strategy [30]. The most commonly used antibiotics are azithromycin, doxycycline, amoxicillin, and sulfamethoxazole/trimethoprim. Ideally, the choice of antibiotics should take into account pervious culture and sensitivity data, as well as local antibiotic resistance patterns. The benefits of prolonged use of prophylactic antibiotics need to be weighed against the risk of drug resistance and other adverse effects. In the setting of breakthrough infection, one may need to use a different class of antibiotics, broader antimicrobial coverage, and different routes of administration (e.g., intravenous or nebulized).

Many studies have demonstrated the utility of IgR therapy in SID due to rituximab [22, 31, 32], and IgR is a commonly used strategy in this setting [30]. Much like the variability in screening and diagnosis of SID, there is significant variability in the initiation of IgR in the setting of SID due to rituximab. As shown by Edgar et al. [30], most clinicians take multiple factors into account when considering IgR therapy. These include the number of bacterial infections, particularly life-threatening bacterial infections and those requiring hospitalization, IgG level, presence of bronchiectasis, microbiological data, and on the number of previously prescribed antibiotic courses. Interestingly, few clinicians used vaccine responses when deciding on the initiation of IgR. Many clinicians started with prophylactic antibiotics for infection prophylaxis and moved to IgR only in the setting of continued infections. To date, there is no consensus on when to initiate IgR in SID. The majority of clinicians prescribing IgR in the UK start with a dose of 400 mg/kg/month and assess the response based on future infections. Goal IgG levels during IgR therapy are not well defined in SID, and this is especially challenging since many patients start with normal to near-normal IgG levels but significant humoral dysfunction as defined by poor vaccine responses. Some have therefore advocated monitoring IgG levels and antibody titers to specific antigens, such as *Streptococcus pneumoniae* [33]. As with PIDD, it is important to titrate doses of IgR to a level that successfully decreases non-neutropenic bacterial infections. Additionally, although the majority of patients treated with IgR receive intravenous infusions, there is increasing literature showing similar efficacy between intravenous IgR and subcutaneous IgR [34, 35]. Compagno et al. presented a case series of patients with SID treated with subcutaneous IgR, many of whom had previously been on IV IgR. Both routes of administration of IgR led to decreased infection and decreased reliance on antibiotics. Patients switching to subcutaneous IgR reported less adverse effects as compared to when they were on IV IgR, including fever, diffuse skin reactions, dyspnea, and anaphylaxis. Patients used less premedications while on subcutaneous IgR as compared to IV IgR. Additionally, patients on subcutaneous IgR also reported improved health-related quality of life parameters [32]. Lastly, there remains uncertainty regarding the duration of IgR in the setting of SID due to rituximab [36]. Given the variable recovery of B-cell function following the discontinuation of rituximab, periodic reevaluation of humoral immunity appears to be a prudent and worthwhile approach.

Case Presentation 1 Revisited

The patient in case 1 presents with recurrent infections, absent B cells, hypogammaglobulinemia, and poor vaccine responses, all consistent with SID due to rituximab. Given his immune evaluation along with an episode of life-threatening pneumonia, he was started on subcutaneous IgR at a dose of (100 mg/kg/week). Subcutaneous IgR replacement was chosen over intravenous IgR for several reasons, most notably the patient's preference to self-administer the infusions at home rather than at a medical facility. The patient was taught to self-administer subcutaneous Ig with three home nursing visits and continued once weekly dosing, with each infusion taking approximately 60 min. He denied any adverse effects and did not require use of a premedication regimen. Three months after the initiation of IgR, his IgG increased from 487 mg/dL to 790 mg/dL, and his specific antibodies also improved (diphtheria = 1.1 IU/mL, tetanus = 1.7 IU/mL). His *Streptococcus pneumoniae* IgG improved into a protective range (>1.3 μg/ml) for 11/23 serotypes, as compared to the baseline of 1/23 serotypes. He clinically has not experienced any additionally infectious complications requiring therapy with antibiotics.

Case Presentation 2

A 68-year-old gentleman with past medical history of Grave's disease, status post ablation and on thyroid replacement, and chronic lymphocytic leukemia (CLL) presents for evaluation of chronic coughing for the last 2 years. The cough is sometimes productive of clear to yellow sputum and associated with occasional difficulty breathing without wheezing or chest tightness. The cough is not exacerbated by exertion but significantly worsens with upper respiratory tract infections. The patient reports profound nasal congestion and postnasal drip, but no rhinorrhea, sneezing, or itchy/watery eyes. The patient also reports a decreased sense of smell. He denies heartburn and tolerates NSAIDs without difficulty. He is diagnosed with one to two sinus infections annually, which are marked with fever, sinus pressure, and increased nasal drainage. Each sinus infection is typically treated with antibiotics with eventual improvement, but not complete resolution of symptoms. The patient has tried proton pump inhibitors, inhaled corticosteroids, and inhaled beta agonists for the cough, all with minimal relief. The patient was also diagnosed with a chest x-ray-documented pneumonia about a year and a half ago that required inpatient hospitalization. He otherwise denies a history of recurrent infections. He denies chronic diarrhea.

The patient was diagnosed with CLL 7 years ago when he presented with incidental lymphadenopathy found on imaging for musculoskeletal complaints. Additional evaluation led to a diagnosis of stage 0 CLL (13q deletion) using the Rai-Sawitsky staging system. The patient has been closely observed to date with stable blood work and has not been on any therapy. He does not use any supplements or over-the-counter medications. He does not smoke cigarettes. Physical exam is largely unremarkable, with minimally erythematous nasal turbinates. There is no evidence of polyps, no oropharyngeal erythema, no lymphadenopathy, no adventitious breath sounds, and no hepatosplenomegaly. A previous CT sinus showed mild ethmoid and maxillary inflammation, with patent osteomeatal complexes.

Diagnosis/Assessment

Much like the first case, this case once again highlights the importance of obtaining a detailed history when evaluating individuals for immunodeficiency. A history consistent with recurrent bacterial sinusitis along with a community-acquired pneumonia requiring inpatient hospitalization raises the possibility of underlying immunodeficiency. The patient in case 2 is at risk for developing SID due to having CLL. Hematological malignancies such as CLL, multiple myeloma, and lymphoma are commonly associated with hypogammaglobulinemia and SID. Multiple myeloma has an annual incidence of approximately 6 per 100,000 individuals in the United States [37] and accounts for roughly 1/5 of hematological malignancies in the USA [38]. Patients with multiple myeloma are at significantly increased risk of infection, particularly during the first months of induction therapy and in the setting of relapsed disease [38]. Additionally, SID occurs in 45–83% of patients with multiple myeloma at some point during their disease [39], leading most commonly to infections with encapsulated bacteria. Despite significant advancements in therapy, infections remain a leading cause of morbidity and mortality in multiple myeloma.

CLL is a B-cell neoplasm and the most common adult leukemia [40] diagnosed in approximately 15,000 patients each year in the USA. Patients with CLL are at increased risk of infections compared to age-matched controls [41]. Up to one-half of patients with CLL experience an infectious complication at some point during their disease, with up to 17–50% of infections being fatal [42]. Infections are typically bacterial in nature and affect the sinopulmonary tract. The primary cause of increased susceptibility to infections in CLL is due to hypogammaglobulinemia, which is present in up to 85% of these patients, due to both disease progression and the use of anti-neoplastic agents [43]. Due to defective functioning of non-clonal CD5 negative B cells, CLL decreases the ability of B lymphocytes to produce immunoglobulins and also increases apoptosis of normal Ig-producing plasma cells [44]. Possible mutations in the immunoglobulin heavy chain variable region may also contribute to abnormal Ig levels, although there is conflicting data on the clinical consequences of these mutations. Additionally, abnormal function of B lymphocytes can also adversely affect crosstalk with T-helper cells, thus further decreasing the appropriate immune response.

Much like hypogammaglobulinemia secondary to biologics like rituximab, checking Ig levels initiates the evaluation of SID in CLL. To date, there are no consensus guidelines on when and how to best evaluate patients with CLL for humoral immunity. Although the risk of infection in CLL is felt to generally increase with IgG levels below 400–600 mg/dL, not all patients with hypogammaglobulinemia will experience infectious complications. Conversely, there is a subset of individuals with CLL who experience increased infectious episodes despite having normal or near-normal IgG levels. The latter clinical scenario is potentially explained by normal levels of IgG with monoclonality of nonfunctional Ig [45–47]. For this reason, much like in PIDD, checking vaccine responses to peptide and polysaccharide antigens should be considered to help evaluate functional status of Ig in CLL and other B-cell malignancies. Previous studies in CLL have shown suboptimal vaccine response to polysaccharide and conjugated vaccines [48–50], with conjugated vaccines potentially leading to a more robust humoral response as compared to polysaccharide vaccines [51]. The role of vaccine responses in CLL and the ability of these patients to respond to newer, potentially more immunogenic vaccines warrants additional research, since this may be superior to Ig levels alone in risk stratifying individuals for risk of infectious complications.

Case Presentation 2 Revisited

This patient is at risk for SID due to his history of CLL and presents with recurrent sinopulmonary infections. He therefore warrants evaluation for SID. The patient's laboratory evaluation is as follows:

- CBC and chemistry panel normal
- IgG = 559 mg/dL (650–1600 mg/dL)
- IgM = 48 mg/dL (50–300 mg/dL)
- IgA = 98 mg/dL (40–350 mg/dL)
- Pre-vaccination diphtheria IgG = 0.04 IU/mL, post-vaccination diphtheria IgG = 0.05 IU/mL
- Pre-vaccination tetanus IgG = 0.61 IU/mL, post-vaccination tetanus IgG = 0.72 IU/mL
- Pre-vaccination *Streptococcus pneumoniae* IgG > 1.3 µg/ml for 4/23 serotypes
- Post-vaccination *Streptococcus pneumoniae* IgG > 1.3 µg/ml for 6/23 serotypes

Normal vaccine responses are defined as follows:

- Diphtheria: twofold increase and must be into the protective range
- Tetanus: twofold increase and must be in the protective range
- *Streptococcus pneumoniae* (based on response to PPV23):
  - If < 1.3 µg/ml, twofold increase to > 1.3 µg/ml OR fourfold increase.
  - If > 1.3 µg/ml, twofold increase.
  - For adults, responses must be demonstrated by 70% of serotypes.

Although there remains debate and a lack of consensus of what constitutes an adequate response to vaccination with *Streptococcus pneumoniae*, an impaired vaccine response is generally defined as an abnormal response to any of the above antigens. The patient's laboratory evaluation reveals mild to moderate hypogammaglobulinemia affecting IgG with preserved levels of IgM and IgA. Very importantly, the patient demonstrates poor vaccine responses to both peptide (diphtheria and tetanus) and polysaccharide (*Streptococcus pneumoniae*) antigens, consistent with humoral immunodeficiency that is consistent with his increased burden of non-neutropenic bacterial infections.

Management/Outcome

Given the known risks of increased morbidity and mortality with recurrent infections in the setting of CLL, the patient warrants consideration of prophylactic therapy aimed at decreasing infections. Management options for his SID include prophylactic vaccination, prophylactic antibiotics, or IgR therapy.

Despite having well-documented suboptimal vaccine responses, particularly to polysaccharide vaccines such as *Streptococcus pneumoniae*, routine vaccination with non-live vaccines is recommended for patients with CLL and other B-cell malignancies like multiple myeloma [52, 53]. If possible, vaccines may generate a more robust humoral response if administered early in disease and prior to initiation of B-cell depleting therapies. In addition, if possible, conjugated vaccines (e.g., pneumococcal 13 valent conjugate vaccine) are preferable to polysaccharide vaccines (e.g., pneumococcal polysaccharide 23), since they may elicit a more robust immune response due to concurrent T-cell immunity. Live vaccines are generally avoided in the setting of significant immunodeficiency but can be considered on a case by case basis for patients with CLL and other B-cell malignancies [54]. Influenza vaccine should be administered on an annual basis given the ongoing changes in viral antigenic composition.

Although no clinical studies have rigorously evaluated the use of prophylactic antibiotics, this strategy is recommended for first-line prophylaxis against infections for patients with CLL [55]. Antibiotic prophylaxis may be particularly helpful in patients with bronchiectasis. The choice of antibiotic is similar to the previous discussion for case 1.

IgR is the best-studied strategy for infection prophylaxis in CLL, and its use is universally supported in patients with CLL with hypogammaglobulinemia and associated infections [56–62]. As demonstrated by the international survey by Na et al., roughly 30% of patients with CLL are treated with IgR at some point during their disease management, and this proportion is similar to other hematological malignancies such as multiple myeloma and non-Hodgkin's lymphoma [23]. There remains heterogeneity in practice of when clinicians initiate IgR therapy in CLL, and guidelines vary from country to country [39]. Given that Ig products are derived from collecting normal IgG antibodies from a large number of healthy donors, Ig therapy is a limited resource and should be used with a thoughtful, individualized approach, rather than for routine management of CLL or other B-cell malignancies. Important factors in initiating IgR include clinically meaningful bacterial infections (particularly severe or life-threatening infection) and the degree of humoral dysfunction as assessed by not only the degree of hypogammaglobulinemia but also the ability to mount an antibody response to polysaccharide and peptide antigens, along with additional considerations of comorbidities, life expectancy, presence of other immune defects such as neutropenia, and efficacy and/or failure of alternative therapies, such as vaccination and/or prophylactic antibiotics. Benefits of IgR should be carefully weighed against potential adverse effects. Once the decision has been made to initiate IgR, the dose and route of administration should be decided through shared decision making with the patient. The efficacy of intravenous IgR is similar to subcutaneous IgR, and there are increasing reports of the use of subcutaneous IgR in the setting of CLL and other SIDs [63, 64]. There are pros and cons to both routes of administration (Table 21.4), with subcutaneous IgR having a better safety profile along with potential cost-effectiveness, compared to IV administration [65, 66]. Regardless of the formulation of IgR, there should be periodic reevaluation of therapy. Although immune dysfunction typically progresses during the course of CLL, the concurrent use of chemotherapeutics may change immune function over time, and thus reevaluation may be warranted with changes in therapy. Additional research is necessary on IgR in the setting of CLL and other hematologic malignancies since the current literature largely dates back more than a decade, and presently there have been vast advances in therapeutic options and life expectancy for patients with CLL and other B-cell malignancies.

Table 21.4 Pros and cons of intravenous versus subcutaneous immunoglobulin replacement

	Intravenous IgR	Subcutaneous IgR
Efficacy	Similar in decreasing infections	Similar in decreasing infections
Access	Intravenous	Subcutaneous (~1–4 sites)
Nursing requirement	Yes	No
Patient/family training	Not required	Required
Location of therapy	Typically at a medical facility but can be at home	Home
Dosing	Large doses can be administered	Typically smaller doses
Duration of therapy	~4 h (dose dependent)	~1 h (dose dependent)
Frequency of therapy	Typically q3–4 weeks	Typically q1 week (flexible dosing can be daily up to q28 days)
IgG levels	Peaks and troughs	Steady
Local side effects	Rare	Common but mild
Systemic side effects	More common, may benefit from premedication	Infrequent, premedication rarely required
Costs	Loss of work, travel, nursing fees, facility fees, product, equipment	Product, equipment

Case Presentation 2 Revisited

The patient presented with recurrent sinopulmonary infections in the setting of CLL and had hypogammaglobulinemia with poor vaccine responses, consistent with SID secondary to CLL. Unlike the patient in case 1, this patient has never experienced a life-threatening infection. After a discussion of pros and cons of all management options, the patient decided to proceed with a trial of prophylactic azithromycin 250 mg twice weekly. Although he tolerated the regimen without difficulty, he continued to experience bacterial sinus infections every 4 months, requiring additional antibiotic therapy and significantly impacting his ability to work and maintain his desired level of activity. The patient was then started on subcutaneous IgR at a dose of 100 mg/kg/week to be administered at home. Prophylactic azithromycin was discontinued, and the patient did very well. Three months after the initiation of IgR, his IgG increased from 559 mg/dL to 916 mg/dL, and his specific antibodies also improved (diphtheria = 0.8 IU/mL, tetanus = 2.6 IU/mL). Most notably, his *Streptococcus pneumoniae* IgG improved into a protective range (>1.3 μg/ml) for 14/23 serotypes, compared to baseline of 4/23 serotypes. He clinically has not experienced any additional infectious complications requiring therapy with antibiotics and reported an improved quality of life.

Patients with B-cell malignancies are routinely managed with a multidisciplinary approach, with the care team involving oncologists, nursing support, social workers, and psychologists, among others. As evidenced by the two cases, a significant percentage of patients experience infectious complications due to SID. Allergists/

clinical immunologists have a unique opportunity to partner with their hematology/oncology colleagues to assist in the management of this patient population, given their expertise in immune deficiency, and their proficiency in utilizing subcutaneous IgR. Allergists/clinical immunologists can assist in a more sophisticated immune evaluation including not only immunoglobulin levels but also vaccine responses. Allergists/clinical immunologists can also be a part of shared decision making for patients with SID pursuing IgR, since they may be more familiar and better suited to discuss various routes and doses of immunoglobulin administration. A partnership between allergists/clinical immunologists and hematology/oncology colleagues has the potential to lead to improved patient-centered outcomes in SID.

Conclusion

As demonstrated by these cases, malignancy and treatment with biologic therapies are a risk factor for SID, which is a leading cause of both morbidity and mortality in this group of individuals. Patients typically present with increased infections, most commonly involving the sinopulmonary tract. Laboratory evaluation reveals varying degrees of hypogammaglobulinemia, with evidence of humoral dysfunction defined by suboptimal vaccine responses. To date, there is a lack of consensus guidelines on optimal management of infectious complications, and there is significant variation in global clinical practice. Therapeutic options include prophylactic vaccination, particularly with peptide-based vaccines, prophylactic antibiotics, and IgR, either with IV or subcutaneous formulations. Additional research on diagnosis and management of SID is needed to provide a more uniform clinical approach leading to reduced morbidity and mortality in the setting of these increasingly common conditions.

> **Clinical Pearls and Pitfalls**
> - SID is more common than PIDD.
> - Patients with B-cell malignancy (multiple myeloma, chronic lymphocytic leukemia, non-Hodgkin's lymphoma) are at significant risk of SID.
> - Patients treated with biologic therapies aimed at B-cell depletion, most commonly rituximab, are at significant risk of SID.
> - Although Ig levels may be helpful in evaluating humoral immunity, they can be normal and near-normal, and evaluating vaccine responses may increase diagnostic sensitivity of immune dysfunction.
> - Response to prophylactic vaccination, particularly polysaccharide-based vaccines, may be impaired in the setting of SID.
> - Despite minimal studies, prophylactic antibiotics are routinely used for infection prophylaxis in the setting of SID.
> - There is significant literature to support the use of IgR in SID.
> - There are increasing reports of using subcutaneous IgR in SID, which has similar efficacy to IV IgR, but a superior safety profile.

References

1. Bourke CD, Berkley JA, Prendergast AJ. Immune dysfunction as a cause and consequence of malnutrition. Trends Immunol. 2016;37(6):386–98.
2. Chinen J, Shearer W. Secondary immunodeficiencies, including HIV infection. J Allergy Clin Immunol. 2008;121:S388–92.
3. Blore J, Haeney MR. Primary antibody deficiency and diagnostic delay. Br Med J. 1989;298:516–7.
4. Quinti I, Soresina A, Spadaro G, Martino S, Donnanno S, Agostini C, et al. Long term follow-up and outcome of a large cohort of patients with common variable immunodeficiency. J Clin Immunol. 2007;27(3):308–16.
5. Chapel H, Lucas M, Lee M, Bjorkander J, Webster D, Grimbacher M, et al. Common variable immunodeficiency disorders: division into distinct clinical phenotypes. Blood. 2008;112:277–86.
6. Boyle JM, Buckley RH. Population prevalence of diagnosed primary immunodeficiency diseases in the United States. J Clin Immunol. 2007;27:497–502.
7. Gathmann B, Mahlaoui N, Gerard L, Oksenhendler E, Warnatz K, Schulze I, et al. Clinical picture and treatment of 2212 patients with common variable immunodeficiency. J Allergy Clin Immunol. 2014;134(1):116–26.
8. Duraisingham SS, Buckland M, Dempster J, Lorenzo L, Grigoriadou S, Longhurst HJ. Primary vs. secondary antibody deficiency: clinical features and infection outcomes of immunoglobulin replacement. PLoS ONE. 2014;9(6):e100324.
9. MacIsaac J, Siddiqui R, Jamula E, Li N, Baker S, Webert KE, et al. Systematic review of rituximab for autoimmune diseases: a potential alternative to intravenous immune globulin. Transfusion. 2018;58(11):2729–35.
10. Thiel J, Rizzi M, Engesser M, Dufner AK, Troili A, Lorenetti R, et al. B cell repopulation kinetics after rituximab treatment in ANCA-associated vasculitides compared to rheumatoid aerthritis, and connective tissue diseases, a longitudinal observational study on 120 patients. Arthritis Res Ther. 2017;19(1):101–8.
11. Venhoff N, Niessen L, Kreuzaler M, Rolink AG, Hassler F, Rizzi M, et al. Reconstitution of the peripheral B lymphocyte compartment in patients with ANCA-associated vasculitides treated with rituximab for relapsing or refractory disease. Autoimmunity. 2014;47(6):401–8.
12. Kelesidis T, Daikos G, Boumpas D, Tsiodras S. Does rituximab increase the incidence of infectious complications? A narrative review. Int J Infect Dis. 2011;15(1):e2–16.
13. Christou EA, Giardino G, Worth A, Ladomenou F. Risk factors predisposing to the development of hypogammaglobinemia and infections post-rituximab. Int Rev Immunol. 2017;36(6):352.
14. Casulo C, Maragulia J, Zelenetz AD. Incidence of hypogammaglobinemia in patients receiving rituximab and the use of intravenous immunoglobulin for recurrent infections. Clin Lymphoma Myeloma Leuk. 2013;13(2):101–11.
15. Van Vollenhoven RF, Emery P, Bingham CO, Keystone EC, Fleischmann R, Furst DE, et al. Longterm safety of patients receiving rituximab in rheumatoid arthritis clinical trials. J Rheumatol. 2010;37(3):558–67.
16. Cabanillas F, Liboy I, Pavia O, Rivera E. High incidence of non-neutropenic inefctions induced by rituximab plus fludarabine and associated with hypogammaglobinemia: a frequently under recognized and easily treatable complication. Ann Oncol. 2006;17:1424–7.
17. Roberts DM, Jones RB, Smith RM, Alberici F, Kumaratne DS, Burns S, et al. Rituximab-associated hypogammaglobinemia: incidence, predictors, and outcomes in patients with multisystem autoimmune disease. J Autoimmun. 2015;57:60–5.
18. Marco H, Smith RM, Jones RB, Guerry MJ, Catapano F, Burns S, et al. The effect of rituximab therapy on immunoglobulin levels in patients with multisystem autoimmune disease. BMC Musculoskelet Disord. 2014;15:178.
19. Otremba MD, Adam SI, Price CC, Hohuan D, Kveton JF. Use of intravenous immunoglobulin to treat chronic bilateral otomastoiditis in the setting of rituximab induced hypogammaglobinemia. Am J Orolaryngol. 2012;33(5):619–22.

20. Ruchlemer R, Ben-Ami R, Bar-Meir M, Brown JR, Malphettes M, Mous R, et al. Ibrutinib associated invasive fungal diseases in patients with CLL and non-Hodgkin lymphoma: an observational study. Mycoses. 2019;62(12):1140–7.
21. Gottenberg JE, Ravaud P, Bardin T, Cacoub P, Cantagrel A, Cobe B. Risk factors for severe infections in patients with rheumatoid arthritis treated with rituximab in the autoimmunity and rituximab registry. Arthritis Rheum. 2010;62(9):2526–632.
22. Makatsori M, Kiani-Alikhan S, Manson AL, Verma N, Leandro M, Gurugama NP, et al. Hypogammaglobinemia after rituximab treatment-incidence and outcomes. Q J Med. 2014;107(10):821–8.
23. Na I, Buckland M, Agostini C, Edgar JD, Friman V, Michallet M, et al. Current clinical practice and challenges in the management of secondary immunodeficiency in hematologic malignancies. Eur J Hematol. 2019;102:447–56.
24. Pescovitz MD, Torgerson TR, Ochs HD, Ocheltree E, McGee P, Krause-Steinrauf H, et al. Effect of rituximab on human in vivo antibody immune responses. J Allergy Clin Immunol. 2011;128(6):1295–302.
25. Van Assen S, Holvast A, Benne CA, Posthumus MD, Van Leeuwen MA, Voskuyl AE, et al. Humoral responses after influena vaccination are severely reduced in patients with rheumatoid arthritis treated with rituximab. Arthritis Rheum. 2010;62(1):75–81.
26. Bingham CO, Looney RJ, Deodhar A, Halsey N, Greenwald M, Codding C, et al. Immunization responses in rheumatoid arthritis patients treated with rituximab: results from a controlled clinical trial. Arthritis Rheum. 2010;61(1):64–74.
27. Mustafa SS, Jamshed S, Ramsey A. Rituximab-associated antibody dysfunction in B cell non-Hodgkin's lymphoma. Abstract. ACAAI Annual Meeting 2018.
28. Orange JS, Ballow M, Stiehm ER, Ballas ZK, Chinen J, De La Morena M, et al. Use and interpretation of diagnostic vaccination in primary immunodeficiency: a working group report of the basic and clinical immunology interest section of the American Academy of Allergy, Asthma, and Immunology. J Allergy Clin Immunol. 2012;130(3 suppl):S1–S24.
29. Svensson M, Dahlin U, Kimby E. Better response with conjugate vaccine than with polysaccharide vaccine 12 months after rituximab treatment in lymphoma patients. Br J Hematol. 2011;156:402–14.
30. Edgar JD, Richter AG, Huissoon AP, Kumararatne DS, Baxendale HE, Bethune CA, et al. Prescribing immunoglobulin replacement therapy for patients with non-classical and secondary antibody deficiency: an analysis of the practice of clinical immunologists in the UK and the Republic of Ireland. J Clin Immunol. 2018;38:204–13.
31. Spadoro G, Pecoraro A, De Renzo A, Della Pepa R, Genovese A. Intravenous versus subcutaneous immunoglobulin replacement in secondary hypogammaglobulinemia. Clin Immunol. 2016;166-167:103–4.
32. Compagno N, Cinetto F, Semenzato G, Agostini C. Subcutaneous immunoglobulin in lymphoproliferative disorders and rituximab-related secondary hypogammaglobulinemia: a single center experience in 61 patients. Haematologica. 2014;99(6):1101–6.
33. Sorenson RU, Edgar D. Specific antibody deficiencies in clinical practice. J Allergy Clin Immunol Pract. 2019;7:801–8.
34. Ochs HD, Gupta S, Kiessling P, Nicolay U, Berger M, Subcutaneous Ig GSG. Safety and efficacy of self-administered subcutaneous immunoglobulin in patients with primary immunodeficiency disease. J Clin Immunol. 2006;26:265–73.
35. Wasserman RL, Melamed I, Nelson RP, Knutsen AP, Fasano MB, Stein MR, et al. Pharmacokinetics of subcutaneous IgPro20 in patients with primary immunodeficiency. Clin Pharmacokinet. 2011;50:405–14.
36. Barmettler S, Price C. Continuing IgG replacement therapy for hypogammaglobulinemia after rituximab—for how long? J Allergy Clin Immunol. 2015;136(5):1407–9.
37. National Cancer Institute. Cancer stats facts: myeloma. Available online at https://seer.cancer.gov/statfacts/html/mulmy.html.
38. Blimark C, Holmberg E, Mellqvist UH, Landgren O, Björkholm M, Hultcrantz M, et al. Multiple myeloma and infections: a population-based study on 9253 multiple myeloma patients. Haematologica. 2015;100(1):107–13.

39. Patel SY, Carbone J, Jolles S. The expanding field of secondary antibody deficiency: casuses, diagnosis, and management. Front Immunol. 2019;10(33):1–22.
40. Siegel RL, Miller KD, Jemal A. Cancer statistics 2019. Cancer J Clin. 2019;69(1):7–34.
41. Twomey JJ. Infections complicating multiple myeloma and chronic lymphocytic leukemia. Arch Intern Med. 1973;132:562–5.
42. Morra E, Nosari A, Montillo M. Infectious complications in chronic lymphocytic leukemia. Hematol Cell Ther. 1999;41:145–51.
43. Dhalla F, Lucas M, Schuh A, Bhole M, Jain R, Patel SY, et al. Antibody deficiency secondary to chronic lymphocytic leukemia: should patients be treated with prophylactic replacement immunoglobulin? J Clin Immunol. 2014;34(3):277–82.
44. Sampalo A, Navas G, Medina F, Segundo C, Cámara C, Brieva JA. Chronic lymphocytic leukemia B cells inhibit spontaneous Ig production by autologous bone marrow cells: role of CD95-CD95L interaction. Blood. 2000;96(9):3168–74.
45. Martin W, Abraham R, Shanafelt T, Clark RJ, Bone N, Geyer SM, et al. Serum-free light chain—a new biomarker for patients with B-cell non-Hodgkin lymphoma and chronic lymphocytic leukemia. Transl Res. 2007;149:231–5.
46. Bernstein ZP, Fitzpatrick JE, O'Donnell A, Han T, Foon KA, Bhargava A. Clinical significance of monoclonal proteins in chronic lymphocytic leukemia. Leukemia. 1992;6(12):1243–5.
47. Deegan MJ, Abraham JP, Sawdyk M, Van Slyck EJ. High incidence of monoclonal proteins in the serum and urine of chronic lymphocytic leukemia patients. Blood. 1984;64(6):1207–11.
48. Sinisalo M, Aittoniemi J, Oivanen P, Käyhty H, Olander RM, Vilpo J. Response to vaccination against different types of antigens in patients with chronic lymphocytic leukaemia. Br J Haematol. 2001;114(1):107–10.
49. Hartkamp A, Mulder AH, Rijkers GT, van Velzen-Blad H, Biesma DH. Antibody responses to pneumococcal and haemophilus vaccinations in patients with B-cell chronic lymphocytic leukaemia. Vaccine. 2001;19(13–14):1671–7.
50. Mustafa SS, Jamshed S, Ramsey A. Humoral immunodeficiency in patients with chronic lymphocytic leukemia. Abstract. ACAAI Annual Meeting 2019.
51. Svensson T, Kättström M, Hammarlund Y, Roth D, Andersson PO, Svensson M, et al. Pneumococcal conjugate vaccine triggers a better immune response than pneumococcal polysaccharide vaccine in patients with chronic lymphocytic leukemia A randomized study by the Swedish CLL group. Vaccine. 2018;36(25):3701–7.
52. Terpos E, Kleber M, Engelhardt M, Zweegman S, Gay F, Kastritis E, et al. European myeloma network guidelines for the management of multiple myeloma-related complications. Haematologica. 2015;100(10):1254–66.
53. Rubin LG, Levin MJ, Ljungman P, Davies EG, Avery R, Tomblyn M, et al. 2013 IDSA clinical practice guideline for vaccination of the immunocompromised host. Clin Infect Dis. 2014;58(3):309–18.
54. National Center for Immunization and Respiratory Diseases. General recommendations on immunization—recommendations of the Advisory Committee on Immunization Practices (ACIP). MMWR Recomm Rep. 2011;60(2):1–64.
55. Oscier D, Dearden C, Eren E, Fegan C, Follows G, Hillmen P, et al. Guidelines on the diagnosis, investigation and management of chronic lymphocytic leukaemia. Br J Haematol. 2012;159(5):541–64.
56. Gale RP, Chapel HM, Bunch C, Rai KR, Foon K, Courter SG, et al. Cooperative Group for the Study of Immunoglobulin in Chronic Lymphocytic Leukemia. Intravenous immunoglobulin for the prevention of infection in chronic lymphocytic leukemia. A randomized, controlled clinical trial. N Engl J Med. 1988;319:902–7.
57. Jurlander J, Geisler CH, Hansen MM. Treatment of hypogammaglobulinaemia in chronic lymphocytic leukaemia by low dose intravenous gammaglobulin. Eur J Haematol. 1994;53:114–8.
58. Chapel H, Dicato M, Gamm H, Brennan V, Ries F, Bunch C, et al. Immunoglobulin replacement in patients with chronic lymphocytic leukaemia: a comparison of two dose regimes. Br J Haematol. 1994;88:209–12.
59. Sklenar I, Schiffman G, Jonsson V, Verhoef G, Birgens H, Boogaerts M, et al. Effect of various doses of intravenous polyclonal IgG on in vivo levels of 12 pneumococcal antibodies in patients with chronic lymphocytic leukaemia and multiple myeloma. Oncology. 1993;50:466–77.

60. Griffiths H, Brennan V, Lea J, Bunch C, Lee M, Chapel H. Crossover study of immunoglobulin replacement therapy in patients with low-grade B-cell tumors. Blood. 1989;73:366–8.
61. Boughton BJ, Jackson N, Lim S, Smith N. Randomized trial of intravenous immunoglobulin prophylaxis for patients with chronic lymphocytic leukaemia and secondary hypogammaglobulinaemia. Clin Lab Haematol. 1995;17:75–80.
62. Molica S, Musto P, Chiurazzi F, Specchia G, Brugiatelli M, Cicoira L, et al. Prophylaxis against infections with low-dose intravenous immunoglobulins (IVIG) in chronic lymphocytic leukemia. Results of a crossover study. Haematologica. 1996;81:121–6.
63. Ochs HD, Gupta S, Kiessling P, Nicolay U, Berger M, Subcutaneous Ig GSG. Safety and efficacy of self-administered subcutaneous immunoglobulin in patients with primary immunodeficiency diseases. J Clin Immunol. 2006;26:265–73.
64. Compagno N, Malipiero G, Cinetto F, Agostini C. Immunoglobulin replacement therapy in secondary hypogammaglobinemia. Front Immunol. 2014;5(626):1–6.
65. Ducruet T, Levasseur MC, Des Roches A, Kafal A, Dicaire R, Haddad E. Pharmacoeconomic advantages of subcutaneous versus intravenous immunoglobulin treatment in a Canadian pediatric center. J Allergy Clin Immunol. 2013;131:585–7.
66. Martin A, Lavoie L, Goetghebeur M, Schellenberg R. Economic benefits of subcutaneous rapid push versus intravenous immunoglobulin infusion therapy in adult patients with primary immune deficiency. Transfus Med. 2013;23:55–60.

Chapter 22
Immunodeficiency Secondary to Prematurity, Pregnancy, and Aging

Irina Dawson and Mark Ballow

Abbreviations

BCG	Bacille Calmette–Guérin
CVID	Common variable immune deficiency
DBS	Dried blood spot
GVHD	Graft-versus-host disease
HSCT	Hematopoietic stem cell transplantation
Ig	Immunoglobulin
IgRT	Immunoglobulin replacement therapy
IV	Intravenous
NBS	Newborn screen
NICU	Neonatal intensive care unit
NK	Natural killer
PCR	Polymerase chain reaction
PHA	Phytohemagglutinin
PI	Primary immunodeficiency
PIDD	Primary immune deficiency disease
PJP	Pneumocystis jiroveci pneumonia
PWM	Pokeweed mitogen
RNaseP	Ribonuclease P
RT-qPCR	Real-time polymerase chain reaction
SCID	Severe combined immunodeficiency
SCIg	Subcutaneous immunoglobulin
TCL	T-cell lymphopenia
TCR	T-cell receptor

I. Dawson · M. Ballow (✉)
Division of Allergy and Immunology, Johns Hopkins All Children's Hospital/USF Department of Pediatrics, St. Petersburg, FL, USA
e-mail: mballow@usf.edu

TMP-SMX	Trimethoprim-sulfamethoxazole
TREC	T-cell receptor excision circle
VDJ	Variable, diversity, and joining

Abnormal Newborn T-Cell Receptor Excision Circle (TREC) Screening

Introduction

T-cell receptor excision circle (TREC) screening, currently utilized in all 50 states in the USA as part of newborn screening (NBS), is able to identify infants with absent or low T-cell numbers [1]. TRECs can be quantified using real-time quantitative polymerase chain reaction (RT-qPCR) from Guthrie card dried blood spots (DBS) [2, 3]. T-cell receptor (TCR) gene rearrangement is an important aspect of normal T-cell development in the thymus. This rearrangement leads to the generation of a diverse T-cell repertoire. TCR gene rearrangement involves the cutting and splicing of DNA encoding the alternative variable, diversity, and joining (VDJ) segments. TRECs are DNA by-products generated during TCR recombination. Therefore, absent or low TRECs indicate either an absent or low production of T cells [4].

TREC newborn screen (NBS) was initially designed to identify newborns with severe combined immunodeficiency (SCID) [1]. In 2008, Wisconsin was the first state to adopt TREC newborn screening for SCID [5]. SCID is a true pediatric medical emergency, manifesting with severe and recurrent infections, chronic diarrhea, and failure to thrive, which can be fatal in the first 2 years of life if left untreated [6, 7]. Early recognition and treatment with hematopoietic stem cell transplantation (HSCT) in the first 3.5 months of life is essential for better infant survival and improved HSCT outcomes [8]. Aside from SCID, TREC NBS can also identify other T-cell disorders associated with T-cell lymphopenia (TCL). Such disorders include DiGeorge syndrome, CHARGE (coloboma, heart, atresia of the choanae, retardation of growth and development, genital and urinary anomalies, and ear anomalies) syndrome, ataxia-telangiectasia, and secondary TCL such as intestinal lymphangiectasis, hydrops, gastroschisis, congenital heart disease, chylothorax, or neonatal leukemia (Table 22.1) [9].

Since 2008, millions of newborn infants have participated in TREC NBS. A review of 6,093,942 subjects identified 1533 infants with low TRECs on initial screening. Of those identified, 611 infants were confirmed to have primary immune deficiency disease (PIDD) (40%) [11]. The remaining 60% of infants proved to have no diagnosed immune defects or secondary cause of TCL. In this cohort of infants, the most common diagnosis was prematurity and low birth weight. It is not uncommon to observe TCL in preterm infants specifically in extremely preterm (less than 28 weeks) and very preterm (28–32 weeks) infants [4, 12–15]. Preterm infants frequently have complicated newborn courses. Stress induced by sepsis, bacteremia, and respiratory failure can negatively impact T-cell production,

Table 22.1 Most common secondary conditions associated with T-cell lymphopenia

Syndromes with T-cell impairment
CHARGE syndrome (coloboma, heart defects, atresia choanae, growth retardation, genital abnormalities, and ear abnormalities)
DiGeorge syndrome (complete DiGeorge syndrome congenital heart defects, hypoparathyroidism, and athymia)
VACTERL (vertebral defects, anal atresia, cardiac defects, tracheoesophageal fistulas, renal and limb abnormalities)
Trisomy 21 (Down syndrome)
Trisomy 18 (congenital heart defects, multiple anomalies)
Jacobsen syndrome (developmental delay, dysmorphic facies, abnormal bleeding, attention-deficit/hyperactivity disorder, frequent ear, sinus infections)
CLOVES (congenital lipomatous [fatty] overgrowth, vascular malformations, epidermal nevi and scoliosis)
Nijmegen breakage (microcephaly, hypogammaglobulinemia, decrease T cells, increased cancer risk, abnormal DNA breakage repair)
Fryns (associated with congenital diaphragmatic hernia, dysmorphic features)
Ectrodactyly ectodermic dysplasia syndrome
Rac2 defect (neutrophil killing defects)
Noonan (dysmorphic facies, short neck, short stature, congenital heart defects)
Renpenning (short stature, intellectual disability, dysmorphic)
Barth syndrome (cardiomyopathy at birth, neutropenia, mostly males)
TAR syndrome (thrombocytopenia, absent radius)
Ataxia-telangiectasia
Other cytogenetic abnormalities (including metabolic diseases)
T-cell loss or destruction
Cardiac defects
Gastrointestinal anomalies (gastroschisis, omphalocele, intestinal lymphangiectasia)
Third spacing (anasarca, hydrops)
Neonatal leukemia
Other conditions
Idiopathic CD4 lymphopenia

Table adapted from Kobrynski [10]

function, and quantities [16]. Preterm infants are also more likely to have congenital anomalies often requiring surgery which can lead to secondary T-cell loss [17].

Case Presentation 1

A 1-month-old male born at 27-weeks gestation was found to have low TRECs on initial NBS that was concerning for severe combined immunodeficiency. The infant was born prematurely due to maternal complications of chorioamnionitis, preeclampsia, and prolonged labor. Postnatal complications have included respiratory distress syndrome and bronchopulmonary dysplasia requiring mechanical ventilation. The infant completed a 2-week course of IV antibiotics for treatment of suspected sepsis. A pathogen was never identified from blood, urine, or endotracheal cultures. He was successfully extubated to room air after 1 week of mechanical ventilation and 3 weeks of positive pressure ventilation. He is currently tolerating trophic feeds through a nasogastric tube and gaining appropriate weight.

Family history is negative for any recurrent infections, failure to thrive, primary immunodeficiency, autoimmune disorders, miscarriages/stillbirths, or sudden infant deaths. Parents and two siblings are healthy.

An initial CBC at birth was normal including the WBC and absolute lymphocyte counts for corrected gestational age. The patient did not have any dysmorphic features, congenital anomalies, or significant electrolyte abnormalities including a normal serum calcium.

Diagnosis/Assessment

The first step in analyzing any abnormal NBS is to evaluate the testing result for artifact or sampling error. TRECs can be artificially low due to inadequate blood sampling, failure to obtain a sufficient quantity of DNA from the dried blood spot (DBS), or the presence of polymerase chain reaction (PCR) inhibitors such as heparin. In parallel to TREC quantification, NBS screening includes the measurement of a housekeeping gene, e.g., β-actin or RNaseP, as a positive control. Low or abnormal β-actin or RNaseP levels signify an inconclusive NBS suggesting a lab error and warrant retesting.

Cutoff values for abnormal TRECs vary among referral centers and states [18]. If a NBS is flagged for low TRECs, all infants are "presumed" to have SCID and must undergo a diagnostic and confirmatory workup. First, the TREC assay should be repeated to rule out a sampling error and confirm the results of the initial abnormal screening test. The next step is to assess the infant for TCL with lymphocyte enumeration using flow cytometry for major lymphocyte subpopulations (i.e., $CD3^+/CD4^+$ T cells and $CD3^+/CD8^+$ T cells with CD45RA (naïve) versus CD45RO (memory) $CD4^+$ and $CD8^+$ subsets to assess naïve versus memory cells ratios, $CD19^+$ B cells, and $CD56/CD16^+$ NK cells). Lymphocyte immunophenotyping is helpful for confirming SCID, and genetic evaluation should be done to establish the type of SCID.

In an otherwise healthy full-term infant, a low TREC with TCL is treated as SCID until proven otherwise. However, in preterm infants and infants with secondary underlying medical conditions such as severe sepsis or congenital defects, flow cytometry can be delayed until the underlying condition is treated or resolves. Certain states and referral centers delay lymphocyte flow cytometry in preterm infants until they have reached full-term corrected gestational age. Instead, the infant's clinical status is closely monitored and the TREC assay is repeated every 2 weeks until reaching 37 weeks gestational age [18]. New York State and Wisconsin mandate a repeat DBS prior to referral in neonates born < 37 of gestational age with an abnormal TREC screening. California requires a repeat DBS for any neonatal intensive care unit (NICU) patient with an abnormal screen [19].

IF TCL is confirmed, additional testing is indicated including T-cell proliferation to mitogens (e.g., PHA, concanavalin A) to assess the function of T-cells, immunoglobulin levels, and T-cell chimerism to assess for maternal engraftment. In the case of severe TCL and high suspicion for SCID, genetic sequencing for SCID-causing genes may be pursued to establish a genetic diagnosis. DNA duplication/deletion array may be utilized to rule out DiGeorge syndrome and CHARGE syndrome caused by deletions and other chromosomal anomalies [18]. In T- B+ SCID or when the diagnosis is unclear the presence of a thymus should be assessed using imaging modalities such as ultrasound, chest x-ray, or CT scan [20]. However, these imaging tests can be misleading since stress can shrink the thymus.

Aside from an immunologic workup, baseline infectious disease assessment is imperative in all infants suspected of SCID regardless of presence of infectious symptoms [21]. Infants are screened for HIV-1 infection using PCR. Other serologic assays are often not obtained, as these infants may have impaired or absent antibody production depending on the SCID immunophenotyping. The frequency for infectious surveillance may increase depending on the clinical status and suspicion for new infection. Infectious workup should include blood PCR for viral pathogens including CMV, EBV, HHV6, adenovirus, HSV1/2, HIV-1, hepatitis B, and hepatitis C. Nasopharyngeal swabs for viral PCR and viral culture regardless of symptoms should be obtained to influenza A and B; parainfluenza 1, 2, and 3; RSV; adenovirus; and human metapneumovirus. Further evaluation may include imaging such as chest x-ray and CT scans of head, neck, chest, abdomen, and pelvis to evaluate for infection [18].

Management

Infants with presumed SCID should be initiated on prophylactic antimicrobials to prevent bacterial, fungal, and viral infections. For pneumocystis jiroveci pneumonia (PJP) prophylaxis infants can be started on trimethoprim-sulfamethoxazole (TMP-SMX) orally at 1 month of age. Monthly nebulized pentamidine remains another alternative. Acyclovir can be initiated at the time of diagnosis for protection against herpes simplex virus (HSV) and vesicular stomatitis virus (VSV). For fungal prophylaxis, fluconazole can be initiated at 1 month of age. Palivizumab may be used during the peak respiratory syncytial virus (RSV) season for the prevention of RSV infection. All blood products including platelets and erythrocytes should be irradiated to prevent the risk of transfusion-associated graft-versus-host disease (GVHD) [22]. In addition, all blood products need to be cytomegalovirus (CMV) seronegative, leukodepleted, or both to prevent transmission of CMV, which can lead to fatal viremia [23]. Infants who test positive for viral infection at baseline or on subsequent infectious surveillance should be promptly hospitalized and treated with antiviral therapy.

Immunoglobulin replacement therapy in the form of intravenous or subcutaneous immunoglobulin can be initiated to help prevent general bacterial and viral infections. Immunoglobulin G troughs should be monitored every 6 months and the serum IgG maintained >600 mg/dl [18]. While on prophylactic antimicrobials and antibody replacement, liver and kidney functions should be monitored frequently. Live viral vaccines (oral poliovirus, measles, mumps, rubella, varicella, yellow fever, herpes zoster, smallpox, rotavirus, or live attenuated influenza virus) and live bacterial vaccines (BCG or S typhi, Ty21a) should be strictly avoided in all patients with SCID or complete DiGeorge Anomaly. Routine vaccinations are also withheld while on immunoglobulin replacement. Close contacts and family members should receive annual influenza vaccines and routine vaccinations. Although the transmission of a virus from a close contact receiving a live-attenuated vaccine is highly unlikely, the literature is mixed on avoiding certain live vaccines in close contacts such as oral polio and varicella [18, 24].

The goal of such vigorous infectious disease surveillance, prophylaxis, and treatment is to minimize infections and infectious complications prior to undergoing bone marrow transplant [25]. Contact precautions are needed to minimize exposure to pathogens. These include strict hand washing, limited contact with young children, and avoidance of public places and daycares. Strict isolation is not warranted. However, depending on social circumstances, isolation may be necessary. Hospitalization may be indicated for SCID evaluation or even the period prior to transplant. Recommendations regarding breastfeeding remains controversial. CMV can be transmitted from the mother to infant through breastfeeding. Many institutions recommend immediately discontinuing breastfeeding in any newborn with an abnormal TREC until the mother's CMV status is established through serology. If the mother is CMV seropositive, breastfeeding is discouraged due to the risk of transmission [18].

Case Presentation Continued

A repeat DBS sample was obtained and the TREC assay was repeated confirming the initial abnormal NBS. Lymphocyte flow cytometry was obtained and revealed moderate T-cell lymphopenia including CD3, C4, and C8 counts. The ratio of naïve to memory CD4 and CD8 was around 90% (normal range 70–90%). B and NK cells and immunoglobulin levels were borderline low for age. Lymphocyte proliferation studies to mitogens were inconclusive due to insufficient quantity of T cells (Table 22.2). Infectious workup at the time of evaluation was entirely negative. The infant was monitored clinically. On routine blood work the absolute lymphocyte counts gradually continued to increase. Upon reaching 37 weeks gestational age, lymphocyte studies were repeated, including flow cytometry and proliferation, and all were within normal limits.

Table 22.2 Summary of initial and full-term gestation evaluation

	Initial evaluation (31 weeks gestation)	37 weeks gestation
WBC	1.68×10^3/mL	17.90×10^3/mL
Hb	14.0 g/dL	13.9 g/dL
Platelet	$33.4 \cdot 10^3$/mL	$90 \cdot 10^3$/mL
Lymphocytes, absolute	$0.80 \times 10^3/\mu L$	$6.9 \times 10^3/\mu L$
Neutrophils, absolute	$0.01 \times 10^3/\mu L$	$9.65 \times 10^3/\mu L$
CD3	$455 \times 10^{-3}/\mu L$	$2550 \times 10^{-3}/\mu L$
CD4	$368 \times 10^{-3}/\mu L$	$1889 \times 10^{-3}/\mu L$
CD8	$256 \times 10^{-3}/\mu L$	$735 \times 10^{-3}/\mu L$
CD56	$118 \times 10^{-3}/\mu L$	$430 \times 10^{-3}/\mu L$
CD19	$773 \times 10^{-3}/\mu L$	$1200 \times 10^{-3}/\mu L$
CD4 naive	$331 \times 10^{-3}/\mu L$	$1705 \times 10^{-3}/\mu L$
CD8 naive	$230 \times 10^{-3}/\mu L$	$662 \times 10^{-3}/\mu L$
Lymphocyte viability	QNS	75.1%
Lymph proliferation CD45, PWM	QNS	41.1
Lymph proliferation CD3, PWM	QNS	48.7
Lymph proliferation CD19, PWM	QNS	13.9
Lymph proliferation CD45, PHA	QNS	88.6
Lymph proliferation CD3, PHA	QNS	90.8
IgG	270 mg/dL	691 mg/dL
IgA	35 mg/dL	102 mg/dL
IgM	39 mg/dL	47 mg/dL
TREC	14.3 (>25)	Within normal limits
BACTIN	25,400 (>10,000)	Within normal limits

PWM pokeweed mitogen, *PHA* phytohemagglutinin

Clinical Pearls and Pitfalls
- Every abnormal TREC assay should be assessed for artifact and sample error. Repeat the assay if necessary, in case of inconclusive testing, preterm infants, NICU patients, or infants with secondary medical conditions.
- Treat every abnormal NBS as a "presumed" SCID until proven otherwise, and evaluate the infant promptly for TCL and immunophenotyping to establish prompt diagnosis and management.
- Conduct thorough infectious evaluation and initiate antimicrobial prophylaxis as soon as possible.
- Minimize risk of infection with appropriate contact precautions and avoidance of live and routine vaccination.

Common Variable Immune Deficiency Treatment with Immunoglobulin Replacement Therapy During Pregnancy

Introduction

Common variable immune deficiency (CVID) is a heterogenous disease characterized by hypogammaglobulinemia and poor specific antibody response often manifesting as recurrent infections. In addition to recurrent infections, most commonly involving the respiratory and gastrointestinal tracts, immune dysregulation including autoimmune disease, enteropathy, lymphoproliferation, granulomatous disease, and malignancy is seen in a significant portion of CVID patients [26, 27]. The exact prevalence of CVID is unknown; however it remains the most frequent symptomatic antibody immune deficiency diagnosed in adulthood with an estimated prevalence of 1:1200 in the USA [28–31]. The etiology of CVID is polygenic and multifocal, although several monogenic forms of CVID and disease-modifying polymorphisms have been identified [29]. Treatment for CVID is well established, starting with immunoglobulin replacement therapy (IgRT), antibiotic prophylaxis, and the use of immunomodulating therapies such as glucocorticoids, rituximab, and azathioprine for various immune dysregulation manifestations [32]. For women of childbearing years with CVID, issues pertaining to pregnancy, including risk of infection, infertility, and fetal loss, are an additional burden for management and long-term sequelae.

Case Presentation 2

A 28-year-old female with CVID presents to your office for routine follow-up. She was diagnosed with CVID at 19 years of age. Immune workup was prompted by a history of recurrent sinopulmonary infections which began around 6 years of age. Throughout her lifetime she estimates 10–12 episodes of otitis media, at least eight episodes of sinusitis, and three episodes of chest x-ray-confirmed community-acquired pneumonia, one of which required hospitalization and IV antibiotics. Immune workup identified low levels of immunoglobulins including low IgG and IgA (measured at least twice; <2 standard deviations of the normal levels for their age), as well as poor vaccine responses to tetanus, diphtheria, and pneumococcus (Table 22.3). Lymphocyte studies, including flow cytometry and proliferation to antigen and mitogens, were unremarkable. She was initiated on intravenous immunoglobulin (IVIG) replacement therapy shortly after the diagnosis of CVID was made. She was transitioned to subcutaneous immunoglobulin 2 years later. The frequency of infections has dramatically improved with the initiation of immunoglobulin replacement therapy (IgRT). She has no history of enteropathy, cytopenias, chronic lung diseases, or signs of lymphoproliferation.

Table 22.3 Summary of initial and post-vaccination lab results

	Initial	Post-vaccination
IgG	245 mg/dL	294 mg/dL
IgA	23 mg/dL	25 mg/dL
IgM	87 mg/dL	82 mg/dL
Tetanus	0.01 IU/mL	0.04 IU/mL
Diphtheria	0.05 IU/mL	0.08 IU/ml
Streptococcus Pneumoniae	3/23 serotypes protective	6/23 serotypes protective
Isohemagglutinins	Absent	

Table 22.4 Revised European Society for Immunodeficiencies – ESID (2014) diagnostic criteria for common variable immune deficiency (CVID)

At least one of the following:
Increased susceptibility to infection
Autoimmune manifestations
Granulomatous disease
Unexplained polyclonal lymphoproliferation
Affected family member with antibody deficiency
And marked decrease of IgG and marked decrease of IgA with or without low IgM levels (measured at least twice; <2 SD of the normal levels for their age)
And at least one of the following:
Poor antibody response to vaccines (and/or absent isohemagglutinins); i.e., absence of protective levels despite vaccination where defined
Low switched memory B cells (<70% of age-related normal value)
And secondary causes of hypogammaglobulinemia have been excluded
And diagnosis is established after the fourth year of life (but symptoms may be present before)
And no evidence of profound T-cell deficiency, defined as two out of the following (y = year of life):
CD4 numbers/microliter: 2–6 y < 300, 6–12 y < 250, >12 y < 200
% Naive CD4: 2–6 y < 25%, 6–16 y < 20%, >16 y < 10%
T-cell proliferation absent

From http://esid.org/Working-Parties/Registry/Diagnosis-criteria

During this visit the patient reports that she is 2 months pregnant. As this is her first pregnancy, she has many concerns regarding possible complications during pregnancy. These include the risk of miscarriage, maternal and fetal infections, the chance of her offspring being born with an immunodeficiency, and treatment of her underlying disease.

Diagnosis

The diagnostic criteria for CVID, based on the European Society for Immunodeficiencies, fulfills the following criteria (Table 22.4) [32]. Genetic studies are generally not required to establish the diagnosis. However, genetic testing should be considered in patients with more severe disease and immune dysregulation. Identification of a single gene defect can provide disease prognosis and may be amendable to more targeted biologic therapy.

Management During Pregnancy

During the third trimester of pregnancy maternal IgG is transported across the placenta from mother to fetus. Transplacental transfer of IgG is critical for newborn passive immunity during the first 6 months of life when newborn IgG levels are relatively low. The levels of immunoglobulin decrease in pregnancy due to plasma dilution (expansion of vascular space) and increased IgG consumption by the fetus during the third trimester. Any patient with CVID not on IgRT remains at increased risk of serious and recurrent bacterial and viral infections. During pregnancy, the risk of infection is further enhanced and correlates with increased risk of fetal loss [33, 34]. Newborn infants born to mothers with CVID, who are not receiving IgRT, have lower levels of IgG at birth. Lower IgG levels have been associated with higher rates of infection and antibiotic use in the newborn period [34]. Several studies have shown that untreated symptomatic patients with CVID can give birth to healthy newborns [35–38]. Rates of infertility and spontaneous pregnancy loss in patients with CVID are on par with the general US population [31]. However, the literature also suggests a connection between abortion and miscarriage in untreated women with CVID [39, 40]. The frequency of infections and antibiotic use is also highest in symptomatic untreated CVID females [41].

Therefore, it remains imperative that clinical immunologists adjust immunoglobulin (Ig) dosing during the third trimester of pregnancy to account for the physiological effects of transplacental transfer, plasma expansion, and weight gain. The dose of IgRT, whether IVIG or subcutaneous immunoglobulin (SCIg), should be adjusted. However, a consensus is lacking on the standard dose increase with recommendations ranging anywhere from 10% to 50% [33, 42, 43]. Many clinical immunologists adhere to standard weight-based dosing 0.4–0.6 mg/kg/month for IVIG or SCIg. Readjustment of IgRT dose based on postpartum weight is also common in clinical practice [31].

Case Presentation Continued

Our 28-year-old female with CVID developed complications of gestation diabetes during pregnancy which was controlled with diet and close monitoring. Her dose of SCIg was increased from 8 g weekly (500 mg/kg/month) to 10 g weekly (500 mg/kg/month). She was advised to avoid the abdomen for administration of SCIg and instead to use the outer thighs or hips. She remained infection-free throughout the entirety of her pregnancy. At 38-week gestation she gave birth to a healthy baby girl. At the time of birth, the newborn's cord blood revealed an IgG level of 850 mg/dL. Three months postpartum the dose of SCIg was adjusted for weight loss and reduced back to 8 g weekly (500 mg/kg/month).

> **Clinical Pearls and Pitfalls**
> - During pregnancy, the risk of infection is enhanced in women with CVID due to physiological drops in serum IgG.
> - The dose of IgRT therapy should be weight adjusted in the third trimester to account for plasma expansion and transplacental IgG transfer from mother to fetus.
> - The lack of IgRT dose adjustment can lead to suboptimal maternal IgG levels, putting the mother at increased risk for infection, fetal loss, and lower baseline IgG levels in newborn.
> - Postpartum IgRT should be readjusted to account for diuresis and weight loss and the decrease in plasma volume.

Switching from the Intravenous Route to the Subcutaneous Route in Elderly Primary Immunodeficiency (PI) Patients on Platelet Inhibitors

Introduction

There is very little information on treating elderly PI patients with SCIg [44]. These patients may experience difficulty performing SCIg infusions unless they have a caretaker. Elderly patients often have other medical conditions such as cardiovascular, renal, or live disease and receive medications that could increase the potential for side effects, particularly with the IV route. As we get older the skin and subcutaneous tissues change which could affect the pharmacokinetics of SCIg. Most importantly, older patients may lack the cognitive skills and dexterity for self-administration of SCIg [45].

Case Presentation 3

RM is a 72-year-old male with a history of CVID diagnosed since age 45. Initially he was receiving RTIg therapy by the intravenous route. However, as he aged his veins started to collapse, and he was switched to a 20% SCIg product every 2 weeks at age 67. He did well with this regimen, but as he got older he developed other medical problems including type 2 diabetes and osteoarthritis. At age 72 he developed paroxysmal arterial tachycardia. Because of an episode of atrial fibrillation, he was started on Plavix (clopidogrel bisulfate) to reduce the risk of stroke. The patient was very concerned that he was on SCIg and now needed to take a "blood thinner."

Diagnosis/Assessment

With better management of RTIg and earlier diagnosis of patients with primary antibody deficiency, patients are living longer into the sixth and seventh decades of life. Approximately, 15% of patients are over 65 years of age. Elderly patients have critical issues affecting their lifestyle in choosing Ig replacement therapy. Many elderly patients are retired and, therefore, do not have the time constraints that younger working patients have. Although going to a hospital base or community infusion center takes travel time and 4–6 h of infusion time, elderly patients often choose this scenario because they feel uncomfortable infusing at home and prefer the social benefits of an infusion center. However, others choose to infuse by vein at home because a nurse will come to the home, particularly if they and their spouse do not drive. SCIg has not been as popular a choice by elderly patients because of the "mechanics" of administering Ig by the subcutaneous route, e.g., tubing, pump, preparation, etc. While SCIg may be convenient for some, it may present special problems for many elderly individuals who have physical limitations. Self-infusions require a number of preparatory steps to infuse, some of which may not be possible if they have arthritis, poor eyesight, muscle weakness, or other frailties. Often a caregiver is required to assist with SCIg infusions. However, with cardiovascular comorbid conditions that may limit intravenous fluids and "poor" veins, SCIg becomes a viable choice. Other comorbid conditions such as heart disease, renal compromise, arthritis, and concomitant medications may place elderly patients at higher risk of adverse events with the intravenous route. Furthermore, lymphoproliferative disease, e.g., leukemia, myeloma, and lymphoma, may complicate diagnosis and treatment, especially with chemotherapy and biologics.

Aging leads to worsening of other diseases including diabetes mellitus, kidney disease, neuropathies, dementia, arthritis, Parkinson's disease, and hypertension. Many of these diseases or disorders may have profound implications on how Ig therapy will be given. This includes dose, frequency and route of administration, product selection, and site of care. Less rapid administration and lower doses in older individuals are important in geriatric individuals, especially in those with renal disease. Furthermore, this age group has a higher risk for blood clots including phlebitis (inflammation of the blood vessels), myocardial infarct, stroke, and pulmonary embolism. This risk is higher in individuals with previous thrombotic conditions or blood clotting diseases, particularly for those with limited mobility.

Management/Outcome

Hospitals are "pushing" patients out of their infusion centers, and PI patients may also be competing with cancer and autoimmune cytopenia patients for IVIG products in an infusion center. Physicians must discuss the benefits and issues with each of the routes of Ig replacement therapy. A spouse or caregiver should also be included in the discussion since they have to feel comfortable with the route of Ig treatment at home. Medicare does not pay for nursing support for self-infusion, and the absence of a caregiver presents formidable obstacles. Finally, our patient was taking a platelet inhibitor for the risk of atrial fibrillation and the risk of thrombotic episodes. Stein and colleagues [46] reviewed the charts of elderly with PI to evaluate the safety and practicality of home-based SCIg infusions. Forty-seven of 111 elderly PI patients elected to receive SCIg at home. Most received weekly infusions. There were no serious systemic adverse events. Local injection site reactions were considered mild or moderate and resolved within 24 h. There was no evidence from the serum IgG levels to suggest that there were any differences in the absorption from the subcutaneous space or in the pharmacokinetics of SCIg in elderly patients. No bruising or bleeding occurred in those 21 patients (45%) on concomitant anticoagulant or platelet inhibitors. Although many patients were on other medications for organ system disease, no apparent drug interactions occurred while on SCIg. This limited data suggests that SCIg treatment can be safely administered in patients on a platelet inhibitor or other anticoagulant.

Because of "poor" veins, SCIg has become an important choice for our patient. He started on a 20% SCIg with infusions every 2 weeks that he tolerated well. He experienced no excessive bruising and no bleeding despite being on a platelet inhibitor. He was happy with his choice of switching to the SCIg therapy in part because he did not have to travel to get his infusion in the hospital.

Clinical Pearls and Pitfalls
- SCIg is an option for elderly PI patients who may have comorbid conditions and receive concomitant medications.
- SCIg may be beneficial for elderly patients by switching from a hospital base or infusion center to home care.
- The flexibility of SCIg can tailor the Ig replacement therapy for the elderly patient and improve quality of life.
- SCIg appears to be safe for elderly patients on anticoagulants or platelet inhibitors.

References

1. IDF SCID Newborn Screening Campaign. Towson: Immune Deficiency Foundation; 2018. Available at: https://primaryimmune.org/idf-advocacy-center/idf-scid-newborn-screening-campaign. Accessed 27 Sept 2019.
2. Puck JM. Laboratory technology for population-based screening for severe combined immunodeficiency in neonates: the winner is T-cell receptor excision circles. J Allergy Clin Immunol. 2012;129:607–16.
3. Chan K, Puck JM. Development of population-based newborn screening for severe combined immunodeficiency. J Allergy Clin Immunol. 2005;115:391–8.
4. Hannon WH, Abraham RS, Kobrynski L, Vogt RF Jr, Adair O, Aznar C, et al. Newborn blood spot screening for severe combined immunodeficiency by measurement of T-cell receptor excision circles; approved guideline. CLSI document NBS06-A. Wayne: Clinical and Laboratory Standards Institute; 2013.

5. Routes JM, Grossman WJ, Verbsky J, Laessig RH, Hoffman GL, Brokopp CD, et al. Statewide newborn screening for severe T-cell lymphopenia. JAMA. 2009;302:2465–70.
6. Dvorak CC, Cowan MJ, Logan BR, Notarangelo LD, Griffith LM, Puck JM, et al. The natural history of children with severe combined immunodeficiency: baseline features of the first fifty patients of the primary immune deficiency treatment consortium prospective study 6901. J Clin Immunol. 2013;33:1156–64.
7. Buckley RH, Schiff RI, Schiff SE, Markert ML, Williams LW, Harville TO, et al. Human severe combined immunodeficiency: genetic, phenotypic, and functional diversity in one hundred eight infants. J Pediatr. 1997;130:378–87.
8. Pai S, Logan B, Griffith L, Buckley R, Parrott R, Dvorak C, et al. Transplantation outcomes for severe combined immunodeficiency, 2000–2009. N Engl J Med. 2014;371:434–46.
9. Kwan A, Abraham RS, Currier R, et al. Newborn screening for severe combined immunodeficiency in 11 screening programs in the United States [published correction appears in JAMA. 2014;312(20):2169. Bonagura, Vincent R [added]]. JAMA. 2014;312(7):729–38.
10. Kobrynski LJ. Identification of non-severe combined immune deficiency T-cell lymphopenia at newborn screening for severe combined immune deficiency. Ann Allergy Asthma Immunol. 2019. pii: S1081-1206(19)30582-4.
11. Mauracher AA, Pagliarulo F, Faes L, Vavassori S, Güngör T, Bachmann LM, et al. Causes of low neonatal T-cell receptor excision circles: a systematic review. J Allergy Clin Immunol Pract. 2017;5:1457–60.
12. Kwan A, Abraham RS, Currier R, Brower A, Andruszewski K, Abbott JK, et al. Newborn screening for severe combined immunodeficiency in 11 screening programs in the United States. JAMA. 2014;312:729–38.11.
13. Verbsky J, Thakar M, Routes J. The Wisconsin approach to newborn screening for severe combined immunodeficiency. J Allergy Clin Immunol. 2012;129:622–7.
14. Vogel BH, Bonagura V, Weinberg GA, Ballow M, Isabelle J, DiAntonio L, et al. Newborn screening for SCID in New York state: experience from the first two years. J Clin Immunol. 2014;34:289–303.
15. Amatuni GS, Currier RJ, Church JA, Bishop T, Grimbacher E, Nguyen AA, et al. Newborn screening for severe combined immunodeficiency and T-cell lymphopenia in California, 2010–2017. Pediatrics. 2019;143:e20182300.
16. Hotchkiss RS, Moldawer LL, Opal SM, Reinhart K, Turnbull IR, Vincent JL. Sepsis and septic shock. Nat Rev Dis Primers. 2016;2:16045. Published 30 Jun 2016.
17. Honein MA, Kirby RS, Meyer RE, Xing J, Skerrette NI, Yuskiv N, et al. National Birth Defects Prevention Network. The association between major birth defects and preterm birth. Matern Child Health J. 2009;13:164–75.
18. Thakar MS, Hintermeyer MK, Gries MG, Routes JM, Verbsky JW. A practical approach to newborn screening for severe combined immunodeficiency using the T cell receptor excision circle assay. Front Immunol. 2017;8:1470. Published 8 Nov 2017.
19. van der Spek J, Groenwold RH, van der Burg M, van Montfrans JM. TREC based newborn screening for severe combined immunodeficiency disease: a systematic review. J Clin Immunol. 2015;354:416–30.
20. McWilliams LM, Dell Railey M, Buckley RH. Positive family history, infection, low absolute lymphocyte count (ALC), and absent thymic shadow: diagnostic clues for all molecular forms of severe combined immunodeficiency (SCID). J Allergy Clin Immunol Pract. 2015;3(4):585–91.
21. Dorsey MJ, Dvorak CC, Cowan MJ, Puck JM. Treatment of infants identified as having severe combined immunodeficiency by means of newborn screening. J Allergy Clin Immunol. 2017;139(3):733–42. https://doi.org/10.1016/j.jaci.2017.01.005.
22. Ruhl H, Bein G, Sachs UJH. Transfusion-associated graft-versus-host disease. Transfus Med Rev. 2009;23:62–71.
23. Alter HJ, Klein HG. The hazards of blood transfusion in historical perspective. Blood. 2008;112:2617–26.

24. Medical Advisory Committee of the Immune Deficiency Foundation, Shearer WT, Fleisher TA, et al. Recommendations for live viral and bacterial vaccines in immunodeficient patients and their close contacts. J Allergy Clin Immunol. 2014;133(4):961–6.
25. Heimall J, Puck JM, Tepas E. Severe combined immunodeficiency (SCID): specific defects. In: UpToDate, Post, TW (Ed), UpToDate. Waltham; 2019.
26. Resnick ES, Moshier EL, Godbold JH, Cunningham-Rundles C. Morbidity and mortality in common variable immune deficiency over 4 decades. Blood. 2012;119:1650–7.
27. Quinti I, Soresina A, Spadaro G, Martino S, Donnanno S, Agostini C, et al. Long-term follow-up and outcome of a large cohort of patients with common variable immunodeficiency. J Clin Immunol. 2007;27:308–16.
28. Boyle JM, Buckley RH. Population prevalence of diagnosed primary immunodeficiency diseases in the United States. J Clin Immunol. 2007;27(5):497–502.
29. International Union of Immunological Societies Expert Committee on Primary, Notarangelo LD, et al. Primary immunodeficiencies: 2009 update. J Allergy Clin Immunol. 2009;124(6):1161–78.
30. Cunningham-Rundles C. How I treat common variable immune deficiency. Blood. 2010;116(1):7–15.
31. Gundlapalli AV, Scalchunes C, Boyle M, Hill HR. Fertility, pregnancies and outcomes reported by females with common variable immune deficiency and hypogammaglobulinemia: results from an internet-based survey. J Clin Immunol. 2015;35(2):125–34.
32. http://esid.org/Working-Parties/Registry/Diagnosis-criteria. Accessed 12 Nov 2019.
33. Gardulf A, Andersson E, Lindqvist M, Hansen S, Gustafson R. Rapid subcutaneous IgG replacement therapy at home for pregnant immunodeficient women. J Clin Immunol. 2001;21:150–4.
34. Sacher RA, King JC. Intravenous gammaglobulin in pregnancy: a review. Obstet Gynecol Surv. 1988;44:25–34.
35. Laursen HB, Christensen MF. Immunoglobulins in normal infant born of severe hypogammaglobulinaemic mother. Arch Dis Child. 1973;48:646–8.
36. Williams PE, Leen CL, Heppleston AD, Yap PL. IgG replacement therapy for primary hypogammaglobulinaemia during pregnancy: report of 9 pregnancies in 4 patients. Blut. 1990;60:198–201.
37. Zak SJ, Good RA. Immunochemical studies of human serum gamma globulins. J Clin Invest. 1959;38:579–86.
38. Bridges RA, Condie RM, Zak SJ, Good RA. The morphologic basis of antibody formation development during the neonatal period. J Lab Clin Med. 1959;53:331–57.
39. Shalev E, Ben-Ami M, Peleg D. Common variable hypogammaglobulinemia in pregnancy. Br J Obstet Gynaecol. 1993;100:1138–40.
40. Holland NH, Holland P. Immunological maturation in an infant of an agammaglobulinaemic mother. Lancet. 1966;2:1152–5.
41. Kralickova P, Kurecova B, Andrys C, Krcmova I, Jilek D, Vlkova M, et al. Pregnancy outcome in patients with common variable immunodeficiency. J Clin Immunol. 2015;35:531–7.
42. Brinker KA, Silk HJ. Common variable immune deficiency and treatment with intravenous immunoglobulin during pregnancy. Ann Allergy Asthma Immunol. 2012;108:464–5.
43. Cunningham-Rundles C. Key aspects for successful immunoglobulin therapy of primary immunodeficiencies. Clin Exp Immunol. 2011;164:16–9.
44. Verma N, Thaventhiran A, Gathmann B, Thaventhiran J, Grimbacher B. Therapeutic management of primary immunodeficiency in older patients. Drugs Aging. 2013;30(7):503–12.
45. Cornett A, Kobayashi R. Moving aging Ig patients into nursing homes. IG Living. 2017;(Oct–Nov):18–20.
46. Stein MR, Koterba A, Rodden L, Berger M. Safety and efficacy of home-based subcutaneous immunoglobulin G in elderly patients with primary immunodeficiency diseases. Postgrad Med. 2011;123(5):186–93.

Chapter 23
Vaccinations in Primary and Secondary Immunodeficiencies Including Asplenia

Lauren Fine and Nofar Kimchi

Introduction

Infectious diseases have been a major cause of death worldwide since the beginning of documented history. The development of the flu vaccine quickly followed the isolation of the influenza virus in 1933 [1]. Even now, despite further developments in medicine and research, lower respiratory infections are the fourth leading cause of death worldwide and are the most common cause of death for low-income developing countries worldwide [2]. Acute respiratory infections including influenza and pneumonia take 4 million lives per year globally. These deaths, as well as many other vaccine-preventable deaths, could be avoided by a more widely accessible distribution of vaccines. While individuals with a normally developed immune system should be able to mount a healthy immunologic protection following routine vaccinations, those with certain immunodeficiency diseases are not able to respond appropriately to vaccines. Vaccinations are used in the evaluation and diagnosis of certain primary immunodeficiency disorders such as common variable immunodeficiency (CVID), specific antibody deficiency (SAD), and other related humoral immunodeficiencies. Individuals with these immunodeficiencies are vulnerable to respiratory infections, especially lower respiratory infections with encapsulated bacteria [3]. However, these immunodeficiencies also preclude the use of certain vaccinations which could prove dangerous due to the risk of transferring infection rather than protection. Like humoral immunodeficiencies, asplenia carries with it an increased risk of infection with encapsulated bacteria. However, the underlying pathophysiology behind this secondary immunodeficiency differs from that of the antibody deficiency disorders. Nevertheless,

L. Fine (✉)
Department of Medicine, VA Medical Center Miami, Miami, FL, USA

N. Kimchi
Ruth and Bruce Rappaport Faculty of Medicine, Technion Israel Institute of Technology, Haifa, Israel

© Springer Nature Switzerland AG 2021
J. A. Bernstein (ed.), *Primary and Secondary Immunodeficiency*,
https://doi.org/10.1007/978-3-030-57157-3_23

both conditions require prudent use of vaccinations that maximize protection while minimizing risk. In this chapter we will review the use of vaccinations in two common immunodeficiencies, CVID, and asplenia.

Case Presentation 1

A 19-year-old female with a history of recurrent bronchitis, chronic sinusitis, and recurrent pneumonia presented to the immunology clinic for an evaluation of possible immunodeficiency. Her birth was an at term vaginal delivery and she was breast-fed until 12 months of age. She was vaccinated throughout her childhood by following the age-appropriate schedule which included Prevnar 13, meningococcal, and Tdap (booster given at age 12) as well as the annual influenza vaccine. She had no significant health problems until around age 8 when she began to have recurrent bronchitis several times per year. She developed pneumonia at the age of 12 and again at ages 14 and 15. She was also treated for bacterial sinusitis twice in the past year. Both times the sinusitis required a lengthy course of two different antibiotics due to a failure to adequately respond to the first course. She had only one episode of otitis media at age 2. She had no atopic history including asthma, chronic rhinitis, or eczema.

Review of systems at the time of presentation was unremarkable including a lack of nasal or conjunctivitis symptoms. She also lacked lower respiratory symptoms when she was not being treated for active infections such as bronchitis. Her past medical history included only recurrent infections as mentioned. She was hospitalized once for pneumonia at age 12 but had no other hospitalizations or surgeries. Her only regular medication was a daily multivitamin. Her family history was notable for a 14-year-old brother with celiac disease and a maternal uncle with IgA deficiency. She has no family history of atopy, other immunodeficiencies, or autoimmune disease.

Physical examination revealed unremarkable findings of the skin, head and neck, lymphatics, pulmonary, cardiac, and gastrointestinal systems.

Her lab evaluation included a urinalysis, CBC with differential, and complete metabolic panel which were all within normal limits. Flow cytometry demonstrated normal numbers of NK cells, T cells, and B cells. Immunoglobulin levels were as follows: IgG 252 mg/dL, IgA 12 mg/dL, IgM 20 mg/dL, and IgE 2 mg/dL. The immunoglobulin levels were repeated and found to be similar to the initial tests. Both times the levels were drawn when she was feeling well and was not on any glucocorticoids or other immunosuppressants. Baseline titers of tetanus and diphtheria were at undetectable levels. Pneumococcal 23 titers were also obtained and all undetectable below <1.3 ug/ml.

Pulmonary function testing demonstrated an irreversible moderate obstructive defect.

Chest CT showed bronchial wall thickening, mucus plugging, and bronchiectasis most prominent in the lower lobes bilaterally but also present in the right middle lobe to a lesser extent.

She was diagnosed with CVID and started on weekly subcutaneous immunoglobulin replacement therapy. She tolerated the infusions well and over the next 12 months she had one episode of bronchitis but no sinusitis, pneumonia, or other infections requiring antibiotics.

Clinical Presentation

CVID patients typically present with recurrent sinopulmonary infections, often with encapsulated bacteria such as *Haemophilus influenzae*, *Streptococcus*, and others, reflecting the lack of humoral immunity. Although there is likely a genetic component to this immunodeficiency, most cases are sporadic and the age at presentation varies widely, with the mean age of presentation occurring in the fourth decade of life [3]. Patients may present with not only recurrent sinopulmonary infections with common bacteria but may also develop less common infections, autoimmune disease (i.e., immune thrombocytopenia purpura [ITP], inflammatory bowel disease [IBD], systemic lupus erythematosus [SLE]), allergic disease, lymphoid hyperplasia, and malignancy.

Diagnosis/Assessment

This case highlights the importance of both clinical history and laboratory evaluation in the diagnosis of CVID. Although there is no consensus on the exact criteria for the diagnosis of CVID, most agree that diagnosis is based on a combination of clinical presentation of recurrent sinopulmonary infections as well as laboratory evidence of both hypogammaglobulinemia (IgG + IgA and/or IgM) and a lack of response to vaccinations. The vaccines that are used in the evaluation of CVID are usually the PPSV23 (Pneumovax 23, US) and the tetanus-diphtheria vaccines. PPSV23 is an inactivated vaccine with no risk of infection to immunodeficient patients where the tetanus vaccine contains tetanus toxoid and the diphtheria vaccine contains diphtheria toxoid, neither of which pose a risk of patient infection. All three of these vaccinations should prompt a robust immune response in any individual with a normal immune system. However, in the case of CVID where there is a lack immunoglobulins, there is also a failure to respond to both infections and vaccinations with specific antibody production. Thus, the immune defect that causes the clinical picture of recurrent infections is also used in the diagnosis of CVID. In this case, the patient had been given the recommended childhood vaccinations and should have had some baseline protection to tetanus, diphtheria, and pneumococcal antigens. However, as evidenced by her undetectable baseline titers she either never responded or lost protection earlier than expected (Table 23.1).

Table 23.1 Clinical presentation and diagnosis of CVID

Common clinical findings in CVID	Diagnosis of CVID

Recurrent infections:
  Bacterial infections (commonly encapsulated bacteria): sinusitis, pneumonia, otitis media
  Viral infections: bronchitis, bronchiolitis
	Clinical manifestations (at least 1): recurrent infections, autoimmunity, lymphoproliferation

Abnormal pulmonary function testing Obstruction, restriction, and/or poor diffusion	Onset of immunodeficiency at >2 years age

Imaging
High-resolution CT scan:
  Bronchial findings including: bronchiectasis, bronchial wall thickening, mucus plugging, and air trapping
  Interstitial findings including nodules, ground glass opacities, honeycombing, emphysema
	Marked decrease of IgG ($\geq$SD below mean) *and* marked decrease of IgM, IgA, or both
	Lab values should be seen on at least 2 measurements more than 3 weeks apart unless the levels are very low, other characteristic features are present, and it is in the best interest of the patient to start

	Poor response to T-cell-dependent or T-cell-independent antigens. Can be deferred if IgG is <100 mg/dL

Based on Refs. [3, 4]

Treatment of CVID Including Use of Vaccinations for Protection and Vaccination Precautions

The treatment of CVID has as its core goal the reduction in risk of infection. This is achieved through either intravenous immunoglobulin (IVIG) or subcutaneous immunoglobulin (SCIG) administration. While the decision on which route is most appropriate for the patient depends on several factors that are usually based on patient independence, frequency of infusions, and tolerance of side effects, the goal is to reach a level of IgG that results in a reduced frequency of infections. Infused immunoglobulin products are produced by combining plasma from a combination of blood and plasma donors, each pool consisting of up to 100,000 donors [5].

The antibodies in this pool of plasma therefore contain IgG representing the humoral immune system of all of the donors. Specific IgG produced from exposure to viral, bacterial, and fungal antigens as well as vaccinations will therefore be transmitted from donor to recipient as a form of natural passive immunity. This means that CVID patients who have a protective level of IgG after either IVIG or SCIG administration also have a certain degree of specific immunity conferred by the specific IgG from the donor pool.

Because pneumococcal, diphtheria, and tetanus vaccines are commonly administered to those in the general population who make up the donor pool, CVID patients on immunoglobulin replacement likely do not need to be given the respective vaccinations although a higher trough level of IgG may need to be maintained to provide sufficient levels of specific IgG [3, 6]. Furthermore, as lack of response to these particular vaccines is part of the criteria for diagnosis, it is unlikely that they would respond to the vaccines with protective titers even if the vaccines were administered.

Some vaccinations, such as influenza, provide T-cell-mediated protection such that even if there is poor antibody production in a patient with CVID, the cellular immune response may provide a desired level of protection worthy of vaccination [7]. In general, those with CVID should only be given inactivated or subunit vaccines. Live viral vaccines such as yellow fever, smallpox, live attenuated influenza, and oral polio vaccine (OPV) are contraindicated [8]. The data for varicella safety is insufficient to provide a clear safety recommendation. If a live attenuated vaccine is given to an individual with CVID, even if on immunoglobulin replacement, it could result in an active infection. Even exposure to close contacts such as family members who have been given the live oral polio vaccine may transmit infection to immunocompromised patients, so caution should be taken for individuals who live with young children undergoing routine vaccinations with OPV. However, there is little evidence to support the risk of infection of close contacts of immunodeficient patients and vaccination of family members provides additional protection and should not necessarily be avoided altogether, with the exception of the smallpox vaccine [9, 10]. On the other hand, the MMR and varicella vaccinations could be considered as they may provide some protection depending on the level of immune response. It should be noted that specific IgG in immunoglobulin replacement neutralizes the antigens in the measles, mumps, rubella, and varicella vaccinations so the efficacy of these vaccinations may be reduced in those on immunoglobulin replacement [11]. However, those on immunoglobulin replacement are often adequately protected from these viruses through the pool of immunoglobulin donors who transmit immunity passively. In fact, the US Food and Drug Administration (FDA) has set a minimum measles virus antibody titer that must be present in immunoglobulin used in the USA in order to aid in protection against infection [12, 13]. In the case of influenza, many patients with CVID can demonstrate a response to the vaccine with the production of IgG, although production of specific IgA seems to be lacking [14]. As protection from the current season's influenza strain may be lacking in plasma pools, and because the additional protection provided by a patient's own humoral and cellular immune response could augment the protection of immunoglobulin, many recommend annual vaccination of CVID patients with the seasonal killed influenza vaccine [11].

In general, in addition to the seasonal killed influenza vaccine arguably the most important vaccinations to give to a patient with CVID are the pneumococcal vaccines. There are currently two types of pneumococcal vaccine in the USA, both which provide protection against *Streptococcus pneumoniae*, an encapsulated bacteria that commonly causes infection in those with humoral immunodeficiency such as CVID. Prevnar (PCV13) is part of the routine childhood vaccinations and therefore is not usually given to older children or adults under 65 years old who completed their childhood vaccinations. However, it is recommended for certain populations, such as those with immunodeficiency. Therefore, any patient with an immunodeficiency who is at least 2 months of age should be given the PCV13 vaccine. Pneumovax (PPSV23) is typically recommended for those 65 and older, but like Prevnar is also recommended for those with immunodeficiency. It can be given starting at the age of 2 years but it should be noted that certain recommendations exist for the order and timing of this vaccine when given along with Prevnar. Table 23.2 provides a summary of the vaccine recommendations for those with CVID and Table 23.3 outlines the recommendations for provision of both pneumococcal vaccinations.

Table 23.2 Use of vaccinations in patients with CVID

Recommended vaccines	Contraindicated vaccines	Special considerations
Pneumococcal (a) 8 10 30 HIB (12–59 months age) 10 30 Inactivated influenza 10	OPV 8 10 30 Smallpox 8 30 Live-attenuated influenza 8 10 30 BCG 8 10 30 Live typhoid 8 10 30 Yellow fever 8 10 30 MMR/MMRV 10 30 Varicella 30	IVIG may interfere with efficacy of measles and varicella vaccines 10 30 but may consider measles 8 11 and varicella vaccines 8

Table based on recommendations from Refs. [8, 10, 11, 15, 16]
Note: There are two types of pneumococcal vaccination. See Table 23.3 for recommendations on administration of each with respect to timing, age, and indications

Table 23.3 Use of pneumococcal vaccinations in adults ≥ 19 years

Prevnar (PCV13)	Pneumovax (PPSV23)	Special considerations
Routine for all children 2 months–59 months and adults ≥ 65 years	Recommended for adults ≥ 65 years of age	Adults: Both PCV 13 and PPSV 23 should be given to adults ≥ 65 but should not be given on the same office visit When both PCV 13 and PPSV 23 are indicated, give PCV13 before PPSV 23 when possible Give PCV13 at age ≥ 19, then ≥ 8 weeks later give PPSV 23 Repeat PPSV 23 ≥ 5 years after first dose of PPSV 23 if given at age < 65 years.
Individuals 6–64 years *not* previously vaccinated, who have immunodeficiency or other increased risk of infection such as certain chronic diseases	Individuals 2–64 years with immunodeficiency or other increased risk of infection such as certain chronic diseases	

Table based on recommendations from Refs. [10, 17]

In summary, vaccinations in those with humoral immunodeficiencies such as CVID should avoid provision of live vaccinations, whether viral or bacterial. The exceptions include varicella and measles which some experts believe confer some protection with minimal risk. The risks and benefits for each patient considering their immunization history, exposure status, and immunoglobulin replacement regimen should be weighed when considering these vaccines. The seasonal killed influenza vaccine may be the single most important vaccination in those with humoral immunodeficiency and although its efficacy cannot be truly measured, the risks of not obtaining this vaccination may outweigh the benefits. Lastly, the pneumococcal vaccines should be strongly considered, but the vaccination status of the patient and the order of vaccination should be given attention. With these vaccinations, a protective dose of SCIG/IVIG and the benefit of herd immunity, most patients with CVID and other severe antibody deficiencies are much less likely to present with a severe viral or bacterial infection than without them.

Case Continued

The patient presented in the last vignette was started on subcutaneous immunoglobulin (SCIG) with an excellent tolerance to the treatment. She had no side effects and her randomly checked IgG was consistently in the 800–900 mg/dL range. She continued on treatment for 3 years without any bacterial sinusitis or pneumonia. She did suffer from bronchitis on two occasions, both which were mild and self-limiting. At the age of 22 she presented to her primary care physician for a routine annual examination and noted that she had been feeling fatigued over the past couple of months. For the prior 6 months she had experienced heavier than usual menstrual flow and at a dental hygiene appointment a week ago she inquired about her gums bleeding easily while brushing. No gum or dental disease was noted although some petechiae were seen on the hard palate.

On examination she had a couple of bruises on her legs that were not associated with any particular trauma that she could recall. She had notable petechiae on the hard palate and pallor of the skin and conjunctivae. There was no active bleeding of her gums or other mucosal areas. Her head and neck, cardiac, and pulmonary examinations were otherwise unremarkable. On the gastrointestinal exam there were no masses and no splenomegaly or hepatomegaly. There was no lymphadenopathy of the head and neck, axillae, or femoral regions.

Lab studies were drawn: An ANA was negative. CBC with differential revealed a Hgb of 11.0 g/dL and a platelet count of 40,000/mL. Her white blood cell count was 7000/mL and the differential was normal. Her peripheral smear did not reveal any abnormalities suggestive of a secondary cause of thrombocytopenia.

She was diagnosed with secondary immune thrombocytopenia (ITP) and started on high-dose dexamethasone while her SCIG was continued at the usual dose. She responded well to the glucocorticoid course and successfully remained in remission for a few months. However, over the next 3 years she continued to have recurrence of severe thrombocytopenia and required high-dose IVIG on several occasions to induce remission. The option of rituximab and thrombopoietin receptor agonists were weighed against the option of splenectomy and she chose to pursue an elective splenectomy. Her vaccination history was reviewed and it was determined that she was up to date on all recommended vaccinations for her age with the exception of the flu vaccine that was pending release for the year and vaccination against meningococcal disease. She received the PCV 13 at age 19 and the first dose of PPSV 23 8 weeks after that. Her second dose of PPSV23 was given at the age of 24. She underwent a successful splenectomy at the age of 25 years and had complete remission of her ITP. She continued on immunoglobulin replacement with SCIG without incident of side effect or infection and has not had any other autoimmune manifestations or complications.

Clinical Presentation

The second part of this case highlights the natural course of CVID. Although CVID is an immunodeficiency, it is somewhat counterintuitive that these patients also have autoimmune tendencies as well as poor immune surveillance and an increased risk of malignancy such as lymphoma [18]. Inflammatory and hematological complications include secondary ITP, autoimmune hemolytic anemia, Evans syndrome, irritable bowel disease, rheumatoid arthritis, and pernicious anemia. In a recent report from 2017, the USIDNET registry calculated that 10.2% of 990 CVID patients developed an autoimmune cytopenia. This is significantly higher vs the general population in which the prevalence of ITP is roughly 8–12 in 100,000 [19]. Of these, the prevalence of ITP is roughly 10–18% of the CVID population and often leads to splenic dysfunction and ultimately functional asplenia. Other patients with CVID may have splenomegaly as a result of lymphoid expansion which may require treatment with splenectomy. Thus, those with CVID and ITP may ultimately develop either a functional asplenia due to ITP or anatomic asplenia as a result of surgical management of complications of CVID [20].

Diagnosis/Assessment

ITP is an autoimmune bleeding disorder that affects 1 in 20,000 individuals. It may occur without a preceding medical condition, or as secondary ITP, as is seen in this patient [21]. Depending on the severity of the decrease in platelet count, the patient may be asymptomatic or may present as our patient with mucocutaneous hemorrhages, petechiae, ecchymoses, heavy menstruation, and oral mucosal bleeds. Other than bleeding, the most pronounced symptom of ITP may be fatigue in 20–40% of cases. In some cases, severe fatigue due to ITP, without the presence of bleeding, may be reason enough to treat a patient [21]. This patient was presented with both medical options and surgical options for treatment of the ITP.

Medical treatment of ITP is typically attempted prior to proceeding to surgery and includes the use of glucocorticoids such as prednisone, methylprednisolone, or dexamethasone in high doses during acute exacerbations with or without the use of high-dose IVIG at 1 g/kg to maintain platelet counts above 50,000/μL [22, 23]. Our patient failed such efforts to manage her ITP with medical therapy, and due to the presence of the CVID as a comorbid condition she elected to proceed with splenectomy.

Since the early 1900s, splenectomy has been the treatment of choice for ITP. However, more recently there have been newer drugs developed, such as TPO mimetics and B-cell targeted treatments, which allow for deferral of surgical management in some patients (Table 23.4) [21–23].

While over 25,000 surgical splenectomies are done in the United States yearly, the option to continue with medical treatment should be discussed with the patient, especially since splenectomies present with their own set of complications [15]. These complications include increased risk of venous thromboembolism, splanchnic vein thrombosis, bleeding during the operation, and sepsis that can be fatal in up to 50% of cases. In addition to the complications associated with surgical splenectomy, the chance for spontaneous remission within the 3 years of disease should be encouraging support for a trial of medical therapy [15, 21, 22, 24, 25]. On the other hand, splenectomy offers the best long-term remission without the need of continuous treatment, with the lowest cost to the patient. The sustained-response rate is 70%, and the early response is similar to the other treatment modalities (85%) as seen in Table 23.4 [21, 22].

Table 23.4 Response rates to treatment for ITP

	Splenectomy	Thrombopoietin receptor agonists	Rituximab
Early response rate	80–85%	70–80%	50–60%
Long-term response rate	60–70%	70–80% while remaining on treatment	20% attain long-term benefits off treatment
Remission rate	60–70%	30–40%	20%
Associated side effects	Perioperative and postoperative complications, sepsis, VTE, and increased risk of malignancy	Dizziness, nausea, vomiting, headaches, hepatotoxicity, myalgia, bone marrow fibrosis, rebound thrombocytopenia after stopping treatment	Infusion reaction, B-cell depletion and infections, progressive multifocal leukoencephalopathy, delayed neutropenia

Based on recommendations from Refs. [21, 22]

Vaccinations in Asplenic Patients

The spleen is a critical organ in conferring immunity as it clears encapsulated and IgG-coated bacteria [26]. Asplenic patients also may have decreased levels of peripheral IgM memory B cells [27]. Taken together, asplenic patients have defects in humoral immunity that put them at an increased risk of infection, especially by encapsulated bacteria [28]. Of these, *Streptococcus pneumoniae*, *H. influenzae* type B, and *Neisseria meningitidis* are the most common pathogens causing sepsis in asplenic patients [29, 30]. Therefore, it is recommended for individuals undergoing elective splenectomy to complete the recommended doses of the pneumococcal, meningococcal, and *Haemophilus influenzae* type B vaccines prior to splenectomy. In addition, patients should receive the annual flu vaccine as early as clinically available [15, 29, 30]. If splenectomy is planned and can be delayed for administration of vaccinations, PCV13 and PPSV23 should be given prior to elective splenectomy. Our patient already completed both the PCV13 and the PPSV23 so no further pneumococcal protection is needed. Although she has already been given the *H. influenza* B vaccine, a one-dose booster is recommended at least 2 weeks prior to elective splenectomy as titers tend to decline over time [30]. Typically MMR and varicella vaccines are given at least 2 weeks prior to elective splenectomy. However, in the case of our patient, being on immunoglobulin replacement will likely reduce or eliminate the efficacy of the measles and varicella vaccines, although administration could still be attempted if not otherwise clinically contraindicated. In any patient with a suspected combined B- and T-cell defect, or a T-cell defect, the use of attenuated vaccines such as MMR and varicella should be strongly cautioned, although they may be safe and effective in those with mild T-cell defects. It should be noted that the phenotypic range of CVID is very broad and can include T-cell deficiencies as well [31]. Therefore, the entire clinical picture must be taken into consideration when recommending vaccinations in patients with CVID. This can be further complicated in the case of the patient with anatomical or functional asplenia and gives further weight to the importance of vaccinating prior to splenectomy whenever possible. Notably, in cases where splenectomy is not planned, indicated vaccines can be given 2 weeks postoperatively.

Of course, as was done in the case of our patient, the vaccination record should be reviewed before administering the vaccines. Table 23.5 outlines the recommended vaccinations for asplenic patients due to splenectomy. As mentioned, the order in which the pneumococcal vaccines are given is important as the sequence recommended allows for a higher antibody response [15].

Table 23.5 Use of vaccinations in asplenic patients

Vaccine	Before elective splenectomy	Following unexpected splenectomy	Special considerations in CVID
Pneumococcal vaccines	If patient is not vaccinated: PCV 13 followed by PPSV23 8 weeks later and at least 2 weeks prior to surgery. Administer second dose of PPSV23 5 years after the first PPSV23 dose	If patient is not vaccinated, administer PCV13 2 weeks post-splenectomy, followed by PPSV23 8 weeks later. If patient has received only PCV13 in the past according to the regimen, administer PPSV23 at least 2 weeks after splenectomy	Usually given at time of CVID diagnosis. Give as per asplenia recommendations if not yet given or recommendations are incomplete for CVID
Hib vaccine	If patient is not vaccinated, administer 1 dose. Consider repeat vaccination in those previously vaccinated	If patient is not vaccinated, administer 1 dose 2 weeks post-splenectomy	Recommended vaccine in CVID patients. Administer per asplenia recommendations if not already immunized
Meningococcal vaccines	If no previous vaccine in patient ≥2 years age: Administer one single dose of MenACWY, repeat 8–12 weeks later. Booster dose every 5 years Meningitis B vaccine. Two doses at least 2 months apart. If not possible to give both doses before splenectomy, give one dose 2 weeks prior to splenectomy and second dose 2 months later	If no previous vaccine in patient older than 2 years old, at least 2 weeks post-splenectomy: Two-dose series of MenACWY. Allow an 8–12-week interval between each dose. Booster dose every 5 years Meningitis B at least 2 weeks postoperatively	Not indicated as a risk-specific vaccine for CVID. Consider giving as per routine vaccination schedule
Influenza vaccines	Administer killed vaccine annually Live attenuated influenza vaccine is contraindicated	Administer killed vaccine annually Live attenuated influenza vaccine is contraindicated	Administer killed vaccine annually Live attenuated influenza vaccine is contraindicated
Other vaccines	Note that pneumococcal, Hib, and meningococcal vaccines are the most important risk-specific vaccinations to provide in asplenia Live-attenuated influenza vaccine is the essential contraindicated vaccine to avoid Other vaccines should be given according to recommendations according to comorbid conditions and coexisting immunodeficiency		

Table adapted from Refs. [16, 30]

Clinical Pearls and Pitfalls
- CVID is a humoral immunodeficiency with a variable phenotype. Nevertheless, vaccine recommendations should be followed with care to provide protection from disease but also take into consideration any contraindications.
- The recommended vaccines for patients with CVID overlap with those recommended for asplenia significantly, reflecting the overlap in the mechanism of immunodeficiency that results for both conditions.
- A major difference in the recommended vaccinations for CVID and asplenia is that the meningococcal vaccine is strongly recommended in patients with asplenia and conditionally for CVID depending on the patient's age and risk factors.
- The live attenuated flu vaccine is contraindicated in both CVID and asplenia. Other contraindicated vaccines exist for those with CVID, although some could be considered on a case-by-case basis, such as MMR and varicella.

References

1. Hannoun C. The evolving history of influenza viruses and influenza vaccines. Expert Rev Vaccines. 2013;12(9):1085–94. https://doi.org/10.1586/14760584.2013.824709.
2. Ferkol T, Schraufnagel D. The global burden of respiratory disease. Ann Am Thorac Soc. 2014;11(3):404–6. https://doi.org/10.1513/AnnalsATS.201311-405PS.
3. Bonilla FA, Barlan I, Chapel H, Costa-Carvalho BT, Cunningham-Rundles C, de la Morena MT, et al. International consensus document (ICON): common variable immunodeficiency disorders. J Allergy Clin Immunol Pract. 2016;4(1):38–59. https://doi.org/10.1016/j.jaip.2015.07.025.
4. Gregersen S, Aaløkken TM, Mynarek G, Kongerud J, Sukrust P, Froland SS, et al. High resolution computed tomography and pulmonary function in common variable immunodeficiency. Respir Med. 2009;103(6):873–80. https://doi.org/10.1016/j.rmed.2008.12.015.
5. Afonso AFB, João CMP. The production processes and biological effects of intravenous immunoglobulin. Biomol Ther. 2016;6(1). https://doi.org/10.3390/biom6010015.
6. Chua I, Lagos M, Charalambous BM, Workman S, Chee R, Grimbacher B. Pathogen-specific IgG antibody levels in immunodeficient patients receiving immunoglobulin replacement do not provide additional benefit to therapeutic management over total serum IgG. J Allergy Clin Immunol. 2011;127(6):1410–1. https://doi.org/10.1016/j.jaci.2011.01.035.
7. Cox RJ, Brokstad KA, Ogra P. Influenza virus: immunity and vaccination strategies. Comparison of the immune response to inactivated and live, attenuated influenza vaccines. Scand J Immunol. 2004;59(1):1–15. https://doi.org/10.1111/j.0300-9475.2004.01382.x.
8. Committee on Infectious Diseases, American Academy of Pediatrics. Redbook: 2012 report of the Committee on Infectious Diseases. Elk Grove Village: American Academy of Pediatrics; 2012.
9. Kamboj M, Sepkowitz KA. Risk of transmission associated with live attenuated vaccines given to healthy persons caring for or residing with an immunocompromised patient. Infect Control Hosp Epidemiol. 2007;28(6):702–7. https://doi.org/10.1086/517952.

10. Kroger A, Duchin J, Vázquez M. General best practice guidelines for immunization. Best practices guidance of the advisory committee on immunization practices (ACIP). Cdc, Ncird. 2017. https://www.cdc.gov/vaccines/hcp/acip-recs/general-recs/downloads/general-recs.pdf.
11. Medical Advisory Committee of the Immune Deficiency Foundation, Shearer WT, Fleisher TA, Buckley RH, Ballas Z, Ballow M, et al. Recommendations for live viral and bacterial vaccines in immunodeficient patients and their close contacts. J Allergy Clin Immunol. 2014;133(4):961–6. https://doi.org/10.1016/j.jaci.2013.11.043.
12. Farcet MR, Karbiener M, Rabel PO, Schirmer A, Ilk R, Kreil TR. Measles virus neutralizing antibodies in immunoglobulin lots produced from plasma collected in Europe or the United States. Vaccine. 2019;37(24):3151–3. https://doi.org/10.1016/j.vaccine.2019.04.022.
13. Modrof J, Tille B, Farcet MR, McVey J, Schreiner JA, Borders CM, et al. Measles virus neutralizing antibodies in intravenous immunoglobulins: is an increase by revaccination of plasma donors possible? J Infect Dis. 2017;216(8):977–80. https://doi.org/10.1093/infdis/jix428.
14. Zhan W, Yue F, Liu J, Lee JK, Ho J, Moir S, et al. Response to influenza immunization in patients with common variable immunodeficiency. Allergy Asthma Clin Immunol. 2011;7(S2). https://doi.org/10.1186/1710-1492-7-s2-a28.
15. Rubin LG, Schaffner W. Care of the asplenic patient. N Engl J Med. 2014;371(4):349–56. https://doi.org/10.1056/NEJMcp1314291.
16. Centers for Disease Control and Prevention (CDC), War W, Ii WW, et al. CDC pink book. Epidemiol Prev Vaccine-Preventable Dis. 13th ed. 2015;1302(9):31–44. https://doi.org/10.1016/B978-1-4377-2702-9.00226-9.
17. Centers for Disease Control and Prevention. Pneumococcal vaccine timing for adults. Centers Dis Control Prev. 2018:11–4. https://www.cdc.gov/vaccines/vpd/pneumo/downloads/pneumo-vaccine-timing.pdf?fbclid=IwAR2fMH6JiqsbZdZy9tnRVmwoMs3OJX1C50N8BfgjRV7hN47lxK2aE7FIdRU (Accessed 8/30/2020).
18. Cunningham-Rundles C, Bodian C. Common variable immunodeficiency: clinical and immunological features of 248 patients. Clin Immunol. 1999;92(1):34–48. https://doi.org/10.1006/clim.1999.4725.
19. Feuille EJ, Anooshiravani N, Sullivan KE, Fuleihan RL, Cunningham-Rundles C. Autoimmune cytopenias and associated conditions in CVID: a report from the USIDNET registry. J Clin Immunol. 2018;38(1):28–34. https://doi.org/10.1007/s10875-017-0456-9.
20. Cunningham-Rundles C. The many faces of common variable immunodeficiency. Hematology Am Soc Hematol Educ Program. 2012;2012:301–5. https://doi.org/10.1182/asheducation.v2012.1.301.3798316.
21. Al-Samkari H, Kuter DJ. Immune thrombocytopenia in adults: modern approaches to diagnosis and treatment. Semin Thromb Hemost. 2019; https://doi.org/10.1055/s-0039-1700512.
22. Stasi R, Newland A, Thornton P, Pabinger I. Should medical treatment options be exhausted before splenectomy is performed in adult ITP patients? A debate. Ann Hematol. 2010;89(12):1185–95. https://doi.org/10.1007/s00277-010-1066-2.
23. Bussel JB. Therapeutic approaches to secondary immune thrombocytopenic purpura. Semin Hematol. 2009;46(suppl. 2). https://doi.org/10.1053/j.seminhematol.2008.12.003.
24. Cirasino L, Robino AM, Cattaneo M, Pioltelli PE, Pogliani EM, Terranova L, et al. Appropriate hospital management of adult immune thrombocytopenic purpura patients in major Italian institutions in 2000–2002: a retrospective analysis. Blood Coagul Fibrinolysis. 2010;21(1):77–84. https://doi.org/10.1097/MBC.0b013e328332dbb6.
25. Di Sabatino A, Carsetti R, Corazza GR. Post-splenectomy and hyposplenic states. Lancet. 2011;378(9785):86–97. https://doi.org/10.1016/S0140-6736(10)61493-6.
26. Brousse V, Buffet P, Rees D. The spleen and sickle cell disease: the sick(led) spleen. Br J Haematol. 2014;166(2):165–76. https://doi.org/10.1111/bjh.12950.
27. Cameron PU, Jones P, Gorniak M, Dunster K, Paul E, Lewin S, et al. Splenectomy associated changes in IgM memory B cells in an adult spleen registry cohort. PLoS ONE. 2011;6(8). https://doi.org/10.1371/journal.pone.0023164.

28. Azar S, Wong TE. Sickle cell disease: a brief update. Med Clin North Am. 2017;101(2):375–93. https://doi.org/10.1016/j.mcna.2016.09.009.
29. Davies JM, Lewis MPN, Wimperis J, Rafi I, Ladhani S, Bolton-Maggs PHB. Review of guidelines for the prevention and treatment of infection in patients with an absent or dysfunctional spleen: prepared on behalf of the British Committee for Standards in Haematology by a working party of the Haemato-Oncology task force. Br J Haematol. 2011;155(3):308–17. https://doi.org/10.1111/j.1365-2141.2011.08843.x.
30. Bonanni P, Grazzini M, Niccolai G, Paolini D, Varone O, Bartoloni A, et al. Recommended vaccinations for asplenic and hyposplenic adult patients. Hum Vaccin Immunother. 2017;13(2):359–68. https://doi.org/10.1080/21645515.2017.1264797.
31. Bonilla FA. Update: vaccines in primary immunodeficiency. J Allergy Clin Immunol. 2018;141(2):474–81. https://doi.org/10.1016/j.jaci.2017.12.980.

Index

A
Abatacept, 5
Activated PI3Kδ mutations, 74
Activation induced cytidine deaminase (AID), 50
Adenoidectomy, 65
Adenosine deaminase deficiency, 119
Agammaglobulinemia
    febrile seizures, 37, 38
        diagnosis/assessment, 38–40
        management/outcome, 41, 42
    recurrent otitis and fevers, 42
        diagnosis/assessment, 42–44
        management/outcome, 45
    types of, 44
Antibody deficiencies, 15, 16
Antibody-dependent cellular cytotoxicity (ADCC), 336
Antigen-presenting cells (APCs), 257, 258, 265
Anti-IgA antibodies, 80
Apoptosis, 192, 194–196
Aspergillus fumigatus, 292
Asplenia, 397, 398, 404, 406
Asthma, 22, 23
    clinical presentation, 23
    gastrointestinal disease, 24
    respiratory disease, 23, 24
Atopic dermatitis, 60
    diagnosis/assessment, 61, 62
    management/outcome, 62, 63
Atopy, 59, 65
Autoimmune cytopenia, 190, 194–196
Autoimmune disease, 3, 24, 25, 79
Autoimmune hemolytic anemia (AIHA), 207, 211
Autoimmune lymphoproliferative syndrome (ALPS), 192, 233
    apoptosis, 189
    clinical manifestations, 189, 190
    differential diagnosis, 195, 196
    idiopathic thrombocytopenic purpura, 187
    laboratory findings, 191, 193, 194
    management, 196–198
    pathogenesis, 189
Autoimmune-polyendocrinopathy-candidiasis-ectodermal dystrophy (APECED), 243, 356
Autoimmune regulator, 229
Autoinflammation, 302
Autoinflammatory syndromes
    combined variable immunodeficiency, 204
    diagnosis, 206, 207, 209, 214
    enteropathy, 203
    immune dysregulation, 203
    innate immunity, 203
    management, 210, 211, 215, 216
    polyendocrinopathy, 203
    recurrent fevers, 204
    symptoms/clinical presentation, 212–214
    whole exome sequencing, 204
    X-linked, 203
Autosomal dominant (AD)-HIES, 150
Autosomal recessive (AR), 51
Autosomal recessive agammaglobulinemia (ARA), 43, 44
Autosomal recessive hyper IgM, 54

B
Bacillus Calmette–Guérin (BCG), 81, 256
Bare lymphocyte syndrome, 264
Baricitinib, 357
B-cell activating factor (BAFF), 28

B-cell development, 43
B-cell immunodeficiency, 2
B-cell receptors (BCR), 21, 39
B-cell sub-population surface markers, 22
Belatacept, 5
Bilateral tympanic membranes, 60
Bloom syndrome, 172
Bone marrow failure syndromes, 272
Bronchiectasis, 23, 69
    diagnosis/assessment, 70–74
    management/outcome, 75, 76
    monitoring control, 76
    symptoms and comorbidities, 74, 75
    testing, 75
Bruton tyrosine kinase (Btk), 38, 39

C

Calcium release activated channel (CRAC), 339
Cancer, 51, 53, 55
Candida albicans, 142
CARD11, 152, 163
Causative mutation, absence of diagnostic criteria in, 98–100
CD4, 139, 141–143
CD4 lymphopenia, 139–145
CD8 count, 139, 141
CD40, 50
CD40L, 53, 54
Celiac disease, 76, 77
    comorbidities, 79
    diagnosis/assessment, 77, 78
    management/outcome, 81, 82
    symptoms, 78, 79
    testing, 79–81
Centromeric instability, 176
Cerebral spinal fluid (CSF), 37
Cernunnos deficiency, 172
CHARGE syndrome, 173
Chediak-Higashi syndrome, 273
Chronic diarrhea, 24
Chronic granulomatous disease, 273, 294, 304
    acute infections, 298, 299
    clinical pearls, 306
    diagnostic testing, 295, 302
    dihydrorhodamine assay, 296
    epidemiology, 291
    gene therapy, 305
    genetics, 292
    genetic testing, 297
    hematopoietic cell transplantation, 303
    infections, 294, 295
    inflammatory complications, 300, 301
    neutrophils dysfunction, 290, 291
    primary immunodeficiency, 289
    prophylaxis, 297, 298
    X-linked carriers, 301, 302
Chronic lymphocytic leukemia (CLL), 371–373
Chronic mucocutaneous candidiasis, 352
    AIRE, 351
    autoimmune polyendocrinopathy syndrome type 1, 356
    CANDF1, 356
    CANDF3, 356
    Candida albicans, 351
    dectin pathway, 352
    diagnosis, 356
    IGE syndrome, 353
    IL12B, 355
    IL17F, 355
    management, 357
    STAT1, 355
    Th17, 351
    TH17, 355
Chronic rhinitis, 22, 23
    clinical presentation, 23
    gastrointestinal disease, 24
    respiratory disease, 23, 24
Class switch defects
    failure to thrive, 53, 54
        diagnosis/assessment, 54, 55
        management/outcome, 55
    otitis media, episodes of, 49, 50
        :management/outcome, 52, 53
        diagnosis/assessment, 50–52
Class switching, 49
Cohen syndrome, 173
Combined variable immunodeficiency (CVID), 3, 15, 195, 388
    asthma and chronic rhinitis, 22, 23
        clinical presentation, 23
        gastrointestinal disease, 24
        respiratory disease, 23, 24
    autoimmune disease, 24, 25
    diagnosis, 389
    flow cytometry, 26, 28
    genetic testing, 28, 29
    infectious features, 16
    intermittent asthma and controlled allergic rhinitis, 17
        clinical presentation, 17, 18
        diagnostic criteria, 18–20
        laboratory findings, 20
        vaccine response, 20–22

Index

lymphoproliferative disease, 25
malignancies, 25, 26
management, 30, 31
prevalence, 15
prognosis, 31
Comel-Netherton syndrome, 153
Common variable immunodeficiency
   disorders-like disorders, 94, 95, 208
   absence of causative mutation, 98–100
   B-cell subsets in, 27
   and CVID-like disorders, 96
   diagnostic criteria, 99
   genetics of, 95–97
   genetic diagnosis, advantages of, 97
   genetic mutations in, 29–30
   noninfectious complications of, 16
   presentation of index patient, 91
   sarcoidosis/granulomatous variant of
      CVID, 93, 94
   TNFRSF13B/TACI and *TCF3* genes, 92
   TNFRSF13B/TACI C104R mutation,
      discordant segregation of, 92, 93
Complement pathway, 320
Controlled allergic rhinitis, 17–22
Cryptococcus neoformans, 142
CTLA-4, 211
CVID disease severity score (CDSS), 96
Cyclic neutropenia, 273
Cytomegalovirus (CMV), 233, 385
Cytopenias, 93

D

Dendritic cells, 258, 259, 261
   antigen-presenting cells, 257, 258
   classfication, 259
   GATA2, 263, 264
   immunodeficiency, 261
   interferon regulatory factor 8, 262
   IRF8, 263, 264
   K108E, 256
   mutation of GATA-binding factor 2,
      262, 263
   primary immunodeficiency disease, 255
   T80A, 257
DiGeorge syndrome, 173
DOCK8, 152
Double-negative T cells, 189, 191–195

E

Eculizumab, 325
Encapsulated bacteria, 397, 399
Enteropathy X-linked (IPEX), 208, 243

Epstein-Barr virus (EBV), 195, 221
EUROclass classification, 26
EXTL3 deficiency, 174

F

Facial dysmorphism syndrome, 176
Failure to thrive, 53, 54
   diagnosis/assessment, 54, 55
   management/outcome, 55
Familial Mediterranean Fever
   (FMF), 206
FAS ligand (FASL), 189
FAS pathway, 189
Fas-associated protein with death domain
   (FADD), 230
Febrile seizures, 37, 38
   diagnosis/assessment, 38–40
   management/outcome, 41, 42
Flow cytometry, 26–28
Fluorescence in situ hybridization, 272
Forkhead box P3 (FOXP3), 230, 243, 245
Functional flow cytometric 107a assays, 4

G

Gait instability, 94
Gastrointestinal disease, 24
GATA binding protein 2, 255
GATA2, 333
Gene editing, 4, 5, 108, 130
Gene therapy, 53
Genocopy, 96
Giardia, 81
Giardia lamblia, 78
GP130, 152, 153
Graft versus host disease (GVHD), 110,
   211, 385
Granulomatous and lymphocytic interstitial
   lung disease (GLILD), 23, 212
Granulomatous variant of combined variable
   immunodeficiency
   (GVCVID), 94, 98
Griscelli syndrome, 174

H

Hematopoietic stem cell transplant (HSCT), 5,
   41, 42, 107, 123, 124
Hemolytic uremic syndrome, 319
Hemophagocytic lymphohistiocytosis
   (HLH), 4, 221
HSCT gene therapy (HSC-GT), 130
Human papillomavirus (HPV), 337

Hyper IgE Syndrome
    AD-HIES, 151
    clinical features, 151–153
    clinical pearls, 162
    C-reactive protein, 149
    diagnosis, 156, 161
    DOCK8, 159, 162
    laboratory features, 154, 155, 161
    management/outcome, 156, 157
    peripheral blood mononuclear cells, 150
    STAT3, 153
    Streptococcus pneumoniae, 149
Hyper IgM phenotype, 55
Hypergammaglobulinemia, 190
Hypogammaglobulinemia, 17, 19, 59
Hypogammaglobulinemia of infancy (THI), 19

I
IL6 receptor, 152
IL6R, 163
IL6ST, 163
Immune dysregulation, 2
    ALPS, 233
    APDS, 236
    APECED, 242
    B cell receptor, 225
    CD25 deficiency, 241
    clinical history, 237
    combined variable immunodeficiency, 236
    CTLA4 haploinsufficiency, 234
    forkhead box P3, 243, 244
    hypomorphic SCID, 241
    IL10R, 242
    interferons, 232
    IPEX, 244–246
    laboratory evaluation, 238
    patient diagnosis, 236
    PI3Kδ, 235
    self-tolerant immune system, 221
    STAT1 GOF, 243
    STAT3 GOF, 235
    STAT5B LOF, 242
    T cell receptor, 225, 229, 232
    treatment, 238, 240
Immune thrombocytopenia (ITP), 403
Immunodeficiency, 142, 143, 176
    CHARGE, 178
    clinical pearls, 179
    diagnosis/assessment, 384, 385
    facial dysmorphism syndrome, 176
    hemophagocytic lymphohistiocytosis, 169
    Kabuki syndrome, 170
    KDM6A, 170

KMT2D, 170
    management, 385, 386
    NK cell, 177
    PIDD, 382
    Pneumocystis jirovecii, 176, 178
    pregnancy, management during, 390
    T-cell receptor excision circle, 382
Immunodeficiency comorbidities, 3
Immunodeficiency laboratories, transplant
        centers with, 7–11
Immunoglobulin, 41
    IgA deficiency, 77, 81
    IgG, 59–61
    IgG subclass deficiency, 15, 71, 74
    IgG2 deficiency, 77
    IgM deficiency, 74
Immunoglobulin replacement therapy, 55
Immunoreceptor tyrosine-based activation
        motifs (ITAMs), 38
Inborn errors of immunity (IEI), 4
Inflammatory bowel disease, 242, 299, 300
Innate immune defects, 2
    Chediak-Higashi syndrome, 272, 281, 282
    complete blood cell count with
            platelets, 272
    congenital neutropenia, 272
    cyclic neutropenia, 272
    diagnosis, 277
    leukocyte adhesion deficiency 1, 283–285
    management, 282
    myeloperoxidase, 278, 279
    Shwachman-Diamond Syndrome, 272,
            276, 277
Innate immunity, 203, 331, 339
Interferon regulatory factor 8 (IRF8), 255, 261
Intermittent asthma, 17–22
International Union of Immunological
        Societies (IUIS), 169
Intravenous immunoglobulin, 370
Isohemagglutinin, 22

J
JAGN1 deficiency, 174
Jakinib, 357

K
Kabuki syndrome, 170, 171, 175

L
Late onset antibody failure (LOAF), 94
Leukocyte adhesion deficiency, 274

Leukocyte adhesion deficiency 1
  (LAD1), 283
Lipopolysaccharide-responsive beige-like
  anchor protein (LRBA), 29, 230
Locus heterogeneity, 96
Lymphadenopathy, 18, 94
Lymphoma, 196
Lymphoproliferative disease, 25

M
Malignancies, 2, 25, 26
Maternal IgG, 19
Membrane attack complex/perforin
  (MACPF), 317
Membranoproliferative glomerulonephritis
  (MPGN), 319
Meningococcus, 317
Mevalonate kinase deficiency (MKD), 206
Molecular technology, 4
Molluscum contagiosum, 160
Monogenic defects, 1, 4, 6
Mononuclear phagocyte system
  (MPS), 259
Mu heavy chain deficiency, 42
Mutations of the T-cell activator, 95
Myeloperoxidase (MPO), 278, 279
Myeloperoxidase deficiency, 272, 274

N
Natural killer (NK) cells, 334
  CD56, 331
  cytotoxicity, 331
  environmental effects, 342
  GATA2, 333, 335
  innate lymphocytes, 331
  primary immunodeficiency
    diseases, 337–341
  Primary immunodeficiency disorders, 332
  primary NK cell disorders, 336
  primary NK Cell disorders, 332, 333,
    336, 337
Netherton syndrome, 173
Neutropenia, 53
Neutrophil specific granule deficiency,
  272, 278
Newborn screening, 382
Next Generation Sequencing (NGS), 64, 93
NF-kB essential modulator (NEMO), 4, 52
Nijmegen breakage syndrome, 55, 175
Non-Hodgkin's lymphoma, 363
NZ hypogammaglobulinemia study
  (NZHS), 98

O
Omenn syndrome, 153, 208
Opportunistic infections, 52, 53, 55,
  140, 142–144
Organomegaly, 18
Otitis media, episodes of, 49, 50
  diagnosis/assessment, 50–52
  management/outcome, 52, 53

P
Pathogen-associated molecular patterns
  (PAMPs), 258
Pattern recognition receptors (PRRs), 257–258
PGM3, 152, 163
Phosphoglucomutase-3 (PGM3), 161
Phosphoinositide 3-kinase (PI3K), 54
Pitt-Hopkins syndrome, 264
Platelet inhibitors, 393
Pneumococcal vaccines, 21
Pneumococcus, 318
Pneumocystis jirovecii, 171, 178
Pneumovax vaccine, 77
Pokeweed mitogen (PWM), 111
Polyendocrinopathy, 243, 246
Precision targeted therapies, 5
Pregnancy, in CVID patient, 390
Primary Immune Deficiency Consortium
  (PIDTC), 109
Primary immune deficiency disease
  (PIDD), 382
Primary immune regulatory disease
  (PIRD), 28
Primary Immunodeficiencies, 1, 2, 94, 169,
  177, 179, 203, 208, 210, 230,
  365, 367
  AH50, 313, 314
  C1q, 315, 316, 328
  C3, 314
  C4, 314
  CH50, 313, 314
  complement pathway, 316–319
  CSF protein, 315
  diagnosis/assessment, 320, 321
  immunodeficiency comorbidities, 3
  laboratory testing, 322, 323
  managmnet/outcome, 323–325
  meningococcus, 317
  novel therapeutic advancements, 4–6
  pneumococcus, 318
  targeted therapies for, 5
  technologic advancements in, 3, 4
Primary immunodeficiency disorders
  (PIDDs), 332

R

RAG1 deficiency, 79
Recurrent fevers, 204
Recurrent otitis, 42
  diagnosis/assessment, 42–44
  management/outcome, 45
Recurrent respiratory tract infections, 63
  diagnosis/assessment, 64
  management/outcome, 64, 65
Regulator of telomere elongation helicase I deficiency (RTEL1), 336
Regulatory T cells, 216
Respiratory disease, 23, 24
Reticular dysgenesis, 264
Retropharyngeal abscess, 54
Rituximab, 30, 365–369, 372
Ruxolitinib, 357

S

Sarcoidosis, 93, 94
Schimke immunoosseous dysplasia, 175
Secondary immunodeficiency (SID), 364, 368
  chronic lymphocytic leukemia, 363, 371–375
  diagnosis, 365–367
  heterogeneous group, 363
  managment, 369, 370
  multiple myeloma, 363
  non-Hodgkin's lymphoma, 364
  subcutaneous immunoglobulin, 370
Selective IgA deficiency, 71, 72, 75, 76, 78–80
Selective IgG subclass deficiency, 70
Selective IgG3 deficiency, 72
Selective IgM deficiency, 73, 74
Selective immunoglobulin deficiency, 70
Selective isotype immunodeficiency
  autoimmune conditions associated with selective IgG deficiencies, 72
  bronchiectasis and recurrent sinusitis, 69
    diagnosis/assessment, 70–74
    management/outcome, 75, 76
    monitoring control, 76
    symptoms and comorbidities, 74, 75
    testing, 75
  celiac disease, 76, 77
    comorbidities, 79
    diagnosis/assessment, 77, 78
    management/outcome, 81, 82
    symptoms, 78, 79
    testing, 79–81
  IgG subclass levels by age, 71
  selective IgA deficiencies, 79
  selective IgM deficiencies, 74
  serum immunoglobulin levels, 70
Severe combined immunodeficiencies (SCID), 338, 382
  adenosine deaminase, 126
  autoimmunity, 129
  CD45RA, 108
  classification, 120
  clinical presentation, 114, 115
  diagnosis, 109, 110
  enzyme replacment therapy, 127, 128
  gene editing, 130
  genetic classification, 121
  heterogeneous group, 107
  HSCT-GT, 130
  immunophenotypic classfication, 118
  initial managment, 121–123
  laboratory testing, 116–118
  newborn screening, 107, 108, 112–114
Severe congenital neutropenia (SCN), 272, 274, 276, 279
Severe hypogammaglobulinemia, 93
Shwachman-Diamond syndrome, 176, 272, 275
Signal transducer and activator of transcription (STAT3), 150
SMARCD2 deficiency, 176
Soluble FAS ligand (sFASL), 193
Somatic hypermutation, 49, 52, 54
Specific antibody deficiency (SAD), 15, 73
  asthma and chronic rhinitis, 22, 23
    clinical presentation, 23
    gastrointestinal disease, 24
    respiratory disease, 23, 24
  autoimmune disease, 24, 25
  flow cytometry, 26, 28
  genetic testing, 28, 29
  intermittent asthma and controlled allergic rhinitis, 17
    clinical presentation, 17, 18
    diagnostic criteria, 18–20
    laboratory findings, 20
    vaccine response, 20–22
  lymphoproliferative disease, 25
  malignancies, 25, 26
  management, 30, 31
  prognosis, 31
Specific granule defect, 275
SPINK, 163
Splenectomy, 404–406
Splenomegaly, 195
Staphylococcal pneumonia, 158
Staphylococcus aureus, 54, 151
Stem cell transplantation, 53
Streptococcus pneumoniae, 149, 365
Subcutaneous immunoglobulin (SCIg), 30, 375, 391, 403

Index

diagnosis/assessment, 392
management/outcome, 393
Switched memory B cells, 26–28
Syk, 38
Syndromic immunodeficiencies, 169
Syndromic primary
   immunodeficiencies, 169

T
T regulatory cells, 229
T-cells, 140–142
T-cell receptor excision circle (TREC), 337, 382–384
T-cell subsets, enumeration of, 64
TCF3 genes, 92
TNFRSF13B/TACI C104R mutation, discordant segregation of, 92, 93
Tonsillectomy, 65
Transient hypogammaglobulinemia of infancy (THI), 15, 19, 59
   atopic dermatitis, 60
      diagnosis/assessment, 61, 62
      management/outcome, 62, 63
   clinical features, 61
   recurrent respiratory tract
      infections, 63
      diagnosis/assessment, 64
      management/outcome, 64, 65
Transmembrane activator and CAML interactor (TACI), 28, 78
Trimethoprim-sulfamethoxazole (TMP-SMX), 385
Tympanostomy, 65

U
Unspecified hypogammaglobulinemia, 19
Uracyl-N-glycosylase (UNG), 50
US Food and Drug Administration (FDA), 401

V
Vaccinations, 20, 314, 324, 325, 398
   combined variable immunodeficiency, 397, 399–401
   encapsulated bacteria, 399
   immune thrombocytopenia purpura, 399
   inflammatory bowel disease, 399
   specific antibody deficiency, 397
   systemic lupus erythematosus, 399

W
Whole exome sequencing (WES), 4, 204
Wiskott Aldrich Syndrome (WAS), 130, 152, 176, 208, 264, 275, 279, 339
Wiskott-Aldrich Syndrome protein (WASp), 160

X
X-linked agammaglobulinemia (XLA), 38–41, 64, 208
X-linked carriers, 301, 302
X-linked hyper IgM, 50

Z
ZNF431, 152, 163